Veterinary Neuroanatomy and Clinical Neurology

ALEXANDER DE LAHUNTA, D.V.M., Ph.D.

Professor of Anatomy
Director, Veterinary Medical Teaching Hospital
New York State College of Veterinary Medicine
Cornell University, Ithaca, New York

*Illustrated by Lewis L. Sadler
and Grant S. Lashbrook*

W. B. SAUNDERS COMPANY • Philadelphia • London • Toronto

W. B. Saunders Company: West Washington Square
Philadelphia, PA 19105

1 St. Anne's Road
Eastbourne, East Sussex BN21 3UN, England

1 Goldthorne Avenue
Toronto, Ontario M8Z 5T9, Canada

Library of Congress Cataloging in Publication Data

de Lahunta, Alexander, 1932–

Veterinary neuroanatomy and clinical neurology.

1. Veterinary neurology.   2. Veterinary anatomy.
   3. Neuroanatomy.   I. Title.

SF895.D44   636.089'68   76–4246

ISBN 0–7216–3024–3

Veterinary Neuroanatomy and Clinical Neurology   ISBN 0-7216-3024-3

Last digit is the print number: 9   8   7   6   5   4   3   2

FOREWORD

This book has been made possible by the willingness of my department head, Dr. Robert E. Habel, to allow me to spend my research time and energy outside the Department of Anatomy in the areas of clinical neurology and neuropathology. The cooperation received from the clinical departments and the Department of Pathology also has made possible the studies that are the basis for this book.

To follow neuroanatomy to its logical conclusion is to explore its function. For a veterinarian, the knowledge of normal function is the basis for understanding the pathophysiology of abnormal function. In the nervous system, this is the study of clinical neurology. Neuroanatomy, neurophysiology, neuropathology, and clinical neurology are a logical sequence of studies that are integrated readily into a single course.

With some modification, this is the subject matter that is taught to first-year veterinary students at the New York State College of Veterinary Medicine. The academic year consists of two semesters. During the first semester the students study the gross anatomy of the dog, including the various components of the peripheral nervous system, followed by a dissection of the brain and spinal cord. This anatomy and the dissection procedure are described in *Miller's Guide to the Dissection of the Dog*, by H. E. Evans and A. de Lahunta. A complete preserved dog brain is provided for each pair of students. Following the dissection each pair of students sections another preserved dog brain transversely, and relates the gross features of the transverse sections to their dissection to obtain a three-dimensional orientation.

In the second semester, the neuroanatomy course is taught in a vertically integrated manner according to functional systems. For each functional system the anatomy of the major components is described, along with its normal function. This is followed by a consideration of the clinical signs that occur if the function of the system is disturbed, and a description and differential diagnosis of the diseases that typically affect this system. Films of clinical cases are used to demonstrate the clinical signs produced by the various diseases. Slides of gross and microscopic lesions are shown to emphasize the clinical-neuroanatomic relationships and to stress characteristic features of some of the diseases.

Clinical diagnoses of disease of the nervous system probably depend more on the understanding of the anatomy of the system than any other diagnoses. The first-year student is in a unique position to study both simultaneously. The direct application of the anatomic study to the disease process and clinical diagnosis is not only logical for this system, but permits the first-year veterinary student the opportunity to work with the clinical patient. Not only does this approach stimulate the student to learn, but it is equally exciting for the professor to teach in this manner.

This book has been written primarily to complement this method of teaching at the New York State College of Veterinary Medicine. It is not intended to be a complete treatise on all aspects of veterinary neuroanatomy, clinical neurology, and neuropathology. It is hoped that its organization will permit the book to be of special use to the practitioner in arriving at a clinical diagnosis. Some of the specialized ancillary diagnostic procedures and therapeutic techniques that are not considered in this book in any depth are described amply in *Canine Neurology*, by B. F. Hoerlein. Similarly, a more detailed account of canine neuroanatomy may be found in *Anatomy of the Dog*, by M. E. Miller, G. C. Christensen, and H. E. Evans, and in *Functional Mammalian Neuroanatomy*, by T. W. Jenkins.

If errors or omissions are found, or the reader has a strong difference of opinion, the author would like to be informed. This book is the result of the cooperation of knowledgeable individuals. Its improvement depends on continued cooperation, so that the information presented is as accurate as possible.

Many thanks are extended to my former students, whose enthusiasm and expertise kept urging me to learn more about each clinical patient and disease process. Special thanks go to Dr. John Cummings, whose excellence in neuroanatomy and neuropathology continually contributed to my better understanding of the nervous system. There are many others throughout the veterinary college who could be singled out for mention, but all are part of this institution's cooperative academic environment that provides the stimulus to pursue knowledge.

Special thanks are given to Karen Allaben-Confer for her secretarial expertise, and to Esther Wilcox for her excellent histologic preparation of neuropathologic specimens.

The outstanding artistic work of the first five chapters was done By Lewis L. Sadler, who was medical illustrator for the Department of Anatomy at the New York State College of Veterinary Medicine. The remaining chapters were illustrated by Grant Lashbrook, Art Director for the Health Sciences at W. B. Saunders Co. This excellent work is greatly appreciated.

ALEXANDER DE LAHUNTA

CONTENTS

Chapter 1

INTRODUCTION 1

Chapter 2

THE DEVELOPMENT OF THE NERVOUS SYSTEM 8

Chapter 3

CEREBROSPINAL FLUID AND HYDROCEPHALUS............................ 33

Chapter 4

LOWER MOTOR NEURON—GENERAL SOMATIC EFFERENT
SYSTEM.. 57

Chapter 5

CRANIAL NERVE—LOWER MOTOR NEURON: GENERAL
SOMATIC EFFERENT SYSTEM, SPECIAL VISCERAL
EFFERENT SYSTEM... 89

Chapter 6

LOWER MOTOR NEURON—GENERAL VISCERAL
EFFERENT SYSTEM.. 110

Chapter 7

UPPER MOTOR NEURON SYSTEM................................... 125

Chapter 8

GENERAL PROPRIOCEPTION SYSTEM—GP..................... 149

Chapter 9

GENERAL SOMATIC AFFERENT SYSTEM—GSA.............. 160

Chapter 10

SPINAL CORD DISEASE.. 169

Chapter 11
VESTIBULAR SYSTEM—SPECIAL PROPRIOCEPTION........................ 221

Chapter 12
CEREBELLUM 238

Chapter 13
VISUAL SYSTEM—SPECIAL SOMATIC AFFERENT SYSTEM.............. 257

Chapter 14
AUDITORY SYSTEM—SPECIAL SOMATIC AFFERENT SYSTEM 281

Chapter 15
VISCERAL AFFERENT SYSTEMS..................................... 288

Chapter 16
NONOLFACTORY RHINENCEPHALON: LIMBIC SYSTEM................... 296

Chapter 17
SEIZURES—CONVULSIONS 303

Chapter 18
DIENCEPHALON.. 318

Chapter 19
DIAGNOSIS AND EVALUATION OF TRAUMATIC LESIONS
OF THE NERVOUS SYSTEM 333

Chapter 20
SMALL ANIMAL AND EQUINE NEUROLOGIC EXAMINATIONS........... 344

Chapter 21
CASE DESCRIPTIONS 373

Appendix... 405

Index 423

Chapter 1

INTRODUCTION

ACCURATE DIAGNOSIS
THE NEURON
FUNCTIONAL SYSTEMS
SENSORY (AFFERENT)
SOMATIC AFFERENT
General Somatic Afferent (GSA)
Special Somatic Afferent (SSA)
VISCERAL AFFERENT
General Visceral Afferent (GVA)
Special Visceral Afferent (SVA)

PROPRIOCEPTION
General Proprioception (GP)
Special Proprioception
MOTOR (EFFERENT)
SOMATIC EFFERENT
General Somatic Efferent (GSE)
VISCERAL EFFERENT
General Visceral Efferent (GVE)
Special Visceral Efferent (SVE)

ACCURATE DIAGNOSIS

The primary objective of this textbook is to teach the morphologic and physiologic features of the nervous system in order to provide a basis for the student to diagnose the location of lesions that occur in this system. An additional goal is to teach the student some of the features and causes of the different kinds of diseases that affect the nervous system. An intelligent diagnosis of disease of the nervous system is entirely dependent upon a firm knowledge of the anatomy, physiology, and pathology of this system. Rational prognosis and treatment can be based only on accurate diagnosis. To perform an accurate neurologic diagnosis, it is necessary to be able to answer the following questions: Where is the disease process located, and what is its nature? The answer to the first question is dependent on the examiner's knowledge of the anatomy and physiology of the nervous system. The answer to the question on the pathogenesis of the lesion depends on a knowledge of pathology and the various basic sciences concerned with the causes of disease, such as microbiology and virology.

Although mortality is high in diseases of the nervous system in which regenerative capabilities are limited, it is the obligation of the diagnostician to diagnose the disease accurately so that transient neurologic disturbances can be recognized and appropriate therapy can be offered when it is applicable. The medical and surgical equipment for the treatment of neurologic disease is improving continually. A firm basis in the interpretation of neurologic examinations increases the confidence of the practitioner.

Proper application and interpretation of the neurologic examination should show the diagnostician where the lesion is located. In considering the various kinds of lesions that occur in the nervous system, the following general list should be reviewed to avoid overlooking a disease.

Inflammation.   Inflammation is a pathologic process involving a reaction of blood vessels and tissues to physical, chemical, and biologic agents—the reaction of tissues to an irritant. In the consideration of neurologic disease, it usually refers to the tissue reaction to a microorganism.

SUPPURATIVE INFLAMMATION.   This is an inflammation characterized by a neutrophilic response and the products of necrosis of tissue and inflammatory cells, usually caused by bacteria, protozoa, or fungi.

NONSUPPURATIVE INFLAMMATION.   This type of inflammation is characterized by a lymphocytic or monocytic response and usually is caused by a viral agent.

Degeneration.   Degeneration is the deterioration of cells from abnormal cellular metabolism caused by an inherited cellular defect, by abnormalities of other systems (nephritis-uremia, hepatitis, hypoxia), or by intoxicants. Abiotrophy is cell degeneration due to an intrinsic defect in essential metabolism necessary for survival and function.

Trauma.   Trauma is physical injury to the nervous system.

Malformation.   Malformation is developmental abnormality of the nervous system.

Neoplasia.   Primary neoplasia is the uncontrolled, continuous proliferation of a cell belonging to the nervous system, while a metastatic neoplasm is the uncontrolled growth of a malignant neoplastic cell which spreads to the nervous system from a primary neoplasm in another organ by metastasis. Such growths have no orderly structure or useful function.

THE NEURON

In this book the neuron is defined as consisting of a dendritic zone, axon, cell body, and telodendron. The dendritic zone is the "receptor" portion in which the stimulus of the internal or external environment becomes converted into an impulse in the neuron. The axon is the cell process that courses from the dendritic zone to the telodendron. The telodendron is the ending of the neuron at which the impulse leaves the neuron; it is often referred to as the synapse. The cell body consists of the nucleus and major organelles, and may be located anywhere along the axon.

For example, a sensory neuron in the peripheral nervous system for proprioception may have its dendritic zone in a neuromuscular spindle in a skeletal muscle of the limb. The axon courses toward the spinal cord through a specific peripheral nerve, a branch of one spinal nerve, its dorsal root, and into the dorsal grey column of that spinal cord segment to synapse in a nucleus within that column. The telodendron is the end of the neuron at the synapse in that nucleus. The cell body is located in the spinal ganglion associated with the dorsal root that the axon courses through. It is actually intercalated in the axon at this point.

The dendritic zone and cell body of a motor neuron of the peripheral nervous system are closely associated in the ventral grey column of one segment of the spinal cord. The axon leaves the cell body, and courses through the white matter to leave the spinal cord in a ventral root. It continues into that segment's spinal nerve, then travels to a branch of the spinal nerve, and by way of a specific peripheral nerve it reaches the skeletal muscle to be innervated. It ends in a telodendron at the neuromuscular ending in a motor end-plate.

TABLE 1–1. FUNCTIONAL CLASSIFICATION OF THE NERVOUS SYSTEM

System	Innervation
I. Afferent (A) — sensory	
Somatic (S)	
General (GSA)	"Pain," temperature, touch — spinal nerves, CN V
Special (SSA)	Vision — CN II; hearing — CN VIII
Visceral (V)	
General (GVA)	Organ content and distention, chemical changes; splanchnic — spinal nerves CN VII, IX, X
Special (SVA)	Taste — CN VII, IX, X; smell — CN I
Proprioception (P)	
General (GP)	Muscle and joint movement — spinal nerves, CN V
Special (SP)	Vestibular balance — CN VIII
II. Efferent (E) — motor	
Somatic (S)	
General (GSE)	Striated skeletal muscle associated with somite and somatic mesoderm origin — spinal nerves, CN III, IV, VI, XII
Visceral (V)	
General (GVE)	Smooth muscle, cardiac muscle, glands, sympathetic — spinal and splanchnic nerves, parasympathetic — CN III, VII, IX, X, XI
Special (SVA)	Striated muscle from branchial arch mesoderm — CN V, VII, IX, X, XI

Within the central nervous system, a neuron of the dorsal spinocerebellar tract is an example of a sensory or afferent neuron to the cerebellum. Its dendritic zone and cell body are closely associated in a nucleus in the dorsal grey column of the spinal cord. The impulse is initiated here by synapse with a sensory proprioceptive neuron of the peripheral nervous system. The axon moves across the grey and white matter to join a tract on the dorsal superficial surface of the lateral funiculus. The axon continues rostrally in this dorsal spinocerebellar tract, traversing the length of the spinal cord and caudal medulla; at the caudal medulla it enters the cerebellum through the caudal cerebellar penduncle. It courses through the cerebellar medulla and white matter of a folium, and ends in a telodendron in the granular layer of the cerebellum; here it synapses with the dendritic zone of a granular cell neuron.

Within the central nervous system, the Purkinje cell of the cerebellum is an example of an efferent or motor neuron. Its dendritic zone is located in the molecular layer of the cerebellar cortex. Telodendria of granular cell neurons synapse on these processes to initiate the impulse in the Purkinje cell. The cell body is located in the Purkinje cell layer of the cerebellar cortex. The axon travels from the cell body through the granular layer, into and through the white matter of that cerebellar folium, and into the white matter of the cerebellar medulla. Here it ends in a telodendron on the dendritic zone of another motor neuron located in a nucleus in the cerebellar medulla.

FUNCTIONAL SYSTEMS

This book is organized along the lines of functional systems rather than by regions of the nervous system. Some of these functional systems are derived from a classification of the peripheral nervous system based on its functional components. The sensory portion has components that continue in the central nervous system. The classification is as follows:

SENSORY (AFFERENT)

The afferent or sensory portion of the peripheral nervous system is classified on the basis of the location of the dendritic zone (the origin of the impulse) in the body.

SOMATIC AFFERENT

The somatic afferent system has its dendritic zone on or near the surface of the body, derived from the somatopleure where it receives the various stimuli from the external environment.

General Somatic Afferent (GSA)

The general somatic afferent system comprises the neurons distributed by the fifth cranial nerve and all the spinal nerves to the surface of the head, body, and limbs, respectively, that are sensitive to touch, temperature, and noxious stimuli.

Special Somatic Afferent (SSA)

The special somatic afferent system involves specialized receptor organs limited to one area deep within the body surface, but stimulated by changes in the external environment. These include light to the eyeball (cranial nerve II) and air waves indirectly to the membranous labyrinth of the inner ear (cranial nerve VIII, cochlear divison).

VISCERAL AFFERENT

The visceral afferent system has its dendritic zone in the wall of the various viscera of the body. This is tissue derived mostly from splanchnopleure and stimulated by changes in the internal environment.

General Visceral Afferent (GVA)

The general visceral afferent system is composed of neurons distributed by the seventh, ninth, and tenth cranial nerves to visceral structures of the head, and by the tenth cranial nerve and the spinal nerves to the viscera of the body cavities and blood vessels throughout the trunk and limbs. This widely distributed system is stimulated primarily by the distention of visceral walls and chemical changes.

Special Visceral Afferent (SVA)

The special visceral afferent system contains the neurons in the seventh, ninth, and tenth cranial nerves whose dendritic zones are limited to the specialized receptors for taste. The specialized receptor neuron for olfaction or cranial nerve I is also a component of this system.

PROPRIOCEPTION

The modality of proprioception is sometimes included in the general somatic afferent system. Here it will be considered as a separate functional system because of its clinical significance. It is the system responsible for detecting changes in the position of the trunk, limbs, and head.

General Proprioception (GP)

The general proprioceptive system is distributed widely throughout all the spinal nerves and the fifth cranial nerve, with receptors located in muscles, tendons, and joints derived from somatopleure deep within the surface of the body. The receptors respond to changes in length and position of the structures at points where they are located.

Special Proprioception (SP)

The special proprioceptive system is composed of the receptors specialized to respond to movements of the head located in the membranous labyrinth of the inner ear. These neurons, concerned with the orientation of the head in space, are in the vestibular division of the vestibulocochlear nerve (cranial nerve VIII).

MOTOR (EFFERENT)

The efferent or motor portion of the peripheral nervous system is classified on the basis of where the neuron terminates, or the site of its telodendron. This peripheral motor system also is referred to as the lower motor neuron, because it is the final neuron that innervates the muscle cell. Its cell body and dendritic zone are in the spinal cord grey matter (brain stem), and its axon is in the ventral root, spinal (cranial) nerve, and peripheral nerve. It terminates in a muscle cell at the neuromuscular ending.

SOMATIC EFFERENT

The somatic efferent system has its telodendria in voluntary striated muscles derived from somites and somatic mesoderm (skeletal), and head myotomes.

General Somatic Efferent (GSE)

The general somatic efferent system is made up of neurons in the third, fourth, sixth, and twelfth cranial nerves and all the spinal nerves that innervate the extraocular and tongue muscles, and the muscles of the axial and appendicular skeletons.

VISCERAL EFFERENT

The visceral efferent system has its telodendria in involuntary smooth muscle of viscera (splanchnic mesoderm), in blood vessels, cardiac muscle, and glands, and in voluntary muscles in the head associated with visceral function.

General Visceral Efferent (GVE)

The general visceral efferent system is the lower motor neuron of the autonomic nervous system. It is a two neuron–lower motor neuron system that includes neurons in the third, seventh, ninth, tenth and eleventh cranial nerves and all of the spinal nerves. It is distributed widely throughout the head and body, and has both sympathetic and parasympathetic divisions.

Special Visceral Efferent (SVE)

The special visceral efferent system is composed of efferent neurons in the fifth, seventh, ninth, tenth, and eleventh cranial nerves that innervate the striated muscle derived from the branchial arch mesoderm. These muscles are associated with visceral structures and functions in the head: jaw, face, palate, pharynx, larynx, and the esophagus in the neck and thorax.

A prerequisite for the use of this textbook is the knowledge and understanding of the gross anatomy of the peripheral and central nervous systems of domestic animals. This can be obtained by dissection of a dog as described in *Miller's Guide to the Dissection of the Dog*, by H. E. Evans and A. de Lahunta. The last section of this book, entitled the nervous system, specifically describes a dissection of the dog brain and spinal cord that should provide the student with the basic knowledge needed for the successful use of this textbook.

The following references may be useful adjuncts to the study of neuroanatomy, clinical neurology, and neuropathology. For neuroanatomy the textbook by T. W. Jenkins on *Functional Mammalian Neuroanatomy* is especially recommended. It is based on the dog and provides some clinical application of the functional anatomy. For clinical neurology and especially therapy, the textbook by B. F. Hoerlein, *Canine Neurology, Diagnosis and Treatment,* is recommended.

Throughout this text the anatomic descriptions are based on the dog unless otherwise stated. Major species differences of clinical importance are described.

REFERENCES

1. Adams, R. D., and Sidman, R. L.: Introduction to Neuropathology. New York, McGraw-Hill, 1968.
2. Blackwood, W., McMenemey, W. H., Meyer, A., Norman, R. M., and Russell, D. S.: Greenfield's Neuropathology. Baltimore, Williams & Wilkins, 1963.
3. Brain, Walter R.: Diseases of the Nervous System. 6th ed., London, Oxford University Press, 1962.
4. Crosby, E. C., Humphrey, T., and Lauer, E. W.: Correlative Anatomy of the Nervous System. New York, Macmillan, 1962.
5. Curtis, B. A., Jacobson, S., and Marcus, E. M.: An Introduction to the Neurosciences. Philadelphia, W. B. Saunders Co., 1972.
6. Evans, H. E., and de Lahunta, A.: Miller's Guide to the Dissection of the Dog. Philadelphia, W. B. Saunders Co., 1971.
7. Fankhauser, R., and Luginbühl, H.: Pathologische Anatomie des zentralen und peripheren Nervensystems der Haustiere. Berlin, Verlag Paul Parey, 1968.
8. Frauchiger, E., and Fankhauser, R.: Vergleichende Neuropathologie des Menschen und der Tiere. Berlin, Springer-Verlag, 1957.
9. Gilroy, J., and Meyer, J. S.: Medical Neurology. London, The Macmillan Co., 1969.
10. Hoerlein, B. F.: Canine Neurology. Diagnosis and Treatment. 2nd ed., Philadelphia, W. B. Saunders Co., 1971.
11. House, E. L., and Pansky, B.: A Functional Approach to Neuroanatomy. New York, McGraw-Hill, 1960.
12. Innes, J. R. M., and Saunders, L. Z.: Comparative Neuropathology. New York, Academic Press, 1962.

13. Jenkins, T. W.: Functional Mammalian Neuroanatomy. Philadelphia, Lea & Febiger, 1972.
14. McGrath, J. T.: Neurologic Examination of the Dog with Clinicopathologic Observations. 2nd ed., Philadelphia, Lea & Febiger, 1960.
15. Merritt, H. H.: A Textbook of Neurology. 4th ed., Philadelphia, Lea & Febiger, 1967.
16. Miller, M. E., Christensen, G. C., and Evans, H. E.: Anatomy of the Dog. Philadelphia, W. B. Saunders Co., 1964.
17. Minckler, J.: Pathology of the Nervous System. New York, McGraw-Hill, 1968.
18. Nickel, R., Schummer, A., and Seiferle, E.: Lehrbuch der Anatomie der Haustiere. Band IV Nervensystem, Sinnesorgane, Endokrine Drüsen. Berlin, Verlag Paul Parey, 1975.
19. Palmer, A. C.: Introduction to Animal Neurology. Philadelphia, F. A. Davis, 1965.
20. Papez, J. W.: Comparative Neurology. New York, T. Y. Crowell Co., 1929.
21. Peele, T. L.: The Neuroanatomic Basis of Clinical Neurology. 2nd ed., New York, McGraw-Hill, 1961.
22. Ranson, S. W., and Clark, S. L.: The Anatomy of the Nervous System. 10th ed., Philadelphia, W. B. Saunders Co., 1959.
23. Singer, M.: The Brain of the Dog in Section. Philadelphia, W. B. Saunders Co., 1962.

Chapter 2

THE DEVELOPMENT OF THE NERVOUS SYSTEM

THE NEURAL TUBE
CELL DIFFERENTIATION
SPINAL CORD
Neural Crest
MYELENCEPHALON – MEDULLA
   OBLONGATA
METENCEPHALON – CEREBELLUM
   AND PONS
MESENCEPHALON – MIDBRAIN
DIENCEPHALON – INTERBRAIN
TELENCEPHALON – CEREBRUM

MALFORMATIONS
BRAIN MALFORMATIONS
Hydrocephalus
Hypoplasia of the Prosencephalon
Hydranencephaly
*CEREBELLAR DEGENERATION AND
   HYPOPLASIA*
SPINAL CORD MALFORMATIONS
Meningomyelocele
Myelodysplasia

THE NEURAL TUBE

The central nervous system is a tubular structure originating from a proliferation of ectoderm referred to as neuroectoderm, which is situated dorsal to the notochord along the axis of the embryo. The thickened ectoderm, known as the neural plate, invaginates along this axis until the lateral extremities of the original plate, the neural folds, meet centrally and fuse over the neural groove to form a neural tube and canal. The margins of the nonneural ectoderm fuse dorsal to the neural tube and the two layers of ectoderm separate. As this fusion and separation of ectodermal layers occurs, a longitudinal column of cells arises from the junction of nonneural and neural ectoderm and separates from these two structures when the neural tube is formed. These two bilateral columns, situated dorsolateral to the neural tube throughout its length, are the columns of neural crest cells (Fig. 2–1).

Closure of the neural tube progresses rostrally and caudally from the level of the site of development of the rhombencephalon, the most caudal division of the brain. The rostral opening, or rostral neuropore, closes as the brain vesicles develop. The caudal opening at the caudal extremity of the spinal cord closes later or not at all. In some animals it communicates with the subarachnoid space of the leptomeninges at the level of the cauda equina (Fig. 2–2).

The rostral end of the neural tube develops rapidly and produces three vesicles: the prosencephalon, mesencephalon, and rhombencephalon, moving from rostral to caudal (Fig. 2–3). Early in its development the prosencephalon has a lateral enlargement, the optic vesicle, which grows out to contact the adjacent ectoderm. The further development of this primordial eyeball is considered in the

8

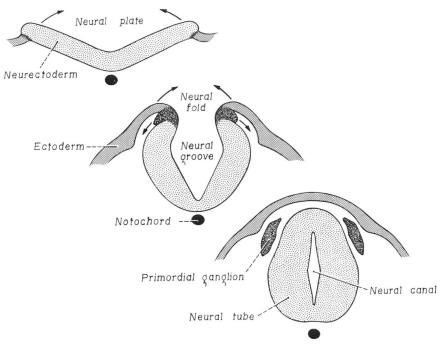

Figure 2–1. Development of the neural tube.

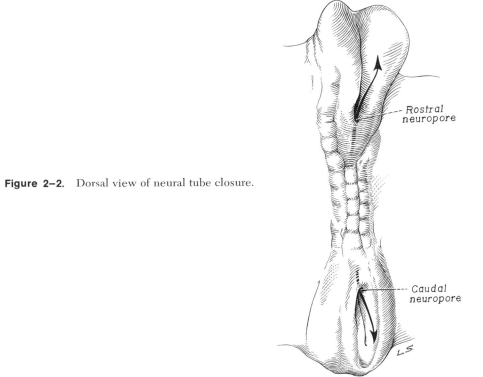

Figure 2–2. Dorsal view of neural tube closure.

section on the visual system. Two additional swellings from the rostral prosencephalon grow laterally and dorsally out of the neural tube. These telencephalic vesicles completely overgrow the original vesicular system and form the cerebral hemispheres. The portion of the prosencephalon that remains at the rostral end of the neural tube is the diencephalon. The optic vesicles remain associated with the diencephalon. The lumen of the diencephalon, the third ventricle, communicates rostrolaterally with the lumen of each telencephalon by the interventricular foramina. The latter lumina are the lateral ventricles of the cerebral hemispheres. The nuclei of the thalamus and hypothalamus develop in the diencephalon. The neurohypophysis is a ventral outgrowth of the diencephalon.

The lumen of the mesencephalon is reduced to a narrow tubular structure, called the mesencephalic aqueduct.

From the rostral rhombencephalon, the cerebellum or dorsal metencephalon develops dorsally. Concomitant developmental changes in the neural tube form the ventral metencephalon or pons. The caudal rhombencephalon forms the myelencephalon or medulla oblongata. The fourth ventricle is the lumen of the neural canal in the rhombencephalon. It communicates with the meningeal spaces that develop around the neural tube by way of openings that arise in the wall of the neural tube. These openings are called lateral apertures and are located caudal to the cerebellum (Fig. 2–3).

CELL DIFFERENTIATION

In the first stage of development within the wall of the neural tube, the cells commonly referred to as neuroepithelial or neuroectodermal cells are organized in a pseudostratified arrangement (Fig. 2–4). The cell membrane of each cell connects to both sides of the wall of the neural tube, but the nuclei are at different levels. These cells are all actively mitotic, increasing the size and thickness of the tube. The nuclei migrate within the wall of the tube, and their position depends upon the cell's stage of mitosis.

During interphase the nuclei are located on the external surface of the tube. DNA or chromosomal duplication occurs in that position. As the nucleus enters mitosis it migrates through its cytoplasm to the luminal surface. The cytoplasm and peripheral cell membrane also retract to that position where cell division is completed. The two new daughter cells extend their cell membrane to the periphery, and the nucleus migrates to the external surface again. Since the nucleus is at the outer surface during interphase, when cell division ceases in any one neuroepithelial cell and differentiation begins, it occurs on the surface of the neural tube. Thus in a short time a new layer of differentiated cells appears on the external surface of the actively mitotic layer.[12]

The cells that are differentiated are of two types. Immature neurons, the parenchymal cells, usually are referred to as neuroblasts, but this is misleading because once a neuron is formed it will not divide again, as is inferred in the term neuroblast. The differentiated neuron grows extensively to become a mature, functioning cell, but it does not divide further. Spongioblasts are the second type of cell. These are the progenitors of the neuroectodermal supporting cell for the nervous system, the neuroglia (glue). Two of the three forms of glial cells are derived from these spongioblasts: astrocytes and oligodendrocytes (Fig. 2–4).

As more primitive neurons and spongioblasts are differentiated and grow and produce processes, the neural tube is arranged into three concentric layers (Fig. 2–5). Adjacent to the neural tube is the germinal layer of proliferating neuroepi-

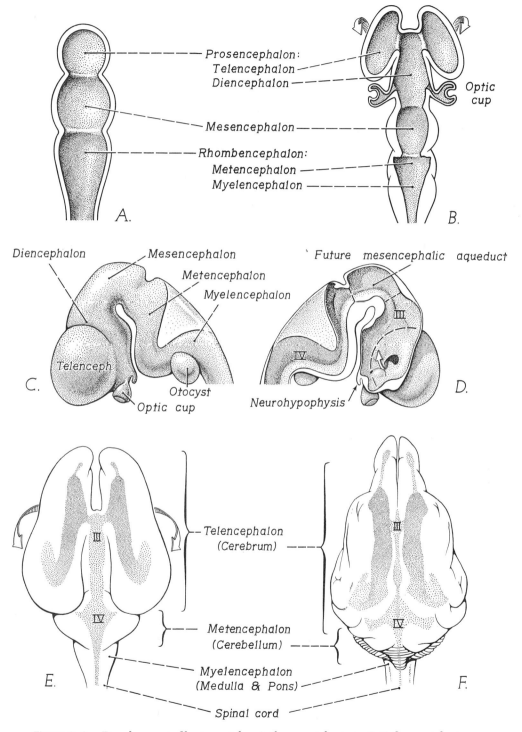

Figure 2–3. Development of brain vesicles. *A:* three vesicle stage; *B–F:* five vesicle stages.

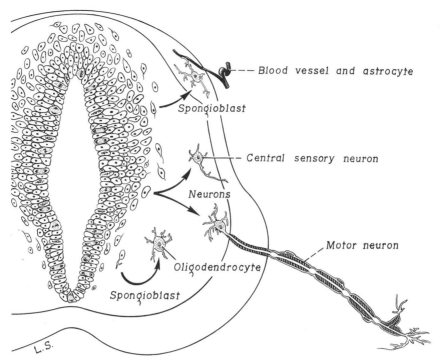

Figure 2–4. Mitosis and differentiation of neuroepithelial cells.

thelial cells. This proliferative function ultimately is exhausted and the multi-cellular layer is reduced .to a single layer of cells, ranging from squamous to columnar, called ependymal cells. The ependymal cells line the entire lumen of the neural tube, which includes the ventricular system in the brain and the central canal of the spinal cord. Peripheral to the germinal layer in the embryonic neural tube is the thick layer of differentiated cell bodies, mostly composed of primitive neurons and spongioblasts. This is the mantle layer that becomes the grey matter of the definitive spinal cord and nuclei of the brain stem. After migration to the external surface of the neural tube, this layer becomes the cerebral cortex of the telencephalon. The external layer in the neural tube is the marginal layer composed mostly of the growing processes of the cell bodies in the mantle layer. These are the tracts of the white matter.

From the mesencephalon caudally, a longitudinal groove, the sulcus limitans, is apparent in the lateral wall of the neural canal. The neural canal can be divided into dorsal and ventral portions by a dorsal plane at the level of this sulcus. The dorsal portion is called the alar plate, and the ventral portion the basal plate. Functionally, the alar-plate mantle layer is concerned predominantly with sensory systems and the basal-plate mantle layer with motor systems (Fig. 2–5).

SPINAL CORD

The spinal cord provides the best example of the symmetric development of the neural tube by layers. Ventral growth of the two basal plates and associated marginal zones leaves a separation between the two sides—the ventral median fissure. The mantle and marginal layers of the alar plates grow dorsally. The dor-

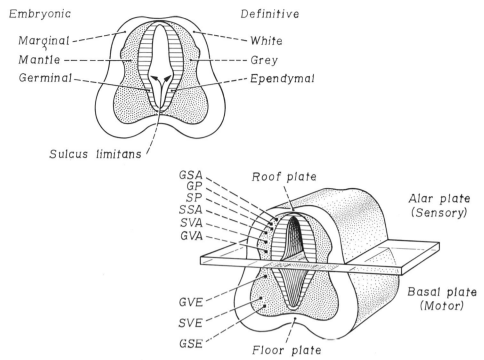

Figure 2–5. Functional organization of neural tube.

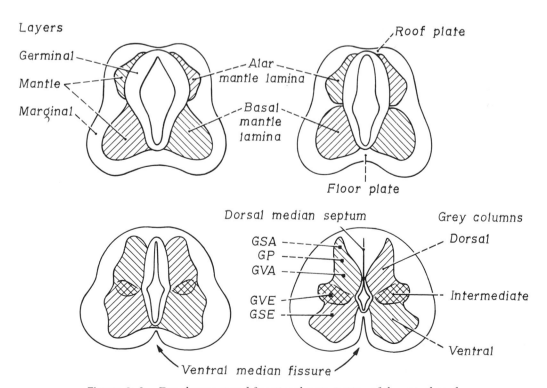

Figure 2–6. Development and functional organization of the spinal cord.

sal marginal layers fuse medially to form the dorsal median septum. The mantle layer of the alar plate becomes the dorsal grey column, and that of the basal plate the ventral grey column. The mantle zone at the plane of the sulcus limitans is the intermediate grey column (Fig. 2–6).

Not only is there a gross topographic differentiation of function of primitive neurons between the alar and basal plates, but within the mantle layer of each plate neurons are arranged in functional columns. The general visceral afferent and general visceral efferent columns are located adjacent to each other on either side of the dorsal plane through the sulcus limitans. The general somatic afferent and general proprioception columns are located dorsally in the alar plate of the mantle layer, and the general somatic efferent column is located ventrally in the basal plate of the mantle layer. Because the relative size of the components of each spinal cord segment depends on the volume of tissue to be innervated, at the levels of the limbs the spinal cord segments responsible for their innervation are enlarged, forming the cervical and lumbosacral intumescences. Studies have shown that the ultimate growth to maturity of a neuron in the peripheral nervous system depends on its appropriate innervation of a muscle cell or formation of a peripheral receptor.[7] The lack of such innervation results in degeneration of the neuron. In the cervical and thoracolumbar regions where appendages are not innervated, the immature primitive neurons in the basal-plate mantle layer and the spinal ganglion that fail to innervate structures will degenerate. The shape of the ventral grey column depicts this phenomenon, and shows further anatomic subdivision of the mantle layer. In the basal-plate mantle layer the general somatic efferent neurons located medially innervate axial skeletal musculature. Those located laterally innervate appendicular skeletal muscles. Within these areas neuronal cell bodies can be grouped further according to the specific peripheral nerve that contains the axon of these cell bodies, and specific muscle innervation.[1]

The growth of axons of the basal-plate neurons through the adjacent marginal layer and outside the neural tube forms the ventral root and part of the spinal and peripheral nerves. This includes the general somatic efferent neurons located in the ventral grey column and the general visceral efferent neurons (preganglionic neurons of the autonomic nervous system lower motor neuron) located in the intermediate grey column adjacent to the sulcus limitans. This intermediate grey column is only evident in the thoracic, part of the lumbar, and the sacral spinal cord segments. In the other segments it was present in the embryo but subsequently degenerated. These general visceral efferent neurons terminate in ganglia in the peripheral nervous system that contain the cell bodies of the postganglionic axons in this two neuron — lower motor neuron system (Fig. 2–8).

Neural Crest

The neural crest cells are the cell bodies in the longitudinal column of cells dorsolateral to the spinal cord. These provide the neurons that form the spinal ganglia at each segment. Adjacent to each somite the neural crest cells proliferate and the cell bodies form the spinal ganglia (Fig. 2–7). The axon that grows centrally into the alar-plate dorsal grey column forms the dorsal root. Distally it forms the sensory component of the spinal and peripheral nerves. The point of penetration of the marginal layer of white matter by axons of the dorsal and ventral roots divides the spinal cord white matter into three regions called funiculi. These are dorsal, lateral, and ventral on each side of the spinal cord. The formation of spinal ganglia is only one of the many outcomes of the neural crest cells. Prior to its

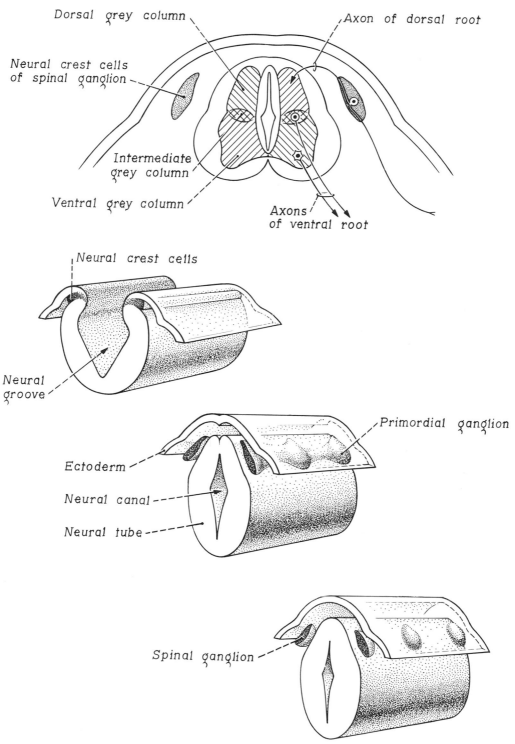

Figure 2–7. Spinal ganglia development from neural crest.

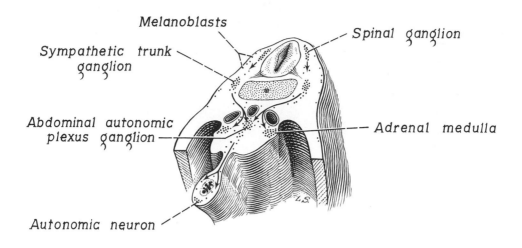

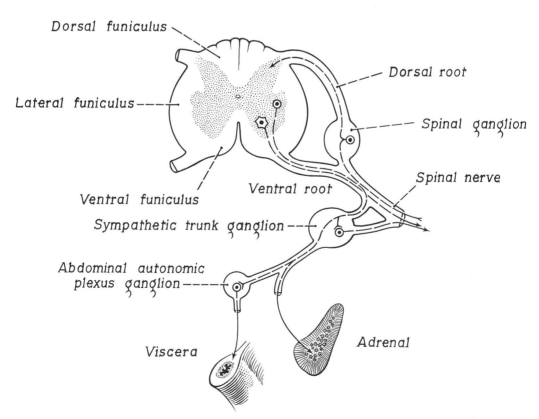

Figure 2–8.   Neural crest contribution to development of general visceral efferent neuron.

segregation into ganglia, an early migration of cells from this column provides melanoblasts to the epidermis and the cell bodies of postganglionic axons in the two neuron–general visceral efferent system. These cell bodies form the ganglia of the sympathetic trunk and the abdominal plexus autonomic ganglia, as well as the cells of the adrenal medulla (Fig. 2–8). These latter cells do not grow processes but synthesize and elaborate into the blood stream the same endocrine substance — norepinephrine — that is the neurotransmitter at the telodendron of the postganglionic axon derived from the neural crest cells. The general visceral efferent neurons located in the wall of the viscera also may be derived from the neural crest. Although melanoblasts and these general visceral efferent neurons seem to be unrelated, their common denominator is the unique metabolism of tyrosine, which provides melanin for the melanoblast and norepinephrine for the neuron. In addition to these cells, the neural crest differentiates into cells found in branchial arch cartilage, thyroid parafollicular (C) cells, odontoblasts, and possibly part of the leptomeninges and the lemmocytes (Schwann cells) that form the myelin of the peripheral nervous system.

MYELENCEPHALON — MEDULLA OBLONGATA

The basic formation of the medulla oblongata involves only a slight modification of the development described for the spinal cord. The potential roof-plate region in the neural tube is expanded extensively instead of being displaced by proliferating alar-plate and marginal layer tissue as it is in the spinal cord. This relegates the entire alar and basal plates of the neural tube to a lateral and ventral position. The region of the ventral median fissure is filled in by neural tissue. This enlarges the lumen of the central canal to form the fourth ventricle, which is covered dorsally only by the thin, single cell layer of ependyma, the roof plate. The sulcus limitans present on the ventrolateral wall of the fourth ventricle provides the plane of division of the medulla into a ventromedial basal plate and a dorsolateral alar plate having the same functional significance as in the spinal cord. Throughout the brain stem the mantle layer of the neural tube is broken up into nuclei that are collections of cell bodies with a common purpose, interspersed with neuronal processes. Some nuclei are more distinct than others. The functional columns described in the spinal cord have a similar location in the brain stem. In addition, there are added neurons organized into functional columns that have components only in cranial nerves (Fig. 2–9).

Cranial nerves VI through XII are associated with the medulla of domestic animals. The sixth and twelfth cranial nerves contain general somatic efferent neurons whose cell bodies are located in an interrupted column along the median plane adjacent to the fourth ventricle. The preganglionic neurons of the general visceral efferent system have axons in the seventh, ninth, and tenth cranial nerves and the cell bodies are located in an interrupted column medial to the sulcus limitans. This relationship of the general somatic efferent and general visceral efferent columns is comparable to that found in the spinal cord. The cell bodies of the special visceral efferent system form a nuclear column which was originally located between the GSE and GVE columns, but migrated to a ventrolateral position closer to the source of their stimulus for sensory neurons in the trigeminal nerve. This phenomenon of migration is called neurobiotaxis. As a result of this migration, the axons from this nucleus course toward the ventricle before coursing ventrolaterally and into their respective cranial nerves — VII, IX, X, and XI.

The sensory components of cranial nerves associated with the medulla arise

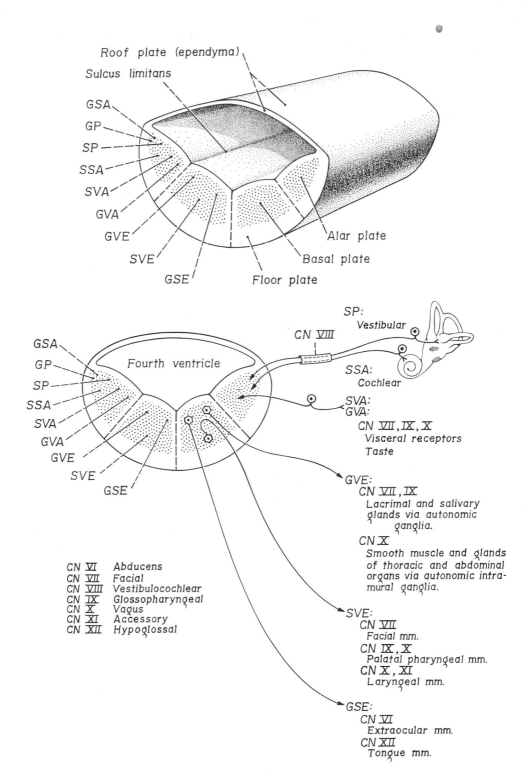

Figure 2–9. Functional organization of cranial nerves VI to XII in the myelencephalon.

from primitive neurons that develop from neural crest cells, with some contribution from ectodermal cells that proliferate from branchial groove ectoderm. These latter are referred to as cranial placodes. These two sources form the sensory ganglia of cranial nerves VII, IX, and X concerned with general and special visceral afferent (taste) function, and of cranial nerve VIII concerned with special proprioception (vestibular) and special somatic afferent (auditory) function. The centrally situated axons grow into the alar-plate region of the medulla to synapse on cell bodies comparable to the dorsal grey column cell bodies in the spinal cord (Fig. 2–9).

The leptomeninges that surround the entire central nervous system form from neural crest cells and adjacent mesodermal cells. These meninges are vascularized. Dorsal to the roof plate of the fourth ventricle, the capillary blood vessels proliferate to form a plexus that extends the adjacent pia mater and ependymal layer into the lumen of the fourth ventricle. This entire structure is referred to as the choroid plexus, although by definition the plexus is the proliferated network of blood vessels. This proliferation occurs in two symmetric sagittal lines parallel to the median plane, from the caudal part of the fourth ventricle rostrally to the level of the cerebellar peduncles, where the plexuses turn laterally. At this point there is an opening in the roof plate called the lateral aperture. At the level of the lateral aperture these choroid plexuses protrude from the lumen of the fourth ventricle out through the lateral aperture, where they are visible at the cerebellomedullary angle (Fig. 2–10).

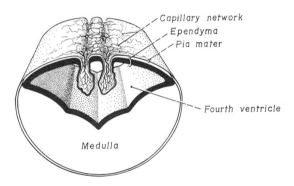

Figure 2–10. Development of roof plate and choroid plexus of fourth ventricle.

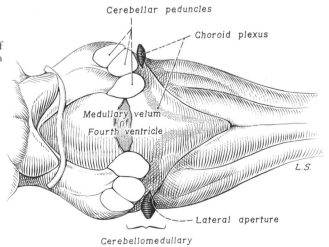

METENCEPHALON—CEREBELLUM AND PONS

The initial development of the metencephalon is comparable to that of the myelencephalon. Cranial nerve V is associated with this division of the brain stem (Fig. 2–11). Its motor neurons function in the special visceral efferent system. Its sensory neurons, whose cell bodies are situated in the trigeminal ganglion, function predominantly in the general somatic afferent system, with some in the general proprioceptive system. The central axons of these neurons grow into the alar-plate region of the metencephalon and course rostrally into the mesencephalon and caudally through the entire myelencephalon to synapse on alar-plate neurons (Fig. 2–11).

The cerebellum, or dorsal metencephalon, is formed from the proliferation of the germinal neuroepithelial cells of the alar plate. This growth dorsolaterally from each side overgrows the roof plate of the fourth ventricle so that the cerebellum forms the dorsal boundary of the fourth ventricle in the metencephalon. The cerebellum is thus the dorsal metencephalon. The ventral metencephalon is the pons. Migration of alar-plate neurons forms the pontine nucleus on the ventral aspect of the metencephalon. The axons of these neurons course dorsally into the cerebellum producing the transverse fibers of the pons, which demarcate the ventral surface of the pons (Fig. 2–12).

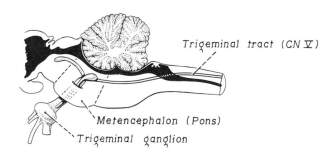

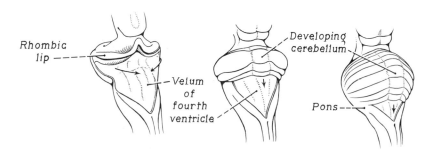

Figure 2–11. Development of the metencephalon: surface view, afferent portion of cranial nerve V.

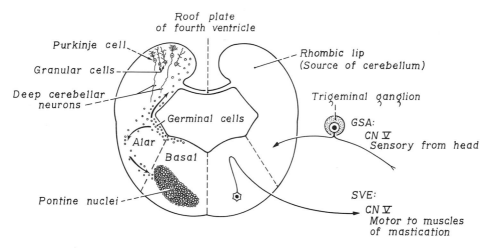

Figure 2–12. Development of the metencephalon: transverse section, pontine nucleus.

MESENCEPHALON—MIDBRAIN

Symmetric proliferation of the walls of the neural tube in the mesencephalon reduces the size of the neural canal to a narrow tube, the mesencephalic aqueduct. This is smaller rostrally at the point where it joins the third ventricle, and larger caudally where it is continuous with the fourth ventricle.

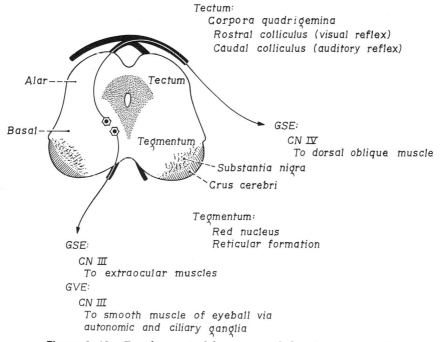

Figure 2–13. Development of the mesencephalon: transverse section.

Cranial nerves III and IV are associated with the midbrain. These contain general somatic efferent axons that innervate extraocular muscles. The cell bodies are in the same topographic nuclear column as those for cranial nerves VI and XII, adjacent to the median plane ventral to the aqueduct. The alar plate proliferates dorsally to form the tectum of the midbrain, which is divided into paired rostral and caudal colliculi. These are associated with visual and auditory reflex functions, respectively. The crus cerebri on the ventral aspect of the midbrain results from the caudal growth of descending telencephalic projection neurons. These are in the internal capsule rostral to the midbrain (Fig. 2–13).

DIENCEPHALON – INTERBRAIN

Rostral to the region of the mesencephalon the sulcus limitans is no longer evident in the primitive neural tube, and the diencephalon and telencephalon are considered to be developments of the alar-plate tissue. The symmetric development of the lateral walls of the neural tube in the diencephalon reduces the neural canal to a vertical slit on the median plane. Adhesion of the developing thalamus in the center forms the interthalamic adhesion, and separates the third ventricle into a small dorsal component and a larger ventral component. These two portions converge caudally at the mesencephalic aqueduct and rostrally at the level of the interventricular foramina. There is only roof plate along the median plane over the small dorsal portion of the third ventricle, and a small choroid plexus is developed along this roof plate on both sides of the median plane. At the interventricular foramina these are continuous with the choroid plexuses of the lateral ventricles (Fig. 2–14).

The dorsal portion of the diencephalon forms the thalamus, which is a complex of numerous nuclei and tracts of neuronal processes. The nervous tissue constituting the walls and floor of the ventral portion of the third ventricle forms the hypothalamus. A ventral outgrowth of the hypothalamus, including an extension of the third ventricle, produces the neurohypophysis. The neurohypophysis becomes associated with the contribution from the oral ectoderm, the hypophyseal (Rathke's) pouch, to form the hypophysis (pituitary gland). The original optic vesicles that grew out of the prosencephalon ultimately become associated with the diencephalon (Fig. 2–3). The axons that grow caudally from the retina (optic cup) in the optic nerve and optic tract enter a nuclear area of the thalamus. These optic nerve axons form cranial nerve II, which is the special somatic afferent or visual system.

TELENCEPHALON – CEREBRUM

The rostral boundary of the brain stem is the lamina terminalis of the diencephalon. It forms the rostral boundary of the third ventricle of the diencephalon. The optic chiasm is located at the ventral portion of this lamina. At this level the telencephalic vesicle grew out of the original prosencephalon, a short distance rostrally and in a large curve caudally and ventrally. The lumen of this vesicle is the lateral ventricle, which communicates with the diencephalic third ventricle by means of the interventricular foramen on either side, at the level of the lamina terminalis (Fig. 2–15).

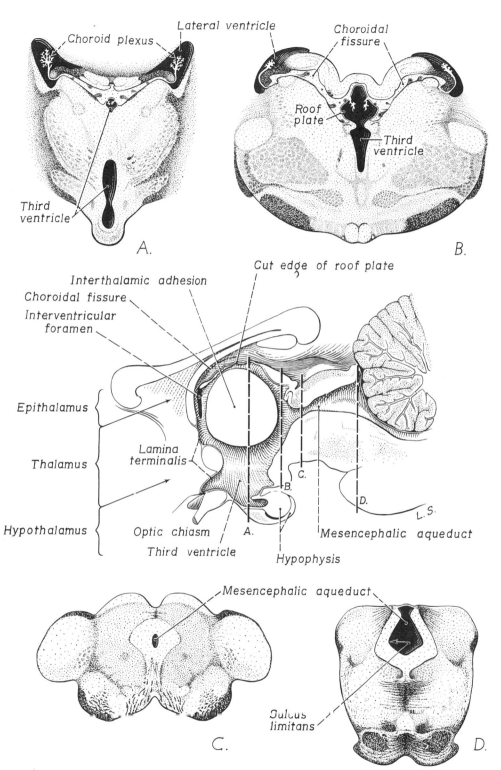

Figure 2–14. Relationship of the diencephalon and mesencephalon. *A:* Transverse section of mid-diencephalon; *B:* transverse section of caudal diencephalon; *C:* transverse section of rostral mesencephalon; *D:* transverse section of caudal mesencephalon.

ventrally by the paleopallium. A small lateral area is the neopallium and the dorsal area is the archipallium. In mammals the neopallium has overgrown the other divisions of the cerebral cortex so that the paleopallium is entirely on the ventral surface of the cerebrum ventral to the rhinal sulcus, and the archipallium is rolled medially into the lateral ventricle as an internal gyrus—the hippocampus. Continual development of the neopallium has resulted in the characteristic gyri and sulci observed over most of the exposed surface of the cerebrum. Although at birth the puppy brain has the primary gyri and sulci present, these undergo extensive development in the first 3 to 6 weeks of life.

The axons of telencephalic cortical neurons form tracts that are classified as association fibers if they course between areas of cortex within one cerebral hemisphere. If the axons leave the cerebrum to enter the brain stem via the internal capsule, they are called projection fibers. Those that cross from the cerebral cortex of one hemisphere to the opposite hemisphere are commissural fibers (Fig. 2–17). All of these axons are intermixed in the centrum semiovale, the mass of white matter in the center of the cerebrum dorsal to the lateral ventricle.

The commissural fibers of the telencephalon originally all develop through the lamina terminalis (Fig. 2–18). The rostral commissure located ventrally in the lamina terminalis courses primarily between paleopallial structures and basal nuclei (amygdala) of each side. Another small group of commissural fibers runs between the archipallium (hippocampus) of either side, forming the hippocampal commissure. The largest group of commissural fibers forms the corpus callosum. This primarily connects the neopallial areas of each hemisphere. Beginning in the lamina terminalis, it extends caudally over the diencephalon as the telencephalic vesicle expands caudally in its development. The corpus callosum forms between the archipallium and neopallium on the medial side of the hemisphere, and thus constitutes the roof of the lateral ventricle dorsal to the hippocampus and the fornix.

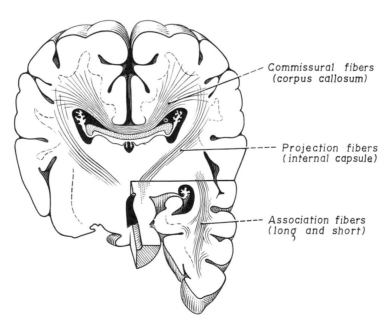

Commissural fibers
(corpus callosum)

Projection fibers
(internal capsule)

Association fibers
(long and short)

Figure 2–17.   Development of neuronal processes in telencephalon.

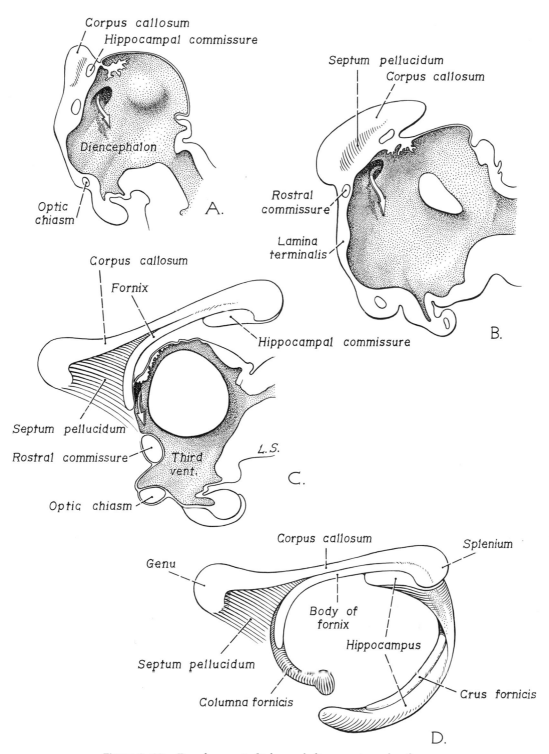

Figure 2–18. Development of telencephalic commissural pathways.

The septum pellucidum develops out of the rostral part of the lamina terminalis, between the genu of the corpus callosum and the body of the fornix (Fig. 2–18).

In the telencephalon the germinal layer ultimately is replaced by the ependyma of the lateral ventricle. Except for the area of the basal nuclei, the mantle and marginal layers reverse their positions by means of the migration of the neuronal cell bodies to the surface of the neural tube and the primary internal (medial) growth of the axons that leave the cerebral cortex. Remnants of this telencephalic germinal layer persist throughout the life of the animal. This is known as the subependymal zone, and consists of a variable-sized collection of small cells that are thought to be a continual source of glia and small neurons.

MALFORMATIONS[10]

BRAIN MALFORMATIONS

Hydrocephalus

Many circumstances can cause the ventricular cerebrospinal fluid pressure to elevate and dilate the lateral ventricles, at the expense of the telencephalon. This hypertensive hydrocephalus causes extensive degeneration of the telencephalon, especially its neopallium. The subject of hydrocephalus is considered in the discussion of cerebrospinal fluid.

Hypoplasia of the Prosencephalon

Failure of the telencephalic vesicles to develop has been observed in calves with cranioschisis, which is a separation of the calvaria and meningoencephalocele (a sac of protruding meninges and brain tissue).[22] These cases of prosencephalic hypoplasia do not have cerebral hemispheres, and show a malformed diencephalon and a relatively normal caudal brain stem with a misshapen cerebellum. The animals have been noted to be able to stand and to live for a few days, but they are obtunded and have no vision. At times these cases have been referred to erroneously as anencephaly, which is a complete failure of brain development.[5]

Cerebral meningocele and meningoencephalocele have been reported in pigs, with a variety of associated brain malformations.[26] Cranium bifidum and exencephaly occurred in a kitten exposed in utero to griseofulvin being used to treat ringworm infection in its dam.[25]

Hydranencephaly—A Model for Viral-Induced Cerebral Malformation in Animals

Hydranencephaly is the condition in which each cerebral hemisphere has been reduced to a cerebrospinal fluid-filled membranous sac within a relatively normal sized cranial cavity. The wall of the sac consists of leptomeninges, a glial membrane, and ependymal remnants with no remains of cortical parenchyma.[6]

In some instances the cause of the malformation is a viral agent that destroys the developing telencephalon.[8, 9] The malformation is the result of necrosis of already differentiated nervous tissue, and aplasia caused by the necrosis of still actively mitotic germinal neuroectodermal tissue. Cells from the latter usually migrate outward from the mantle layer to form the glia and neurons of the cerebral cortex. Interference with the blood supply of this germinal layer, causing ischemic necrosis of these precursor cells, also produces this lesion.

The bluetongue virus has been shown to produce this lesion in both clinical and experimental studies.[19, 20, 24] This virus causes systemic disease in sheep that is characterized by fever, lameness, and erosions and ulcerations of the oral and nasal mucosae. The live-virus vaccine produced to establish immunity in sheep was found to cause brain malformations, including hydranencephaly in lambs born from ewes immunized during gestation. These lambs were referred to as "dummy lambs" because of their depressed sensorium and lack of response. They were also blind. Experimental studies of direct inoculation of this vaccine into fetal sheep have demonstrated that inoculation between 50 and 58 days' gestation consistently produced a severe necrotizing encephalitis that presented at term as hydranencephaly. Inoculation between 75 and 78 days' gestation produced multifocal encephalitis, which presented at term as porencephaly. This consists of congenital cystic cavities in the cerebrum that often communicate with the lateral ventricle. Inoculation after 100 days' gestation caused mild focal encephalitis with no resulting malformation. Thus the nature of the malformation depended on the gestational age at which infection of the fetus occurred.

The germinal cells of the telencephalon are especially susceptible to this infection, and are most abundant at the end of the first trimester in the lamb fetus. Necrosis of these cells in the first trimester prevents their contributing to the cerebral cortex, and, along with the necrosis of the already differentiated cortical plate, leads to the cavitation typical of the malformation. By birth the inflammation has resolved, leaving the malformed tissue as the "scar" from the in utero infection.

Hydranencephaly also has been reported in calves; in these cases circumstantial evidence has incriminated the bluetongue virus as the cause.[23] Visual deficit, dullness ("dummy calves"), ataxia, and inability to suckle were the clinical signs. There was no history of clinical illness in the pregnant cattle, but the dams of the affected calves had high serum antibody titers to this virus, as did the affected calves that had not received colostrum. Elevated serum antibody levels in neonatal calves that did not receive colostrum is indicative of in utero infection which stimulated the production of specific antibodies.

Hydranencephaly sometimes associated with arthrogryposis has been observed in Japan, Israel, and Australia.[4, 14, 18, 28] Recently the Akabane virus has been implicated as the cause.[29, 30]

Unilateral hydranencephaly was found in an 8-month-old miniature poodle whose only clinical sign was a visual deficit. No data were available to establish an in utero infection as the cause. In studying the pathogenesis of this malformation in human neurology, considerable emphasis has been placed on prenatal occlusion or agenesis of the carotid artery, and this has been produced experimentally in puppies.

CEREBELLAR DEGENERATION AND HYPOPLASIA

Abnormalities of the development of the cerebellum are discussed in the section on that organ system.

SPINAL CORD MALFORMATIONS

Meningomyelocele

Spina bifida (the failure of closure of one or more vertebral arches) associated with meningocele or meningomyelocele has been observed in Manx cats and brachiocephalic breeds of dogs, especially the English bulldog.[2, 11, 13, 15, 17, 21] This usually involves the sacral or last few lumbar vertebrae and the associated spinal cord. The owner's chief complaint usually is that the animal lacks control of its excretions. The tail, anus, and perineum are usually analgesic and may be atonic and areflexic. The pelvic limb gait may be normal or weak and ataxic. Cranial to the meningomyelocele various median plane–spinal cord abnormalities (myelodysplasia) are often found, with or without signs of abnormal pelvic limb function.

Myelodysplasia

Various forms of myelodysplasia have been observed in calves, sometimes associated with a malformed vertebral column. The myelodysplasia has included bizarre overgrowth of spinal cord tissue, varying from a doubled or tripled dorsal grey column in one segment of spinal cord, to two complete spinal cord segments side by side. The latter is referred to as diplomyelia. This usually has involved the caudal thoracic and lumbar spinal cord segments. Hydromyelia (dilated central canal), syringomyelia (cavitated white matter), or both, may accompany this. These conditions present with a nonprogressive difficulty in the use of the pelvic limbs from birth characterized by a marked, occasionally bizarre, incoordination of the pelvic limbs without obvious paresis. Pain perception and spinal reflexes usually are normal.

Spinal dysraphism has been reported as an hereditary disease in Weimaraner dogs.[16] It is a form of myelodysplasia and is primarily an abnormality in development of the structures of the spinal cord along the median plane. There is no failure of the neural tube to close, as the term dysraphism connotes. The malformation includes aberrations in the dorsal median septum and the ventral median fissure, a dilated central canal (hydromyelia) or an absent central canal, cavitation in the white matter (syringomyelia), usually in the dorsal funiculi, and the abnormal presence of ventral grey column cells across the median plane between the central canal and the ventral median fissure. The signs are apparent by 4 to 6 weeks of age and do not progress. A characteristic symmetric use of the pelvic limbs called "bunny hopping" is observed, along with some proprioceptive deficit. The spinal cord abnormality may be accompanied by scoliosis, abnormal dorsal cervical hair patterns, and a depression of the sternum on the median plane (koilosternia).

A similar dysraphism was observed in 3 of a litter of 9 huskies. Two others had an undefined malformation of the appendicular skeleton. These 3 puppies had shown simultaneous symmetric use of the pelvic limbs ("bunny hopping") since they had been able to walk. The signs had remained static.

The following is a case description to show the value of the history, careful clinical and pathologic examinations, and knowledge of the literature in the understanding of disease. It is an example of an inherited malformation.

Case Report. Hereditary Hereford syndrome with brain, spinal cord, ocular, and muscle dysplasia.

Signalment. A 1-day-old Hereford calf.

Chief Complaint. Recumbent, blind with "white" eyes.

History. Following a normal parturition this calf was unable to get up. According to the owner the calf was representative of a herd problem of 3 years' duration. The herd consisted of 7 cows (6 of which traced back to 1 female) and 1 bull. Of the 7 calves born 2 years ago, 2 had been affected similarly. One year ago 5 out of 7 had been affected. This case was the second calf born this year. The other was normal.

Physical Examination. The calf was severely depressed (obtunded), recumbent, and unable to get up. Voluntary movements could be elicited from the limbs, along with normal spinal reflexes. The calf was blind. There were cataracts in both eyeballs ("white eyes") and the pupils were fixed and unresponsive to light. The eyeballs were deviated ventrally and an abnormal nystagmus could be elicited in some positions of the head.

Necropsy. Multiple lesions of malformations were observed. Both cerebral hemispheres were enlarged owing to the accumulation of an excessive amount of cerebrospinal fluid in widely dilated lateral ventricles (hydrocephalus). The third ventricle also was dilated. The cerebral gyri were smaller and more numerous than normal (polymicrogyria). The cerebellum was malformed and smaller than usual. Cerebellar cortical dysplasia and lack of myelin development were observed microscopically. The brain stem was bent in a sharp dorsal curve at the level of the midbrain. The colliculi were fused and projected caudally. The aqueduct was malformed and stenotic. The optic nerves and chiasm were small and cystic.

There were cataracts bilaterally, along with retinal dysplasia and a cone-shaped detachment of the retina bilaterally.

Muscular dystrophy and spinal cord–white matter dysplasia have been observed in similar Hereford calves reported in the literature. They were not studied in this calf.

Cause. Based on the herd history and previous published studies of a morphologically similar syndrome, it was assumed that the disease was inherited as an autosomal recessive.[3, 27]

REFERENCES

1. Amann, J.: The organization of spinal motoneurons and their relationship to corticospinal fibers in the raccoon(*Procyon lotor*). Ph.D. thesis, Ithaca, NY, Cornell University, 1971.
2. Bailey, C. S.: An embryological approach to the clinical significance of congenital vertebral and spinal cord abnormalities. J. Am. Anim. Hosp. Assoc., *11*:426, 1975.
3. Baker, M. L., Payne, L. C., and Baker, G. N.: The inheritance of hydrocephalus in cattle. J. Hered., 52:135, 1961.
4. Bonner, R. B., Mylrea, P. J., and Doyle, B. J.: Arthrogryposis and hydranencephaly in calves. Aust. Vet. J., *37*:160, 1961.
5. Dennis, S. M., and Leipold, H. W.: Anencephaly in sheep. Cor. Vet., *62*:273, 1972.
6. Halsey, J. H., Jr., Allen, N., and Chamberlain, H. R.: The morphogenesis of hydranencephaly. J. Neurol. Sci., *12*:187, 1971.
7. Jacobsen, M.: Developmental Neurobiology. New York, Holt, Rinehart, and Winston, 1970.
8. Johnson, R. T.: Effects of viral infection on the developing nervous system. N. Engl. J. Med., 287:599, 1972.
9. Johnson, R. T., and Mims, C. A.: Pathogenesis of viral infections of the nervous system. N. Engl. J. Med., *278*:23, 1968.
10. Kalter, H.: Teratology of the Central Nervous System. Chicago, University of Chicago Press, 1968.
11. Kitchen, H., Murray, R. E., and Cockrell, B. Y.: Spina bifida, sacral dysgenesis and myelocele. Am. J. Pathol., *68*:203, 1972.
12. Langman, J., Guerrant, R. L., and Freeman, B. G.: Behavior of neuroepithelial cells during closure of the neural tube. J. Comp. Neurol., *127*:399, 1966.
13. Leipold, H. W., Huston, K. Blauch, B., and Guffy, M. M.: Congenital defects of the caudal vertebral column and spinal cord in Manx cats. J. Am. Vet. Med. Assoc., *164*:520, 1974.
14. Markusfeld, O., and Mayer, E.: An arthrogryposis and hydranencephaly syndrome in calves in Israel, 1969–1970. Epidemiological and clinical aspects. Refuah Vet., *28*:51, 1971.
15. Martin, A. H.: A congenital defect in the spinal cord of the Manx cat. Vet. Path., 8:232, 1971.
16. McGrath, J. T.: Spinal dysraphism in the dog. Pathol. Vet., *2* Suppl.:1, 1965.

17. Michael James, C. C., Lassman, L. P., and Tomlinson, B. E.: Congenital anomalies of the lower spine and spinal cord in Manx cats. J. Pathol., 97:269, 1969.

18. Nobel, T. A., Klopfer, V., and Neumann, F.: Pathology of an arthrogryposis-hydranencephaly syndrome in domestic ruminants in Israel, 1969–1970. Refuah Vet., 28:144, 1971.

19. Osburn, B. I., Johnson, R. T., Silverstein, A. M., Prendergast, R. A., Jochim, M. M., and Levy, S. E.: Experimental viral-induced congenital encephalopathies. II. The pathogenesis of bluetongue vaccine virus infection in fetal lambs. Lab. Invest., 25:206, 1971.

20. Osburn, B. I., Silverstein, A. M., Prendergast, R. A., Johnson, R. T., and Parshall, C. J., Jr.: Experimental viral-induced congenital encephalopathies. I. Pathology of hydranencephaly and porencephaly caused by bluetongue vaccine virus. Lab. Invest., 25:197, 1971.

21. Parker, A. J., Park, R. D., Byerly, C. S., and Stowater, J. L.: Spina bifida with protrusion of spinal cord tissue in a dog. J. Am. Vet. Med. Assoc., 163:158, 1973.

22. Püschner, H., and Fankhauser, R.: Drei seltene Gehirnmissbildungen beim Rind—"Duplicatas palli," einseitige Zystenzephalie und Mikroenzephalie mit Enzephalozele. Schweiz. Arch. Tierheilkd., 110:198, 1968.

23. Richards, W. P. C., Crenshaw, G. L., and Bushnell, R. B.: Hydranencephaly of calves associated with natural bluetongue virus infection. Cornell Vet., 61:336, 1971.

24. Schmidt, R. E., and Panciera, R. J.: Cerebral malformation in fetal lambs from a bluetongue enzootic flock. J. Am. Vet. Med. Assoc., 162:567, 1973.

25. Scott, F. W., de Lahunta, A., Schultz, R. D., Bistner, S. I., and Riis, R. C.: Teratogenesis in cats associated with griseofulvin therapy. Teratology, 11:79, 1975.

26. Trautwein, G., and Meyer, H.: Experimentelle Untersuchungen über erbliche Meningocele cerebralis beim Schwein. II. Pathomorphologie der Gehirnmissbildungen. Pathol. Vet., 3:543, 1966.

27. Urman, H. K., and Grace, O. D.: Hereditary encephalopathy, a hydrocephalus syndrome in newborn calves. Cornell Vet., 54:229, 1964.

28. Whittem, J. H.: Congenital abnormalities in calves: Arthrogryposis and hydranencephaly. J. Pathol. Bacteriol., 73:375, 1957.

29. Hartley, W. J., Wanner, R. A., Della-Porta, A. J., and Snowdon, W. A.: Serological evidence for the association of Akabane virus with epizootic bovine congenital arthrogryposis and hydranencephaly syndromes in New South Wales. Aust. Vet. J., 51:103, 1975.

30. Omori, T., Inaba, T., Kurogi, H., Miura, Y., Nobuto, K., Ohashi, Y., and Matsumoto, M.: Viral abortion, arthrogryposis-hydranencephaly syndrome in cattle in Japan, 1972–1974. Bull. Off. Int. Epix., 81 (5–6):447, 1974.

Chapter 3

CEREBROSPINAL FLUID AND HYDROCEPHALUS

PRODUCTION
CIRCULATION
ABSORPTION
FUNCTION
CLINICAL APPLICATION OF CSF
METHOD TO OBTAIN CSF
*ATLANTO-OCCIPITAL (CEREBELLO-
 MEDULLARY CISTERN) CEREBROSPINAL
 FLUID COLLECTION IN SMALL ANIMALS*
*ATLANTO-OCCIPITAL (CEREBELLO-
 MEDULLARY CISTERN) CSF
 COLLECTION IN THE HORSE*

*LUMBOSACRAL CSF COLLECTION IN
 THE HORSE*
CEREBROSPINAL FLUID
 EXAMINATION
Pressure
Physical
Cytologic-Biochemical
Microbiologic
HYDROCEPHALUS
CLINICAL SIGNS
ANCILLARY EXAMINATION
TREATMENT

Cerebrospinal fluid (CSF) is a clear, colorless fluid that surrounds and permeates the entire central nervous system (CNS) and therefore protects, supports, and nourishes it. In general the CSF is produced by the choroid plexuses, circulates to the subarachnoid space, and is absorbed into the venous sinuses.[18, 67]

PRODUCTION

More specifically, CSF originates from a number of sites. These include the choroid plexuses of the lateral, third, and fourth ventricles, directly from the brain by way of the ependymal lining of the ventricular system, directly from the brain by way of the pial-glial membrane covering its external surface, and from blood vessels in the pia-arachnoid (Fig. 3–1).[43, 44]

One study on total production of CSF in the dog revealed that 35 per cent derived from the third and lateral ventricles, 23 per cent from the fourth ventricle, and 42 per cent from the subarachnoid space. The results of these studies vary with the experimental model that is used.[9, 40]

The method of production is both by ultrafiltration from the blood plasma and by active transport mechanisms that utilize energy. The blood-CSF barrier is composed of the capillary endothelium, which is fenestrated, a thin basement membrane, and the ependymal cells. These cells have the characteristics of cells that function in the transcellular transport of materials: they have microvilli on their luminal surface and infoldings of the basal cytoplasm. The blood-CSF barrier is a semipermeable membrane that selectively and actively transports some materials and inhibits others.[15, 29]

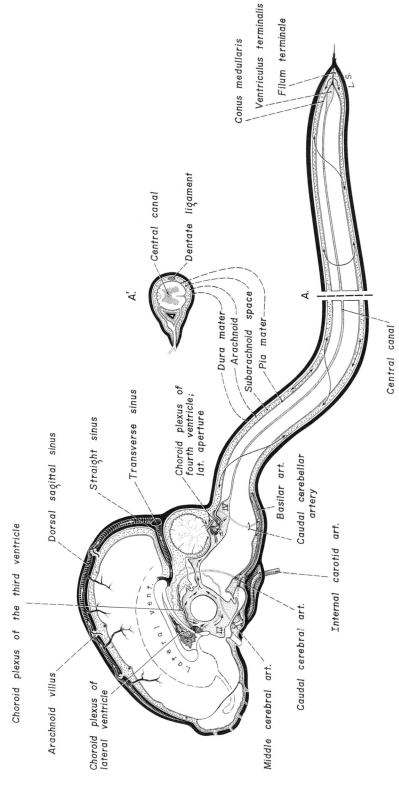

Figure 3–1. Relationship of meninges and subarachnoid space to ventricular system.

Compared to plasma ultrafiltrate the CSF has less potassium and calcium, and more chloride, sodium, and especially magnesium. It has slightly less glucose, about 80 per cent of the blood level, and much less protein. There is less than 25 mg per dl of protein, which is mostly albumin. Products of the breakdown of hemoglobin, bile salts, and penicillin are prevented from entering the CSF from the blood.

The rate of production varies with the species and method of determination. The following rates have been determined: dog—.047 cc per min, cat—.017 cc per min, man—0.5 cc per min.[14] In man this rate is equivalent to 3 to 5 times the total volume per day.

There is a continual turnover of CSF. There is evidence that it is produced at a constant flow rate despite the pressure of CSF in the ventricular system. The rate is independent of the hydrostatic pressure of the blood, but is influenced by the osmotic pressure of the blood. Hypertonic solutions in the blood will reduce the rate of formation. This has clinical application in head injuries with cerebral edema. An osmotic diuretic is administered to decrease the rate of CSF formation and aid in the removal of excessive amounts of interstitial fluid in the CNS. Mannitol, a hypertonic solution of a carbohydrate, is used at the rate of 1 gm per lb intravenously of a 20 per cent solution.[33]

CIRCULATION

The CSF circulates from the ventricular system to the subarachnoid space by way of the lateral apertures of the fourth ventricle (Fig. 3–2). In some individuals there is a similar passage between the central canal and subarachnoid space at the conus medullaris (Fig. 3–1).[64] Much of the CSF passes dorsally over the cerebrum to the dorsal sagittal sinus. It covers the entire surface of the brain and spinal cord, and penetrates the parenchyma, along with the larger blood vessels in the perivascular spaces.[68] These spaces are extensions of the subarachnoid space to the point at which the pia mater reflects onto the wall of the blood vessel. This is not a distinct point, and for some distance the cells of the leptomeninges and the adventitia of the blood vessel may be indistinct, and the perivascular space reduced to small clefts between the cells. At the capillary level the blood-brain barrier consists of a nonfenestrated capillary endothelium, a thick basement membrane, and the processes of astrocytes.[34]

The flow of the CSF is thought to be due to the pulsation of the blood in the choroid plexuses. With each pulsation the CSF pressure rises and surges towards the lateral apertures. The cilia on the ependymal cells may contribute to the flow.

In man there is evidence that despite the erect posture, CSF tends to flow cranially as well as caudally. Radioiodinated serum albumin injected into the lumbar cistern can be followed by scanning radiographic procedures of the dorsum of the hemisphere in 12 to 24 hours. Radiopharmaceuticals injected into the lateral ventricle appear in the thoracolumbar subarachnoid space in 30 to 40 minutes.[70] Comparison of cerebellomedullary and lumbosacral CSF in animals with spinal cord disease suggests that there is some caudal flow of CSF in animals.

The cranial cavity is a closed space consisting of brain parenchyma, CSF, and the blood. Any change in the volume of one requires an adjustment in the volume of the others. This sensitive relationship and the continuity of the cranial and spinal subarachnoid spaces can be demonstrated by compressing the external jugular veins and measuring the CSF pressure at the cerebellomedullary cistern and the lumbar cistern. Venous compression causes an increase in venous blood volume

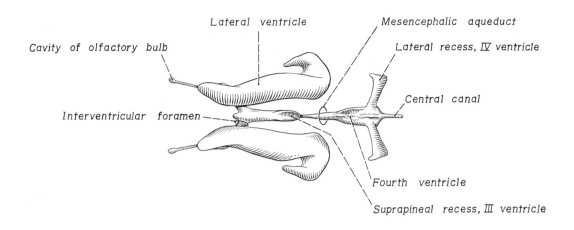

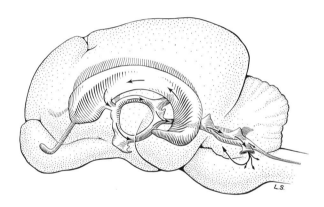

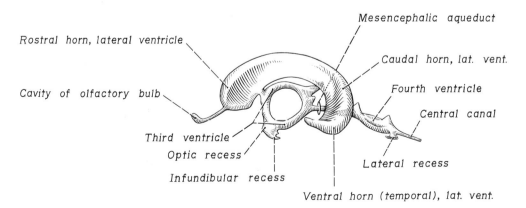

Figure 3–2.   The canine ventricular system.

in the cranial cavity. This requires more space and the CSF space is compressed, causing the pressure in the subarachnoid space to rise. For a similar reason the CSF in the pressure-measuring manometer will rise and fall, with the respirations reflecting the associated changes in thoracic venous pressure. The pressure elevation is reflected at both ends of the spinal subarachnoid space.

If there is a lesion such as a neoplasm or large abscess that obliterates the subarachnoid space along the spinal cord, and the CSF pressure is measured at the lumbar cistern, this pressure will not elevate when the intracranial CSF pressure is elevated by external jugular compression. This is called the Queckenstedt or jugular compression maneuver.

Another practical application of the knowledge that the cranial cavity is a closed space often can be seen following injury. One of the cardinal rules in the emergency room is to be sure the patient has a patent airway. This not only assures the proper oxygenation of blood for tissues, but prevents dilation of cerebral blood vessels. Hypercapnia causes cerebral arterial vasodilation and increases the volume of blood in the cranial cavity. If head injury is part of the syndrome, this augments the already existing problem of cerebral hemorrhage or edema that has taxed the space requirements in the cranial cavity. Similarly, when a dog is positioned for intracranial or cervical spinal cord surgery, the head and neck should be elevated and suspended from a specialized holding device, rather than resting on padding that will compress the external jugular veins. Normal CSF pressure is quite variable and fluctuates widely over a 24-hour period.

ABSORPTION

The major site of CSF absorption is at the arachnoid villus located in a venous sinus or cerebral vein.[2, 48, 49] Collections of villi are known as arachnoid

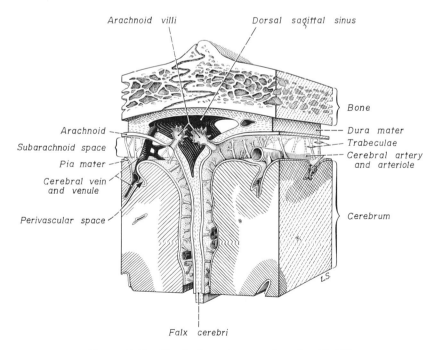

Figure 3–3. Cerebral meninges and arachnoid villi.

granulations.[30] The arachnoid villus is a prolongation of the arachnoid and the subarachnoid space into the venous sinus. The arachnoid tissue is covered by venous endothelium. These are structured and function to act as a "ball valve" so that they are open when the CSF pressure exceeds the venous pressure, which is the normal relationship between these two fluids. If venous pressure exceeds that of the CSF, these villi collapse. Flow is one way, from CSF to blood. These villi are found in the venous sinuses and in some cerebral veins (Fig. 3–3).

Electron-microscopic studies of the endothelial cells lining the arachnoid villi have revealed transient transcellular channels that develop for the passage of materials from CSF to the venous system. These apparently develop only in response to a pressure gradient between the CSF and venous blood, and function as a "one-way valve" system.[61, 62]

Other sites of absorption include the veins and lymphatics found around spinal nerve roots, and the spinal nerves and the first and second cranial nerves at the sites at which they leave the skull.[21] Some CSF may enter directly into the subarachnoid blood vessels. Some CSF may enter the brain parenchyma through the ependyma and be absorbed in blood vessels there. This probably occurs more often when intraventricular CSF pressure is elevated.[45]

Thus CSF is formed and absorbed throughout the ventricles and subarachnoid space, is in constant motion, and progresses generally toward the surface of the cerebral hemisphere and along the spinal cord. With the rate of production being independent of intracranial pressure, absorption is the primary homeostatic mechanism for maintenance of the intracranial pressure.

FUNCTION

CSF has a number of functions, including the protection and nourishment of the parenchyma and the maintenance of homeostasis. The brain is suspended in and buoyed by CSF, and thus is physically protected by it. CSF helps to modulate pressure changes that occur within the cranial cavity. In conjunction with cerebral blood flow, it helps regulate the intracranial pressure.

As a chemical buffer to the central nervous system, CSF helps maintain the proper ionic environment for the parenchyma. Being closely related to the "interstitial fluid" and in close proximity to the parenchyma, it provides a more stable and closely controlled ionic environment than the blood plasma. The pH of CSF has a direct influence on medullary function. A metabolic function may be served by CSF in acting as a medium for transport of metabolites and nutrients between the brain and the blood. It also may serve to transport neuroendocrine substances and neurotransmitters.

A clinical example of the importance of these functions is seen in the remarkable neurologic deficits that can accompany severe inflammation of the leptomeninges without direct involvement of the parenchyma. This is most commonly noted in cryptococcal meningitis of dogs and bacterial meningitis of calves.

CLINICAL APPLICATION OF CSF

CSF may be used in selected radiographic procedures, and may be analyzed for its cellular and chemical constituents.

Radiographic procedures utilizing a radiopaque dye or air are employed to

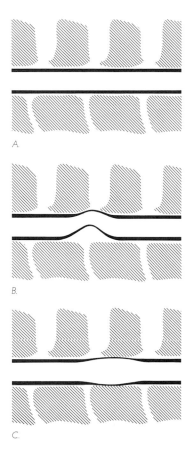

Figure 3–4. Myelographic interpretation. A: normal; B: extradural compression; C: intradural enlargement.

demonstrate the shape of the CSF-containing system and reveal changes caused by disease.

Myelography. A radiopaque water-soluble medium such as methiodal sodium (Skiodan) is injected into the spinal subarachnoid space, usually between L5–L6, to determine if the subarachnoid space has been altered by a space-occupying lesion or abnormality of the vertebral column (Figs. 3–4, 3–5, 3–6).[12] In order to outline the cervical spinal cord the volume of dye injected at L5–L6 needs to be increased by about 50 per cent, and the flow is facilitated if a needle is placed in the cerebellomedullary cistern to let CSF run off. This procedure sometimes causes convulsions, which usually can be controlled by an anticonvulsant, diazepam sodium (Valium). Alternatively, the water-soluble media may be injected in smaller amounts into the cerebellomedullary cistern, but this must be done with caution as they have a toxic effect on medullary vital centers. The head must be kept elevated at all times. Some prefer to inject a radiopaque oil emulsion (iophendylate or Pantopaque) into the cerebellomedullary cistern to outline the cervical spinal cord. This is less toxic and does not produce convulsions, but over a long period of time may produce a foreign-body meningitis. Subsequent CSF evaluations are useless.

Pneumoventriculography. This involves the injection of air directly into the lateral ventricle, allowing it to outline the ventricular system (Fig. 3–2).[25, 32, 69] The site of injection is located by finding the half-way point between the external occipital protuberance and the lateral angle of the eyelids. Trace a line from there medially, perpendicular to the median plane of the skull. Enter the skull on that

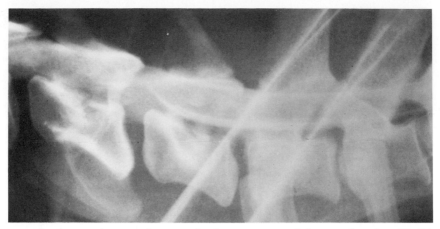

Figure 3–5. Skiodan myelogram of an extradural compression of the spinal cord at C6–C7 articulation in a 5-year-old Doberman pinscher. A protruded-proliferated intervertebral disk was presumed.

perpendicular line 3 to 5 mm from the median plane. A straight, pointed intramedullary bone pin about the size of the spinal needle may be used to bore a hole in the calvaria through which to pass the needle. On a lateral radiograph of the skull measure the depth of the cranial cavity. Do not insert the needle beyond half the distance from the calvaria. The normal ventricle may be difficult to enter. The widely dilated ventricle is entered immediately, but the pressure may be low enough to require aspiration to obtain the CSF. Withdraw a small amount of CSF (1 to 2 cc) and replace it with air. By rotating the patient, the air can be moved in the ventricle so as to define all its borders. This is a safe procedure that can be done routinely on hospital patients with no aftereffects (Fig. 3–7).

   Contrast Ventriculography. This may be performed by the same procedure using small amounts of meglumine iothalamate (Conray), but it is less safe than air. It is especially useful to determine if there is a block in the ventricular system at the aqueduct or lateral aperture of the fourth ventricle. The latter cannot be determined at necropsy. The appearance of contrast medium in the cervical subarach-

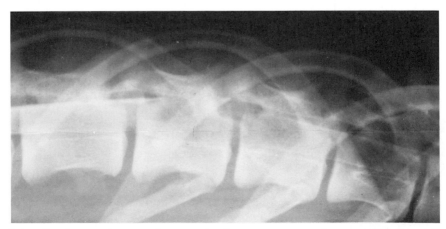

Figure 3–6. Skiodan myelogram of an intradural space-occupying lesion at T13 in a 3.5-year-old German shepherd. A neuroepithelioma was diagnosed.

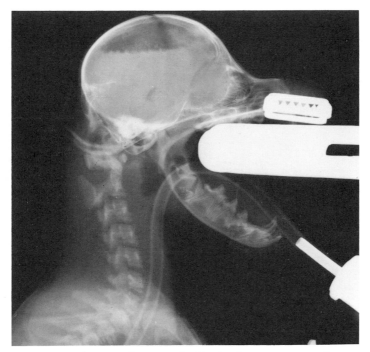

Figure 3–7. Pneumoventriculogram of a 3-month-old Manchester terrier with extensive dilation of the lateral ventricles.

noid space from injection into the lateral ventricle confirms the patency of the system (Fig. 3–8).

Laboratory examination is performed on CSF because it often reflects disease processes that involve the parenchyma or meninges.

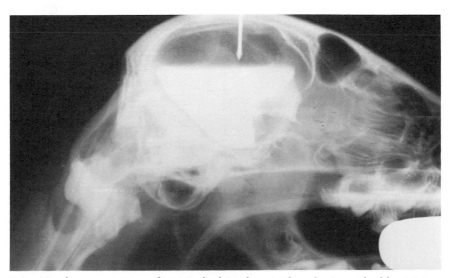

Figure 3–8. Air above contrast medium in the lateral ventricles of a 3-month-old miniature poodle with extensive hydrocephalus. The contrast medium can be visualized in the subarachnoid space in the vertebral canal, indicating the absence of any obstruction to flow through the ventricular system.

METHOD TO OBTAIN CSF

In the dog, the most reliable source of CSF for laboratory analysis is the cerebellomedullary cistern. The L5–L6 site used for myelography is good if an adequate amount of nontraumatized CSF can be obtained.[4] In the horse, cow, sheep, goat, and pig both the atlanto-occipital and lumbosacral sites are useful sources of CSF. The following are detailed descriptions for the dog and horse that are applicable to the other species.

ATLANTO-OCCIPITAL (CEREBELLOMEDULLARY CISTERN) *CEREBROSPINAL FLUID COLLECTION IN SMALL ANIMALS*

With the patient under general anesthesia, surgically prepare the atlanto-occipital area between and caudal to the ears. For the right-handed individual, place the dog in left lateral recumbency with its skull and cervical vertebrae at the edge of the table. Have an assistant elevate the nose slightly so that it is parallel with the vertebral column, and flex the atlanto-occipital joint so that the median axis of the head is about at right angles to the median axis of the cervical vertebrae. Observe respirations continually, because vigorous flexion may bend the endotracheal tube and cause an obstructed airway.

If the tapping site is not palpated and the needle is handled only at the hub, surgical gloves are not necessary. With the left hand, place the thumb on the external occipital protuberance and the first finger on the cranial edge of the right wing of the atlas. From these landmarks draw one imaginary line caudally along the dorsal midline from the external occipital protuberance, and another transversely between the cranial edges of the wings of the atlas. The needle should be inserted where these two lines cross.

A spinal needle with stilette that is 1.5 inches long and 20 gauge is adequate for most dogs and cats.[a] A 3-inch 20-gauge needle may be necessary in some dogs of the larger breeds. With the bevel directed to the side, insert the needle through the skin and into the underlying muscle and fascia. Direct it toward the angle of the jaw. Place the palm of the left hand on the skull for support and grasp the hub of the needle with thumb and first finger; do not release it until the procedure is completed. Remove the stilette with the right hand and observe for fluid. If none is seen, replace the stilette, and without releasing the left hand from the needle, continue to advance the needle 1 to 2 mm at a time. After each advancement remove the stilette and observe for fluid. In many instances a slight sudden loss of resistance may be felt as the atlanto-occipital membrane and dura mater are penetrated simultaneously. Because it is not consistent, do *not* rely on this sign for the depth of your needle. Continual observation for fluid is the safest method. Slight rotation of the needle may produce fluid when the desired level has been reached but no fluid has emerged.

If the needle strikes bone at about the level you would expect fluid to appear, then the point of the needle must be walked gently caudally off the occipital bone or cranially off the atlas to reach the atlanto-occipital space. It is often preferable to withdraw the needle and start again, correcting for the slight error in direction of the first attempt.

----

[a]Becton, Dickinson and Co., Rutherford, N. J. 07070.

At all times maintain a firm grip on the needle with the left hand.

When fluid is observed, place the tip of the 3-way valve of the manometer[a] in the hub and measure the opening pressure when the CSF has reached its maximum height in the tube. Rotate the valve arm to close the connection to the tube and open the syringe. Withdraw 1 to 2 cc of CSF. Reopen the lumen to the manometer tube and measure the closing pressure. When this is determined close off the connection to the tapping needle, and remove the manometer and syringe unit. Replace the stilette and remove the needle in one motion.

In some small breeds of dogs and cats, if measurement of CSF pressure is not essential to the differential diagnosis it may be preferable not to attach the manometer unit to the needle, but to collect the fluid directly with a syringe. If the flow is slow, a direct sample may be collected most readily by letting the CSF drip from the hub into a test tube. Simultaneous jugular vein compression may hasten this flow.

The level at which the subarachnoid space is reached varies with the breed and the individual animal. In toy breeds and some cats it is often very close to the surface and is small. Caution is advised.

ATLANTO-OCCIPITAL (CEREBELLOMEDULLARY CISTERN) CSF COLLECTION IN THE HORSE[42]

The horse is given a general anesthetic of choice and placed in lateral recumbency. An area of the poll and neck (from between the ears to 6 to 8 inches caudally and approximately 3 to 4 inches on either side of the mane) is prepared surgically. The horse's head is flexed so that the median axis of the head is at right angles to the median axis of the cervical vertebrae. Such flexion of the atlanto-occipital joint can result in upper airway obstruction. A sterile fenestrated drape is used to cover the site and sterile surgical gloves may be used to handle the 18- or 20-gauge 3.5-inch spinal needle.[b]

The site of skin penetration is located at the intersection of imaginary lines drawn between the cranial borders of the atlas and along the dorsal midline (Fig. 3–9). Palpate the wings of the atlas and define the site of skin penetration. It is important that the needle traverse the median plane during insertion, as it is possible to pass through the atlanto-occipital space and be too far lateral, thus missing the subarachnoid space. The needle usually is aimed at the lower jaw or lips (perpendicular to the cervical vertebrae), and the wrist of the hand holding the needle must rest on the sterile drape over the occipital area or dorsum of the neck so the needle can be moved slowly and with steady pressure. An initial thrust is often helpful to advance the needle the first inch through the thick skin and funicular part of the ligamentum nuchae. The needle is advanced until the dorsal atlanto-occipital membrane and cervical dura mater are penetrated. These tissues, being stretched with flexion of the head, often give rise to a clear "popping" sensation either of increased or sudden lack of resistance when penetrated. During insertion of the needle the stilette should be withdrawn whenever such a sensation is felt or whenever it is judged that a sufficient depth has been reached. Clear CSF appearing at the hub of the needle indicates a successful procedure. If no spinal

---

[a]Manometer Tray, Pharmaseal Laboratories, Glendale, Calif. 91201.
[b]Becton, Dickinson and Co., Rutherford, N.J. 07070.

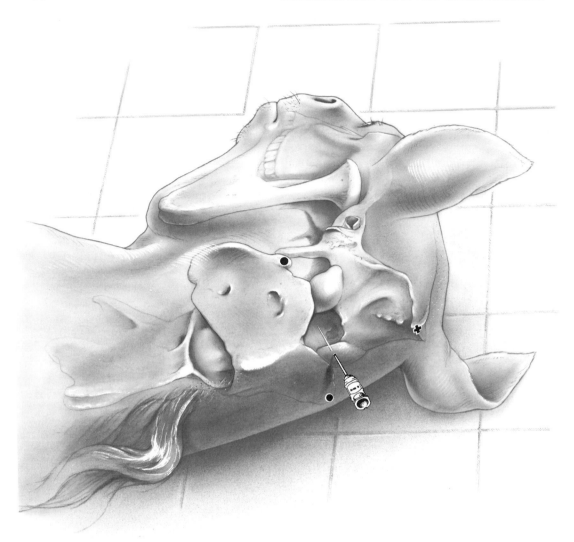

Figure 3–9. Atlanto-occipital cerebrospinal fluid collection from the recumbent horse. Spinal needle in position with stilette removed. Palpable landmarks are the cranial borders of the atlas (●——●) and the external occipital protuberance (+) on the dorsal midline.

fluid appears the needle is rotated 90 degrees, and if this is unsuccessful, the stilette is replaced and the needle advanced further.

The depth at which the subarachnoid space is entered and CSF obtained is normally between 2 and 3 inches. This depends on the size and weight of the horse, the angle of insertion of the spinal needle, and the degree of flexion of the atlanto-occipital joint. The needle must never be advanced without the stilette in place in order to prevent damage to neural tissue and plugging of the needle with tissue.

When CSF is obtained the opening pressure is measured immediately with a manometer, and the sample collected.[a] After measuring the closing pressure the stilette is replaced and the needle withdrawn.

---

[a]Manometer Tray, Pharmaseal Laboratories, Glendale, Calif. 91201.

LUMBOSACRAL CSF COLLECTION IN THE HORSE
(Method of I. Mayhew)[42]

The horse is lightly restrained in a standing position. Only in overtly excitable animals is use of a tranquilizer advised, as this tends to cause the horse to stand with most of the caudal weight supported on one pelvic limb with a resulting displacement of the utilized landmarks. Lumbosacral CSF collection in the laterally recumbent horse (either tetraplegic or under general anesthesia) is generally more difficult than in the standing subject because of the resulting asymmetry of the palpable bony prominences.

The area is surgically prepared; a sterile drape and surgical gloves may be used in the procedure.

The site of skin penetration is found by attempting to correlate many different landmarks. This is because there are considerable individual and sex differences

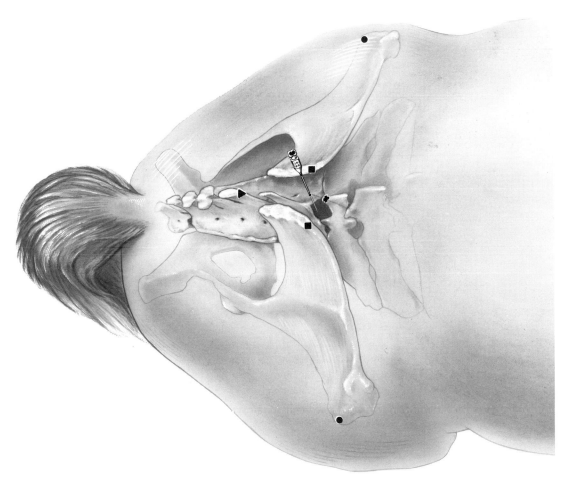

Figure 3–10. Lumbosacral cerebrospinal fluid collection from the standing horse. Spinal needle in position with stilette removed. Palpable landmarks are the caudal borders of each tuber coxae (●——●), the caudal edge of the spine of L6 (+), the cranial edge of the second sacral spine (▲), and the cranial edge of each tuber sacrale (■——■).

and often some of the landmarks cannot be palpated easily. The preferred site of skin penetration is within the depression bordered laterally by the medial rim of the tuber sacrale, cranially by the caudal edge of the sixth lumbar spine, and caudally by the cranial edge of the second sacral spine (Fig. 3–10). It is often one-quarter to one-half inch caudal to the cranial border of this depression and at the point of intersection of a line drawn between the cranial edge of each tuber sacrale and the dorsal midline. The first estimate of this site is the intersection at a line joining the caudal border of each tuber coxae with the dorsal midline. This often is between the highest points of the gluteal region. Palpate the lumbar spines and by moving caudally, the caudal edge of the spines of the fifth (L5) and sixth (L6) lumbar vertebrae can be palpated. Because the spine of L6 usually is shorter than that of L5, there is often palpable depression at the caudal edge of L5, and this is occasionally mistaken for the site. The first sacral spine is usually too short to palpate. The tuber sacrale of each side can be palpated a variable distance from the dorsal midline on a sagittal plane. The exact position and distance between each tuber sacrale vary. Generally these are more prominent and further apart in mares.

Following appropriate local analgesia, a small stab incision is made with a sterile surgical blade through the skin at this site. It is advisable to have a twitch available or lightly applied to the horse's upper lip. However, it is usually only during penetration of the dura mater that there is any response on the part of the horse, and generally this is restricted to a local response of tail movement, slight flexion of the pelvic limbs, and slight axial muscle contraction with evidence of conscious perception. An occasional horse will react with sudden violent movements, and if these cannot be predicted and prevented, an appropriate sedation or general anesthesia may be necessary.

A 3.5-inch 18- or 20-gauge spinal needle can be used in ponies and foals up to approximately 12 hands tall, and a 6.0-inch 18-gauge thin-wall needle with fitted stilette can be used on horses up to approximately 17 hands tall.[a] Occasionally, a special 8- or 9-inch spinal needle is required on very tall horses.

A right-handed person should stand on the horse's right side and rest the wrist of the right hand on the dorsal midline of the horse cranial to the site of the previously made small skin incision. Holding the stilette firmly in place, advance the spinal needle along the median plane toward the lumbosacral space. The average depth of penetration of the needle to reach the subarachnoid space in a 450-kg horse is approximately 5 inches, and the diameter of the lumbosacral space is approximately 1.0 inch (Fig. 3–11).

The needle usually can be moved forward without much resistance. Penetration of the lumbosacral interarcuate ligament (ligamentum flavum) often is felt as a sudden loss of a slightly increased resistance, and the dura mater and arachnoid may be entered at the same time; otherwise, these membranes may be penetrated by advancing the needle a few millimeters, and this usually is accompanied by some local response on the part of the horse, as described. If CSF is not obtained, the needle can be advanced to the floor of the vertebral canal and then withdrawn, slowly rotating it a millimeter or less at a time. In this situation, the needle passes through the dorsal dura mater and subarachnoid space and conus medullaris, then through the ventral subarachnoid space and dura mater. It is im-

[a]Becton, Dickinson and Co., Rutherford, N. J. 07070.

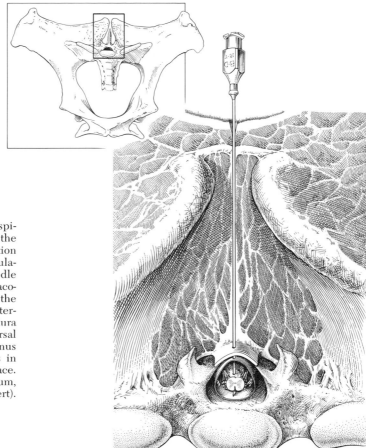

Figure 3–11. Lumbosacral spinal fluid collection from the horse. Transverse dissection through lumbosacral articulation, cranial view. Spinal needle passes through the skin, thoracolumbar fascia adjacent to the interspinous ligaments, interarcuate ligament, dorsal dura mater and arachnoid, dorsal subarachnoid space, and conus medullaris. Needle point is in ventral subarachnoid space. Cranial view of pelvis, sacrum, and area of dissection (insert).

L. Sadler

perative that the hand holding the hub of the spinal needle rests very firmly on the horse whenever the needle is held or manipulated, and the stilette always must be in place during movement of the needle.

At each stage when the stilette is withdrawn to determine if the subarachnoid space is entered, several different efforts should be made to obtain CSF before the stilette is replaced and the needle advanced or withdrawn. First, an assistant should occlude both jugular veins to increase intracranial and thus intraspinal pressure. Then, the needle can be rotated up to 180° to stop any of the meninges or nerve roots from lying across and occluding the bevel of the needle point. Finally a small (5-ml) syringe can be applied to the needle hub and gentle suction pressure intermittently applied. (A heavy syringe tends to force the needle down further, and continuous strong suction pressure also tends to promote hemorrhage and often occludes the needle with meninges or cauda equina. If the horse moves during collection, the jugular veins still can be readily occluded and CSF often can be aspirated from within the hub of the needle without connecting the syringe to it, thus reducing the chances of dislodging the needle from the subarachnoid space or initiating hemorrhage.

CEREBROSPINAL FLUID EXAMINATION[3, 14, 19, 22, 23, 47, 57, 58]

Pressure

The pressure is only significant if it is elevated above normal. Occasionally in the normal animal there is insufficient pressure to cause the CSF to rise in the manometer. Although most dogs have a pressure of less than 170 mm under general anesthesia, some animals of the larger breeds have a higher normal pressure. This may be augmented by some gas anesthetics, especially if the anesthesia is prolonged prior to the pressure determination. Some of the conditions that cause an elevated CSF pressure are: (1) Space-occupying lesions—neoplasm, abscess, hemorrhages, noncommunicating hypertensive hydrocephalus. These compress the venous sinuses and prevent CSF absorption from the arachnoid villi. (2) Cerebral edema usually associated with brain injury. (3) Communicating hydrocephalus (occasionally), and (4) meningitis.

Physical

Normal CSF is clear and colorless. A red tinge appears if hemorrhage occurs during the tap. This should disappear as further aliquots of CSF are withdrawn. Centrifugation should leave a clear fluid. If the discoloration persists, then there has been previous hemorrhage into the CSF. In general, contamination by blood during the tapping procedure provides 1 mg of protein and 1 white blood cell (WBC) per 500 red blood cells (RBCs). It is more accurate to calculate the ratio of white blood cells to red blood cells in a blood sample to determine if the WBC count of the CSF is elevated significantly. With massive contamination, this ratio becomes inadequate. The tap can be repeated in 24 hours to obtain a fresh sample. Whole blood may be obtained from epidural veins without entering the subarachnoid space. Repeat the procedure with a clean needle until CSF is obtained.

Xanthochromic yellow CSF usually is caused by free bilirubin of previous subarachnoid hemorrhage. Extremely high CSF total protein (more than 400 mg per 100 cc) or severe prolonged systemic icterus may cause xanthochromia. Centrifugation does not remove this color.

Turbidity is caused by an increase in the cell count (WBC or RBC or both) greater than 500 per cmm.

Foam that persists on the surface of the sample is indicative of an elevated protein content.

Fibrin clots occur with increased protein levels when fibrinogen is present, as in suppurative meningitis or profuse hemorrhage. This may be prevented by using an anticoagulant in the sampling tube.

TABLE 3–1. TABLE OF NORMAL VALUES

Species	Pressure (mm H_2O)	Protein (mg/dl)	Cells/cmm
Dog	<170	<25	<5
Cat	<100	<20	<5
Ox	<200	<40	<5
Sheep	<270	<40	<5
Pig	<145	<40	<5
Horse	<400	<70	<5

**TABLE 3–2.   CSF DETERMINATIONS AND DISEASES
OF THE NERVOUS SYSTEM**

Determination	Meningitis Bacterial Disease (suppurative inflammation)	Disease Parenchymal Disease Tissue Necrosis: Neoplasia, Degenerations Viral Disease (nonsuppurative inflammation)
Physical	turbid, clot	clear, colorless
Cytologic (WBC)[51]		
Quantitative	large increase greater than 100/cmm	small increase less than 100/cmm
differential	mostly neutrophils	mostly mononuclear cells
Chemical		
Protein		
quantitative (total)	large increase greater than 100 mg/dl	small increase less than 100 mg/dl
qualitative (globulins)		
Pándy (phenol)	plus 2–4	0 to plus 1
Nonne Apelt (NH_3SO_4)	plus 2–4	0 to plus 1
Glucose—normally about 80% of blood level	normal or decreased to below 50% of the blood level	normal

Cytologic-Biochemical

The following guidelines relate the physical, cytologic, and chemical determinations in CSF with diseases of the nervous system. There are many exceptions. The CSF study must be evaluated in relation to the patient's history and the physical and neurologic examinations.

The CSF protein may increase without a concomitant increase in cells. This is sometimes called an albuminocytologic dissociation, and occurs under the following circumstances:

1. Extensive noninflammatory degeneration of brain parenchyma with tissue necrosis.

2. Vascular lesions with hemorrhage, or transudation from diseased blood vessels, or both.

3. Neoplasms that produce protein, interfere with blood vessel integrity, or produce necrosis of the adjacent parenchyma.

4. Some instances of nonsuppurative encephalitis caused by the canine distemper virus. In these cases the globulin fraction of protein is increased.[17, 39]

The enzymes glutamic-oxaloacetic transaminase (GOT) and creatine phosphokinase (CPK) may increase in CSF when extensive myelin degeneration has occurred.[65] Lactic dehydrogenase (LDH) is increased in lymphosarcoma that directly involves the nervous system parenchyma.

Microbiologic

The fungus *Cryptococcus neoformans* is the only agent that can be identified consistently in CSF. India ink staining of CSF may enhance its visibility. Bacteria may be observed in white blood cells in suppurative meningitis. Such cells should be Gram stained. All fluid that is turbid or any clots should be Gram stained and cultured. All fluid with neutrophils, or with moderate elevations of WBC, or both, should be cultured.

HYDROCEPHALUS[5, 6, 54]

In the broad sense of the term, hydrocephalus is an increase in the volume of CSF. Terms often used in reference to hydrocephalus are:

Internal—Ventricular dilation.
External—Dilation of subarachnoid space.
Communicating—Extraventricular obstruction or compensatory hydrocephalus.
Noncommunicating—Intraventricular obstruction preventing communication of the entire ventricular system with the cerebellomedullary cistern of the subarachnoid space.
Normotensive—Normal CSF pressure.
Hypertensive—Increased CSF pressure.

TABLE 3–3. CLINICAL EXAMPLES OF ABNORMAL CEREBROSPINAL FLUID

Disease Process		Pressure mm H$_2$O	RBC/cmm	WBC/cmm	Protein mg/dl	Other
Inflammation:						
Viral Inflammation:						
Canine distemper encephalitis	1.	120	23	19–66% mononuclear	49	
	2.	65	—	4 mononuclear	88	
	3.	—	26	4 mononuclear	45	
Equine rhinopneumonitis		—	326	11 mononuclear	278	
Feline infectious peritonitis,						
meningoencephalitis	1.	—	—	500 mononuclear	185	
	2.	—	—	66–84% mono-nuclear, 26% neutrophils	404	
	3.	—	410	1144 mononuclear	498	
Fungal Inflammation:						
Canine cryptococcal meningo-encephalomyelitis						
1. Xanthochromic						
Organisms in CSF		too viscid	—	1353–mostly neutrophils	501	glucose–21 mg per dl blood glucose–67 mg per dl
2. Organisms in CSF		364	76	498–92% eosinophils	187	
3. Organisms in CSF		—	4670 (trauma)	280 mononuclear	154	
Protozoal Inflammation:						
Canine toxoplasma encephalitis						
1. Cerebral granuloma		256	2	17 mononuclear, 8 neutrophils	94	
2. Diffuse encephalitis		—	16	18 mononuclear	103	
Equine protozoal myelitis (lumbosacral)		—	—	29 mononuclear	51	
Bacterial Inflammation:						
Suppurative (bacterial) meningoencephalitis—calf		168	—	188–66% neutrophils	110	
Coliform meningoencephalitis–calf		—	650	2800–69% neutrophils	143	

**TABLE 3-3. CLINICAL EXAMPLES OF
ABNORMAL CEREBROSPINAL FLUID—Continued**

Disease Process		Pressure mm H$_2$O	RBC/cmm	WBC/cmm	Protein mg/dl	Other
Listeriosis-(meningo)encephalitis– bovine	1.	—	—	31 mononuclear mostly	79	
	2.	—	—	7 mononuclear mostly	27	
	3.	—	105	29–90% mononuclear	81	
Parasitic Inflammation:						
Cuterebra encephalitis (cat)		—	—	258–mostly neutrophils	89	
Cuterebra encephalitis (dog)		—	10	280–84% neutrophils, 16% mononuclears	98	
		—	24	20–50% neutrophils, 6% eosinophils, 44% mononuclear	38	
Parelaphostrongylus tenuis encephalomyelitis (goat)	1.	—	3340	50–70% mononuclear, 30% neutrophils	63	
	2.	—	2440	650–3% mononuclear, 97% eosinophils	71	
	3.	—	5040	70–61% mononuclear, 34% eosinophils, 5% neutrophils	92	
Neoplasia—Inflammation:						
Canine primary reticulosis	1.	—	—	58 mononuclear	90	
	2.	—	—	324 mononuclear	360	
Neoplasia						
Ependymoma		237	—	13 mononuclear	110	
Choroid plexus carcinoma (lumbosacral roots)		—	5	2 mononuclear	42	
Choroid plexus papilloma (fourth ventricle)		170	30	4 mononuclear	54	
Reticulosarcoma		245	2	1 mononuclear	19	
Astrocytoma		410	—	10 mononuclear	20	
Ependymoblastoma		185	8	3 mononuclear	214	
Prostatic adenocarcinoma		—	—	9 mononuclear	67	
Degeneration						
Polioencephalomalacia–goat,		210	50	8 mononuclear	52	
cow		220	3800	30 mononuclear	135	
Focal myelomalacia (infarct)—dog		—	187	4 mononuclear	57	

Two major categories of hydrocephalus are compensatory and obstructive.

Compensatory. CSF accumulates in space in the cranial cavity not occupied by brain parenchyma. Examples include malformation with hypoplasia of tissue, and destruction of tissue from degeneration associated with ischemia, inflammation, or injury. The bluetongue virus destroys developing cerebrocortical tissue, producing hydranencephaly and a massive accumulation of CSF. The bovine virus diarrhea virus destroys fetal cerebellar tissue, leaving cystic CSF-filled spaces. Thrombosis of the middle cerebral artery in cats causes infarction of a large portion of the cerebrum. CSF accumulates and fills in the area of destroyed tissue. The same occurs in severe polioencephalomalacia (cerebrocortical necrosis) in ruminants.

These are examples of normotensive communicating compensatory hydrocephalus.

Obstructive. Obstruction to flow or absorption of CSF causes ventricular dilation, especially of the lateral ventricles, with loss of the white matter prior to grey matter. The cerebral cortex is relatively spared. The obstruction can be caused by a number of conditions.

1. Neoplasia may interfere directly with flow through the interventricular

foramen, third ventricle, mesencephalic aqueduct, or lateral apertures. This produces a noncommunicating hypertensive hydrocephalus in the lateral ventricles that may be normotensive at the cerebellomedullary site. The degree of hydrocephalus is variable but often minimal.

2. Neoplasia may interfere indirectly with absorption through the arachnoid villi because of its compressive effect on the venous sinuses. CSF pressure is usually hypertensive at the cerebellomedullary cistern. The degree of hydrocephalus is variable.

3. Inflammation of the ependyma of the mesencephalic aqueduct causes obstruction to flow and a noncommunicating hypertensive hydrocephalus of the third and lateral ventricles.[35,36,37,71]

Example: Experimental inoculation of neonatal hamsters or ferrets with human myxoviruses including mumps virus or the type 1 reovirus results in an acute ependymitis, which in the healing stage causes obstruction to CSF flow through the mesencephalic aqueduct, and subsequent noncommunicating hydrocephalus. The signs are observed 2 to 4 weeks after the inoculation. At necropsy there is a loss of ependyma or abnormalities of the ependyma, with partial or complete obstruction. The lesions of active inflammation have disappeared.

Feline infectious peritonitis virus may cause a severe meningitis and ependymitis. The latter may occlude the aqueduct, producing hydrocephalus.[16, 56]

4. Inflammation of the meninges may interfere with flow through the lateral apertures, or with absorption through the arachnoid villi.[13, 31, 56]

5. Malformation of the mesencephalic aqueduct produces a noncommunicating obstructive hydrocephalus.[7, 35, 36, 37, 38, 41, 60] A failure of a continuous aqueduct to develop causes permanent obstruction to flow and a noncommunicating, obstructive hypertensive hydrocephalus with severe dilation of the third and lateral ventricles. This usually is accompanied by a massive expansion of the cranial cavity and large nonossified portions of the calvaria. In puppies it is common to have hydrocephalus with widely dilated lateral ventricles that is normotensive at the lateral ventricle and cerebellomedullary cistern. The cranial cavity may be normal or expanded. Clinical signs are often static. At necropsy no obstruction to flow can be found. It is hypothesized that this condition may result if during a critical period in fetal development the aqueduct is inadequate to accommodate the total flow of CSF produced in the third and lateral ventricles. A partial but critical obstruction occurs, and the lateral ventricles expand against the extremely susceptible fetal cerebral tissue. With growth the aqueduct expands to accommodate the CSF produced rostral to it, and pressures are normalized. However, the damage has been done, and the expanded lateral ventricles covered by attenuated cerebral cortex persist. This hypothesis remains to be proved.

6. Malformation of the arachnoid villi in number or structure or both produces a communicating hydrocephalus. This also may be the critical defect in some dogs that are seen with hydrocephalus early in life. There is a critical point above which CSF pressure will not induce an increase in absorption owing to the lack of function of the absorptive mechanism. There are no more valves to open. This critical point may be within the normal range of physiologic CSF pressures. A functional obstruction exists and the ventricles dilate. The ventricular and cisternal pressures generally are normal. This hypothesis also has not been substantiated.

These two hypothesized mechanisms—inadequate aqueductal flow during a critical period of development, and arachnoid villi malformation—may account for the so-called congenital or constitutional hydrocephalus common among small breeds of dogs with large skulls (Chihuahua, Yorkshire terrier, Manchester terrier, toy poodle) and among the brachiocephalic breeds (Boston terrier, Pekingese, English bulldog).

A syndrome of late-onset hydrocephalus that is referred to as occult or normal pressure hydrocephalus occurs in man.[13, 28, 40] It is a progressive disorder despite the lack of CSF hypertension, and is related to inadequate CSF circulation to the cerebral arachnoid villi for absorption. It is treated readily by surgical shunting procedures. Most hydrocephalic puppies with or without progressive signs have normal CSF cisternal and ventricular pressures. The pathogenesis of these two diseases may be related.

Under all of the preceding circumstances CSF production usually continues at a constant rate regardless of the intraventricular CSF pressure. CSF flow volume is constant regardless of the CSF pressure. Production decreases only when the choroid plexus becomes altered by the hypertension. Intraventricular pressure is not constant but varies continuously.

Numerous studies have been done on the pathophysiology of hydrocephalus.[40, 46, 52, 53, 54, 59] Light and electron-microscopic studies of the cerebrum adjacent to the lateral ventricle indicate that during the hypertensive phase CSF may pass into the parenchyma.[66] There is also evidence that CSF absorption may occur through the choroid plexus.[45]

CLINICAL SIGNS

Clinical signs are variable.[20, 54] They are mostly referable to disturbance of the cerebral hemispheres. No signs may be seen in the presence of considerable ventricular dilatation. The following signs should be looked for.

1. Disturbed consciousness, with lethargy to severe depression (obtundation), tendency to sleep, hypoactivity, propulsive circling, head pressing, convulsions, changes in behavior, dementia.

2. Motor signs include a spastic paresis, especially if the brain stem is involved. With severe cerebral disturbance the gait may be normal if the brain stem is normal. Hypermetric ataxia occurs if the cerebellum is involved. An abnormal position of the eyeballs with a ventral and lateral deviation may occur from pressure on the oculomotor nerve or from a malformation of the orbit owing to changes in the shape of the skull bones. The majority probably are caused by the latter.

3. Sensory signs include ataxia and blindness. A bilateral visual deficit with normal pupillary response is the most common and consistent clinical sign observed in these patients. This reflects the attenuation of the cerebral white matter optic radiation and visual cortex. A mild, general proprioceptive ataxia occasionally occurs. Postural reactions are consistently slow when there is disturbance of the sensorimotor portion of the cerebrum.

4. Abnormal shape of the skull, with an enlarged calvaria with open sutures (fontanelles).

ANCILLARY EXAMINATION

RADIOGRAPHY. Plain radiographs may show a diffuse homogeneous "ground glass" opacity of the cranial cavity from the fluid contents. The gyral pattern of the calvaria may be absent and open sutures may be apparent.

PNEUMOVENTRICULOGRAPHY. This is performed best by direct injection of air into the lateral ventricle, as described under the uses of CSF. Air injected into the cerebellomedullary cistern may pass through the lateral apertures into the ventricular system, but this procedure is not dependable. Contrast ventriculography by direct injection of meglumine iothalamate (Conray) determines the degree of ventricular dilation and the integrity of the aqueduct and lateral apertures.

ELECTROENCEPHALOGRAPHY. The EEG pattern in hydrocephalus is usually consistent and characteristic. In all leads there is a diffuse slowing of the normal pattern with a remarkable increase in amplitude.[11, 20, 50]

TREATMENT

The treatment for hydrocephalus depends on the cause. In cases of obstructive hydrocephalus a direct lateral ventricular tap may confirm the diagnosis and provide temporary relief from some of the signs.[55]

Medical therapy with corticosteroids (1 to 2 mg per lb of dexamethasone or Azium) may provide temporary relief in patients with exacerbated or progressive clinical signs. Lower doses of steroids may be effective (0.25 to 1 mg per day for several or on alternate days).

Surgical therapy for more permanent relief involves a procedure for draining the fluid from the lateral ventricle.[24, 26, 27] Most shunt this fluid into the vascular system such as the jugular vein or right atrium (the ventriculoatrial shunt). Others shunt the CSF into the peritoneal cavity. A one-way valve is installed so that only CSF can flow out of the ventricle.

REFERENCES

1. Adams, R. D., Fisher, C. M., Hakim, S., Ojemann, R. G., and Sweet, W. H.: Symptomatic occult hydrocephalus with "normal" cerebrospinal fluid pressure: A treatable disease. N. Engl. J. Med., 273:117, 1965.
2. Andres, K. H.: Zur Feinstruktur der Arachnoidalzotton bei Mammalia. Z. Zellforsch. Mikrosk. Anat., 82:92, 1967.
3. Averill, D. A., Jr.: Examination of the cerebrospinal fluid. In Kirk, R. W., ed., Current Veterinary Therapy, V. Small Animal Practice. Philadelphia, W. B. Saunders Co., 1974, 645–648.
4. Bailey, C. S.: Lumbar puncture for collection of CSF. Am. Anim. Hosp. Assoc. Proc., 40:289, 1973.
5. Baker, M. L., Payne, C. A., and Baker, G. N.: The inheritance of hydrocephalus in cattle. J. Hered., 52:135, 1961.
6. Banks, W. C., and Monlux, W. S.: Canine hydrocephalus. J. Am. Vet. Med. Assoc., 121:453, 1952.
7. Barlow, R. M., and Donald, L. G.: Hydrocephalus in calves associated with unusual lesions in the mesencephalon. J. Comp. Pathol., 73:410, 1963.
8. Benson, D. F., LeMay, M., Patten, D. H., and Rubens, A. B.: Diagnosis of normal-pressure hydrocephalus. N. Engl. J. Med., 283:609, 1970.
9. Bering, E. A., Jr., and Sato, O.: Hydrocephalus: Changes in formation and absorption of cerebrospinal fluid within the cerebral ventricles. J. Neurosurg., 20:1050, 1963.
10. Bowster, D.: Cerebrospinal Fluid Dynamics in Health and Disease. Springfield, Ill., Charles C Thomas, 1960.
11. Brass, W., and Horzinek, I.: I.: Klinik und Elektronenencephalogramm des Hydrocephalus internus beim Hund. Deutsch Tiererztl. Wochenschr., 78:42, 1971.
12. Bullock, L. P., and Zook, B. C.: Myelography in dogs using water-soluble contrast mediums. J. Am. Vet. Med. Assoc., 151:321, 1967.
13. Cammermeyer, J.: The frequency of meningocephalitis and hydrocephalus in dogs. J. Neuropathol. Exp. Neurol., 20:386, 1961.
14. Coles, E. H.: Cerebrospinal fluid. In Keneko, J. J., and Cornelius, C. E., eds., Clinical Biochemistry of Domestic Animals. 2nd ed., vol. II, New York, Academic Press, 1970.
15. Cserr, H. F.: Physiology of the choroid plexus. Physiol. Rev., 51:273, 1971.
16. Csiza, C. K., Scott, F. W., de Lahunta, A., and Gillespie, J. H.: Feline viruses. XIV. Transplacental infections in spontaneous panleukopenia of cats. Cor. Vet., 61:423, 1971.

17. Cutler, R. W. P., and Averill, D. R., Jr.: Cerebrospinal fluid gamma globulins in canine distemper encephalitis. Neurology, *19*:1111, 1969.
18. Davson, H.: Physiology of the Cerebrospinal Fluid. London, J. & A. Churchill, 1967.
19. de Lahunta, A.: Examination of the cerebrospinal fluid. *In* Kirk, R. W., ed., Current Veterinary Therapy, III. Philadelphia, W. B. Saunders Co., 470–472. 1970.
20. de Lahunta, A., and Cummings, J. F.: The clinical and electroencephalographic features of hydrocephalus in three dogs. J. Am. Vet. Med. Assoc., *146*:954, 1965.
21. DiChiro, G., Stein, S. C., and Harrington, T.: Spontaneous cerebrospinal fluid rhinorrhea in normal dogs. Radioisotope studies of an alternate pathway of CSF drainage. J. Neuropathol. Exp. Neurol., *31*:447, 1972.
22. Fankhauser, R.: The cerebrospinal fluid. *In* Innes, J. R. M., and Saunders, L. S., eds., Comparative Neuropathology. New York, Academic Press, 1962.
23. Fedotov, A. I.: Cerebrospinal fluid of domestic animals. Russian Scientific Translation Program, Division of General Medical Services. National Institute of Health, Washington, D.C., U.S. Department of Health, Education, and Welfare, 1960.
24. Few, A. B.: The diagnosis and surgical treatment of canine hydrocephalus. J. Am. Vet. Med. Assoc., *149*:286, 1966.
25. Fitzgerald, T. C.: Anatomy of cerebral ventricles of domestic animals. Vet. Med., *56*:38, 1961.
26. Gage, E. D.: Surgical treatment of canine hydrocephalus. J. Am. Vet. Med. Assoc., *157*:1729, 1970.
27. Gage, E. D., and Hoerlein, B. F.: Surgical treatment of canine hydrocephalus by ventriculo-atrial shunting. J. Am. Vet. Med. Assoc., *153*:1418, 1968.
28. Geschwind, N.: The mechanism of normal pressure hydrocephalus. J. Neurol. Sci., *7*:481, 1968.
29. Gomez, D. G., and Potts, D. G.: The choroid plexus of the dog. Anat. Rec., *181*:363, 1975.
30. Gomez, D. G., Potts, D. G., and Deonarine, V.: Arachnoid granulations of the sheep. Arch. Neurol., *30*:169, 1974.
31. Green, H. J., Leipold, H. W., and Vestwebor, J. E.: Experimentally induced hydrocephalus in calves. Am. J. Vet. Res., *35*:945, 1974.
32. Hoerlein, B. F., and Petty, M. F.: Contrast encephalography and ventriculography in the dog—preliminary studies. Am. J. Vet. Res., *22*:1041, 1961.
33. Hooshmand, H., Dove, J., Houff, S., and Suter, C.: Effects of diuretics and steroids on CSF pressure. Arch. Neurol., *21*:499, 1969.
34. Iida, T.: Elektronenmikroskopiche Untersuchungen am Oberflächlichen Anteil des Gehirns bei Hund und Katze. Arch. Histol. Jap., *27*:267, 1966.
35. Johnson, R. T., and Johnson, K. P.: Hydrocephalus as a sequela of experimental myxovirus infections. Exp. Mol. Pathol., *10*:68, 1969.
36. Johnson, R. T., and Johnson, K. P.: Hydrocephalus following viral infection. The pathology of aqueductal stenosis developing after experimental mumps virus infection. J. Neuropathol. Exp. Neurol., *27*:591, 1968.
37. Johnson, R. T., Johnson, K. P., and Edmonds, C. J.: Virus-induced hydrocephalus: Development of aqueductal stenosis in hamsters after mumps infection. Science, *157*:1066, 1967.
38. Kilham, L., and Margolis, G.: Hydrocephalus in hamsters, ferrets, rats and mice following inoculations with reovirus type I. I. Virologic studies. Lab. Invest., *21*:183, 1969.
39. Long, J. F., Jacoby, R. O., Olson, M., and Koestner, A.: Beta-glucuronidase activity and levels of protein and protein fractions in serum and cerebrospinal fluid of dogs with distemper-associated demyelinating encephalopathy. Acta Neuropathol. (Berlin), *25*:179, 1973.
40. Lorenzo, A. V., Page, L. K., and Watters, G. V.: Relationship between cerebrospinal fluid formation, absorption, and pressure in human hydrocephalus. Brain, *93*:679, 1970.
41. Margolis, G., and Kilham, L.: Hydrocephalus in hamsters, ferrets, rats, and mice following inoculations with reovirus type I. II. Pathologic studies. Lab. Invest., *21*:189, 1969.
42. Mayhew, I. G.: Collection of cerebrospinal fluid from the horse. Cor. Vet., *65*:500, 1975.
43. Milhorat, T. H.: The choroid plexus and cerebrospinal fluid production. Science, *166*:1514, 1969.
44. Milhorat, T. H., Hammock, M. K., Fenstermacher, J. D., Rall, D. F., and Levin, V. A.: Cerebrospinal fluid production by the choroid plexus and brain. Science, *173*:330, 1971.
45. Milhorat, T. H., Mosher, M. B., Hammock, M. K., and Murphy, C. F.: Evidence for choroid-plexus absorption in hydrocephalus. N. Engl. J. Med., *283*:286, 1970.
46. Oppelt, W., Patlack, C., and Rall, D.: Effect of certain drugs on cerebrospinal fluid production in the dog. Am. J. Physiol., *206*:247, 1964.
47. Parker, A. J.: The diagnostic uses of cerebrospinal fluid. J. Small Anim. Pract., *13*:607, 1972.
48. Pollay, M., and Welch, K.: The function and structure of the canine arachnoid villi. J. Surg. Res., *2*:307, 1962.
49. Potts, D. G., and Deonarine, V.: Effect of positional changes and jugular vein compression on the pressure gradient across the arachnoid villi and granulations of the dog. J. Neurosurg., *38*:722, 1973.
50. Prynn, R. B., and Redding, R. W.: Electroencephalogram in occult canine hydrocephalus. J. Am. Vet. Med. Assoc., *152*:1651, 1968.
51. Roszel, J. F.: Membrane filtration of canine and feline cerebrospinal fluid for cytologic evaluation. J. Am. Vet. Med. Assoc., *160*:720, 1972.

52. Russell, D. S.: Observations on the pathology of hydrocephalus. London, England, Medical Research Council Report No. 265, 1949.
53. Sahar, A., Hochwald, G. M., and Ranschoff, J.: Experimental hydrocephalus: Cerebrospinal fluid formation and ventricular size as a function of intraventricular pressure. J. Neurol., Sci., *11*:81, 1970.
54. Sahar, A., Hochwald, G. M., Kay, W. J., and Ranschoff, J.: Spontaneous canine hydrocephalus: Cerebrospinal fluid dynamics. J. Neurol. Neurosurg. Psychiatry, *34*:308, 1971.
55. Savell, C. M.: Cerebral ventricular tap: An aid to diagnosis and treatment of hydrocephalus in the dog. Am. Anim. Hosp. Assoc. Proc., 532, 1974.
56. Slauson, D. O., and Finn, J. P.: Meningoencephalitis and panophthalmitis in feline infectious peritonitis. J. Am. Vet. Med. Assoc., *160*:729, 1972.
57. Slesingr, L., and Hrazdira, C. L.: Untersuchungen der Zerebrospinalflüssigkeit von Hunden und Pferden. Zentralbl. Veterinaer Med., *17*:338, 1970.
58. Steinberg, S.: Cerebrospinal fluid. *In* Medway, W., Prier, J. E., and Wilkinson, J. S., eds., Textbook of Veterinary Clinical Pathology. Baltimore, Williams & Wilkins, 1969.
59. Strecker, E. P., Bush, M., and James, A. E., Jr.: Cerebrospinal fluid imaging as a method to evaluate communicating hydrocephalus in dogs. Am. J. Vet. Res., *34*:101, 1973.
60. Timmonds, G. D., and Johnson, K. D.: Aqueductal stenosis and hydrocephalus after mumps encephalitis. N. Engl. J. Med., *283*:1505, 1970.
61. Tripathi, B. J., and Tripathi, R. C.: Vascular transcellular channels as the drainage pathway of cerebrospinal fluid. J. Physiol. (London), 239:195, 1973.
62. Tripathi, R.: Tracing the bulk outflow of cerebrospinal fluid by transmission and scanning electron microscopy. Brain Res., *80*:503, 1974.
63. Urman, H. K., and Grace, O. D.: Hereditary encephalomyopathy. A hydrocephalus syndrome in newborn calves. Cor. Vet., *54*:229, 1964.
64. Vermeulen, H. A.: Über den Conus Medullaris der Haustiere sein besonders verhalten beim Pferd und desen Bedeutung. Berl. Munch. Tierarztl. Wochenschr., 2:13, 1916.
65. Wakim, K. G., and Fleisher, G. A.: The effect of experimental cerebral infarction on transaminase activity in serum, cerebrospinal fluid and infarcted tissue. Mayo Clin. Proc., *31*:391, 1956.
66. Weller, R. O., Wisniewski, H., Shulman, K., and Terry, R. D.: Experimental hydrocephalus in young dogs. Histological and ultrastructural study of the brain tissue damage. J. Neuropathol. Exp. Neurol., *30*:613, 1971.
67. Wolstenholme, G. E. W., and O'Connor, C. M., eds., The Cerebrospinal Fluid. Boston, CIBA Symposium, Little Brown Co., 1958.
68. Woolam, D. H. M., and Miller, J. W.: The perivascular spaces of the mammalian central nervous system and their relation to the perineuronal and subarachnoid spaces. J. Anat., *89*:193, 1955.
69. Yaghmai, J., Deonarine, V., Deck, M. D. F., and Potts, D. G.: Air ventriculography in the dog brain, utilizing tomography. Am. J. Vet. Res., *32*:319, 1971.
70. Di Chiro, G., Hammock, M. K., and Bleyer, W. A.: Spinal descent of cerebrospinal fluid in man. Neurology, 26:1, 1976.
71. Johnson, Richard T.: Hydrocephalus and viral infections. Review article. Dev. Med. Child Neurol., *17*:807, 1975.

Chapter 4

LOWER MOTOR NEURON – GENERAL SOMATIC EFFERENT SYSTEM

LOWER MOTOR NEURON
GENERAL SOMATIC EFFERENT
SYSTEM (GSE)
SPINAL NERVE DIVISION
*SPINAL CORD SEGMENTS – VERTEBRAL
COLUMN*
FUNCTION
Thoracic Limb Reflexes
Pelvic Limb Reflexes
LOWER MOTOR NEURON DISEASE
ELECTRODIAGNOSTIC TECHNIQUES

IN NEUROMUSCULAR DISEASE
*DISEASES OF THE GSE LOWER MOTOR
NEURON*
Neuromusclar Ending
Peripheral Nerve
Spinal Roots and Nerves
Spinal Roots and/or Nerves and
Peripheral Nerves
Spinal Cord
Muscle Disease
Episodic Weakness

LOWER MOTOR NEURON

This is the efferent neuron of the peripheral nervous system that connects the central nervous system with the muscle to be innervated. The entire function of the central nervous system is manifested through the lower motor neuron. The lower motor neuron system (LMN) includes three components: the general somatic efferent system (GSE), the general visceral efferent system (GVE), and the special visceral efferent system (SVE).

GENERAL SOMATIC EFFERENT SYSTEM (GSE)

This system of the lower motor neuron includes neurons that innervate striated voluntary skeletal muscle derived from somites, somatic mesoderm of body wall (limb buds), and head myotomes. These neurons are located in all the spinal nerves and cranial nerves III, IV, VI, and XII.

SPINAL NERVE DIVISION

The cell bodies are located in the ventral grey column throughout the entire spinal cord. The shape and size of the ventral grey column reflect the number of neurons present. The ventral grey column is topographically organized.[3] The GSE neurons innervating the axial musculature populate the medial portion of the column. The GSE neurons that innervate the appendicular musculature are located laterally and cause the lateral bulge of the ventral grey column that is evi-

57

dent at the cervical and lumbosacral intumescences (Fig. 4–1). These lateral portions of the ventral grey column can be subdivided further into motonuclear columns representative of muscle groups, or the peripheral nerves present in the limbs. Neurons that innervate proximal limb muscles are located in the ventral portion of the lateral part of the ventral grey column. Those to the distal limb muscles are in the dorsal portion. These motonuclear columns have been identified by sectioning peripheral nerves or ablating specific muscles, and then observing in the spinal cord ventral grey column the retrograde chromatolysis of the cell bodies whose axons were destroyed by the experimental procedure.

The dendritic zone of the multipolar general somatic efferent neuron is confined to the grey matter of the spinal cord. The axon courses through the white matter between lateral and ventral funiculi to leave the spinal cord as part of a ventral rootlet. It continues in a ventral root, through the spinal nerve, and into the limbs as part of a specific peripheral nerve, which is distributed to a specific group of muscles (Fig. 4–2).

At the level of the muscle cells each axon of a general somatic efferent neuron divides into several branches. Each of these axonal branches ends on a muscle cell at a motor end-plate. Each muscle cell is usually only innervated by the axon of one neuron. The number of muscle cells innervated by one motoneuron is called the motor unit. It varies from 100 to 150 cells in the proximal appendicular muscles to 3 to 4 cells in extraocular muscles. Muscles involved in functions that require a large degree of coordination are innervated by motoneurons with small

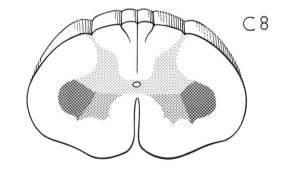

C 8

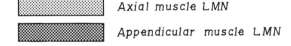

Axial muscle LMN

Appendicular muscle LMN

Figure 4–1. Spinal cord topography depicted at the cervical (C8) and lumbar (L7) intumescences.

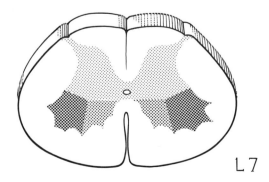

L 7

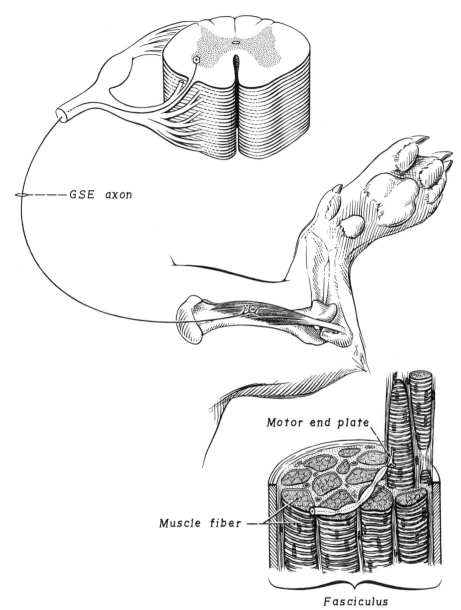

GSE axon

Motor end plate

Muscle fiber

Fasciculus

Figure 4–2. Lower motor neuron—GSE innervation of the medial head of the triceps brachii.

motor units (only a few muscle cells per neuron). The strength of a muscle contraction depends on the number of motor units activated in a muscle.

At the motor end-plate the myelin is lost and the axon terminates in several small branches that form a cluster in a localized area near the longitudinal center of the muscle cell. Each of these branches terminates on a specialized modification of the sarcolemma. This terminal is called the neuromuscular ending (junction) or synapse (Fig. 4–3).

The neuromuscular ending consists of a distended axonal terminal covered by a nonmyelinated lemmocyte (Schwann cell) up to the point at which the axon extends into a sarcoplasmic trough on the surface of the muscle cell. The endoneurium of the neuron and the endomysium of the muscle cell are continuous outside the trough. Inside the trough the axolemma and sarcolemma are jux-

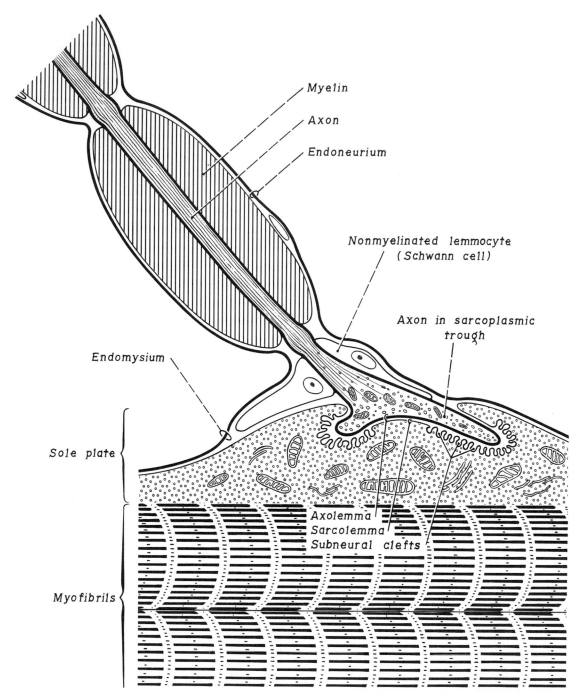

Figure 4–3.   Neuromuscular junction of a motor end-plate.

taposed. The axon terminal contains numerous mitochondria and synaptic vesicles that are presumed to be the source of the neurotransmitter substance, acetylcholine.

The sarcoplasmic trough is located on an area of the muscle cell at which the
sarcoplasm has accumulated. This is called the sole plate, and abounds with
muscle-cell nuclei and mitochondria. The sarcoplasmic trough is extended further
by invaginations of the sarcoplasm to form postsynaptic membrane folds (sub-

neural clefts) that probably contain a glycoprotein. This is the site at which the acetylcholine causes depolarization of the muscle cell membrane and is degraded by the enzyme acetylcholinesterase. The synaptic cleft between the presynaptic membrane (axolemma) and postsynaptic membrane (sarcolemma) is about 200Å.

SPINAL CORD SEGMENTS — VERTEBRAL COLUMN

For clinical purposes it is important to know in which segments of the spinal cord the cell bodies of general somatic efferent motor neurons are found whose axons are in specific peripheral nerves.

In the dog the spinal cord is composed of about 36 segments: 8 cervical, 13 thoracic, 7 lumbar, 3 sacral, and usually 5 caudal. Each segment has a number of dorsal and ventral rootlets that arise from the dorsolateral and ventrolateral aspects of each of its sides. They join to form a dorsal and ventral root on each side. The segmental spinal ganglion is found in the dorsal root at the level of the intervertebral foramen. Just beyond this, the dorsal and ventral roots join to form the spinal nerve. Thus, each spinal cord segment is connected to the tissues of the body by a spinal nerve on each side.

The development of the spinal cord segments and the vertebral column in the embryo are closely related events, which accounts for the manner in which the roots of each spinal cord segment are distributed between the vertebrae. The roots of the first cervical spinal cord segment leave the canal through the lateral vertebral foramina in the arch of the atlas. The roots of the second to the seventh cervical segments leave the canal through the intervertebral foramina cranial to the vertebrae of the same number. The roots of the eighth cervical segment exit cranial to the first thoracic vertebra. All the remaining roots leave the canal through the intervertebral foramina caudal to the vertebrae of the same number. Because of the greater growth in length of the vertebral column the relationship of the spinal cord segments and vertebrae is somewhat altered. In the dog only the first and occasionally second cervical spinal cord segments, and the last two thoracic and first two or three lumbar segments lie in the vertebral column within the vertebrae of the same number, but all the remaining segments reside in the canal cranial to the vertebrae of the same number (Figs. 4–4, 4–5).

The more cranial the location of a spinal cord segment is from its corresponding vertebra, the longer the roots are to reach the appropriate intervertebral foramina. This is particularly evident in the lumbosacral region of the spinal cord of the dog, in which the last three lumbar segments reside approximately over the fourth lumbar vertebral body and the three sacral segments are within the fifth lumbar vertebra. The spinal cord usually ends within the cranial half of the seventh lumbar vertebra. In small breeds of dogs these relationships may shift caudally by one half of a vertebra. Each species varies in this relationship.[37] In the mature cat the three sacral segments may be found in the vertebral canal over the body of L6 or at the articulation of L5 and L6.

FUNCTION

The general somatic efferent portion of the lower motor neuron comprises the motor component of the spinal reflexes that are tested in the neurologic examina-

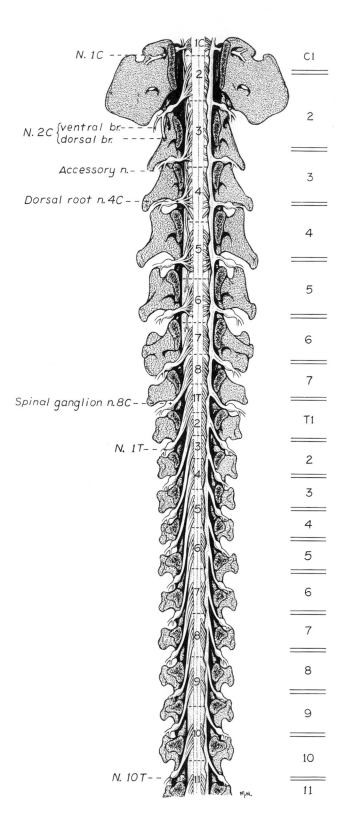

Figure 4–4. Spinal cord segmental relationship to vertebral bodies. From C1 to T11 the spinal cord, roots, ganglia, and nerves have been exposed by removal of the vertebral arches. The dura mater has been removed except on the right side. The numbers on the right represent the levels of the vertebral bodies. (From Miller, M. E., Christensen, G. C., and Evans, H. E., Anatomy of the Dog. Philadelphia, W. B. Saunders Co., 1964. Drawn by M. Newsom.)

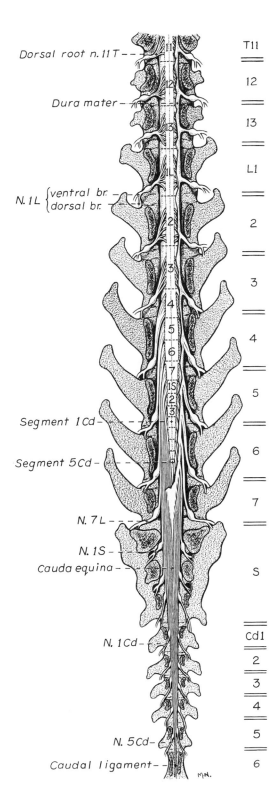

Figure 4–5. Spinal cord segmental relationship to vertebral bodies. From T11 through the caudal segments the spinal cord, roots, ganglia, and nerves have been exposed by removal of the vertebral arches. The dura mater has been removed except on the right side. The numbers on the right represent the levels of the vertebral bodies. (From Miller, M. E., Christensen, G. C., and Evans, H. E., Anatomy of the Dog. Philadelphia, W. B. Saunders Co., 1964. Drawn by M. Newsom.)

tion. Knowledge of the anatomy of this system is helpful in localizing lesions to portions of the peripheral nervous system or spinal cord. The general somatic afferent (GSA) or general proprioceptive (GP) system contains the sensory component of these reflexes. It consists of a dendritic zone (receptor) in the skin or neuromuscular spindle, and an axon that courses through a specific peripheral nerve, spinal nerve, and dorsal root, entering the dorsal grey column of the corresponding spinal cord segment, and terminating in a telodendron on a second neuron, usually in the dorsal grey column. The cell body of the general somatic afferent neuron is located in the respective spinal ganglion at the distal end of the dorsal root.

In the patellar tendon reflex the sensory neuron terminates directly on the GSE neuron in the ventral grey column. For most other spinal reflexes the sensory neuron telodendron is on an interneuron in the grey matter that in turn terminates on the GSE neuron (Fig. 4–6).

Spinal reflexes need only the peripheral components and involved segments of the spinal cord to function. They will function even if the spinal cord segments have been cut off and isolated from the rest of the central nervous system.

In order to interpret the spinal reflexes properly, their anatomic components must be understood.

Thoracic Limb Reflexes

The thoracic limbs are innervated primarily from the sixth cervical (C6) to the first thoracic (T1) segment. A small contribution comes from the C5 and T2 segments. The spinal nerves from these segments intertwine to form the brachial plexus, out of which course the specific peripheral nerves of the thoracic limbs. The flexor reflex is performed by pinching a toe. This may be done with the fingers, but a pair of forceps applied to the base of the nail is more reliable. The subsequent prompt flexion or withdrawal of the limb requires the integrity of the roots and grey matter of the spinal cord from C6 to T1. The axillary, musculocutaneous, median, ulnar, and part of the radial peripheral nerves function in this reflex (Fig. 4–7).

Two tendon reflexes can be tested in the thoracic limbs. They are not always present in normal animals. The biceps reflex is elicited by ballottement of the first finger placed on the distal end of the biceps brachii and brachialis on the medial side of the elbow. Contraction of these muscles may be palpated and flexion of the elbow observed. This reflex is mediated entirely by the musculocutaneous nerve (C6, 7, 8). The triceps reflex tests the radial nerve (C7, 8, T1, 2), and is elicited by tapping the triceps tendon just proximal to its insertion on the olecranon. Extension of the elbow is observed.

The panniculus reflex may involve a much larger portion of the spinal cord segments. Light irritation or pricking the skin of the trunk with a pin causes contraction of the cutaneous trunci and a quick movement of the skin. This reflex is mediated through the segmental sensory neurons, in which the stimulus is elicited. The impulse enters the corresponding segment of the spinal cord and through interneurons is passed cranially through the spinal cord white matter to the T1 and C8 spinal cord segments, where the general somatic efferent neurons of the lateral thoracic nerve are located. Stimulation of these causes contraction of the cutaneous trunci muscle.

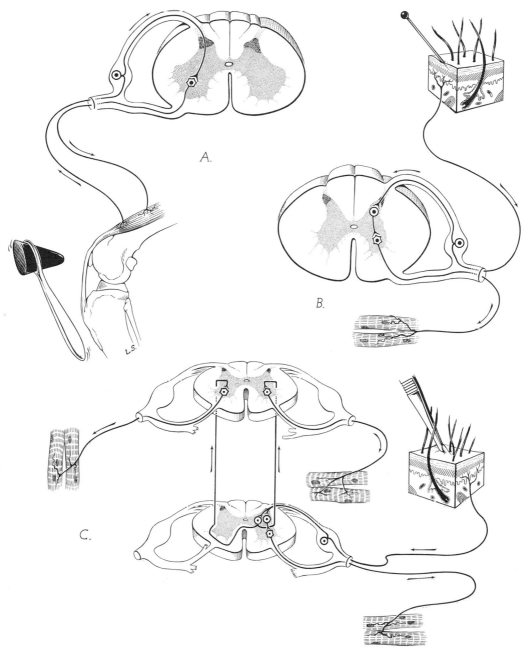

Figure 4–6. Spinal segmental reflexes: *A:* monosynaptic myotatic—patellar reflex; *B:* polysynaptic flexor reflex to a noxious stimulus; *C:* polysynaptic flexor reflex with intersegmental transmission of impulses.

Pelvic Limb Reflexes

The pelvic limbs are innervated from the L4 to S1 segments of the spinal cord.[26] Muscles that flex the hip joint receive innervation from as far cranial as the L1 segment. The spinal nerves from the L4 to S3 segments join to form the lumbosacral plexus. The peripheral nerves to the perineum and pelvic limbs are

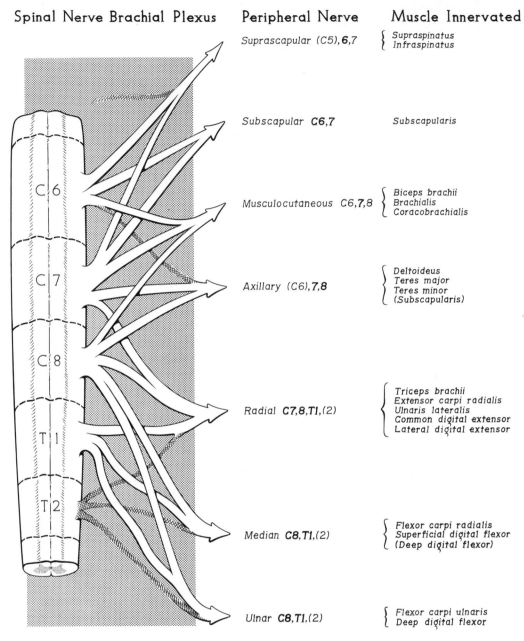

Figure 4–7.   Segmental innervation from cervical intumescence of thoracic limb muscles in the dog.

derived from this plexus. The flexor reflex of the pelvic limbs depends on the integrity of the sciatic nerve, whose roots and cell bodies are located from the L6 to S1 segments of the spinal cord. The patellar reflex is the only reliable tendon reflex. When the patient is relaxed, a light tap of the patellar tendon elicits a brisk

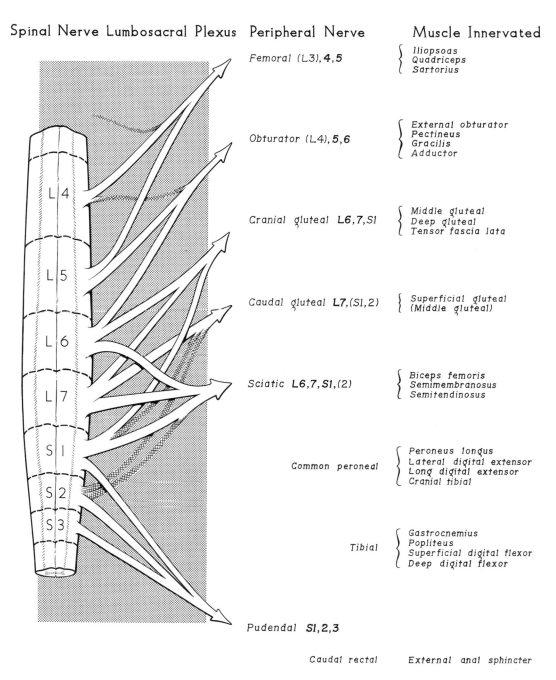

Spinal Nerve Lumbosacral Plexus   Peripheral Nerve   Muscle Innervated

Femoral (L3),**4,5**
  { Iliopsoas
  { Quadriceps
  { Sartorius

Obturator (L4),**5,6**
  { External obturator
  { Pectineus
  { Gracilis
  { Adductor

Cranial gluteal **L6,7**,S1
  { Middle gluteal
  { Deep gluteal
  { Tensor fascia lata

Caudal gluteal **L7**,(S1,2)
  { Superficial gluteal
  { (Middle gluteal)

Sciatic **L6,7,S1**,(2)
  { Biceps femoris
  { Semimembranosus
  { Semitendinosus

Common peroneal
  { Peroneus longus
  { Lateral digital extensor
  { Long digital extensor
  { Cranial tibial

Tibial
  { Gastrocnemius
  { Popliteus
  { Superficial digital flexor
  { Deep digital flexor

Pudendal **S1,2,3**

Caudal rectal   External anal sphincter

Flexor reflex: Sensory and Motor: Sciatic nerve
Patellar reflex: Sensory and Motor: Femoral nerve
Perineal reflex: Sensory and Motor: Pudendal nerve

Figure 4–8.   Segmental innervation from lumbosacral intumescence of pelvic limb muscles in the dog.

extension of the stifle. If present, the reflex can be observed for its briskness, degree of activity, or the presence of clonus. The peripheral nerve controlling this reflex is the femoral nerve, whose roots and cell bodies are located in the L3 to L5 spinal cord segments. The patellar reflex is graded plus 2 for normal, plus 1 for depressed, 0 for absent, plus 3 for hyperactive, and plus 4 for clonus (Fig. 4–8).

The perineal reflex is elicited by light stimulation of the perineum with a pin or forceps. The normal response is a sharp contraction of the anal sphincter and flexion of the tail. This reflex depends on the integrity of the sacral and caudal segments of the spinal cord.

LOWER MOTOR NEURON DISEASE

Abnormalities of any part of the general somatic efferent lower motor neuron cause signs of muscle weakness—paresis or paralysis, along with hyporeflexia or areflexia, hypotonia or atonia, and neurogenic atrophy.

Spinal reflexes are depressed or absent when there is a loss of the motor component of the reflex arc. Muscle tone is dependent on a continual contraction of a small, regulated number of muscle cells. When their motor innervation is lost, there can be no contraction to maintain muscle tone. This condition is ascertained best by passive manipulation of the limb of the recumbent animal. Palpation of the anus and manipulation of the tail also help to detect hypotonia or atonia.

Muscle cells that are denervated degenerate. Muscle protein is lost rapidly, and over a long period of time the cell eventually dies and is replaced by connective tissue. As the cell degenerates and loses protein, it atrophies. This occurs rapidly—within 1 week of denervation—and is referred to as neurogenic atrophy. The rate and degree of atrophy vary with the species and the muscle that is denervated. Denervated muscles may be atrophic for weeks and return to normal size when reinnervated. A good example of this phenomenon is coonhound paralysis (acute polyradiculoneuritis).

The clinical presentation depends on how much of the general somatic ef-

TABLE 4–1. TOPOGRAPHIC ANATOMY OF SPINAL REFLEX TESTING IN DOGS

	Reflex	Peripheral Nerve	Spinal Cord Segments	Level in Vertebral Canal
Thoracic Limb	Biceps	Musculocutaneous	C6–8	C5–7
	Triceps	Radial	C7–T2	C6–T1
	Flexor	All peripheral nerves of thoracic limb	C6–T2	C5–T1
Pelvic Limb	Patellar	Femoral	L3–5	L3–4
	Flexor	Sciatic	L6–S1	L4–5
	Perineal	Pudendal	S1–3	L5

ferent lower motor neuron is affected. The abnormality may occur at any point along the lower motor neuron: at the cell body in the ventral grey column, in the ventral root, spinal nerve, or peripheral nerve, or at the neuromuscular ending. Ischemic necrosis of the ventral grey column, segmental demyelinization of the ventral roots, traumatic avulsion of selected dorsal and ventral roots, neoplasia of a spinal nerve, contusion to a peripheral nerve, inflammation of the peripheral nerves, and ineffective transmission at the neuromuscular ending are all examples of diseases of the GSE lower motor neuron that produce the characteristic signs, but with differing degrees of severity. The dysfunction owing to destruction of an entire peripheral nerve exceeds that caused by destruction of an entire root or spinal nerve. This is because the peripheral nerve supplies the total innervation of a specific muscle, whereas a ventral root or spinal nerve contributes a few neurons to many peripheral nerves and muscles but not the entire innervation of that muscle.

When the axon of any neuron is destroyed at some point along its course, the part of the axon that courses away from the cell body will degenerate completely. This is because the axon needs the axoplasmic flow of cytoplasmic materials from the cell body for its survival. Waller described this degeneration for the peripheral nerves; therefore it is called Wallerian degeneration (Fig. 4–9).

Wallerian degeneration is a trophic degeneration that occurs in the neuron from the lesion distally from the cell body, as follows: (1) The axon disintegrates by a process of swelling and subsequent granulation that takes about 3 to 4 days. (2) The myelin disintegrates simultaneously with the axonal degeneration. This demyelination includes the formation of swellings along the internodes called ellipsoids, and the fragmentation of myelin into droplets. (3) The motor end-plate disintegrates. (4) The lemmocytes proliferate within their endoneurial covering and fill up the space previously occupied by the axon and myelin, thus retaining the anatomic boundary of the original neuron.

In addition to these changes that occur distal to the lesion, because of the loss of the trophic influence of the cell body other changes occur proximal to the lesion. (1) The trauma of the injury produces degeneration over a few internodes proximal to the lesion in a manner similar to the trophic degeneration distal to the lesion. (2) A reaction occurs in the cell body called the axonal reaction, in which there is a swelling of the cell body, a displacement of the nucleus to one side of the cytoplasm (eccentric), and partial dispersal of the granular endoplasmic reticulum (Nissl substance) in the region around the nucleus and center of the cell body, or central chromatolysis.

Regeneration begins in about 7 days, starting at the site of the axonal degeneration where normal axonal material exists. Each axon grows out a number of processes called axonal buds, which develop into the existing cords of proliferated lemmocytes and the endoneurium that provides a pathway for them. The rate of growth is approximately 1 to 4 mm per day. This process is dependent on the proximity of the severed stumps of the neurons and the absence of any impediment to the growth of these axonal buds, such as the proliferation of fibrous connective tissue secondary to the tissue destruction that destroyed the neurons.

When the axonal buds cannot find a pathway to the distally located bands of lemmocytes they grow in a haphazard manner and form an observable swelling known as a neuroma. These are often a sequel to the neurectomies that are performed in the distal extremities of horses and may be a source of irritation to the patient.[23]

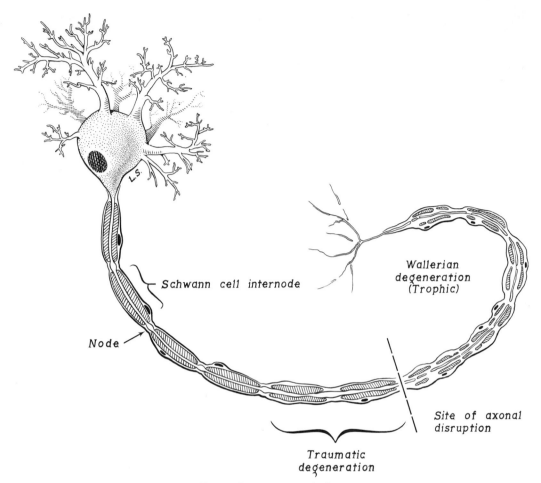

*Wallerian
degeneration
(Trophic)*

— *Schwann cell internode*

Node

*Site of axonal
disruption*

*Traumatic
degeneration*

Figure 4–9.   Wallerian degeneration of a lower motor neuron.

ELECTRODIAGNOSTIC TECHNIQUES IN NEUROMUSCULAR DISEASE

Electromyography (EMG) is the study of the electrical activity of muscle by insertion of a recording electrode into the muscle and recording the electrical activity by means of an amplifier on an oscilloscope.[9, 12, 13, 50] An audible signal accompanies this recording. It is used clinically to determine if the lower motor neuron or the muscle fibers themselves are the site of the lesion. Like any other ancillary procedure, it is used to confirm a clinical observation of neuromuscular disease.

Normal resting muscle does not show observable electrical activity on the electromyograph once the electrode placement is stabilized. There also is no audible signal given. This is the resting potential. In lower motor neuron disease muscle cells become denervated. About 5 days following such denervation in the dog continuous spontaneous potentials called fibrillations develop, with amplitudes usually less than 100 μv. They are biphasic, of 1 to 2 msec in duration, and produce a sound like eggs frying. They may occur as often as 2 to 30 per sec.

Fibrillations are said to represent the spontaneous action potential or contraction of a single denervated muscle cell. Denervation disturbs the muscle cell metabolism that is thought to account for its spontaneous activity. The prevalence of fibrillations in denervated muscle may decrease after a 3-week period. Positive sharp waves (potentials) also accompany the denervation of lower motor neuron disease and are characterized by an initial low voltage sharp deflection with a slow return to the baseline. Voltage is variable, ranging from 50 to 1000 μv. These waves last up to 100 msec and have a dull sound. Spontaneous contraction of single motor units is often visible on the muscle surface and is called a fasciculation. It varies from 300 to 2000 μv in amplitude and lasts from 4 to 10 msec. This also may accompany the denervation of lower motor neuron disease. It occasionally occurs in normal muscle.

Nerve conduction can be determined by the same electromyographic instruments, and the evoked potential of the muscle can be observed.[43] For practical purposes this usually is performed in the thoracic limb by stimulating the ulnar nerve at the elbow and in the carpal canal, and recording from the interosseous muscles. Normal conduction time varies between 50 and 60 m per sec. Nerves that have been injured and avulsed and have undergone Wallerian degeneration (from 4 to 5 days) will not conduct an impulse.[2][69] Decreased conduction times occur only in severely compromised nerves. The evoked potential resulting from motor nerve stimulation is the summated motor unit potential recorded on the oscilloscope. Normally it is a smooth bi- or triphasic wave, 5 to 10 msec in duration, varying in amplitude but often greater than 3000 μv. In lower motor neuron disease the evoked potential may be polyphasic and prolonged if some nerve fibers are conducting slowly. Loss of some motor units prevents smooth summation of response. Polyphasic potentials of decreased amplitude also may occur in myositis. If the inflammation involves the neuromuscular ending, denervation potentials may accompany this.

Myotonia is defined as the continued active contraction of a muscle that persists after the stimulation or voluntary effort has stopped. On the electromyograph, it is stimulated by the needle insertion and appears as a repetitive, high frequency discharge that initially increases in amplitude and frequency and then decreases. On the loudspeaker this produces a distinct sound that waxes and wanes and is described as the "dive-bomber sound" because of the resemblance. This is a nonspecific change that occurs with many forms of muscle disease. It presumably results from a hyperexcitable muscle-cell membrane.[35,75]

DISEASES OF THE GSE LOWER MOTOR NEURON

The following examples of general somatic efferent lower motor neuron disease are organized topographically starting with the neuromuscular ending and progressing proximally toward the spinal cord. Some include other systems of the lower motor neuron and others include lesions of the peripheral sensory neurons as well. They are discussed here because of the recognizable deficit of GSE function.

Neuromuscular Ending

Botulism, tick paralysis, and myasthenia gravis all are diseases that affect the function of the neuromuscular ending. Myasthenia gravis is characterized by

TABLE 4–2. DISEASES OF THE GSE LOWER MOTOR NEURON

Neuromuscular ending
    Botulism
    Tick paralysis
    Myasthenia gravis
Peripheral nerve
    Trauma
    Neoplasia
    Ischemia—caudal aortic embolism
Spinal roots and nerves
    Trauma—root avulsion
    Neoplasia—neurofibroma
    Inflammation
Spinal roots and/or nerves and peripheral nerves
    Inflammation:
        Acute polyneuritis—coonhound paralysis, brachial plexus neuritis
        Chronic canine polyneuritis
        Chronic equine polyneuritis
Spinal cord
    Focal myelopathy from compression
    Acute ischemic myelopathy—fibrocartilaginous emboli
    Diffuse myelomalacia
    Inflammations—viral, protozoal
    Hereditary abiotrophy
Muscle disease
    Myopathy—myositis:
        Masticatory
        Polymyositis
    Myotonia:
        Adult polymyopathy
        Hereditary polymyopathy in puppies
        Myotonia congenita

episodic occurrences of lower motor neuron weakness associated with exercise, and is responsive to anticholinesterase therapy. Botulism and tick paralysis are rapidly progressive, sometimes fatal, lower motor neuron paralytic diseases that are not significantly responsive to such therapy.

Botulism. Botulism is a LMN paralysis caused by the toxin produced by the bacterium *Clostridium botulinum.* The toxin may be ingested in feed in which this organism is growing, or the agent may infect a wound and produce toxin that presumably gains entrance to the blood stream and ultimately reaches neuromuscular endings, in which it is thought to interfere with acetycholine release and function.[48] There are significant species differences in susceptibility to botulism. Some are dependent on the type of toxin to which the animal is exposed. Dogs and pigs are the most resistant to this disease. Ruminants are most susceptible to type C and D toxins.[58]

At the New York State College of Veterinary Medicine, botulism has been diagnosed presumptively as a herd problem in cattle and in individual horses. In neither situation has it been possible to prove the diagnosis. Usually, once the signs are recognized the disease is fatal.

Cattle assumed to have this disease show a weak, unsteady gait without ataxia and often become recumbent in 24 to 48 hours.[7, 25] It is important to recognize the lack of ataxia in order to differentiate this condition from a spinal cord lesion. All muscles are hypotonic and weak. This includes the tail, anus, limbs, ears, eyelids, lips, tongue, and pharynx. Palpation of facial muscles and testing tongue strength by pulling it from the mouth are helpful in determining the signs of diffuse lower motor neuron disease. Dysphagia, or difficulty in swallowing, is a prominent sign. Death is caused by respiratory paralysis.

Some forms of organophosphate poisoning may mimic botulism, except that pelvic limb weakness may be more apparent than thoracic limb weakness before the animal becomes recumbent.[49] The tail may be carried slightly elevated, and the animal constantly is dribbling urine. Diffuse neuromuscular paresis prevails, including cranial nerves with lower motor neuron function. Cattle become recumbent and die from respiratory paralysis. Careful study of spinal cord and peripheral nerves may reveal degeneration of axons, myelin, and cell bodies. The neuropathy is described as a dying back of the axon. Triorthocresyl phosphate and triorthotolyl phosphate can produce these lesions.[11, 53]

A similar rapidly progressive neuromuscular paralysis is seen occasionally in individual adult horses, with no lesions found in the central or peripheral nervous systems. It is usually fatal after a few days, death occurring from respiratory paralysis. Botulism is the presumptive diagnosis.

A diffuse neuromuscular paresis occurs in young foals about 2 to 8 weeks old.[55] The signs resemble those of experimental botulism and the condition is characterized by a sudden onset of severe weakness and prostration. These foals have been referred to as "shaker foals" because of the way they shake while trying to remain standing with weak muscles. Dysphagia is common. Death occurs from respiratory paralysis, often as soon as 72 hours after the onset. In some instances vigorous continual therapy with anticholinesterases (2 mg of neostigmine every 2 hours for 4 to 7 days) has resulted in recovery. Pathologic studies have not revealed significant lesions. No toxin has been isolated from the foal or the mare's milk. The pathogenesis remains unknown.

Tick Paralysis. Tick paralysis, most commonly observed in dogs and children, can affect all species in those areas in which the appropriate tick is located. The common wood tick, *Dermacentor variabilis,* is incriminated most often. The tick is presumed to elaborate a salivary neurotoxin that circulates and interferes with acetylcholine synthesis or liberation at the neuromuscular ending. Signs occur 5 to 7 days after tick infestation, with a rapid onset of lower motor neuron paresis. Dogs often first appear weak in the pelvic limbs, and then become recumbent in 48 to 72 hours. Spinal reflexes are depressed or absent. Pain is perceived normally. The lower motor neurons of the cranial nerves are not affected significantly. Death may occur in 1 to 5 days from respiratory paralysis. Direct removal of the tick or ticks or dipping the animal in an insecticide solution to kill them is followed by recovery in 24 to 72 hours.

In eastern Australia *Ixodes holocyclus* produces a severe lower motor neuron paralysis that rapidly progresses from pelvic to thoracic limbs. Signs often include sialosis, emesis, and mydriasis. Death from respiratory paralysis may occur despite insecticide dips and tick removal. Antiserum is administered intravenously.[76]

Myasthenia Gravis. Myasthenia gravis (grave muscle weakness) is a common disease in man. A similar syndrome occasionally has been reported in the dog.[27, 46, 52] Dogs of all ages are susceptible, but the syndrome appears to be more common in young adults. This is an episodic weakness associated with exercise. The stride may be shortened, followed by collapse in the pelvic or all four limbs. This disease should be considered in dogs that fatigue excessively. The lower motor neuron paresis may be as severe in muscles innervated by cranial nerves as in those innervated by spinal nerves. In one case, exercise produced laryngeal paresis causing a severe inspiratory dyspnea and hypoxic cyanosis. This was accompanied by facial paresis, dysphagia, and continual drooling of saliva. Mega-esophagus commonly is observed on thoracic radiographs. Postprandial vomiting also may be associated with this disease. In some instances repeated nerve stimulation has caused a decrement in muscle response.

The clinical signs are responsive to a test dose of anticholinesterase. One or two intramuscular injections of neostigmine methylsulfate (0.02 to 0.03 mg per lb) given 10 minutes apart in a dog pretreated with atropine (0.025 mg per lb) is usually sufficient to achieve a response. Edrophonium chloride may be used intravenously at 0.5 to 1.0 mg per lb. This produces an immediate response that lasts from 3 to 8 minutes. Oral therapy with 0.25 mg per lb of neostigmine bromide 3 times daily usually prevents the clinical signs. In dogs the therapy can be discontinued after 2 to 4 weeks and the signs do not recur.

The pathogenesis of this disease in man still is not understood fully. It is thought at present that it is an immunopathologic disease, with antibodies produced against a portion of the neuromuscular ending that interfere with acetylcholine function. In some individuals steroid therapy has been found to be effective.

Peripheral Nerve

Trauma.   Individual nerves or groups of peripheral nerves are susceptible to injury.[40, 41, 63, 67] The following is an enumeration of these nerves and the signs to be expected. These signs include the general somatic afferent deficit as well as loss of function of the general somatic efferent lower motor neuron.

THORACIC LIMB

Radial Paralysis—Distal Brachium.   The limb can support weight, but often only on the dorsum of the paw. The carpus and digits do not extend properly, occasionally causing the paw to be placed on the ground on its dorsal surface (knuckled). The dog may compensate by flipping the paw forward when the elbow is quickly flexed. There is analgesia of the cranial and lateral antebrachium and dorsal paw. This injury often follows fractures of the distal humerus.[28, 39, 60]

Radial Paralysis—Proximal Brachium.[54]   The limb cannot support weight, and collapses on the dorsal surface of the paw. Initially the elbow is "dropped," a position more ventral than normal owing to the loss of shoulder flexion function of the long head of the triceps. The limb often is carried off the ground with the elbow flexed (musculocutaneous). There is analgesia of the cranial and lateral antebrachium and dorsal paw. In the calf there also may be difficulty in advancing the limb.

Radial, Axillary, and Thoracodorsal Paralysis.   In addition to the signs of a proximal radial paralysis, the elbow is permanently in a posture more ventral than normal (dropped) because of the paralysis of almost all the flexors of the shoulder.[40, 41] There is analgesia of the dorsal paw, cranial and lateral antebrachium (radial), and lateral brachium (axillary).

Median and Ulnar Paralysis.   The gait is normal, but the carpus is more extended than usual and therefore slightly closer to the ground surface as a result of the lack of contraction in the flexors of the carpus and digits.

There is analgesia of the caudal antebrachium, lateral paw, and possibly the palmar paw. The latter area may have innervation from the branch of the musculocutaneous nerve that joins the median nerve near the elbow.

In the calf, the gait appears slightly stiff owing to the extension of the carpus, fetlock, and pastern joints.

Musculocutaneous Paralysis.　The gait is normal in the dog. The elbow may be slightly straight (overextended), and the paralysis of elbow flexion may make it difficult to raise the paw to a table surface. There is analgesia of the medial antebrachium.

Suprascapular Paralysis.　No clinical signs are evident in the dog. In the horse complete paralysis causes abduction of the shoulder on bearing weight. In the calf only slight abduction of the limb occurs, causing a slight circumduction of the limb.

Pectoral Paralysis.　In the horse the elbow abducts when weight is born by the affected limb.

PELVIC LIMB

Femoral Paralysis.　There is inability to support weight, and the limb collapses. The dog learns to walk bearing most of its weight on the normal limb and only making a short stride on the affected limb. In the horse when the stifle collapses (flexes), the tarsus and digit automatically suddenly flex.

There is analgesia of the medial side of the thigh, leg, and paw (saphenous). The horse rests with all the joints of the affected limb flexed, and the affected hip region appears more ventral than normal. Femoral nerve paralysis has been observed in calves born following dystocia caused by a hip or stifle lock position that resulted in a stretching of the femoral nerve.[61]

Peroneal Paralysis.　The paw often is placed with its dorsal surface on the ground (knuckled) and the tarsus is overextended—straighter than normal. There is analgesia of the cranial leg and dorsal paw areas.

This occurs in cattle that are recumbent and lie with pressure on the lateral side of the tibia, where this nerve courses subcutaneously. Peroneal nerve compression has been documented.[14]

Tibial Paralysis.　On bearing weight the paw sinks and is closer to the ground owing to the lack of tarsal extension. There is analgesia of the caudal leg and plantar paw area. In the calf the fetlock also is "knuckled forward."

Sciatic Paralysis.　The limb can support weight, but the tarsus is overflexed and sinks close to the ground surface, and the paw is dragged on its dorsum and placed with the dorsum on the ground surface. Hip flexion and stifle extension are normal. There is analgesia of the limb distal to the stifle, except for the medial surface.

The sciatic nerve is subject to fractures of the ilium at the greater sciatic notch and fractures of the femur with caudal displacement of a fractured portion. It is susceptible to injury by closed intramedullary bone pinning through the trochanteric fossa. Intramuscular injections of drugs into this nerve caudal to the femur cause varying degrees of sciatic paralysis that usually is transient but may be permanent.

Obturator Paralysis.　The paralyzed limb slides out or abducts on a smooth surface. The gait is normal on a surface that provides a grip for the dog. Similar signs occasionally are seen in cattle following dystocia.

In the calf, unilateral or bilateral obturator nerve section causes no alteration in the standing posture, but on walking or running the affected limb or limbs are noticeably abducted. In the adult cow, unilateral obturator nerve section causes slight abduction when the animal is standing or walking. The limb often slides laterally when the cow stands up. Bilateral neurectomy causes total abduction and collapse of the cow; it is unable to stand unassisted.

Cranial Gluteal Paralysis. In the supporting-propulsive phase of the stride, as all the weight is borne on the affected limb and this phase is completed, the stifle is observed to abduct or rotate so that its cranial surface is directed laterally.

Neoplasia. Nonneural neoplasms may compress one or more peripheral nerves, causing lower motor neuron paresis. In parakeets renal adenocarcinoma may compress the sciatic or femoral nerves that course dorsal to the kidney. Sciatic paralysis in the bird prevents the normal perching mechanism from functioning, and causes hyporeflexia, atrophy, and hypalgesia.

An osteogenic sarcoma of the ventral aspect of the sacrum may compress the sacral nerves and caudal lumbar nerves that form the sciatic nerve. Paralysis of the anus, bladder and rectum, and caudal thigh and leg muscles results. The tail is spared if the vertebral canal is not invaded by the mass. Such a lesion can be diagnosed by rectal examination.

Ischemic Neuropathy. Caudal aortic thrombosis or embolism is common in cats and occasionally is observed in dogs and horses.[10] There is complete pelvic limb paralysis (paraplegia), except for hip flexion in some patients. The pelvic limbs are cold; the affected muscles may be firm on palpation and no femoral pulse is present. In addition to the lack of muscle function owing to the interference with their circulation, the peripheral nerves also become ischemic. This can be determined by the sensory deficit that is also present. The spinal cord is not ischemic in these cases unless the thrombosis is proximal to the renal arteries.

Spinal Roots and Nerves

Trauma. The spinal roots are susceptible to injury by fractured vertebrae. Usually the signs observed reflect the damage done to the spinal cord. The exceptions to this are caudal lumbar, sacral, and caudal fractures that injure the roots of the cauda equina caudal to the end of the spinal cord. For example, a fracture and luxation of L7 may spare the spinal cord parenchyma or only affect the caudal segments, and yet may severely injure the roots of L6 and L7 and all the sacral and caudal roots that pass through the displaced vertebral foramen of L7. This could produce a denervated tail, anus, bladder, and rectum, and sciatic nerve paralysis bilaterally. The dog can stand and walk by hip flexion and stifle extension, but bears weight on the dorsal surface of the paws. The tail and anus are atonic, unresponsive to the perineal reflex, and analgesic. The pelvic limb paws are analgesic except for the medial side, which is innervated by the saphenous nerve (L3, L4, L5). Noxious pressure applied to digits 2, 3, and 4 elicits no pain response or flexor reflex. Similar stimulation of the first digit produces pain and hip flexion, but no flexion of the stifle, tarsus, or digits.

Root Avulsion Avulsion of the roots of the brachial plexus is the most common cause of the ipsilateral thoracic limb paralysis that occurs following an animal's being struck by a car.[31, 32] When the proximal thoracic limb is forced caudally along the trunk strain is put on the spinal roots, especially at C8 and T1. Excessive strain causes them to rip off of the cord or pull apart intrinsically.

The signs vary depending on the severity of the lesion and the number of roots involved. Usually for signs to occur the roots of two or more spinal cord segments must be involved. In total dysfunction, the roots of segments C6 through T1 are involved. In the latter case all muscles are paralyzed and the limb is dragged constantly along the ground on the dorsal surface of the paw, completely unable to be moved or support weight. Analgesia is variable but may be present over all aspects of the paw, antebrachium, and the distal half of the brachium. With incomplete involvement of these roots the area of analgesia does not correspond to specific peripheral nerves, but is probably dermatomal in distribution.

If the roots of the more caudal segments (C8 and T1) are avulsed, sparing C6 and C7, shoulder and elbow function may be spared and the motor signs are similar to those of proximal radial paralysis.

The ipsilateral panniculus reflex is absent in all cases with the C8 and T1 roots avulsed. A contralateral response is observed. Normally, sensory stimulation of the skin over the thorax or abdomen induces a bilateral contraction of the cutaneous trunci. The impulses enter the spinal cord at the level of the stimulus. They are passed cranially through the white matter to the grey matter at T1 and C8, where the neurons of the lateral thoracic nerve are activated to cause the cutaneous trunci to contract.

Avulsion of the T1 roots also causes ipsilateral miosis (partial Horner's syndrome).

Avulsion of the lumbosacral roots is rare. One case was observed in a cat in which the roots of L5, L6, L7, and S1 were avulsed traumatically from the spinal cord on one side or severely contused. There were associated femoral and sciatic paralyses of the ipsilateral limb.

Neoplasia.   Neurofibroma may affect one spinal root without producing significant neurologic deficit. Clinical signs usually occur when the spinal cord becomes compressed by the mass lesion.

Inflammation.   Occasionally, a neuritis occurs in the spinal roots, caused by the protozoa *Toxoplasma gondii.*[6] This organism can affect any portion of the central nervous system, as well as the roots of the spinal nerves. The clinical signs reflect the areas in which the most damage has taken place.

Spinal Roots and/or Nerves and Peripheral Nerves

Acute Polyneuritis

IDIOPATHIC   POLYRADICULONEURITIS.   Acute   idiopathic   polyradiculoneuritis, the lesion of coonhound paralysis, is the most common inflammation of multiple portions of the peripheral nervous system.[15, 18] It usually predominates in the ventral spinal roots, but can affect any portion of the nervous system covered by peripheral myelin, including cranial nerves. A description of this disease follows.

Signalment.   Dogs of any age, sex, or breed that are in territory inhabited by raccoons are susceptible.

Chief complaint.   Progressive weakness.

History and Clinical Course.   The patient has been exposed to a raccoon and presumably has been bitten, usually 7 to 14 days prior to the onset of signs. Signs begin with a variable degree of paresis in the pelvic limbs. At that time the owner may note that the dog's voice is altered in quality. The paresis progresses in severity in the pelvic limbs and subsequently involves the thoracic limbs. Typically, the patient becomes totally recumbent with tetraplegia 7 to 10 days after the onset of signs. This interval is variable and on occasion has been as brief as 72 hours. In some instances the signs begin with the thoracic limbs and later involve the pelvic limbs. At the height of the disease the head cannot be raised, and occasionally even the tail is paralyzed. The patient is alert and responsive at all times and will eat if supported. Evacuations may be normal or, occasionally for a few days, the bladder may be distended without being evacuated.

During the progressive course of the disease there is a concomitant progressive loss of spinal reflexes in all extremities. Characteristically, pain is perceived when a noxious stimulus is applied to the extremity, but the patient cannot remove the limb from the stimulus. Muscle tenderness may be evident on palpation. Muscle tone is absent. There is decreased resistance to passive manipulation of all extremities. In some instances a facial diplegia may be noted. Dysphagia has not been observed.

The signs may be summarized as a bilaterally symmetric flaccid tetraplegia with areflexia and atonia. Most patients recover, but a few die from respiratory paralysis at the height of the disease.

In the majority of cases recovery begins 5 to 7 days after complete tetraplegia is evident. After 7 to 10 days of slow improvement in muscle strength the limbs may be able to support weight and the patient may take a few cautious steps. Approximately 3 to 4 weeks after the start of signs the patient may be walking again. In a few cases this interval may be as long as 12 to 15 weeks, followed by complete recovery.

Neurogenic atrophy of all muscles, axial and appendicular, becomes evident shortly after tetraplegia occurs and progresses through the recovery period. In addition, following tetraplegia skin erosions appear over the bony prominences and demand rigorous nursing care.

Complete recovery of muscle strength and mass takes place over the following weeks, and the hunting dog may return to hunting. However, reexposure to the bite of a raccoon may precipitate the signs again. There seems to be no acquired immunity to this disease. *Treatment.* There is no specific therapy available. Persistent nursing care is mandatory in order to prevent secondary bacterial infections, particularly of the skin and bladder. A thick bedding of straw is especially helpful in preventing skin ulcerations. Some feel that vigorous corticosteroid therapy at the onset enhances the recovery rate. In fulminating cases mechanical respiratory assistance may be necessary to prevent death.

The cause of this disease remains an enigma. Viral isolation studies on diseased tissue have been unrewarding. The inflammatory component of the lesion varies from only an occasional perivenular lymphocytic cuff to large numbers of perivascular lymphocytes, plasma cells, and mononuclear cells. Nerves that are stained with osmic acid and teased apart to allow study of individual neurons reveal a segmental demyelination that is presumed to be the primary lesion. The ability of these lemmocytes to remyelinate accounts for the often rapid recovery from this disease.

The lesion closely resembles the experimental allergic neuritis produced in laboratory animals by the injection of peripheral nerve emulsified with an adjuvant. A similar experiment was performed on a group of coonhounds raised from parents that had contracted the natural disease and recovered.[38] It produced a peracute polyneuritis with fibrinoid necrosis of vessel walls and severe necrosis of peripheral neurons, with edema and hemorrhage. This suggested a unique susceptibility of this group of dogs. The natural disease often has occurred in coonhounds related to each other. In all dogs that suffer raccoon bites, the critical factor appears to be the unique susceptibility of the dog and not the specific raccoon involved. This remains to be determined. Recently at the New York State College of Veterinary Medicine a clinically identical disease was reproduced by the subcutaneous injection of raccoon saliva into a dog that had previously had the natural disease and recovered.

A few cases of canine polyradiculoneuritis have been recognized in which exposure to a raccoon was not possible.

In man, the comparable disease clinically and pathologically is the acute polyneuritis of the Landry-Guillain-Barré syndrome. The pathogenesis of this disease is also unknown. Virologists recently have related a number of these cases to the presence of the agent that causes infectious mononucleosis, the Epstein-Barr virus.[36]

BRACHIAL PLEXUS NEURITIS-NEUROPATHY. A syndrome has been recognized in the dog similar to brachial plexus neuropathy in man, which in some instances follows prophylactic inoculations such as tetanus antiserum.[1, 19, 62] Such cases have been referred to as serum neuritis. The disease is characterized by a sudden onset of pain and paresis in the thoracic limbs. Signs of paresis progress rapidly and are limited to muscles innervated by the brachial plexus. The prognosis for functional recovery in man is considered good, but it may take up to 3 years or longer for the destroyed axons to regenerate and reinnervate the paralyzed muscles. In many cases of brachial plexus neuropathy there has been no antecedent injection of foreign protein. In some, other illnesses or strenuous exercise preceded the onset of neurologic signs. In others, there has been no history to associate with this disease.

A 9-month-old female Great Dane suddenly developed severe paresis of the thoracic limbs, preceded by 2 allergic episodes with facial edema and generalized urticaria over a 48-hour period. A diet of horse meat had been instituted 2 weeks prior to the first allergic attack. Severe lower motor neuron deficit was found in both thoracic limbs. Flexor reflexes were depressed and neurogenic atrophy developed rapidly in all thoracic limb muscles. The signs were bilateral but not symmetric. Pelvic limb function was essentially normal, but patellar reflexes were depressed. Facial paresis was present on one side. Electromyography showed evidence of denervation. Biopsy of the sensory branches of the radial nerve in the forearm revealed extensive Wallerian degeneration. Skin testing showed hypersensitivity to horse serum. Over a period of 9 weeks no change was noted, and a necropsy was performed. Severe axonal and myelin degeneration had occurred in many of the peripheral nerves, leaving only cords of collagen, fibroblasts, and lemmocytes. The degenerative lesions were limited to the peripheral nerves of the thoracic limbs and could be followed proximally to the level of the spinal nerve component.

Chronic Polyneuritis

CHRONIC CANINE POLYNEURITIS.[15, 16, 17] A number of mature dogs have been observed with a slowly progressive weakness of one or more limbs, and occasionally with facial paresis and a loss of voice volume. Asymmetry of signs is common but not constant. If advanced lesions are present, the animal may be unable to support its weight and its limbs may slide out from under it. In the early stages of chronic canine polyneuritis the resemblance of the lower motor neuron paresis to the lame gait caused by musculoskeletal disease often has confused the diagnosis. Normal joint palpation, the lack of joint or bone pain, the presence of neurogenic atrophy and sometimes hyporeflexia, and the demonstration of paresis on postural reaction testing help to establish the signs as neurogenic. Ataxia generally is not observed in peripheral nerve disorders.

Electromyography, conduction times, and biopsy of nerve tissue help confirm the diagnosis. If there is nerve root involvement, an albuminocytologic dissociation may be present in the CSF.

Pathologic changes are variable and suggest a diverse pathogenesis.[21, 22] In one case the polyneuropathy was associated with chronic uremia. Others have been associated with pituitary chromophobe adenomas and hypothyroidism, at times with facial paresis and occasionally peripheral vestibular signs.

CHRONIC EQUINE POLYNEURITIS (Neuritis of the Cauda Equina in the Horse).[30, 47, 51, 59] The following case report illustrates this disease.

Signalment. A 4-year-old Morgan stallion.

Chief Complaint. Inability to excrete or move the tail.

History. Two months prior to admission the animal rubbed the skin beside the tail. About 1 week later the stallion began to urinate small amounts of urine frequently, and control of the tail was lost. Feces began to be retained. For 5 to 6 weeks prior to admission the animal's bladder was catheterized daily and the rectum was evacuated of feces manually. No obvious abnormality of gait was observed until possibly the last few days before admission.

Physical Examination. The pelvic limb gait was stiff. The right pelvic limb often remained locked in extension, and weight was borne on the dorsum of the hoof. Some mild weakness also was evident in the left pelvic limb, along with proprioceptive deficit.

The tail and anus were flaccid, areflexic, and analgesic. An area of analgesia was apparent up to a line about 3 inches cranial to the base of the tail and 8 to 10 inches laterally. This continued distally on the caudal thigh region and between the legs medially. The bladder was atonic. The biceps femoris lateral to the tail was atrophied slightly. The cranial portion of this muscle and the gluteals constantly fasciculated and seemed hyperesthetic to palpation.

There were no cranial nerve abnormalities.

Laboratory Findings. Lumbosacral spinal fluid contained 14 RBCs and 240 WBCs per cmm with 72 mononuclear and 28 polymorphonuclear cells per 100 and 87 mg of protein per dl.

Cisternal fluid contained 194 RBCs and 2 WBCs per cmm, and 54 mg of protein per dl.

Diagnosis. Neuritis of the cauda equina.

Prognosis. Poor for recovery. No specific therapy is known. The disease usually progresses.

Findings and Necropsy. There was extensive thickening and adhesion of the spinal roots of the cauda equina, predominantly from the point at which they penetrated the dura to the intervertebral foramina. This involved all the caudal nerves, and the sacral nerves except for the first. The S1 and L6 nerves were involved mildly. This fibrous matrix completely filled the epidural space in the vertebral canal around these nerves. The proliferated tissue was composed of a massive collection of inflammatory cells. Most were lymphocytes and plasma cells with numerous eosinophils and macrophages, including giant cells. There were many foci of suppuration in this granulomatous lesion, which contained a center of neutrophils surrounded by the mononuclear inflammation. Collagen was abundant throughout the lesion. It involved the perineurial and epineurial connective tissues primarily, and secondarily infiltrated the endoneurium and was associated with demyelination and axonal degeneration of the neurons.

This is a disease of horses that has been recognized in Europe for many years, but only recently reported in North America. Although the primary lesion and clinical signs involve the cauda equina, in some cases cranial nerve signs and lesions have been reported, as well as a diffuse involvement of the other spinal nerves. There are no brain or spinal cord lesions. Infectious (streptococcal) and allergic etiologies have been proposed for this neuritis. No one etiology has been confirmed.

A second case was examined in which the caudal and sacral nerve paralyses were identical to those of the patient described in the case report, but the gait was unaffected. However, the patient showed a constant left head tilt and mild paresis of all the facial muscles on the left side. The gait was normal except for a slight tendency to drift to the left side.

The lesions of the cauda equina found in the necropsy were similar to those described in the case report, but the proliferative granuloma extended through the sacral intervertebral foramina and invaded the adjacent hypaxial muscles. A similar but milder neuropathy was present in the left facial nerve.

Spinal Cord

Lesions that affect the cell bodies of the general somatic efferent lower motor neuron in the spinal cord produce similar signs of lower motor neuron disease that are specific to the area innervated.

Focal Myelopathy from Compression. A neoplasm, extruded intervertebral disk, or vertebral fracture that compresses spinal cord segments L3, L4, and L5 produces a paresis or paralysis of the pelvic limbs due to the spinal cord dysfunction. This is accompanied by a bilateral femoral nerve paralysis and loss of the patellar reflex as a result of the direct injury to the cell bodies of these femoral nerve neurons.

A similar lesion between T3 and L3 causes paresis and ataxia or paralysis of the pelvic limbs with normal or hyperactive pelvic limb reflexes and no obvious signs of lower motor neuron disease in the neurologic examination. This is because spinal cord segments L4 through S1 are not involved directly with the lesion. There may be destruction of general somatic efferent lower motor neuron cell bodies in one or more segments, but unless they supply limb muscles their region of denervation is difficult to detect except by means of electromyography. EMG of the axial muscles may find the level of the lesion by showing denervation potentials in the affected segment.

Ischemic Myelopathy. Ischemic myelopathy has been associated with fibrocartilaginous emboli in both arteries and veins in the parenchyma and leptomeninges at all levels of the spinal cord.[20, 24, 29, 34, 68] The infarcts that occur may be ischemic or hemorrhagic and usually affect both grey and white matter at the level of the lesion. If the infarction occurs on the right side of the spinal cord from the sixth through the eighth cervical spinal cord segments, the loss of the cell bodies in the lateral portion of the ventral grey columns causes a lower motor neuron paralysis of the ipsilateral thoracic limb. The adjacent white matter lesion causes ataxia and spastic paresis, or paralysis of the ipsilateral pelvic limb.

In some dogs the emboli may cause almost total infarction of the caudal, sacral, and caudal and middle lumbar spinal cord segments. This results in complete lower motor neuron paralysis of the tail, perineum, bladder, rectum, and pelvic limbs. Tone and spinal reflexes are all absent. In addition, there is analgesia of the affected area due to loss of the spinal cord portion of the general somatic afferent neurons entering from the dorsal roots, as well as of the cell bodies of the neurons in the dorsal grey column. Despite the destruction of the spinal cord white matter, the clinical signs reflect the grey matter destruction. Cases such as these with signs of extensive grey matter destruction have a very poor prognosis.

The signs are sudden in onset and usually stabilize within 24 hours. From then on they may remain unchanged or improve, depending on the degree of ischemic compromise of the tissue. Some dogs have returned to nearly normal function.

Usually no pain is felt by the patient on vertebral manipulation. Radiographs are normal, or at the onset slight swelling of the parenchyma may be observed on a myelogram. Within the first few hours cerebrospinal fluid may show an elevated neutrophil count along with mild elevation of protein levels. After 24 to 48 hours cell counts are normal, or there is a slight elevation of mononuclear cells and the protein typically remains elevated. The pathogenesis of the emboli is still unknown. Intervertebral disk material is suspected as the source.[74]

Diffuse Myelomalacia.   A diffuse progressive myelomalacia occasionally can be found following an acute intervertebral disk extrusion at any level of the thoracolumbar vertebral column.[33] It also was observed in one case in which a neurofibroma was compressing the lumbar spinal cord; in two other cases no associated vertebral column lesion could be identified. The lesion is a combination of ischemic and hemorrhagic infarction of the entire parenchyma of the spinal cord, but the roots in the leptomeninges are spared. Hemorrhage often occurs in the subarachnoid space. The spinal cord lesion has been termed hematomyelia, but this is not accurate. The parenchymal bleeding that occurs is secondary to the infarction. Despite the severe ischemic lesion, no significant lesions of the vessels have been observed. Necrosis of the vessels takes place in the infarct, but this is assumed to be secondary to the ischemic lesion.

Careful study of a case from the start shows that the myelomalacia first occurs at the site of the disk extrusion, and then typically descends and ascends from that site. In a few instances a portion of a spinal cord segment is normal between areas of myelomalacia, indicating that this is not just a pressure-induced phenomenon.

Usually, at the cranial extent of the lesion in the cervical spinal cord there is a core of necrosis in the central canal and ventral aspect of the dorsal funiculi.

The typical case of ascending and descending myelomalacia secondary to protrusion of an intervertebral disk at any site along the thoracolumbar vertebral column begins with a sudden onset of complete paraplegia. At the initial examination of the pelvic limbs the reflexes may be intact and hyperactive (spastic). Later examination (48 to 72 hours) reveals a flaccid paraplegia with atonia and total areflexia of the muscles of the pelvic limbs. The tail is flaccid and the anus is dilated and unresponsive to stimuli. There is no pain perception from any of these areas. The abdomen is flaccid. At that time or within the next few days the animal begins to act paretic and ataxic in the thoracic limbs. It prefers to lay in lateral recumbency with the thoracic limbs extended, and demonstrates exquisite pain when handled in the thoracic or cervical region. Reflexes persist in the thoracic limbs at this time. A line of analgesia usually can be located in the cranial thoracic region. Bilateral Horner's syndrome may occur. Respirations progressively become more diaphragmatic. Death often occurs in 7 to 10 days from the onset of signs and is caused by respiratory paralysis. There is no treatment for this condition.

Occasionally the myelomalacia only descends and therefore death does not occur, but no therapy is known that will bring about recovery.

This extensive lower motor neuron disease with analgesia is not difficult to recognize, and patients should not be subject to surgical therapy. The lesion has developed following immediate decompressive laminectomy of the acute extrusion and prior to recognizable signs of progressive myelomalacia; thus it would seem that such surgery is not preventive.

Inflammations.   These may affect focal or diffuse areas of the spinal cord grey matter and produce associated signs of lower motor neuron disease.

Polioencephalomyelitis caused by an enterovirus in young pigs (Teschen's, Talfan's, or Ontario disease) has a predilection for spinal cord grey matter.

Rabies encephalomyelitis also may produce an ascending type of lower motor neuron paralysis, since it destroys more of the spinal cord grey matter. The signs of this disease are extremely variable but one should be on the lookout for it when lower motor neuron signs accompany the ataxia, paresis, and indications of cerebral disturbance. A hypotonic tail often is found in rabid cattle. Horses with rabies often present with spinal cord signs.

Occasionally, the canine distemper virus or *Toxoplasma gondii* in dogs destroys enough spinal cord grey matter to produce lower motor neuron signs along with the signs of destruction of white matter.

Hereditary Abiotrophy.   An autosomal recessive hereditary disease of young Swedish Lapland dogs characterized by neuronal abiotrophy causes tetraplegia, muscle atrophy, and severe limb contractures.[56] The onset is at around 5 weeks of age. The paralysis involves the general somatic efferent lower motor neuron system, especially to appendicular muscles, and is rapidly progressive. The neurogenic atrophy is accompanied by severe limb deformity and arthrogryposis related to the young age and rapid growth of the animal.

Neuronal cell body degeneration occurs in the ventral grey column of the spinal cord. This predominates in the lateral portion at the intumescences, which accounts for the clinical signs. The neuronal degeneration is diffuse, involving spinal ganglion cell bodies, cerebellar Purkinje cells, myelin and axons in spinocerebellar tracts, dorsal funiculi, and the central portions of vestibulocochlear, optic, and trigeminal nerves. Only the loss of general somatic efferent neurons is reflected in the clinical signs.

Muscle Disease

Myopathy-Myositis.   This disease is described here because it has many signs that closely resemble those of lower motor neuron disease.

MASTICATORY MYOSITIS-MYOPATHY.   Bilateral involvement of the muscles of mastication is the more commonly recognized muscle disease, especially in German shepherds. This usually is referred to as eosinophilic myositis because of the abundance of these cells and of lymphocytes and plasma cells, and the occurrence of edema and hemorrhage in the acute phase of the disease when the muscles are swollen and painful. Gamma globulins are elevated significantly in the serum of these patients, and an immunopathologic basis for the disease is suspected. After one or more acute episodes, severe atrophy occurs to the extent that the dog may be unable to open its jaws. At no time does paralysis occur.

In some dogs, including most non-German shepherd breeds, the atrophy of masticatory muscles can be found without evidence of an acute myositis. Biopsies suggest that some of these cases may represent a progressive myopathy.

POLYMYOSITIS.   Polymyositis has been observed mostly in German shepherds with lymphocytes, monocytes, and sometimes eosinophils in the muscle inflammation.[5, 57] A mild to moderately progressive paresis occurs, usually in all limbs but occasionally in just the pelvic limbs. Exertion may exacerbate the paresis.

The gait appears as a significantly short stride in the affected limb, and there is a tendency for the limb to slide out and for the dog to collapse.

Some dogs have decreased voice volume, prehension difficulty, dysphagia, and postprandial vomiting. Facial muscle weakness has not been observed. Spinal reflexes usually are normal, occasionally decreased. Muscle tone appears to be normal but muscle palpation often elicits pain.

Confirmation of the clinical diagnosis may be helped by electromyography, biopsy of muscle tissue, and testing for elevation in levels of one or more of the serum enzymes that may be released with muscle cell necrosis—glutamic-oxaloacetic transaminase, lactic dehydrogenase, creatine phosphokinase, and aldolase. The latter two are specific muscle enzymes and are the most reliable. Only occasionally a mild eosinophilia occurs in the differential count of white blood cells. Thoracic radiographs may reveal an esophageal dilation.

Toxoplasmosis is the most commonly reported myositis in dogs and causes a severe necrotizing myositis. This has not been observed in the muscle biopsies of the cases of polymyositis described here. The mononuclear interstitial myositis with minimal muscle cell necrosis suggests that the disease has an immunologic basis. Autoimmune polymyositis occurs in systemic lupus erythematosus.[72]

The prognosis for these cases is often good. Remarkable improvement in clinical signs occurs in 24 to 48 hours after the administration of corticosteroid therapy. Usually 0.25 mg per lb of prednisolone every 12 hours is sufficient. If no improvement is shown, the dose may be increased until the clinical signs disappear. After the signs are gone and serum enzyme levels are normal, the corticosteroid may be withdrawn gradually over a 7- to 10-day period. In some instances relapses occur and prolonged corticosteroid therapy is necessary.

MYOTONIC POLYMYOPATHY OF ADULT DOGS.   In some instances the canine polymyopathy is associated with a myotonia that was described in the section on electrodiagnostic techniques in this chapter.[4, 8, 35] This muscle disease is characterized by a stiff, stilted gait and varying degrees of paresis. No neurologic abnormalities are apparent. Muscle enzyme levels often are elevated in the serum. Most biopsies have shown varying degrees of muscle cell degeneration without obvious inflammation.

In some cases, percussion of a muscle causes a depression or dimple on the surface that persists after the stimulus is withdrawn. This represents the myotonia that is present. One case was observed that was associated with chronic hyperadrenocorticism. Limited therapy with procainamide and phenytoin has been unsuccessful in a few of these cases.[35]

HEREDITARY MYOTONIC MYOPATHY OF PUPPIES.   An hereditary X-linked recessive myotonic myopathy has been described in male Irish terrier puppies from 8 litters.[64] A similar disease was observed in two male Golden retriever litter mates. All had identical clinical signs, an identical clinical course, and similar lesions. A stiff gait or difficulty in swallowing first was noticed around 6 to 8 weeks of age. By 3 months the gait was significantly abnormal in all dogs. They walked with a stilted, stiff, shuffling gait. They fatigued with exertion and occasionally demonstrated respiratory distress and cyanosis. The limbs of the Irish terriers were stiff when manipulated, but spinal reflexes were normal. There were no neurologic abnormalities in any of the dogs. The neck was stiff but not painful, the jaw was resistant to opening, and the base of the tongue felt enlarged. Muscle atrophy was a prominent early sign in the Irish terriers, but only occurred late in the course of the disease in the Golden retrievers. The disease was slowly progressive, but all the dogs could still ambulate at 6 to 9 months of age, when euthanasia was performed.

Muscle enzyme levels were elevated greatly in the serum. Myotonia was evident on electromyography. A severe degenerative muscle disease was apparent on muscle biopsy or necropsy with necrosis of muscle cells, mononuclear phagocytosis, giant cells, and calcification.

The histologic lesions resembled those caused by vitamin E deficiency, but vitamin E level determinations on the Irish terriers were normal. The necropsy studies, including histochemical and electron-microscopic studies, suggested a primary myopathy in the Irish terriers. Pedigree studies indicated an X-linked recessive inheritance in the Irish terriers. The Golden retriever disease is presumed to be similar, but there were only two litter mates affected. No further genetic studies have been done.

MYOTONIA CONGENITA. Myotonia congenita is a disturbance of neuromuscular function that occurs in goats, in horses, and in man.[42, 65, 71, 73] In man it is known as Thomsen's disease. Inheritance factors have been demonstrated in man and are suspected in goats. The onset is at a variable period after birth in the young animal. A myotonic attack is precipitated at the start of a voluntary movement following rest. It may be aided by excitement or surprise, but these need not be present. Cold may enhance the attack. It lasts from 10 to 20 seconds, during which the limbs suddenly are rigidly extended, preventing any movement. The animal remains motionless or may fall into lateral recumbency with the limbs fully extended. There is no loss of consciousness. As the goat relaxes the signs subside, and they continue to abate as the goat begins to walk. A period of rest is required before the signs can be precipitated again. A focal myotonic reaction, dimpling, may occur in muscle percussion. No lesions have been observed in nervous or muscle tissue. Therapy with quinidine prevents the signs.

The signs of myotonia congenita in the foal may be mild and only reflected by a stiff gait which may be apparent at birth or not until a few months of age. They may improve temporarily with exercise. Focal areas of muscle may protrude under the skin where the myotonia is especially severe. These muscle lumps are most prominent in the proximal caudal thigh area and can be exaggerated by percussion. This is called myotonic dimpling.

In man and goats myotonia congenita is associated with an abnormal chloride conductance across the muscle cell membrane. This conductance is normal in the foal. A myotonic syndrome has been reported in a family of chows.[75]

Episodic Weakness

Episodic weakness waxes and wanes and usually is exacerbated by exercise.[45, 66] When the animal is at rest it may be mild or not apparent. It is a clinical sign of several pathophysiologic conditions. The differential diagnosis primarily involves three major categories of disease: neuromuscular, metabolic, and cardiorespiratory. Some of the following have been described previously in this chapter.

Neuromuscular Diseases

MYASTHENIA GRAVIS. Myasthenia gravis probably is the most classic disease whose signs are characterized by weakness following exertion. In addition to the appendicular weakness that may cause collapse, there may be facial, laryngeal, pharyngeal, and esophageal muscle weakness resulting in sialosis, dysphagia, occasional vomiting, and inspiratory dyspnea. There may be incontinence and a weak voice. Ataxia does not occur in this disease.

POLYMYOSITIS. Some dogs with polymyositis may show exacerbation of their weakness during exercise. The clinical signs may be manifested in the pelvic limbs alone or in all four limbs. The gait may be stiff, short-strided, symmetric or asymmetric, but not ataxic. Other signs of muscle involvement include dysphagia, postprandial vomiting, difficulty in chewing, and a hoarse bark. Proximal limb muscles may be painful on palpation.

Metabolic Disease

HYPOGLYCEMIA.   Weakness, or ataxia and lethargy, or both, may occur with hypoglycemia and be increased by exertion. Hypoglycemia may result from increased utilization of glucose when there are neoplasms of pancreatic beta cells. These usually occur in the older dog.

Decreased synthesis may cause hypoglycemia. This occurs in the glycogen storage diseases of toy breed puppies, in functional hypoglycemia of hunting dogs, in adrenocortical insufficiency, and in hepatic insufficiency.

HYPERKALEMIA.   Hyperkalemia may occur in adrenocortical insufficiency, diabetes mellitus, acute renal failure, or severe acidosis. Weakness that may be episodic results, accompanied by the more characteristic signs of these diseases.

HYPOKALEMIA.   Hypokalemia resulting from severe vomiting, diarrhea, or insulin therapy is uncommon. However, it may produce an episodic weakness.

Cardiorespiratory Disease

Cardiorespiratory diseases may produce episodic weakness, ataxia, lethargy, and syncope. The diseases most commonly implicated are cardiac arrhythmias (atrial fibrillation, ventricular tachycardia), third degree heart block, and heart worms.

A minimum data base should be obtained from laboratory work that includes determinations for fasting blood glucose, serum electrolyte, and enzyme levels, an examination for microfilaria, and an electrocardiogram. In addition, a neostigmine response test and a muscle biopsy should be considered.

REFERENCES

1. Alexander, J. W., de Lahunta, A., and Scott, D. W.: A case of brachial plexus neuropathy in a dog. J. Am. Anim. Hosp. Assoc., *10*:515, 1974.
2. Allam, M. W., Nulsen, F. E., and Lewey, F. H.: Electrical intraneural bipolar stimulation of peripheral nerves in the dog. Am. Vet. Med. Assoc., *114*:87, 1949.
3. Amann, J. F.: The organization of spinal motoneurons and their relationship to corticospinal fibers in the raccoon *(Procyon lotor)*. Ph.D. thesis, Ithaca, N.Y., Cornell University, 1971.
4. Arnold, S.: An endocrine abnormality in a dog. Senior seminar, Flower Library, New York State College of Veterinary Medicine, 1974.
5. Averill, D. A., Jr.: Polymyositis in the dog. *In* Kirk, R. W., ed., Current Veterinary Therapy, V. Small Animal Practice. Philadelphia, W. B. Saunders Co., 1974, 652–655.
6. Averill, D. A., Jr., and de Lahunta, A.: Toxoplasmosis of the canine nervous system: Clinicopathologic findings in four cases. J. Am. Vet. Med. Assoc., *159*:1134, 1971.
7. Bargai, V., Cohen, A., and Benado, A.: An outbreak of botulism in a dairy herd. Refuah Vet., *30*: 135, 1973.
8. Bluvas, P.: Myotonia in a case of canine Cushing's disease. Senior seminar. Flower Library, New York State College of Veterinary Medicine, 1974.
9. Bowen, J. M.: Electrodiagnostic testing and electromyography. *In* Hoerlein, B. F., ed., Canine Neurology. 2nd ed., Philadelphia, W. B. Saunders Co., 1971, 202–216.
10. Butler, H. C.: An investigation into the relationship of an aortic embolus to posterior paralysis in the cat. J. Small Anim. Pract., *12*:141, 1971.
11. Cavanagh, J. B.: Peripheral nerve changes in orthocresyl phosphate poisoning in the cat. J. Pathol. Bacteriol., *87*:365, 1964.
12. Chrisman, C. L.: Electromyography in the localization of spinal cord and nerve root neoplasia in dogs and cats. J. Am. Vet. Med. Assoc., *166*:1074, 1975.
13. Chrisman, C. L., Bunt, J. R., Wood, P. K., and Johnson, E. W.: Electromyography in small animal neurology. J. Am. Vet. Med. Assoc., *160*:311, 1972.
14. Cox, V. S., and Martin C. E.: Peroneal nerve paralysis in a heifer. J. Am. Vet. Med. Assoc., *167*:142, 1975.
15. Cummings, J. F., and de Lahunta, A.: Canine polyneuritis. *In* Kirk, R. W., ed., Current Veterinary Therapy, V. Small Animal Practice. Philadelphia, W. B. Saunders Co., 1974, 655–657.
16. Cummings, J. F., and de Lahunta, A.: Chronic relapsing polyradiculoneuritis in a dog. A clinical, light-, and electron-microscopic study. Acta Neuropathol., *28*:191, 1974.

17. Cummings, J. F., and de Lahunta, A.: Hypertrophic neuropathy in a dog. Acta Neuropathol., 29:325, 1974.
18. Cummings, J. F., and Haas, D. C.: Coonhound paralysis. An acute idiopathic polyradiculoneuritis in dogs resembling the Landry-Gullain-Barré syndrome. J. Neurol. Sci., 4:51, 1967.
19. Cummings, J. F., de Lahunta, A., Lorenz, M. D., and Washington, L. D.: Canine brachial plexus neuritis: A syndrome resembling serum neuritis in man. Cor. Vet., 63:590, 1973.
20. de Lahunta, A., and Alexander, J. W.: Ischemic myelopathy secondary to presumed fibrocartilaginous embolism in nine dogs. J. Am. Animal. Hosp. Assoc., 12:37, 1976.
21. Dyck, P. J., and Lambert, E. H.: Polyneuropathy associated with hypothyroidism. J. Neuropathol. Exp. Neurol., 29:631, 1970.
22. Dyck, P. J., Johnson, W. J., Lambert, E. H., and O'Brien, P. C.: Segmental demyelination secondary to axonal degeneration in uremic neuropathy. Mayo Clin. Proc., 46:400, 1971.
23. Evans, L. H., Campbell, J. H., Pinner-Poole, B., and Jenny, J.: Prevention of painful neuromas in horses. J. Am. Vet. Med. Assoc., 153:313, 1968.
24. Feigin, I., Popoff, N., and Adachi, M.: Fibrocartilaginous venous emboli to the spinal cord with necrotic myelopathy. J. Neuropathol. Exp. Neurol., 24:63, 1965.
25. Fjolstad, M., and Klund, T.: An outbreak of botulism among ruminants in connection with ensilage feeding. Nord. Vet.-Med., 21:609, 1969.
26. Fletcher, T. F.: Lumbosacral plexus and pelvic limb myotomes of the dog. Am. J. Vet. Res., 31:35, 1970.
27. Fraser, D. C., Palmer, A. C., and Senior, J. E. B.: Myasthenia gravis in the dog. J. Neurol. Neurosurg. Psychiatry, 33:431, 1970.
28. Frost, W. W., and Lumb, W. V.: Radiocarpal arthrodesis: A surgical approach to brachial paralysis. J. Am. Vet. Med. Assoc., 149:1073, 1966.
29. Green, C. E., and Higgins, R. J.: Fibrocartilaginous emboli as the cause of ischemic myelopathy in a dog. Cor. Vet., 66:131, 1976.
30. Greenwood, A. G., Barker, J., and McLeish, I.: Neuritis of the cauda equina in a horse. Equine Vet. J., 5:111, 1973.
31. Griffiths, I. R.: Avulsion of the brachial plexus. 1. Neuropathology of the spinal cord and peripheral nerves. J. Small Anim. Pract., 15:165, 1974.
32. Griffiths, I. R.: Avulsion of the brachial plexus. 2. Clinical aspects. J. Small Anim. Pract., 15:177, 1974.
33. Griffiths, I. R.: The extensive myelopathy of intervertebral disc protrusions in dogs (the ascending syndrome). J. Small Anim. Pract., 13:425, 1972.
34. Griffiths, I. R.: Spinal cord infarction due to emboli arising from the intervertebral discs in the dog. J. Comp. Pathol., 83:225, 1973.
35. Griffiths, I. R., and Duncan, I. D.: Myotonia in the dog: A report of four cases. Vet. Rec., 93:184, 1973.
36. Grose, C., Henle, W., Henle, G., and Feorino, P. M.: Primary Epstein-Barr virus infections in acute neurologic diseases. N. Engl. J. Med., 292:392, 1975.
37. Habel, R. E.: Applied Veterinary Anatomy. Ithaca, N. Y., R. E. Habel, 1975.
38. Holmes, D. F., and de Lahunta, A.: Experimental allergic neuritis in the dog and its comparison with the naturally occurring disease; Coonhound paralysis. Acta Neuropathol., 30:329, 1974.
39. Hussain, S., and Pettit, G. D.: Tendon transplantation to compensate for radial nerve paralysis. Am. J. Vet. Res., 28:336, 1967.
40. Knecht, C. D.: Radial-brachial paralysis. In Kirk, R. W., ed., Current Veterinary Therapy, V. Small Animal Practice. Philadelphia, W. B. Saunders Co., 1974, 658–662.
41. Knecht, C. D., and St. Claire, L. E.: The radial-brachial paralysis syndrome in the dog. J. Am. Vet. Med. Assoc., 154:653, 1969.
42. Kolb, L. C.: Congenital myotonia in goats. Bull. Johns Hopkins Hosp., 63:221, 1938.
43. Lee, A. F., and Bowen, J. M.: Evaluation of motor nerve conduction velocity in the dog. Am. J. Vet. Res., 31:1361, 1970.
44. Levin, M.: Paroxysmal hypertonia induced by affect: A symptom in man and animals. Arch. Neurol. Psychiatry, 32:1286, 1934.
45. Lorenz, M. D.: Episodic weakness in the dog. In Kirk, R. W., ed., Current Veterinary Therapy, V. Small Animal Practice. Philadelphia, W. B. Saunders Co., 1974, 648–652.
46. Lorenz, M. D., de Lahunta, A., and Almstrom, D. H.: Neostigmine-responsive weakness in the dog similar to myasthenia gravis. J. Am. Vet. Med. Assoc., 161:705, 1972.
47. Martens, R., Stewart, J., and Eicholtz, D.: Clinicopathologic Conference—University of Pennsylvania. J. Am. Vet. Med. Assoc., 156:478, 1970.
48. Merson, M. H., and Dowell, V. R., Jr.: Epidemiologic, clinical and laboratory aspects of wound botulism. N. Engl. J. Med., 289:1005, 1973.
49. Nicholson, S. S.: Bovine posterior paralysis due to organophosphate poisoning. J. Am. Vet. Med. Assoc., 165:280, 1974.
50. Norris, F. H.: The EMG. New York, Grune & Stratton, 1963.
51. Pallaske, G.: Zur Pathologie der chronischen Neuritis der Cauda Equina. Dtsch. Tieraerztl. Wochenschr., 73:415, 1966.

52. Palmer, A. C., and Barker, J.: Myasthenia in the dog. Vet. Rec., 95:452, 1974.
53. Prineas, J.: The pathogenesis of dying-back polyneuropathies. Part I. An ultrastructural study of experimental triorthocresylphosphate intoxication in the cat. J. Neuropathol. Exp. Neurol., 28:571, 1969.
54. Rooney, J. R.: Radial paralysis in the horse. Cor. Vet., 53:328, 1963.
55. Rooney, J. R., and Prickett, M. E.: The shaker foal syndrome. Mod. Vet. Pract., 48:44, 1967.
56. Sandefelt, E., Cummings, J. C., de Lahunta, A., Bjork, G., and Krook, L.: Hereditary neuronal abiotrophy in the Swedish Lapland dog. Cor. Vet., 63(Suppl. 3):1, 1973.
57. Scott, D. W., and de Lahunta, A.: Eosinophilic polymyositis in a dog. Cor. Vet., 64:47, 1974.
58. Simmons, G. C., and Tammemage, L.: Clostridium botulism type D as a cause of bovine botulism in Queensland. Aust. Vet. J., 40:123, 1964.
59. Stünzi, H., and Pohlenz, J.: Zur Pathologie der Neuritis Caudae Equinae beim Pferd. Schweiz. Arch. Tierheilkd., 116:533, 1974.
60. Swaim, S. F.: Peripheral nerve surgery in the dog. J. Am. Vet. Med. Assoc., 161:905, 1972.
61. Tryphonas, L., Hamilton, G. F., and Rhodes, C. S.: Perinatal femoral nerve degeneration and neurogenic atrophy of quadriceps femoris muscle in calves. J. Am. Vet. Med. Assoc., 164:801, 1974.
62. Tsairis, P., Dyck, P. J., and Mulder, D. W.: Natural history of brachial plexus neuropathy. Arch. Neurol., 27:109, 1972.
63. Vaughan, L. C.: Peripheral nerve injuries: An experimental study in cattle. Vet. Rec., 76:1293, 1964.
64. Wentink, G. H., Van der Linde-Sipman, J. S., Meijer, A. E. F. H., Kamphiusen, H. A. C., Van Vorsteinbosch, C. J. A. H. V., Hartman, W., and Hendricks, H. J.: Myopathy with a possible recessive X-linked inheritance in a litter of Irish terriers. Vet. Pathol., 9:328, 1972.
65. White, G. R., and Plaskett, J.: Nervous, stiff-legged or fainting goats. Am. Vet. Rev., 28:556, 1904.
66. Woods, C. B., and Lorenz, M. D.: Episodic weakness: A problem-oriented case study. J. Am. Anim. Hosp. Assoc., 11:473, 1975.
67. Worthman, R. P.: Demonstration of specific nerve paralyses in the dog. J. Am. Vet. Med. Assoc., 131:174, 1957.
68. Zaki, F., Prata, R. G., and Kay, W. J.: Necrotizing myelopathy in five Great Danes. J. Am. Vet. Med. Assoc., 165:1080, 1974.
69. Griffiths, I. R., and Duncan, I. D.: Some studies of the clinical neurophysiology of denervation in the dog. Res. Vet. Sci., 17:377, 1974.
70. Griffiths, I. R., Duncan, I. D., McQueen, A., Quirk, C., and Miller, R.: Neuromuscular disease in dogs: Some aspects of its investigation and diagnosis. J. Small Anim. Pract., 14:533, 1973.
71. Innes, J. R. M., and Saunders, L. Z.: Comparative Neuropathology. New York, Academic Press, 1962.
72. Lewis, R. M.: Systemic lupus erythematosus. In Kirk, R. W., ed., Current Veterinary Therapy, V: Small Animal Practice. Philadelphia, W. B. Saunders Co., 1974, 375–377.
73. Steinberg, S., and Botelho, S.: Myotonia in a horse. Science, 137:979, 1962.
74. Zaki, F., and Prata, R. G.: Necrotizing myelopathy secondary to embolization of herniated intervertebral disk material in the dog. J. Am. Vet. Med. Assoc., 169:222, 1976.
75. Wentink, G. H., Hartman, W., and Koeman, J. P.: Three cases of myotonia in a family of chows. Tijdschr. Diergeneeskd., 14:729, 1974.
76. Cooper, B. J.: Studies on the pathogenesis of tick paralysis. Ph.D. thesis, University of Sydney, Sydney, Australia, 1976.

Chapter 5

CRANIAL NERVE – LOWER MOTOR NEURON: GENERAL SOMATIC EFFERENT SYSTEM, SPECIAL VISCERAL EFFERENT SYSTEM

GENERAL SOMATIC EFFERENT – GSE
*CRANIAL NERVE XII – HYPOGLOSSAL
NEURONS*
Anatomy
Clinical Signs
*CRANIAL NERVE VI – ABDUCENT
NEURONS*
Anatomy
*CRANIAL NERVE IV – TROCHLEAR
NEURONS*
Anatomy
*CRANIAL NERVE III – OCULOMOTOR
NEURONS*
Anatomy
Function

Clinical Signs
SPECIAL VISCERAL EFFERENT – SVE
*CRANIAL NERVE V – TRIGEMINAL
NEURONS*
Clinical Signs
CRANIAL NERVE VII – FACIAL NEURONS
Clinical Signs
*CRANIAL NERVES IX, X, AND XI –
GLOSSOPHARYNGEAL, VAGUS, AND
ACCESSORY NEURONS*
Clinical Signs
DISEASES
*DIFFERENTIAL DIAGNOSIS OF
PHARYNGEAL PARALYSIS IN THE HORSE*

GENERAL SOMATIC EFFERENT – GSE

The cranial nerve general somatic efferent neurons innervate the striated voluntary musculature derived from occipital somites (tongue muscles) and head myotomes (extraocular muscles). They are found in cranial nerves III, IV, VI, and XII. As is the case with spinal nerves, this is not the only function of these cranial nerves. Cranial nerve III also contains general visceral efferent neurons, and all of these nerves contain sensory neurons, mostly of a proprioceptive nature.

The nuclei that contain the general somatic efferent neurons in the brain stem are located in an incomplete longitudinal column from caudal medulla to rostral midbrain. This column is adjacent to the midline ventral to the floor of the ventricular system. Except for cranial nerve IV, the nerves emerge from the brain stem in a longitudinal row near the ventral median plane (Fig. 5–1).

CRANIAL NERVE XII – HYPOGLOSSAL NEURONS
Anatomy

The general somatic efferent neuronal cell bodies are located in the hypoglossal nucleus in the medulla. The nucleus is adjacent to the midline and floor of

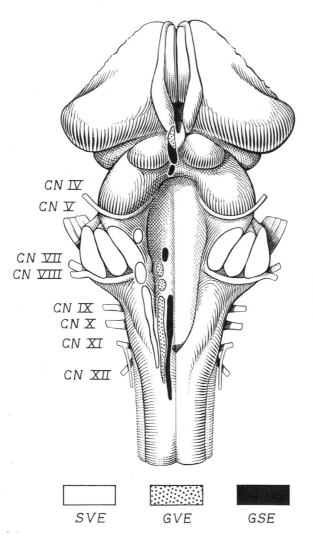

CN IV

CN V

CN VII
CN VIII

CN IX
CN X
CN XI

CN XII

SVE   GVE   GSE

Figure 5–1. Functional organization of cranial nerve nuclei in brain stem: special visceral efferent (SVE), general visceral efferent (GVE), general somatic efferent (GSE).

the fourth ventricle. It is a long nucleus (3 to 5 mm), extending from the obex caudally nearly to the level of the acoustic stria rostrally (Fig. 5–2).

The axons pass directly ventral and slightly lateral through the reticular formation across the lateral portion of the olivary nucleus. They emerge lateral to the pyramid as a longitudinal series of small roots. The row of hypoglossal roots merges at the small hypoglossal canal to form the hypoglossal nerve. The neurons course to the extrinsic tongue muscles (styloglossus, hyoglossus, and genioglossus), the intrinsic tongue muscles, and the geniohyoideus. The hypoglossal nerve is much smaller inside the cranial cavity than outside the skull. This is owing to the increase in myelination and connective tissue that occurs after the nerve emerges from the hypoglossal canal.

Clinical Signs

Lesions of any part of the neurons result in impairment of the function of the tongue in deglutition, prehension, mastication, and speech. With unilateral lesions the tongue, when protruded, deviates toward the side of the lesion. The normally functioning genioglossus and intrinsic muscles protrude the tongue toward the affected side. The weight of the atonic paralyzed half also contributes to this deviation. The animal may be observed to lick its lips only on the paralyzed side. The entire ipsilateral half of the tongue atrophies.

CRANIAL NERVE VI—ABDUCENT NEURONS

Anatomy

The general somatic efferent neuronal cell bodies are located in the abducent nucleus. This is a small nucleus located in the rostral medulla in the GSE neuron column at the level at which the caudal cerebellar peduncles merge with the cer-

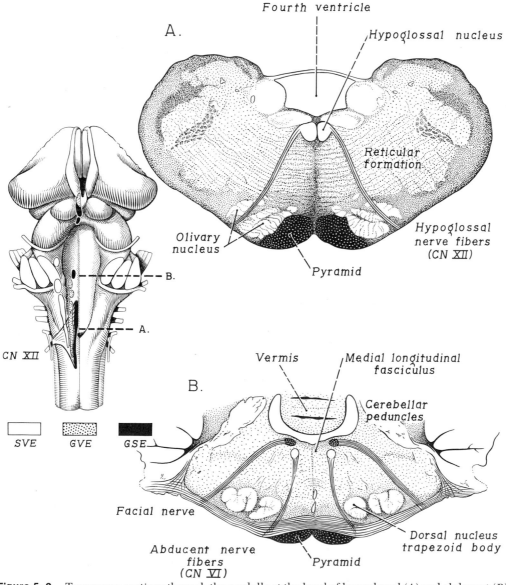

Figure 5–2. Transverse sections through the medulla at the level of hypoglossal (*A*) and abducent (*B*) nuclei.

ebellum. It is adjacent to the midline ventral to the floor of the fourth ventricle. The axons of the genu of the facial special visceral efferent neurons pass over this nucleus (Figs. 5–2, 5–6).

The axons of the cell bodies in the abducent nucleus flow directly ventrally through the reticular formation medial to the distinct dorsal nucleus of the trapezoid body, and emerge through the trapezoid body lateral to the pyramid. The abducent nerve leaves the cranial cavity through the orbital fissure, and within the periorbita innervates the lateral rectus and retractor bulbi muscles.

The clinical signs caused by lesions of these neurons will be discussed after the anatomy of all three cranial nerves to the extraocular muscles is considered.

CRANIAL NERVE IV—TROCHLEAR NEURONS

Anatomy

The general somatic efferent neuronal cell bodies are located in a small nucleus in the caudal mesencephalon at the level of the caudal colliculi. The nucleus is adjacent to the midline in the ventral part of the central grey substance that surrounds the mesencephalic aqueduct. It is caudal to the oculomotor nucleus, which is in the same functional column. The medial longitudinal fasciculus is medial and ventral to the trochlear nucleus (Fig. 5–3).

The axons course dorsally around the central grey substance and caudally to reach the rostral medullary velum between the two caudal colliculi. Here the axons cross to the opposite side and emerge from the velum caudal to the caudal colliculus, where they pass rostroventrally over the side of the mesencephalon to reach the floor of the cranial cavity. These axons leave the cranial cavity through the orbital fissure, and within the caudal periorbita innervate the dorsal oblique muscle.

CRANIAL NERVE III—OCULOMOTOR NEURONS

Anatomy

The general somatic efferent neuronal cell bodies are located in a nucleus in the rostral mesencephalon at the level of the rostral colliculus. The nucleus is adjacent to the midline within the ventral part of the central grey substance that surrounds the mesencephalic aqueduct. In primates this nucleus has been subdivided into the groups of neurons that innervate specific muscles. It extends caudally to the trochlear nucleus and rostrally to the level of the pretectal area. It is dorsal to the red nucleus. The medial longitudinal fasciculus is located ventral and medial to this nucleus. This longitudinal fasciculus serves to interconnect the general somatic efferent nuclei of the neurons innervating the extraocular muscles, and functions in their coordinated conjugate movements (Fig. 5–3).

The axons of the oculomotor neurons move ventrally through the reticular formation of the tegmentum medial to the red nucleus, substantia nigra, and crus cerebri. They emerge on the lateral side of the intercrural fossa and course rostrally lateral to the hypophysis and through the orbital fissure. Within the periorbita they innervate the dorsal and ventral recti, medial rectus, ventral oblique, and levator palpebrae muscles.

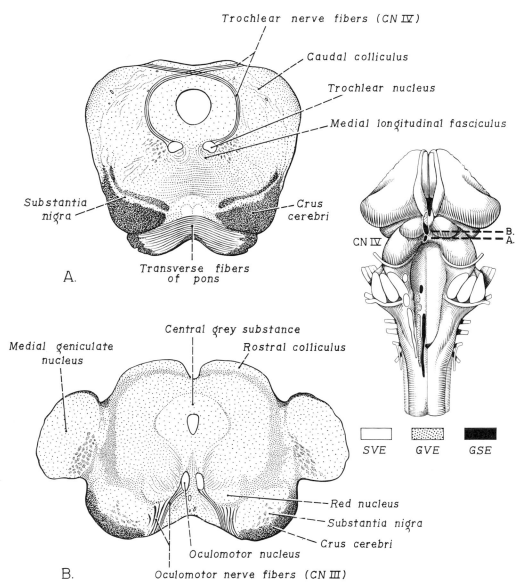

Figure 5–3. Transverse sections through the mesencephalon at level of trochlear (*A*) and oculomotor (*B*) nuclei.

Function

In order to understand the signs that result from lesions of one or more of the three cranial nerves that innervate the extraocular muscles, the normal action of the muscles on the eyeball must be understood. If the eyeball is assumed to have three axes for rotation, the muscles can be grouped into three opposing pairs. Around a horizontal axis through the center of the eyeball the dorsal rectus elevates the eyeball and the ventral rectus depresses it. Around a vertical axis through the center of the eyeball the medial rectus adducts and the lateral rectus abducts the eyeball. Around the anterior-posterior axis through the center of the eyeball the dorsal oblique intorts the eyeball or rotates the dorsal portion medioventrally toward the nose, and the ventral oblique extorts the eyeball or moves the same point lateroventrally away from the nose. These muscles do not function alone, but continually act together in a synergistic or antagonistic manner to provide for conjugate movement of both eyeballs in the same direction at the same time. This is exemplified most easily by the action of the medial and lateral recti in horizontal conjugate movement (Fig. 5–4).

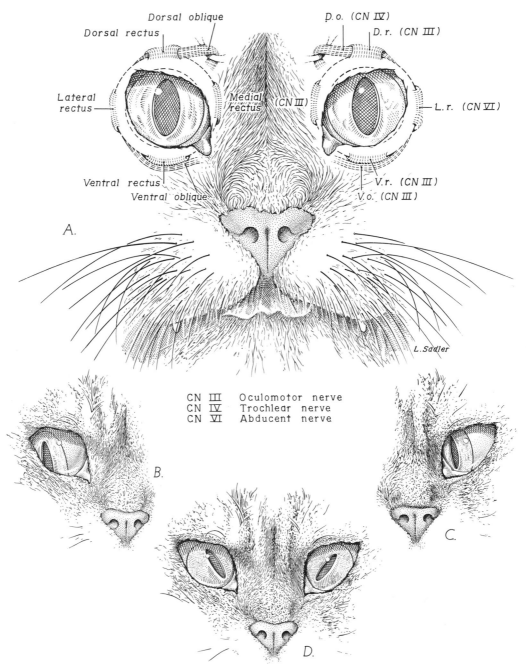

CN III   Oculomotor nerve
CN IV   Trochlear nerve
CN VI   Abducent nerve

Figure 5–4.   Functional anatomy of the extraocular muscles (A). Directions of strabismus following paralysis of the oculomotor (B), abducent (C), and trochlear (D) neurons.

When the eyeballs move conjugately to the right, this requires facilitation of abducent neurons to the lateral rectus of the right eyeball and inhibition to those of the left eyeball, simultaneous with facilitation of the oculomotor neurons to the medial rectus of the right eyeball and inhibition to those of the left eyeball. The medial longitudinal fasciculus functions in this coordinated activity.

The function of any one muscle at a specific time depends on the position of the eyeball. The functions of the extraocular muscles in domestic animals do not compare exactly with those in man because of anatomic differences in the position of the eyeball with respect to the muscle insertion. Discrepancies exist in the published descriptions of the normal and abnormal functions of the extraocular muscles in the dog because of the lack of experimental data for the dog and the reliance upon what is known in man.

Clinical Signs

Strabismus (Fig. 5–4).   Lesions of the abducent nucleus or nerve cause paralysis of the lateral rectus and retractor bulbi muscles. Paralysis of the lateral rectus results in a medial strabismus (squint), an abnormal position of that eyeball resulting in asymmetry. Compared to the normal eyeball, the affected eyeball cannot be abducted fully. This can be detected by moving the head from side to side in a horizontal plane and observing the degree of abduction and adduction of each eyeball.

Lesions of the trochlear nucleus or nerve paralyze the dorsal oblique muscle. In species with a round pupil, no strabismus may be observed; however, ophthalmoscopic examination may show the superior retinal vein deviated laterally from its normal vertical position because of the abnormal rotation caused by the tone in the unopposed ventral oblique muscle. In the calf with a horizontal pupil, the medial aspect of the pupil is deviated dorsally. This is referred to as dorsomedial strabismus, and is seen in ruminants with polioencephalomalacia. It is assumed to be caused by the effects of this disease on the trochlear nucleus.

Lesions of the oculomotor nucleus or nerve produce a lateral and ventral strabismus due to the paralysis of the extraocular muscles, and ptosis due to the paralysis of the levator palpebrae muscle. In addition, the loss of function of the general visceral efferent neurons which are also a component of this nerve results in a dilated pupil that is unresponsive to light stimulus. There is experimental evidence to support the direction of this strabismus, although it is difficult to explain the ventral deviation on the basis of the anatomy of the oblique muscles.

When a strabismus is suspected, the eyeball movements should be tested to verify the paralysis of the extraocular muscles. This can be done by directing the gaze of the patient in different positions, or by moving the head of the patient vertically or horizontally and watching for the symmetry of the eyeball movements. The vestibular and cervical proprioceptive systems exert considerable influence over the nuclei of the cranial nerves innervating extraocular muscles. Movements of the head require a simultaneous conjugate response by the eyeballs to maintain the normal plane of vision. One of the major pathways involved in connecting the vestibular system to these nuclei is the medial longitudinal fasciculus. Lesions of the vestibular system or medial longitudinal fasciculus may cause an abnormal position of an eyeball when the head is in certain positions. This appears as a strabismus, but usually can be corrected by repositioning the head. A general somatic efferent lower motor neuron strabismus persists in all positions of the head.

Normal Nystagmus. Nystagmus is an involuntary rhythmic movement of the eyeballs. It can be induced normally by slowly moving the head from side to side or up and down. Such head movement induces impulses in the vestibular component of the eighth cranial nerve from the stimulus to the receptors in the semicircular ducts. The afferent neuronal pathway that results in nystagmus continues through the vestibular nuclei in the medulla and via the medial longitudinal fasciculus to the brain stem nuclei, whose axons innervate the extraocular muscles. The efferent pathway involves the appropriate facilitation and inhibition of general somatic efferent neurons of cranial nerves III, IV, and VI to move the eyeballs.

This is tested best in domestic animals by slowly moving the head from side to side and observing the limbus to note the nystagmus. This form of nystagmus has a rapid phase in one direction and a slow phase in the opposite direction. The direction of the nystagmus is defined by the direction of the rapid phase.

This form of normal nystagmus is called vestibular nystagmus because it is induced by head movements that initiate activity in the vestibular system. The rapid phase or direction of the nystagmus is in the same direction as the movement of the head. Moving the head to the left causes a left nystagmus. Moving the head ventrally causes a ventral nystagmus. This only occurs as the head is being moved. Both eyeballs are affected similarly and move simultaneously, in conjugate fashion. It is abnormal if a nystagmus persists after the head movement is stopped. If the entire animal is rotated rapidly and then stopped, a brief normal postrotatory nystagmus occurs usually for less than 10 seconds. This nystagmus is opposite to the direction of the rotation. It is assumed that the slow movement is induced by the stimulation of the receptors in the vestibular system. The fast movement is a nonvestibular reflex resetting of the eyeball induced by a pontine reticular formation mechanism.

Lesions that destroy the vestibular system, the medial longitudinal fasciculus, or the neurons of cranial nerves III, IV, and VI cause a loss of normal vestibular nystagmus. In the neurologic evaluation of a patient following intracranial injury, it is important to distinguish between the signs of diffuse cerebral edema and those of brain stem contusion. A loss of the normal vestibular nystagmus indicates a severe lesion in the brain stem affecting the vestibular nuclei, or the medial longitudinal fasciculus, or both.

Observation of the eyeball response in normal vestibular nystagmus also allows evaluation of the function of specific extraocular muscles. In an animal with a right abducent nerve paralysis, there would be a medial strabismus of the right eyeball. In testing for normal vestibular nystagmus, the right eyeball would fail to abduct fully on moving the head to the right.

SPECIAL VISCERAL EFFERENT—SVE

The neurons of the special visceral efferent portion of the lower motor neuron innervate striated voluntary muscle derived from branchial arch mesoderm that is associated with visceral structures of the respiratory and digestive systems. These neurons are found in cranial nerves V, VII, IX, X, and XI. The muscles innervated include the muscles of mastication (V), facial muscles (VII), the muscles of the palate, pharynx, larynx, and esophagus, (IX, X, XI), and the cervical muscles (XI).

The nuclei that contain the SVE neurons in the brain stem are located in an incomplete longitudinal column in a ventrolateral position from the pons to the caudal medulla. In the embryo these are located ventral to the floor of the fourth ventricle between the general somatic efferent and general visceral efferent immature neurons. This SVE column migrates ventrolaterally to a position closer to its main source of afferent stimuli from the trigeminal system. This phenomenon is called neurobiotaxis. An additional special visceral efferent nucleus is located in the ventral grey column of the cervical spinal cord.

CRANIAL NERVE V—TRIGEMINAL NEURONS

The SVE neuronal cell bodies are located in the motor nucleus of the trigeminal nerve in the pons. The nucleus is found at the level of the rostral cerebellar peduncle in the lateral reticular formation, medial to the pontine sensory nucleus of the trigeminal nerve and dorsal to the dorsal nucleus of the trapezoid body. This nucleus lacks a distinct boundary (Fig. 5–5).

The axons pass laterally and slightly ventrally through the middle cerebellar peduncle to join the sensory neurons of the trigeminal nerve. Between the pons and the trigeminal canal these motor neurons often can be seen as a separate

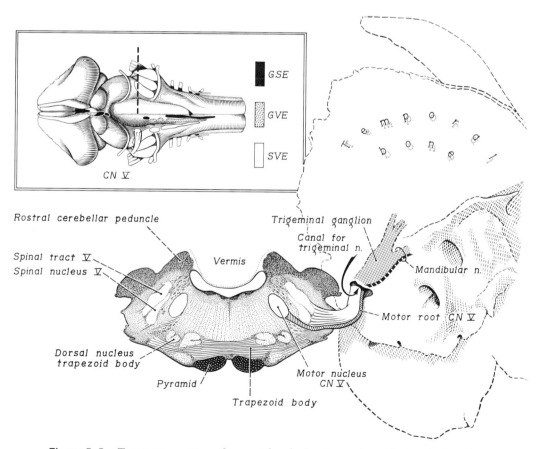

Figure 5–5. Transverse section of pons at level of motor nucleus of trigeminal nerve.

nerve (the motor root) on the medial aspect of the sensory part of the trigeminal nerve. These motor neurons pass through the trigeminal ganglion in the trigeminal canal of the petrosal bone, join the mandibular nerve, and pass through the oval foramen to be distributed to the muscles of mastication: masseter, temporal, pterygoids, rostral digastricus, and mylohyoid.

Clinical Signs

Bilateral disease of these motor neurons causes a dropped jaw that cannot be closed. There is difficulty prehending food or retaining it in the oral cavity. Manipulation of the jaw reveals the muscle atonia. Neurogenic atrophy follows if the paralysis persists. Unilateral disease may be difficult to discover until the muscle atrophy appears. The lower jaw may be directed toward the side of the lesion by the unopposed tone in the normal pterygoids and chewing may be asymmetric, but this is difficult to detect.

CRANIAL NERVE VII—FACIAL NEURONS

These special visceral efferent neuronal cell bodies are located in the facial nucleus in the medulla caudal to the trapezoid body and the level of attachment of the caudal cerebellar peduncle to the cerebellum. The nucleus is ventrolateral in the medulla midway between the pyramid and the spinal tract of the trigeminal nerve. It is caudal to the dorsal nucleus of the trapezoid body and rostral to the olivary nucleus (Fig. 5–6).

The axons pass dorsomedially to the midline of the floor of the fourth ventricle. Here they pass rostrally over the abducent nucleus in the genu of the facial nerve, then course ventrolaterally through the medulla medial to the spinal nucleus and tract of the trigeminal nerve and lateral to the dorsal nucleus of the trapezoid body. The axons emerge through the trapezoid body on the ventral side of the vestibulocochlear nerve. The facial nerve passes into the internal acoustic meatus of the petrosal bone on the dorsal side of the vestibulocochlear nerve. The facial nerve passes through the facial canal in the petrosal bone and emerges through the stylomastoid foramen. Branches of the facial nerve are distributed to the muscles of facial expression, that is, the muscles of the ear, eyelids, nose, cheeks, lips, and the caudal portion of the digastricus muscle.

Clinical Signs

Lesions of the nucleus or the nerve up to the level of its termination into the branches that supply the different muscle groups result in a complete facial paresis or paralysis, with inability to move these muscles normally. The paralysis can be seen in the asymmetric position of the ears, eyelids, lips, and nose. The ear may droop in those animals with a normally erect aural posture. If the ear cartilage is stiff, as in most cats and some dogs, it may keep the ear erect despite the muscular paralysis. The lip may droop on the affected side, allowing saliva to drip from the corner of the mouth. It is helpful to extend the head with a finger between the mandibles and examine the corner of the lips for asymmetry. On the paralyzed side more mucosa is exposed, and drooling may be apparent. The nose may be pulled toward the normal side owing to the unopposed nasal muscles. This

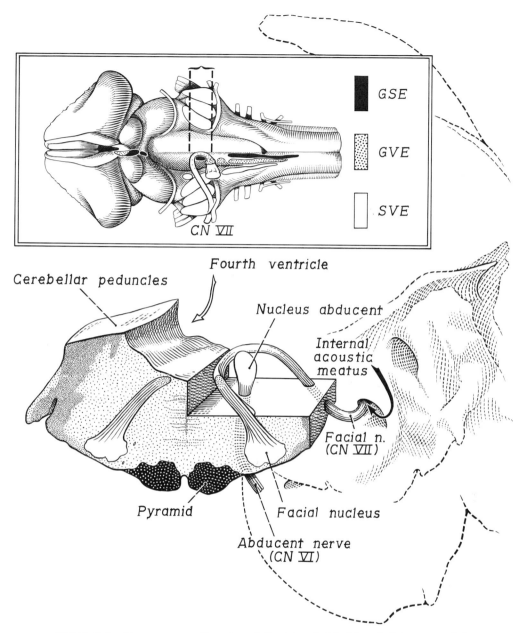

GSE

GVE

SVE

CN VII

Fourth ventricle

Cerebellar peduncles

Nucleus abducent

Internal acoustic meatus

Facial n. (CN VII)

Pyramid

Facial nucleus

Abducent nerve (CN VI)

Figure 5–6. Transverse section of medulla at level of facial and abducent nuclei.

deviation is remarkable in the horse. In the dog there is only a slight deviation of the philtrum from its normally vertical position. During inspiration the nostril may not be opened as wide as usual on the affected side. The palpebral fissure in small animals is often slightly wider than average and fails to close on stimulation of the cornea or eyelids (corneal and palpebral reflexes). In facial paresis this closure is weak. In large animals the loss of tone in the frontalis muscle which contributes fibers that elevate the dorsal eyelid causes slight ptosis. The eyelids of both sides should be palpated simultaneously for strength of closure in examining for asymmetry in cases of facial paresis.

Lesions of the individual branches of the facial nerve along their course to the muscles they innervate produce paresis or paralysis restricted to those muscle groups. Injury to the buccal branches of the facial nerve on the side of the masseter muscle causes the lips to droop and the nose to be pulled toward the normal side. This occurs in horses that are tabled for surgery for a prolonged period of time without proper padding of the head. Eyelid and ear function are normal. Injury to the auriculopalpebral nerve at the zygomatic arch only causes paresis of the ear and eyelid muscles.

Because of the close association of the facial and vestibulocochlear nerves, they often are affected simultaneously by the same lesion. This can happen in or on the medulla or in the petrosal bone.[2] It is important to distinguish between the two locations because of the difference in the therapy and prognosis. Both a medullary neoplasm and otitis media-interna can affect the function of these two cranial nerves. The former usually affects the function of other brain stem structures, which aids in the location of the lesion. These structures include the upper motor neuron, causing tetra- or hemiparesis; general proprioception, producing ataxia; ascending reticular activating system, resulting in signs ranging from depression to coma; and the abducent nucleus, bringing about medial strabismus.

CRANIAL NERVES IX, X, AND XI—GLOSSOPHARYNGEAL, VAGUS, AND ACCESSORY NEURONS

These three will be considered together because their special visceral efferent neuronal cell bodies are all located in one nucleus, nucleus ambiguus.[8] They are topographically organized, with the SVE neuronal cell bodies of the glossopharyngeal nerve the most rostral and those of the accessory nerve the most caudal. Nucleus ambiguus is an ill-defined column of neurons located ventrolateral in the medulla medial to the spinal tract and nucleus of the trigeminal nerve. It extends from the facial nucleus rostrally through the caudal medulla to a level slightly caudal to the obex. It is continued by the motor nucleus of the accessory nerve through the grey matter of the cervical spinal cord segments (Fig. 5–7).

The axons of the neuronal cell bodies in the rostral part of nucleus ambiguus arch slightly dorsally and ventrolaterally, to emerge with the general visceral efferent axons of the glossopharyngeal nerve along the lateral aspect of the medulla caudal to the vestibulocochlear nerve. The glossopharyngeal nerve traverses the jugular foramen and the occipitotympanic fissure. Its special visceral efferent axons innervate the stylopharyngeus and are distributed to other pharyngeal muscles by way of the pharyngeal plexus.

The axons of the SVE cell bodies in the middle portion of nucleus ambiguus take a similar course and emerge with the GVE axons of the vagus nerve on the lateral aspect of the medulla caudal to the glossopharyngeal roots.[11, 20] The SVE axons pass in the vagus nerve through the jugular foramen and occipitotympanic fissure. Some join the pharyngeal plexus with the glossopharyngeal neurons to innervate muscles of the palate and pharynx and cervical esophagus. Others leave the vagus in the cranial laryngeal nerve to innervate the cricothyroid muscle. The recurrent laryngeal nerve and its caudal laryngeal branch innervate all the other muscles of the larynx and cervical esophagus. In the cat and in man, these latter SVE axons have been determined to arise from the caudal portion of nucleus ambiguus, and they pass to the vagus by way of the cranial root of the accessory nerve. As the vagus nerve courses through the neck and thorax, branches supply the stri-

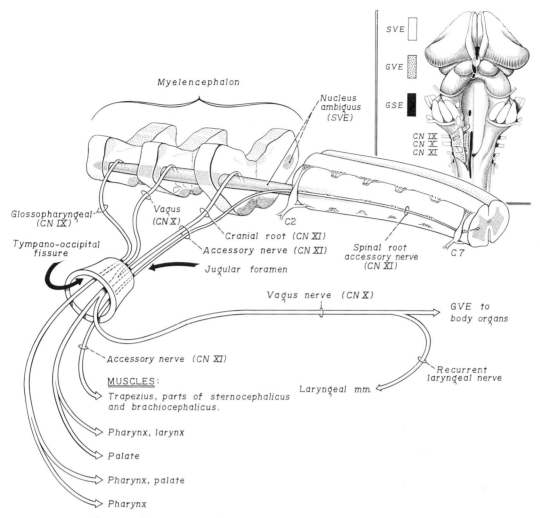

Figure 5–7. Schematic drawing of medulla with nucleus ambiguus and its efferent neurons and cervical spinal cord with spinal root of accessory nerve.

ated esophageal muscle. These branches presumably contain SVE neurons from nucleus ambiguus.

The axons of the SVE neuronal cell bodies in the caudal portion of nucleus ambiguus arch slightly dorsally and course ventrolaterally to emerge from the lateral aspect of the medulla with the GVE axons of the cranial root of the accessory nerve. These are caudal to the vagal SVE and GVE axons. They pass laterally and join the spinal root of the accessory nerve, which courses rostrally along the cervical spinal cord and medulla. For a short distance they form part of the accessory nerve as it enters the jugular foramen. As the accessory nerve traverses the jugular foramen and occipitotympanic fissure, the cranial root leaves the accessory nerve and joins the vagus nerve. The SVE axons of this cranial root are thought to innervate the muscles of the larynx and cervical esophagus by way of the recurrent laryngeal nerve branch of the vagus nerve.[24]

The SVE neuronal cell bodies of the spinal root of the accessory nerve are located in the motor nucleus of the accessory nerve in the lateral portion of the ventral grey column, from the first to sixth or seventh cervical spinal cord segments.

The axons pass laterally to emerge from the lateral side of the spinal cord, where they form a common bundle—the spinal root—which courses cranially dorsal to the denticulate ligament between the segmental dorsal and ventral rootlets. More SVE axons are added to it from each successive cervical segment. The spinal root passes rostrally through the foramen magnum into the cranial cavity. The cranial root joins with it temporarily as it passes through the jugular foramen. The accessory nerve emerging from the occipitotympanic fissure contains only its spinal root. These SVE axons innervate the trapezius and portions of the sternocephalicus and brachiocephalicus muscles.

Clinical Signs

Lesions of the rostral two thirds of nucleus ambiguus or the SVE axons in the glossopharyngeal and vagal nerves cause varying degrees of swallowing difficulty, referred to as dysphagia. With unilateral pharyngeal paralysis partial ability to swallow is retained, but choking, gagging, and loss of food through the nostrils occurs. With bilateral pharyngeal paralysis swallowing cannot be performed, and attempts are accompanied by choking and the appearance of food at the nostrils. The gag reflex is absent.

Lesions of the caudal nucleus ambiguus or the SVE axons in the cranial root of the accessory nerve, vagus nerve, recurrent or caudal laryngeal nerve result in paralysis of the laryngeal muscles.[14] Laryngeal hemiplegia is proposed to occur more frequently in mature, long-necked horses from constant stretching of the longer left recurrent laryngeal nerve.[17, 18] This causes an inspiratory dyspnea (roaring), owing to the failure of the left cricoarytenoideus dorsalis muscle to abduct the vocal fold and dilate the glottis. Similar inspiratory dyspnea generally is seen only in the dog with bilateral disease of the SVE neurons that innervate the laryngeal muscle.

DISEASES

The following are examples of diseases that affect one or more of the cranial nerve general somatic efferent and special visceral efferent lower motor neuron.

Neuromuscular Ending

BOTULISM. The toxin produced by *Clostridium botulinum* affects all the neuromuscular junctions of striated muscle, interfering with the release of acetylcholine. Multiple cranial nerve deficits accompany the generalized GSE spinal nerve deficit. Facial, hypoglossal, and pharyngeal paresis all occur. Extraocular muscle paresis often is not obvious to the examiner. Cattle probably are the most susceptible among domestic animals, and the dog the least susceptible. A more complete description of this disease can be found in Chapter 4.

MYASTHENIA GRAVIS. A clinical syndrome similar to this human disease has been reported in the dog. In this disease there is interference with neuromuscular transmission. This affects both the spinal nerve GSE neurons and the cranial nerve GSE and SVE neurons that elaborate acetylcholine at the neuromuscular junction.

Dysphagia and megaesophagus have been seen most commonly. Facial and hypoglossal paresis with abnormal prehension also have been found. A more complete description of this disease can be found in Chapter 4.

Peripheral Nerves. Peripheral nerves can be injured, involved in inflammatory or neoplastic lesions of adjacent tissue, or undergo degeneration from direct inflammation of the nerve (neuritis) or from metabolic disturbances (neuropathy).

1. A fractured hyoid bone could injure the hypoglossal nerve and cause ipsilateral paresis of the tongue.

2. Strenuous manipulation of the tongue has been reported to produce a temporary paralysis in horses and small dogs.

3. Laryngeal hemiplegia is the cause of the so-called "roarer horse." It is usually more profound on the left side and involves paralysis of all the muscles innervated by the left recurrent laryngeal nerve. Paralysis of the cricoarytenoideus dorsalis causes inability to abduct the vocal fold; on inspiration this interferes with the flow of air, creating an audible sound—roaring. Expiration takes place without an audible sound, since the vocal fold is moved aside passively by the air. The position of the laryngeal ventricle, with its opening cranial to the vocal fold, augments the inspiratory dyspnea.

Pathologic studies on the laryngeal muscles and recurrent laryngeal nerves have confirmed that the muscle lesions are caused by neurogenic atrophy.[9, 10] The most profound peripheral nerve lesions occur at the level of the larynx, with both myelin and axon degeneration.[4] More proximally, in the recurrent laryngeal nerve there is segmental demyelination and remyelination of normal-appearing axons. The cause is still obscure, but chronic stretching of the nerve at the thoracic inlet causing ischemia could interfere with axon flow and produce the most severe neuropathy distally at the larynx. Many subclinical cases have been observed.

Previous explanations have considered the greater intrathoracic course of the left recurrent laryngeal nerve, and therefore its exposure to the inflammatory diseases that affect the adjacent lymph nodes and pleura.[13]

The disease is reported to occur predominantly in the larger breeds or the larger individuals of the light horse breeds (15 to 17 hands).[17, 18] The following hypothesis has been suggested, and remains to be proved.[22, 23]

The left recurrent laryngeal nerve passes caudal to the aortic arch and is longer and further ventral from the vertebral column than the right recurrent laryngeal nerve, which passes around the costocervical artery of the right subclavian artery. If the center of rotation of the head and neck is considered to be the cervicothoracic junction, and both recurrent nerves are fixed cranially at the larynx and caudally at their respective arteries that they pass around, the right recurrent laryngeal nerve is closer to the center of rotation and is more congruent with the axis of the cervical vertebrae. Therefore, when the neck is extended or flexed to the right, greater tension is exerted on the left recurrent laryngeal nerve. Continual tension on this left nerve directly or on its blood supply causes the nerve to degenerate. This happens more commonly in large, mature horses with long necks and deep chests, because the left nerve is displaced further from the cervicothoracic junction and the vertebral axis and is more susceptible to tension in this position.

Laryngeal paresis has been noted in dogs with chronic polyneuritis. Excessive manipulation of the vagal nerves or their fibrosis subsequent to surgery for fenestration of cervical intervertebral disks may cause laryngeal paresis or paralysis and regurgitation due to thoracic esophageal malfunction.[14] In thyroidectomy the recurrent laryngeal nerve is often interrupted or fibrosed. The nerve passes cranially on the dorsal edge of this gland. Bilateral involvement causes laryngeal paralysis with episodes of gagging, cyanosis, and collapse.

    4. Guttural pouch mycosis: In horses, mycotic inflammation of the dorsal wall of the guttural pouch is the most common cause of dysphagia and epistaxis (nosebleed).[5, 6, 7, 16] This pouch is a sac-like ventral diverticulum of the auditory tube that is situated dorsal to the pharynx on each side, ventral to the cranium and atlas (Fig.

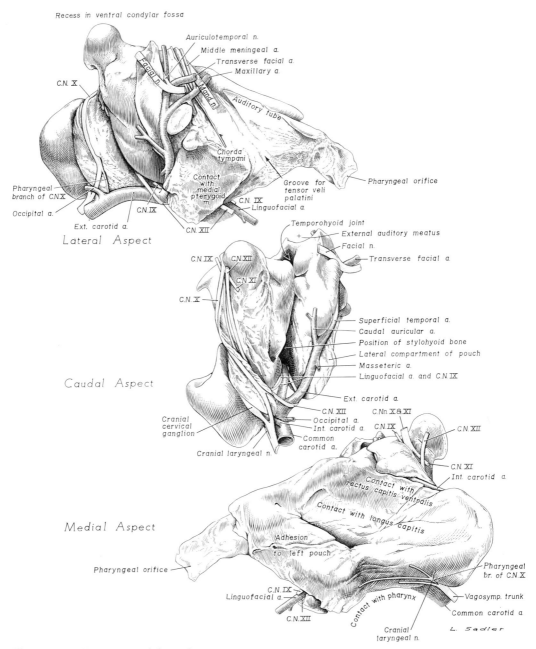

Figure 5–8. Dissection of the right guttural pouch of a horse with its associated cranial nerves and vessels. (From Habel, R. E.: Applied Veterinary Anatomy. Ithaca, N.Y., R. E. Habel, 1975.)

5–8). As they course to the pharyngeal muscles, the glossopharyngeal nerve and pharyngeal branch of the vagus nerve are associated closely with the caudodorsal and lateral walls of the medial compartment of the guttural pouch. Involvement of these nerves in the mycotic inflammation causes ipsilateral dysphagia. If the inflammation erodes the internal carotid artery, which also courses along the caudodorsal and mediodorsal walls of the medial compartment, bleeding occurs into the pouch and out the pharyngeal opening into the nasopharynx. This is the source of the epistaxis. The same lesion that affects the internal carotid artery may involve the associated internal carotid nerve, which consists of postganglionic sympathetic axons passing to structures in the head, including the contents of the orbit. Paralysis of the smooth muscle of the orbit results in Horner's syndrome. Extensive inflammation also can involve the adjacent facial nerve, producing facial paralysis, or the vagus nerve, producing laryngeal hemiplegia. It is hypothesized that the fungus, a species of *Aspergillus* that is normally a harmless contaminant of the guttural pouch, invades the tissues of the wall of the pouch when they are injured by trauma associated with the hyoid bone.

5. Neoplastic involvement of the nerves along their course can affect their function. These neoplasms can be external to the skull, involving only the peripheral nerves, or inside the cranial cavity, involving bone or meninges and the peripheral nerves flowing through them. Signs of involvement of the adjacent brain stem aid in locating the mass within the cranial cavity.

Meningioma of the meninges ventral to the medulla and mostly on the right side resulted in progressive partial hypoglossal paresis (XII), right-sided vestibular signs (VIII), paresis more on the right side of the body (right hemiparesis) with deficient postural reactions (upper motor neuron and general proprioception), and depression (ascending reticular activating system—ARAS) in a 9-year-old spaniel dog.

Osteogenic sarcoma of the right petrous temporal and basioccipital bone caused dysphagia in a 1-year-old German shepherd from involvement of the glossopharyngeal nerve and vagus nerve.

A carotid body neoplasm in a 9-year-old wire-haired fox terrier involved the hypoglossal nerve and produced an ipsilateral paresis of the tongue.[3]

A 4-year-old female Norwegian elkhound developed bilateral paralysis and atrophy of the muscles of mastication, complete inability to move the eyeballs, and blindness with dilated unresponsive pupils. This was caused by a diffuse meningioma in the middle and rostral cranial fossae that destroyed cranial nerves II, III, IV, V, and VI as they coursed to their appropriate foramina.

6. Otitis media in all species occasionally involves the facial nerve as it traverses the facial canal in the petrosal bone.[2] In its course through this canal, a portion of the nerve is separated from the cavity of the tympanic bulla (middle ear) only by a small amount of loose connective tissue. Paresis or paralysis is observed in the entire area of distribution of the facial nerve. These usually are associated with signs of vestibular ataxia caused by the disturbance of the vestibulocochlear nerve in the inner ear.

In rare cases of chronic otitis media, a hypersensitivity of the facial nerve has been reported which causes spasm of the facial muscles on the affected side.[12, 21] These signs are the opposite of those observed with paralysis, and include blepharospasm (eyelids), elevated wrinkled upper lip with caudal displacement of the angle of the mouth, elevation of the ear, and deviation of the nose to the affected side. This hemifacial spasm has been explained as an irritative affect of the lesion on the facial nerve as it passed through the facial canal. No pathologic studies were performed. In all three cases reported there was an ipsilateral Horner's syndrome but no signs of vestibular dysfunction.

One mature dog had episodes of hemifacial spasm and Horner's syndrome every 3 to 4 weeks following head trauma from an automobile that caused rupture of the ipsilateral tympanum.

Hemifacial spasm has been observed in dogs and man as a sequel to facial palsy or as an acute disturbance with no other neurologic deficits. A facial neuritis is presumed to be the cause of the signs. The lack of normal intervals between spasms in dogs has caused speculation that in those cases that follow facial palsy denervation contracture may be involved.

In man hemifacial spasm is reported with intramedullary neoplasms of the mesencephalon, pons, and medulla.[19] It is proposed that the lesion isolates the facial nuclear motoneurons from the upper motor neuron and inhibitory interneuronal activity. Mild hemifacial spasm was noted in a mature horse with a proliferative nonsuppurative focal encephalitis of the medulla thought to be caused by a protozoal agent.

7. Injury to the petrosal bone may cause hemorrhage in the middle and inner ears and bleeding from the external ear canal through a ruptured tympanum. This usually is associated with a fracture of the basioccipital or petrosal bone. Facial nerve function may be sacrificed, along with that of the vestibulocochlear nerve.

8. Facial paresis can accompany the signs of polyneuritis of coonhound paralysis, of brachial plexus neuritis, or of neuropathy. The signs are usually those of paresis, not paralysis.

9. Idiopathic facial paralysis occurs in the dog and the horse. The onset is generally sudden and the course variable. Recovery usually takes place in a few weeks. Complete recovery may never occur. There are no other signs of neurologic disease. Pathologic studies have not been performed. The inability to close the eyelids may lead to secondary corneal lesions from improper lubrication with lacrimal secretions. In man this is referred to as Bell's palsy and is postulated to be a facial neuritis. It is treated with corticosteroids.[1]

Unilateral or bilateral facial paresis or paralysis in dogs may be caused by a neuropathy associated with chronic hypothyroidism, or pituitary neoplasia, or both. Signs of peripheral vestibular disturbance often are associated with this. In experimental studies of hypothyroidism the signs of facial and vestibular nerve disturbance have resolved following thyroid hormone therapy. Results have been less remarkable in clinical cases.

In a few instances bilateral facial paralysis with unilateral or bilateral vestibular signs unrelated to hypothyroidism has resolved spontaneously. Steroid therapy has been used, but its efficacy is unknown. It is suspected that the lesion is a polyneuritis of cranial nerves VII and VIII.

10. Trigeminal neuritis: Bilateral paralysis of the muscles of mastication (motor V palsy) is found in dogs. There is a fairly sudden onset of inability to close the jaw, and it hangs loose with the mouth open. Food cannot be prehended. Swallowing is usually normal, although occasionally some dysphagia has been suspected. No deficit of sensory perception from the head has been observed. Recovery usually occurs in 2 to 3 weeks. The dog may have to be tube-fed during part of this time. Necropsy of one case revealed an extensive bilateral nonsuppurative neuritis of all portions of the trigeminal nerve and ganglion, but no involvement of the brain stem. Demyelination was more prominent than axonal degeneration. The cause is unknown. Recovery is assumed to follow remyelination.

11. Compression of the oculomotor nerve on the ventral surface of the cranial cavity in cases of extensive hydrocephalus involving the lateral ventricles may be

the cause of a ventrolateral strabismus. However, in most instances the apparent strabismus is due to the malformation of the orbits that accompanies the skull deformity.

Brain Stem Neurons. Disease of the brain stem can destroy the cell bodies or the intramedullary axons of these neurons.

1. Listeriosis is a bacterial disease of the brain caused by *Listeria monocytogenes*. It is seen primarily in ruminants and has a predilection for the brain stem, in which it produces foci of necrosis and inflammation. These usually consist of a mixture of mononuclear cells and foci of neutrophils in the parenchyma. Occasionally, it is entirely a mononuclear inflammation.

Multiple neurologic signs are produced that may include unilateral facial paresis or paralysis, abducent paralysis, trigeminal paralysis, especially the motor component, and pharyngeal paralysis. Signs of disturbance to consciousness (ARAS), circling (SP), and paresis to paralysis of the limbs (UMN) indicate that the lesion is confined to the central nervous system. Vestibular signs (SP) often accompany the lesion because of the involvement of the vestibular nuclei in the medulla. CSF is often abnormal, with changes characteristic of nonsuppurative disease despite the fact that this is a bacterial disease, often with many neutrophils in the lesion. (Example: a 2-year-old cow with 31 mononuclear cells per cmm and 79 mg of protein per dl.) The most common signs are facial paresis, head tilt and ataxia, paresis of limbs, and depression.

2. Rabies is caused by a virus that primarily destroys neuronal cell bodies. Although there are textbook descriptions of the furious and dumb forms of this disease, there is nothing typical about the way it presents. Involvement of the cell bodies of these lower motor neurons in the brain stem can cause deficits in their function. Pharyngeal paralysis (nucleus ambiguus) and paralysis of the muscles of mastication with a dropped jaw (motor nucleus of cranial nerve V) are the symptoms most commonly seen.

3. Focal protozoal encephalitis of the medulla of horses may produce signs similar to those of listeriosis in ruminants.

4. Leukoencephalomalacia occurs in horses that feed on moldy corn for an extended period of time. The lesion is primarily in the cerebral white matter, but all parts of the neuraxis can be affected by the necrosis and the edema. Pharyngeal paralysis often accompanies the signs of cerebral disturbance (lethargy, dementia, visual deficit, circling). This dysphagia actually may be caused by the acute disturbance of upper motor neuron control of the brain stem centers for swallowing.

5. Neoplasms of the brain stem may involve the intramedullary portion of these neurons. Other signs of brain stem involvement accompany the lower motor neuron.

6. In polioencephalomalacia in ruminants the only suggestion of cranial neuronal involvement is the strabismus, with the medial aspect of the eyeball deviated dorsally.[15] This is thought to be the result of a peculiar sensitivity of trochlear neurons to this degenerative metabolic disease.

DIFFERENTIAL DIAGNOSIS OF PHARYNGEAL PARALYSIS IN THE HORSE

Pharyngeal paresis or paralysis is a common clinical sign in the horse. The following is a differential diagnosis for this clinical deficit, in order of site of lesion.

Pharyngeal Muscles. There are no accompanying signs to suggest involvement of the brain. Myositis of pharyngeal muscles may be accompanied by myositis of the muscles of the tongue, mastication, or heart. Inflammation of heart muscles causes the patient's sudden demise. Muscle cell enzyme levels may be elevated in the serum.

Pharyngeal Nerves (Glossopharyngeal and Vagus Nerves). There are no accompanying signs to suggest involvement of the brain. Pathogenesis is as follows:

1. Guttural pouch mycosis may lead to pharyngeal hemiplegia, laryngeal hemiplegia, or both, accompanied by an epistaxis. Visual examination of the interior of the pouch may be diagnostic.

2. Polyneuritis with pharyngeal, laryngeal, facial, and hypoglossal nerve involvement may accompany a neuritis of the cauda equina. The latter causes lower motor neuron paresis or paralysis of the tail, anus, bladder, and rectum, with hypalgesia or analgesia of the same areas. Pelvic limb function may be abnormal.

3. In botulism, the dysphagia is associated with other signs of the lower motor neuron–neuromuscular ending dysfunction of cranial and spinal nerves. It is helpful for diagnosis if more than one animal is affected.

4. Polyneuropathy with pharyngeal and laryngeal nerve involvement occurs in chronic lead poisoning.

Nucleus Ambiguus or the Swallowing Center in the Medulla. Pharyngeal paralysis is accompanied by other signs of a focal (medullary) or diffuse (brain stem–cerebral) lesion. Pathogenesis is as follows:

1. Suppurative meningitis around the brain stem or a focal abscess in this area.

2. Encephalitis: rabies, equine viral encephalitides (VEE, EEE, WEE), or protozoal encephalitis.

3. Encephalomalacia: moldy corn poisoning.

4. Acute liver necrosis or chronic liver necrosis in the advanced stages, with encephalopathy.

Pharyngeal paralysis frequently accompanies severe cerebral disease without a specific lesion of the nucleus ambiguus or swallowing center, suggesting that higher centers are involved in this function. This is referred to as a pseudobulbar palsy, for there is no specific lesion in the nuclei in the medulla (bulb). The lesion has destroyed the neurons in the cerebrum that influence the activity of the medullary nuclei, and dysphagia results.

REFERENCES

1. Adoor, K. K., Wingerd, J., Bell, D. N., Manning, J. J., and Hurley, J. P.: Prednisone treatment for idiopathic facial paralysis (Bell's palsy). N. Engl. J. Med., 287:1268, 1972.
2. Blauch, B., and Strafuss, A. C.: Histologic relationships of the facial (7th) and vestibulocochlear (8th) cranial nerves within the petrous temporal bone in the dog. Am. J. Vet. Res., 35:481, 1974.
3. Chrisman, C. L.: Electromyography in the localization of spinal cord and nerve root neoplasia in dogs and cats. J. Am. Vet. Med. Assoc., 166:1074, 1975.
4. Cole, C. R.: Changes in the equine larynx associated with laryngeal hemiplegia. Am. J. Vet. Res., 7:69, 1946.
5. Cook, W. R.: The clinical features of guttural pouch mycosis in the horse. Vet. Rec., 83:336, 1968.
6. Cook, W. R.: Observations on the etiology of epistaxis and cranial nerve paralysis in the horse. Vet. Rec., 78:396, 1966.
7. Cook, W. R., Campbell, R. S. F., and Dawson, C.: The pathology and etiology of guttural pouch mycosis in the horse. Vet. Rec., 83:422, 1968.

8. Dubois, F. S., and Foley, J. O.: Experimental studies on vagus and spinal accessory nerves in the cat. Anat. Rec., 64:285, 1936.
9. Duncan, I. D., and Griffiths, I. R.: Pathological changes in equine laryngeal muscles and nerves. Proc. Am. Assoc. Equine Pract., 19:97, 1973.
10. Duncan, I. D., Griffiths, I. R., McQueen, A., and Baker, G. O.: The pathology of equine laryngeal hemiplegia. Acta Neuropathol., 27:337, 1974.
11. Flieger, S.: The nerve centers of the nervus laryngicus cranialis and caudalis and their participation in the innervation of the larynx. Polskie Archiwum Weterynaryjne, 14:467, 1971.
12. Fox, M. W.: A canine neuropathy resembling facial hemiatrophy and spasms in man. Mod. Vet. Pract., 44:64, 1963.
13. Habel, R. E.: Applied Veterinary Anatomy. Ithaca, N.Y., R. E. Habel, 1975.
14. Higgs, B., and Ellis, F. H., Jr.: The effect of bilateral supranodosal vagotomy on canine esophageal function. Surgery, 58:828, 1965.
15. Howard, J. R.: Neurological examination of cattle. Scope, 13:2, 1968.
16. Leemann, W., and Seiferle, E.: Mykosen des Luftsackes beim Pferd. Schweiz. Arch. Tierheilk., 112:627, 1970.
17. Marks, D., Mackey-Smith, M. P., Cushing, L. S., and Leslie, J. A.: Etiology and diagnosis of laryngeal hemiplegia in horses. J. Am. Vet. Med. Assoc., 157:429, 1970.
18. Marks, D., Mackey-Smith, M. P., Cushing, L. S., and Leslie, J. A.: Observations on laryngeal hemiplegia in the horse and treatment by abductor muscle prosthesis. Equine Vet. J., 2:159, 1970.
19. O'Connor, P. J., Parry, C. B., and Davies, R.: Continuous muscle spasm in intramedullary tumors of the neuraxis. J. Neurol. Neurosurg. Psychiatry, 29:310, 1966.
20. Rethi, A.: Histological analysis of the experimental degenerated vagus nerve. Acta Morphol. (Budapest), 1:221, 1951.
21. Roberts, S. A., and Vainisi, S. J.: Hemifacial spasm in dogs. J. Am. Vet. Med. Assoc., 150:381, 1967.
22. Rooney, J. R.: Autopsy of the Horse. Baltimore, Md., Williams & Wilkins, 1970.
23. Rooney, J. R., and Delaney, F. M.: Laryngeal hemiplegia in horses, a theoretical analysis. Proc. AAEP, 15:13, 1969.
24. Watson, A. G.: Some aspects of the vagal innervation of the canine esophagus. An anatomical study. M. S. thesis, Massey University, New Zealand, 1974.

Chapter 6

LOWER MOTOR NEURON—GENERAL VISCERAL EFFERENT SYSTEM

CONTROL OF PUPILS
SYMPATHETIC GVE LOWER MOTOR NEU-RON INNERVATION OF THE EYEBALL
Clinical Signs
Diseases
PARASYMPATHETIC GVE LOWER MOTOR NEURON INNERVATION OF THE EYEBALL (CRANIAL NERVE III — OCULOMOTOR NEURONS)
Clinical Signs
Diseases Associated with Anisocoria
Pupils in Acute Brain Disease

Protrusion of the Third Eyelid
SACRAL PARASYMPATHETIC GVE LOWER MOTOR NEURON
CONTROL OF MICTURITION
Diseases
PARASYMPATHETIC GVE LOWER MOTOR NEURON OF THE MEDULLA (CRANIAL NERVES VII, IX, X, AND XI-FACIAL, GLOSSOPHARYNGEAL, VAGUS, AND ACCESSORY NEURONS)

This group of lower motor neurons innervates the smooth muscle associated with blood vessels and visceral structures, glands, and cardiac muscle. It is an involuntary system and represents the lower motor neuron for the autonomic nervous system. The autonomic nervous system is a physiologic and anatomic system with central and peripheral components. It includes higher centers situated in the hypothalamus, midbrain, pons, and medulla. The hypothalamus is the primary integrating center for the autonomic nervous system. Nuclei in its rostral portion subserve the parasympathetic division of the general visceral efferent lower motor neuron, whereas the nuclei in its caudal portion subserve the sympathetic division of the general visceral efferent lower motor neuron. These hypothalamic nuclei receive afferents from the cerebrum by way of numerous pathways, from thalamic nuclei, and from ascending general visceral afferent (GVA) pathways. The hypothalamus influences the activity of the metabolic centers in the reticular formation of the midbrain, pons, and medulla. These centers influence visceral smooth muscle, cardiac muscle, and glandular activity by means of the general visceral efferent lower motor neuron located in specific cranial and spinal nerves. This autonomic nervous system is concerned with emergency mechanisms and the repair and preservation of a constant internal environment. The concept of maintaining a steady state in the internal environment for continuous efficient function of the body is referred to as homeostasis. The peripheral part of the autonomic nervous system includes the sensory neurons from the body viscera, the GVA system, and a lower motor neuron, the GVE system.

The GVE lower motor neuron is composed of two neurons interposed between the central nervous system and the organ innervated. The first neuron has its cell body located in the grey matter of the CNS, and its axon courses through a cranial or spinal nerve to a peripheral ganglion, where it synapses with the cell body of the second neuron. The first neuron with its telodendron in a peripheral ganglion is called the preganglionic neuron. The second neuron has its cell body and dendritic zone in a peripheral ganglion and its axon, the postganglionic axon, terminates in the structure to be innervated.

The GVE system is grouped into two divisions physiologically and anatomically. The sympathetic system, the thoracolumbar system, has the cell bodies of the preganglionic neuron located in the intermediate grey column of the spinal cord from approximately the first thoracic to fifth lumbar spinal cord segment. With a few exceptions, the neurotransmitter elaborated at the telodendron of this postganglionic axon is norepinephrine. The parasympathetic system, the craniosacral system, has the cell bodies of the preganglionic neuron located in the sacral segments of the spinal cord and in nuclei of the brain stem associated with cranial nerves III, VII, IX, X, and XI. Acetylcholine is the neurotransmitter released at the telodendron of the postganglionic axon.

CONTROL OF PUPILS

In clinical neurology knowledge of this GVE system is important in the understanding of pupillary size and responsiveness to light and excitement. The parasympathetic GVE innervation of the eyeball responds to the afferent modality of light, whereas the sympathetic GVE innervation is stimulated by the factors that elicit excitement, fear, or anger.

SYMPATHETIC GVE LOWER MOTOR NEURON INNERVATION OF THE EYEBALL

The preganglionic cell bodies are located in the intermediate grey column of the first three or four segments of the thoracic spinal cord. The axons pass through the ventral grey column and adjacent white matter to join the ventral roots of these segments and the proximal portion of the segmental spinal nerve. Before the spinal nerve branches, these preganglionic axons leave the spinal nerve in the segmental ramus communicantes, which joins the thoracic sympathetic trunk inside the thorax ventrolateral to the vertebral column. The axons usually pass cranially without synapse in a trunk ganglion. They pass through the cervicothoracic and middle cervical ganglia and course cranially in the cervical sympathetic trunk, where the latter is part of the vagosympathetic trunk. Medial to the origin of the digastricus muscle and ventromedial to the tympanic bulla, the cervical sympathetic trunk separates from the vagus and terminates in the cranial cervical ganglion, where the preganglionic axons synapse. The cell body of the postganglionic axon is in the cranial cervical ganglion. The axons for ocular innervation in the cat and dog course rostrally through the tympanooccipital fissure with the internal carotid artery, and pass between the tympanic bulla and the petrosal bone into the middle ear cavity, closely associated with the ventral surface of the petrosal bone.[2] The axons continue rostrally between the petrosal bone and

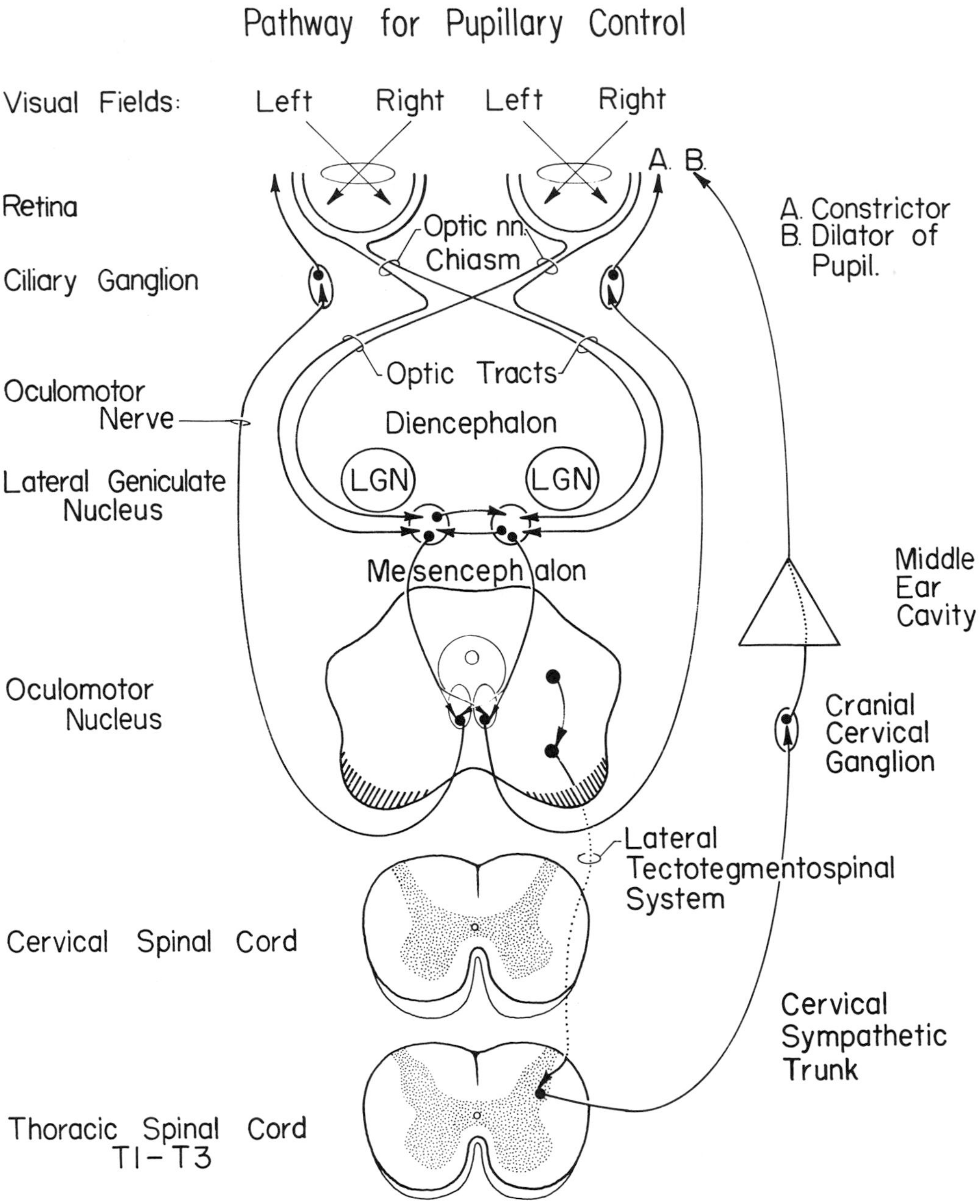

Figure 6–1.   Neuroanatomic pathway for pupillary control.

the basisphenoid to join the ventral surface of the trigeminal ganglion and the ophthalmic nerve. The ophthalmic nerve enters the periorbita through the orbital fissure. The postganglionic sympathetic axons are distributed by way of ophthalmic nerve branches to the smooth muscle of the periorbita, the eyelids, including the third eyelid, and the iris muscles, particularly the dilator of the pupil.[1, 25, 27] In large animals most of these axons follow the internal carotid artery in the internal carotid nerve and reach the orbital smooth muscle by way of its blood vessels.

Normal tone in these muscles keeps the eyeball protruded, the palpebral fissure widened, the third eyelid retracted, and the pupil partially dilated.

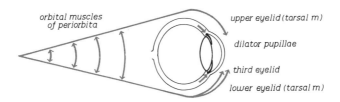

Clinical Signs

Loss of this innervation causes a lack of tone in the periorbital smooth muscle so that the eyeball retracts slightly, producing enophthalmos. Loss of tone in the eyelid muscle results in slight narrowing of the palpebral fissure. Lack of retraction of the third eyelid makes it protrude, and lack of pupillary dilation in response to painful stimuli or stress causes the pupil at rest to be smaller than the opposite normal pupil. A small pupil is referred to as miosis. Changes in the amount of light stimulating the retina alter the size of the pupil by the activation of the pupillary constrictor muscle. In the absence of light a small amount of dilation occurs in the pupil that is miotic from lack of sympathetic innervation. These signs are referred to as Horner's syndrome, and are associated with lesions in any portion of this lower motor neuron pathway from the cranial thoracic spinal cord segments to the orbit.

In addition to these signs of denervation of orbital smooth muscle, peripheral vasodilation takes place and may cause increased warmth, a pink color to the skin that may be observed best in the ear, and congestion of the nasal mucosa on the side of the lesion.

Pre- or postganglionic destruction of the sympathetic innervation of the head of horses is followed immediately by profuse sweating of the ipsilateral half of the face and cranial neck.[24, 28] The same area is hyperthermic and the nasal and conjunctival mucosae are congested. The hyperthermia can best be determined by palpation of the ears. There is a prominent ptosis of the upper eyelid, but only a slight third eyelid protrusion and slight miosis. In cattle, sheep, and goats[28] the most constant signs are the hyperthermia detected on ear palpation and the upper eyelid ptosis. The miosis and third eyelid protrusion are subtle. In cattle there is less sweating visible on the surface of the nose on the denervated side.

Some examples of lesions that disturb this GVE lower motor neuron system follow.

Diseases

1. Injury, infarction, or neoplastic involvement of the cranial thoracic spinal cord causes signs of paresis or paralysis of the pelvic limbs and mild deficits in the thoracic limbs, in addition to ipsilateral Horner's syndrome.

2. Avulsion of the roots of the brachial plexus in dogs and cats commonly results from automobile accidents. The finding of Horner's syndrome on the same side as the paralyzed thoracic limb indicates that the injury to the nerves innervating the thoracic limb is at the level of the vertebral column.

3. Thoracic inlet or cranial mediastinal lesions such as lymphosarcoma that involve the cranial thoracic sympathetic trunk, or caudal cervical sympathetic trunk, or both, may lead to Horner's syndrome.[10]

4. Injury to the cervical sympathetic trunk from a dog bite or from the surgical exposure of the cervical intervertebral disks may result in an ipsilateral Horner's syndrome that usually is transient. Neoplastic involvement of the cervical sympathetic trunk along its course is another cause. Thyroid adenocarcinoma is the most common cause.

5. Mycosis of the guttural pouch in horses may involve the cranial cervical ganglion or internal carotid nerve and produce Horner's syndrome.

6. Otitis media may produce Horner's syndrome, often accompanied by signs of peripheral vestibular disturbance, or facial paresis, or both.

7. Retrobulbar injury, neoplasia, or abscess may cause this syndrome.

The sympathetic GVE lower motor neuron is influenced by pathways descending from the higher centers of the autonomic nervous system in the brain stem. In man such a pathway is described that affects the sympathetic GVE innervation of these orbital smooth muscles. This pathway begins in the rostral colliculus and tegmentum of the midbrain, where it is influenced by the hypothalamus. It descends through the lateral pons, medulla, and lateral funiculus of the cervical spinal cord to the cranial thoracic spinal cord segments, where it synapses in the grey matter, influencing the activity of the cell bodies in the intermediate grey column. This is called the lateral tectotegmentospinal system. Pain stimuli or emotional responses that cause pupillary dilation do so by activating the sympathetic GVE of the cranial thoracic spinal cord by way of the lateral tectotegmentospinal system. This system is activated by ascending spinotectal and spinothalamic (pain) pathways, or direct corticotectal pathways, or both, or indirectly by corticohypothalamic pathways and the dorsal longitudinal fasciculus from the hypothalamus to the tectum.

In man lesions in any part of the lateral tectotegmentospinal system cause a miotic pupil on the affected side that does not respond to stress stimuli, but passively dilates a small amount in response to the reduction of light. In domestic animals lesions in the cervical spinal cord do not affect this system as often to produce Horner's syndrome. It has been observed only for a short period (24 to 48 hours) following severe acute trauma to the spinal cord bilaterally that produced tetraplegia and respiratory embarrassment. Unilateral infarction of the cervical spinal cord lateral funiculus from fibrocartilaginous emboli may cause a persistent Horner's syndrome, along with hemiplegia.[8, 12]

Denervation hypersensitivity is a phenomenon peculiar to smooth muscle innervated by the general visceral efferent system. This involves increased sensitivity of the muscle to circulating neurotransmitters, and is especially evident in smooth muscle innervated by sympathetic neurons when the postganglionic axon is affected. Such denervated muscle shows hypersensitivity to the application of epinephrine or to circulating epinephrine released during emotional excitement. This phenomenon has been studied in the dog with lesions of the sympathetic innervation of the ocular smooth muscles.[3] Greater hypersensitivity is present with

TABLE 6-1. HORNER'S SYNDROME—SUMMARY OF LESIONS

Location	Lesion	Associated Neurologic Deficit
Cervical spinal cord	External injury Focal Leukomyelomalacia (ischemic)	Tetraplegia—spastic Hemiplegia–Ipsilateral, spastic
T1–T3 spinal cord	External injury Neoplasm Focal poliomyelomalacia (ischemic)	Pelvic and thoracic limb paresis or paralysis with lower motor neuron deficit in thoracic limbs and upper motor neuron deficit in pelvic limbs
	Diffuse myelomalacia (ascending and descending)	Lower motor neuron deficit and analgesia of tail, anus, pelvic limbs, abdomen, and thorax with paretic thoracic limbs
T1–T3 ventral roots Proximal spinal nerves	Avulsion of roots of brachial plexus	Brachial plexus paresis or paralysis of the thoracic limb on the same side
Cranial thoracic sympathetic trunk	Lymphosarcoma Neurofibroma	None if confined to the trunk
Cervical sympathetic trunk	Injury from surgical intervention in the area, or from dog bites Neoplasm (thyroid adenocarcinoma)	None if unilateral. Bilateral lesions interfere with laryngeal and esophageal function because of vagal involvement
Middle ear cavity	Otitis media	Signs of peripheral vestibular disturbance: ipsilateral ataxia, head tilt, nystagmus, and sometimes facial palsy, or hemifacial spasm
Retrobulbar	Contusion Neoplasia	Varies with degree of contusion to the optic and oculomotor nerves, which also influences pupillary size

lesions of the postganglionic axons or their cell bodies than with lesions of the preganglionic neurons. Intraocular application of 0.1 cc of 0.001 per cent epinephrine causes pupillary dilation in 20 minutes with lesions of the postganglionic axons or their cell bodies, and in 30 to 40 minutes with lesions of the preganglionic neurons. This test may be useful to determine the location of the lesion responsible for Horner's syndrome.

PARASYMPATHETIC GVE LOWER MOTOR NEURON INNERVATION OF THE EYEBALL (CRANIAL NERVE III— OCULOMOTOR NEURONS)

The cell bodies are located in the parasympathetic oculomotor nucleus rostral to the general somatic efferent component of this nucleus at the level of the rostral part of the rostral colliculus and pretectal area. This portion of the oculomotor nucleus is called the Edinger-Westphal nucleus in man, and is located in the ventral part of the central grey substance next to the midline ventral to the rostral part of the mesencephalic aqueduct. The axons course ventrally with the general somatic efferent axons, and leave the mesencephalon medial to the crus cerebri in the lateral part of the intercrural fossa. The general visceral efferent axons in the canine oculomotor nerve are located superficially on the medial side of the nerve, where they are especially susceptible to disturbance caused by compression of the nerve from midbrain swelling or displacement.[19] The nerve passes through the orbital fissure into the periorbita. At the rostral end of the oculomotor nerve, ventral to the optic nerve, the ciliary ganglion is located. The preganglionic general visceral efferent axons of the oculomotor nerve synapse here with the dendritic zone and cell bodies of the postganglionic axons. The postganglionic axons pass by way of short ciliary nerves along the optic nerve to the eyeball to innervate primarily the ciliary muscle and the constrictor of the pupil.

This system is sensitive to the amount of light received by the retinas of each eyeball. In diminished light its activity is decreased and the pupils dilate. In bright light the system is activated and pupillary constriction (miosis) occurs.

The function of this GVE lower motor neuron can be tested by the pupillary light reflex. Stimulation of the retina of one eyeball with a bright source of light causes constriction of the pupils of both eyeballs. The constriction in the eyeball being stimulated is the direct response. That in the opposite eyeball is the indirect or consensual response. The afferent pathway to the parasympathetic oculomotor nucleus is through the optic nerve to the optic chiasm, where some crossing occurs, through both optic tracts, over the lateral geniculate nuclei without synapse, and ventrally into the region between the thalamus and the rostral colliculus called the pretectal area. Synapse takes place in the pretectal nuclei. Crossing occurs between the pretectal nuclei by way of the caudal commissure. Axons of the pretectal cell bodies course to the parasympathetic oculomotor nucleus of both sides, activating these preganglionic neurons, which causes the bilateral pupillary constriction.

Clinical Signs

Lesions restricted to the visual pathways in the cerebral hemispheres can cause blindness, but pupillary responses remain normal. With a lesion in the right GVE oculomotor neuron the right pupil is dilated widely (mydriasis), and stimulation with light in either eyeball only induces constriction in the left eyeball. A lesion in the right optic nerve causes the pupil to be partially dilated on that side. Stimulation with light in the left eyeball induces constriction of both pupils. Light stimulation of the right eyeball produces no change in either pupil because of the interference with the sensory limb of the reflex at the level of the optic nerve. When evaluating the pupillary light reflex, a strong light source should be directed at the lateral aspect of the retina at the site of the area centralis, and the patient should be as relaxed as possible. Circulating epinephrine may interfere with the rapidity and degree of the response.

Complete oculomotor nerve dysfunction should cause a widely dilated pupil that is unresponsive to light directed into either eyeball (general visceral efferent deficit) and a lateral and ventral strabismus (general somatic efferent deficit).

Diseases Associated with Anisocoria

Anisocoria is the occurrence of unequal or asymmetric pupils. Some of the causes include the following:

1. A unilateral oculomotor nerve lesion produces ipsilateral severe mydriasis, unresponsive to light directed into either eyeball.

2. A unilateral lesion of GVE sympathetic innervation of the pupil causes ipsilateral miosis that dilates slightly in reduced light.

3. Unilateral ocular disorders causing pain, such as keratitis, cause activation of the oculopupillary reflex (V–III) and ipsilateral miosis.

4. Unilateral severe retinal or optic nerve lesions may result in partial ipsilateral mydriasis that only responds to light directed into the opposite eyeball. No miosis occurs in either eyeball from light directed into the affected eyeball.

5. Iritis causes ipsilateral miosis.

6. Iris degeneration with atrophy brings about ipsilateral mydriasis with a variable response to light, sometimes none. It is more common in older dogs.

7. Glaucoma is increased intraocular pressure created by abnormal circulation of aqueous. It may cause ipsilateral mydriasis that is unresponsive to light.

Pupils in Acute Brain Disease

Pupillary abnormalities are common following intracranial trauma, and often accompany severe acute brain lesions such as polioencephalomalacia or lead poisoning in ruminants. These may not necessarily reflect destruction of the general visceral efferent oculomotor neurons, or the origin of the lateral tectotegmentospinal system. Severe bilateral miosis is a sign of acute extensive brain disturbance that in itself is not necessarily of any localizing value. The return of the pupils to normal size and response to light is a favorable prognostic sign and indicates recovery from the brain disturbance, especially following trauma. In cases of trauma, progression from bilaterally miotic to bilaterally mydriatic fixed pupils unresponsive to light indicates that the brain disturbance is advancing and the general visceral efferent oculomotor neurons associated with the midbrain are nonfunctional. This often accompanies severe contusion of the midbrain with hemorrhage, usually along the midline. This may follow brain swelling and herniation of the occipital lobes ventral to the tentorium cerebelli accompanied by compression and displacement of the midbrain, or oculomotor nerve, or both.

The cause of unilateral or bilateral miotic pupils in acute brain disease is not understood clearly. It probably represents facilitation of the oculomotor general visceral efferent neurons that have been released from higher center (prosencephalon) inhibition owing to its functional disturbance. It may represent direct disturbance along the origin of the lateral tectotegmentospinal system, causing lack of facilitation of the sympathetic general visceral efferent lower motor neuron. However, the usual absence of the other signs of Horner's syndrome is evidence against this theory. The rapid recovery of the pupils that follows intracranial injury in patients with only cerebral signs supports the first hypothesis. Pupillary changes may take place hourly following head trauma. Unilateral mydriasis that in some cases may be accompanied by miosis of the opposite pupil is probably brought about by compression of the ipsilateral oculomotor nerve.

Experimental studies in dogs have shown that compression of the brain stem tectum at the level of the rostral colliculus causes miosis.[19] Compression of the third cranial nerve produces mydriasis. Acute cerebral swelling from a unilateral cerebral abscess in a horse resulted in compression of the ipsilateral midbrain and oculomotor nerve and an associated ipsilateral mydriasis. A diagram of pupil size and prognosis in intracranial injury follows.

	Pupil Size		Prognosis
Normal	◯	◯	Good
Unilateral oculomotor nuclear or nerve contusion or compression[a]	◯	◦	Guarded
Compression of midbrain tectum[b]	◦	◦	Guarded
Bilateral oculomotor nuclear or nerve contusion or compression	◯	◯	Grave

[a]Asymmetric interference with cerebral control of oculomotor neurons and/or the sympathetic upper motor neuron system.

[b]Bilateral sympathetic upper motor neuron deficiency or loss of facilitation, bilateral release, of oculomotor GVE neurons from cerebral inhibition.

Protrusion of the Third Eyelid

The third eyelid (membrana nictitans) may protrude for a number of reasons. Except possibly in the cat, this protrusion is a passive event. The third eyelid passively protrudes when the eyeball is retracted actively by the retractor bulbi (VI) and other extraocular muscles (III, IV, and VI). In the cat slips of striated muscle from the lateral rectus and levator palpebrae superiorus attach to the two extremities of the eyelid and may contract and contribute actively to this protrusion.

A constant partial protrusion of the third eyelid occurs in Horner's syndrome because of loss of the sympathetic innervation of the smooth muscle that normally keeps it retracted.

Brief, rapid, passive protrusions (flashing of the third eyelid) occur in tetanus owing to the effect of the tetanus toxin on the neurons that innervate the extraocular muscles. This causes brief contractions of these muscles, especially if the animal is startled. This is most noticeable in the horse with tetanus.

In facial paralysis the eyelids cannot close to blink when the animal is threatened. However, the eyeball is retracted, which causes a brief rapid protrusion of the third eyelid.

Cats with severe systemic disease and depression often have a persistent bilateral protrusion of the third eyelid. The cause is unknown.

Severe atrophy of the muscles of mastication causes enophthalmos and secondarily a protruded third eyelid.

SACRAL PARASYMPATHETIC GVE LOWER MOTOR NEURON

The sacral part of the parasympathetic division of the GVE lower motor neuron has the cell bodies of its preganglionic neurons located in the intermediate grey column of the sacral spinal cord segments (the second and third sacral segments in the dog).[21, 22] The axons course with the ventral roots to the spinal nerves, where they leave as ventral branches that unite ventral to the sacral vertebrae to form the pelvic nerve on each side. The preganglionic neurons of the pelvic nerve to the bladder synapse in ganglia in the pelvic plexus or in the bladder wall. The pelvic nerve is distributed by way of the pelvic plexus to the urogenital organs, rectum and descending colon.

CONTROL OF MICTURITION

The normal control of micturition is an important consideration in clinical neurology. The parasympathetic GVE system in the sacral spinal cord is under the control of centers in the reticular formation of the midbrain, pons, and medulla. Cortical influence on these centers initiates voluntary micturition. Ascending sensory pathways inform the cortex of the distended bladder.

Sensory neurons (general visceral afferent, general proprioception) have stretch receptors in the bladder wall, axons in the pelvic nerve, and cell bodies in the sacral spinal ganglia. Some terminate in the dorsal grey column of the sacral segments on a second group of neurons that enter the lateral funiculus and ascend the spinal cord with the spinothalamic system. Other primary afferents enter the dorsal funiculus without interruption and ascend in the fasciculus gracilis to the medulla, where they synapse in the nucleus gracilis. Both these routes relay through the thalamus to reach the somesthetic cortex. By way of these pathways bladder sensation reaches conscious perception.

Voiding is prevented willfully by the contraction of the striated urethral muscle distal to the bladder. The general somatic efferent neurons that innervate this muscle are in the first two sacral segments of the canine spinal cord. Voluntary micturition requires the influence of descending upper motor neuron pathways facilitory to the sacral general visceral efferent neurons that innervate bladder smooth muscle, and inhibitory to the sacral general somatic efferent neurons that innervate the urethral muscle.

Motor areas of cerebral cortex project to numerous nuclear groups in the

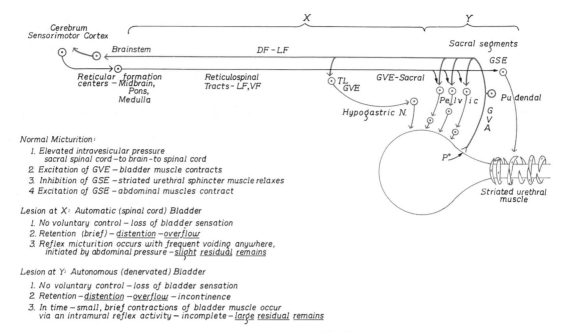

Figure 6–2. Neuroanatomy of bladder function.

midbrain, pons, and medulla concerned with the inhibition and facilitation of the bladder and urethral musculature by way of these lower motor neurons in the sacral spinal cord segments. These brain stem centers project to this area by way of reticulospinal and tectospinal tracts of the lateral and ventral funiculi. Facilitation of the general somatic efferent neurons that innervate the abdominal muscles is an important part of normal micturition.

The smooth muscle fibers of the bladder are oriented in an oblique fashion around the neck, which causes dilation of the opening of the bladder into the urethra when the bladder smooth muscle (detrusor) contracts to empty the bladder. There is no smooth muscle sphincter at this orifice. As the detrusor muscle contracts, receptors are stimulated in the bladder wall that initiate reflex inhibition of the general somatic efferent lower motor neurons to the urethral muscle.

The sympathetic innervation to the bladder arises from the intermediate grey column in the second to fifth lumbar segments of the spinal cord. The preganglionic neurons course from the sympathetic trunk in lumbar splanchnic nerves to the caudal mesenteric ganglion. Synapse occurs here with cell bodies of postganglionic axons that flow to the bladder through hypogastric nerves by way of the pelvic plexus. These provide innervation for the smooth muscle of blood vessels in the bladder wall, and in addition provide an inhibitory effect on some of the bladder smooth muscle. This inhibition is initiated by increasing intravesicular pressure, which is transmitted to the spinal cord by GVA neurons in the pelvic or hypogastric nerves. This information passes cranially to the lumbar segments from which this sympathetic GVE lower motor neuron arises. This reflex inhibitory effect allows the bladder muscle to stretch and increase its volume of urine with less intravesicular pressure. The sympathetic innervation probably has no major role in the smooth muscle contraction for the evacuation of the bladder.

Lesions of the brain stem or spinal cord that disturb the ascending or descending upper motor neuron pathways for normal micturition cause loss of voluntary control over the bladder. For a while urine is retained and the bladder distends and requires manual expression or catheterization to be emptied. If the bladder pressure can overcome the normal elasticity of the urethra and any spasticity there may be in the urethral muscle, then urine overflow occurs and sporadically dribbles from the penis or vulva. The inability to prevent the discharge of excretions is known as incontinence. In about 1 week reflex urination usually takes place, utilizing the sacral segments of the spinal cord. It often can be initiated by abdominal pressure. There is no voluntary control by the animal over when or where this will occur. This kind of a functioning bladder is called an automatic or spinal bladder. Bladder emptying is not complete and a small residual remains.

When a lesion destroys the GVE lower motor neuron at the level of the cell bodies in the sacral spinal cord or in the sacral roots or pelvic nerves, the bladder is denervated. Again, there is complete loss of voluntary control because of the lower motor neuron lesion. Urine is retained, and the bladder distends. Overflow occurs when bladder pressure exceeds the elasticity of the urethral wall. In time some reflex urination may take place as a result of the development of intramural reflexes in the wall of the bladder. Denervated smooth muscle does not degenerate or atrophy. It has the intrinsic capability of contracting. A large residual of urine remains. This kind of a denervated bladder that contracts is known as an autonomous bladder.

For reflex bladder contraction to occur, whether by way of the sacral spinal cord segments or the reflexes in the wall of the bladder, it requires healthy bladder smooth muscle. Excessive prolonged bladder distention eventually causes irreversible atonia of the muscle. Urea breaks down into ammonia in retained urine and is irritating to the bladder mucosa, causing inflammation. Opportunist bacteria often proliferate and augment the cystitis. Severe prolonged cystitis damages the bladder musculature. For these reasons overdistention and infection must be prevented by continual observation, manual evacuation or catheterization, and urinary antiseptic therapy if necessary.

Defecation is dependent on similar brain stem centers, spinal cord tracts and the same sacral spinal cord segments, and the pelvic nerve to the descending colon and rectum. Clinically, spinal cord lesions cranial to the first sacral segment that cause a loss of voluntary control over defecation usually do not result in obstruction to flow of bowel contents. Although some retention may take place, evacuation usually follows involuntarily. Even with lower motor neuron lesions of the pelvic nerve neurons, although retention may be more of a problem, evacuation usually occurs. Occasionally, enemas are necessary to relieve retention. If retention persists and is not attended to, a chronic megacolon may result. Failure to defecate with these lower motor neuron lesions is more of a problem in the horse than in the dog.

Diseases

Severe spinal cord contusion from an extruded intervertebral disk at the T13–L1 articulation interferes with the ascending and descending pathways to and from the brain for micturition, leading to an upper motor neuron paralysis accompanied by incontinence. An automatic bladder results. A fracture and subluxation at the L7-Sl articulation destroys the sacral nerves, resulting in bladder paralysis and incontinence, followed by the development of an autonomous bladder. Neuritis of the cauda equina in horses often destroys all the sacral nerves, bringing about bladder and rectal paralysis. Daily manual evacuation of the rectum and bladder may be necessary.

PARASYMPATHETIC GVE LOWER MOTOR NEURON OF THE MEDULLA (CRANIAL NERVES VII, IX, X, AND XI—FACIAL, GLOSSOPHARYNGEAL, VAGUS, AND ACCESSORY NEURONS)

The nuclear column containing the cell bodies of these general visceral efferent preganglionic neurons is located dorsolateral to the general somatic efferent column, medial to the solitary tract and nucleus, and ventral to the floor of the fourth ventricle from about the level of the special visceral efferent facial nucleus in the rostral medulla to the obex.

Preganglionic GVE axons in the facial nerve synapse in the pterygopalatine ganglion, whose postganglionic axons innervate the lacrimal, palatine, and nasal glands. Other facial nerve preganglionic axons synapse in the mandibular and sublingual ganglia. The postganglionic axons innervate the mandibular and sublingual salivary glands. Preganglionic GVE axons in the glossopharyngeal nerve synapse in the otic ganglion. Postganglionic axons innervate the zygomatic and parotid salivary glands. All of these postganglionic axons pass to the glands to be innervated in branches of the trigeminal nerve.

The parasympathetic vagal nucleus comprises the majority of this nuclear column.[14] It is dorsolateral to the hypoglossal nucleus and slightly longer. It is medial to the solitary tract and nucleus that is part of the general visceral afferent system. The general visceral efferent axons leave the lateral side of the medulla with the special visceral efferent axons from nucleus ambiguus. They course through the jugular foramen and tympanooccipital fissure and descend the neck in the vagal part of the vagosympathetic trunk. They are distributed to organs in the thorax and abdomen, where they synapse on cell bodies of postganglionic axons in the wall of the viscera being innervated. The preganglionic axons of the cell bodies in the caudal part of this nucleus leave the medulla with the cranial root of the accessory nerve, along with its special visceral efferent axons. These join the vagus as they pass through the jugular foramen and are distributed with the vagal general visceral efferent axons.

Recent investigations in the cat have suggested that this parasympathetic nucleus of the vagus is the source of innervation to the glandular structures of the mucosa of the viscera.[18, 20] The cell bodies of the preganglionic axons that innervate the visceral smooth muscle may arise from a nucleus located ventrolateral in the medulla between nucleus ambiguus and the spinal nucleus of the trigeminal nerve.

Some consider the general visceral efferent vagal neurons interneurons because they may not be necessary for direct initiation of smooth muscle activity in the digestive tract, but instead modulate the intrinsic reflex activity of the enteric plexus. The gastrointestinal tract can carry out its major functions without its extrinsic innervation. This is accomplished by the intrinsic neural mechanism in

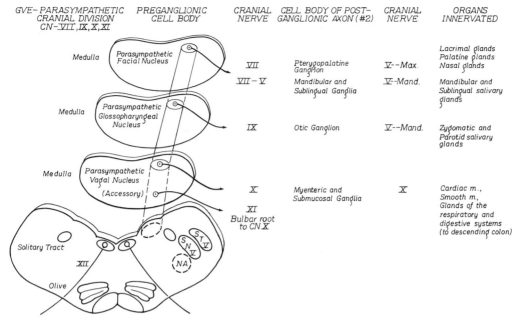

GVE–PARASYMPATHETIC CRANIAL DIVISION CN-VII,IX,X,XI	PREGANGLIONIC CELL BODY	CRANIAL NERVE	CELL BODY OF POST- GANGLIONIC AXON (#2)	CRANIAL NERVE	ORGANS INNERVATED
Medulla	Parasympathetic Facial Nucleus	VII	Pterygopalatine Ganglion	V--Max.	Lacrimal glands Palatine glands Nasal glands
		VII – V	Mandibular and Sublingual Ganglia	V-Mand.	Mandibular and Sublingual salivary glands
Medulla	Parasympathetic Glossopharyngeal Nucleus	IX	Otic Ganglion	V--Mand.	Zygomatic and Parotid salivary glands
Medulla	Parasympathetic Vagal Nucleus (Accessory)	X / XI Bulbar root to CN.X	Myenteric and Submucosal Ganglia	X	Cardiac m., Smooth m., Glands of the respiratory and digestive systems (to descending colon)

Figure 6–3. Parasympathetic general visceral efferent nuclear column in medulla.

the wall of the bowel, which can maintain small intestinal peristalsis and colonic mass movement, and the ability of the smooth muscle cell to contract rhythmically.

Unilateral vagus nerve lesions or vagotomy usually are not associated with clinical signs in dogs. Bilateral cervical vagal disease or vagotomy causes paralysis of the larynx with inspiratory dyspnea and cyanosis, and abnormal esophageal swallowing with regurgitation and megaesophagus.[15, 17] In response to swallowing there is absence of normal esophageal peristalsis and failure of the gastroesophageal junction (sphincter) to relax. Food accumulates in the distal esophagus, which dilates. Bilateral cranial thoracic vagal disease or vagotomy that spares the recurrent laryngeal nerves produces abnormal function of the thoracic esophagus with regurgitation of undigested food and megaesophagus. These signs closely resemble the natural disease in dogs and cats most often referred to as achalasia.

Canine esophageal achalasia, megaesophagus, and esophageal neuromuscular disease are synonyms for a disease that is common in dogs and occasionally occurs in cats.[5, 6, 7, 9, 11, 14, 16, 23, 26] It has been reported in almost all breeds of dogs including mixed breeds, but predominantly in the German shepherd. It is reported as an inherited disease in wire-haired fox terriers. It usually becomes apparent in the young animal when it is weaned, which suggests that it is a congenital disease. It is also acquired in older dogs.

The salient clinical features are postprandial regurgitation of undigested food, with radiographic evidence of megaesophagus to the level of the diaphragm. Contrast radiography demonstrates abnormal esophageal motility, with failure of the gastroesophageal junction to dilate when swallowing is initiated. Often if the dog is stood on its pelvic limbs, the added weight of the esophageal contents aids movement through this junction, which is not hypertonic. In most cases there is no true achalasia or primary failure of the gastroesophageal junction to relax.

The pathogenesis is unknown, but experimental studies suggest that the disturbance is neural, not muscular, and possibly is in the extrinsic innervation. One study demonstrated a lack of the normal number of neuronal cell bodies in nucleus ambiguus.[6] Further investigations of a similar nature are needed. Presumably the striated muscle of the esophagus is innervated by special visceral efferent neurons that course from nucleus ambiguus to the esophagus in the vagus nerves.

REFERENCES

1. Acheson, G. H.: The topographical anatomy of the smooth muscle of the cat's nictitating membrane. Anat. Rec., 71:297, 1938.
2. Barlow, C. M., and Root, W. S.: The ocular sympathetic path between the superior cervical ganglion and the orbit in the cat. J. Comp. Neurol., 91:195, 1949.
3. Bistner, S., Rubin, L., Cox, T. A., and Condon, W. E.: Pharmacologic diagnosis of Horner's syndrome in the dog. J. Am. Vet. Med. Assoc., 157:1220, 1970.
4. Carveth, S. W., Schlegel, J. F., Code, C. F., and Ellis, F. H.: Esophageal motility after vagotomy, phrenicotomy, myotomy, and myomectomy in dogs. Surg. Gynecol. Obstet., 114:31, 1962.
5. Clifford, D. H., and Gyorkey, F.: Myenteric ganglion cells in dogs with and without hereditary achalasia of the esophagus. Am. J. Vet. Res., 32:615, 1971.
6. Clifford, D. H., Pirsch, J. G., and Mauldin, M. L.: Comparison of motor nuclei of the vagus nerve in dogs with and without esophageal achalasia. Proc. Soc. Exp. Biol. Med., 142:878, 1973.
7. Clifford, D. H., Waddell, E. D., Patterson, D. R., Wilson, C. F., and Thompson, H. L.: Management of esophageal achalasia in miniature schnauzers. J. Am. Vet. Med. Assoc., 161:1012, 1972.
8. de Lahunta, A., and Alexander, J. W.: Ischemic myelopathy secondary to presumed fibrocartilaginous embolism in nine dogs. J. Am. Anim. Hosp. Assoc. 12:37, 1976.
9. Diamant, N., Szizepanski, M., and Meci, H.: Manometric characteristics of idiopathic megaesophagus in the dog: An unsuitable animal model for achalasia in man. Gastroenterology, 65:216, 1973.
10. Fox, J. G., and Gutnick, M. J.: Horner's syndrome and brachial paralysis due to lymphosarcoma in a cat. J. Am. Vet. Med. Assoc., 160:977, 1972.
11. Gray, G. W.: Acute experiments on neuroeffector function in canine esophageal achalasia. Am. J. Vet. Res., 35:1075, 1974.
12. Greene, C. E., and Higgins, R. J.: Fibrocartilaginous emboli as the cause of ischemic myelopathy in a dog. Cor. Vet., 66:131, 1976.
13. Harding, R., and Leek, B. F.: The locations and activities of medullary neurons associated with ruminant forestomach motility. J. Physiol., 219:587, 1971.
14. Harvey, C. E., O'Brien, J. A., Durie, V. R., Miller, D. J., and Veenena, R.: Megaesophagus in the dog: A clinical survey of 79 cases. J. Am. Vet. Med. Assoc., 165:443, 1974.
15. Higgs, B., and Ellis, F. H.: The effect of bilateral supranodosal vagotomy on canine esophageal function. Surgery, 58:828, 1965.
16. Hoffer, R. E., Valdes-Dapena, A., and Bane, A. E.: A comparative study of naturally occurring canine achalasia. Arch. Surg., 95:83, 1967.
17. Huang, K., Essex, H., Essex, E., and Mann, F. C.: A study of certain problems resulting from vagotomy in dogs with special reference to emesis. Amer. J. Physiol., 149:429, 1947.
18. Kerr, F. W. L.: Function of the dorsal motor nucleus of the vagus. Science, 157:451, 1967.
19. Kerr, F. W. L., and Hollowell, O. W.: Location of pupillomotor and accommodation fibres in the oculomotor nerve: Experimental observations on paralytic mydriasis. J. Neurol. Neurosurg. Psychiatry, 27:473, 1964.
20. Kerr, F. W. L., Hendler, H., and Bowren, P.: Viscerotopic organization of the vagus. J. Comp. Neurol., 138:279, 1970.
21. Oliver, J. E., Jr., Bradley, W. E., and Fletcher, T. F.: Identification of preganglionic parasympathetic neurons in the sacral spinal cord of the cat. J. Comp. Neurol., 137:321, 1969.
22. Oliver, J. E., Jr., Bradley, W. E., and Fletcher, T. F.: Spinal cord representation of the micturition reflex. J. Comp. Neurol., 137:329, 1969.
23. Osborne, C. A., Clifford, D. H., and Jessen, C.: Hereditary esophageal achalasia in dogs. J. Am. Vet. Med. Assoc., 141:572, 1967.
24. Owen, R. ap R.: Epistaxis prevented by ligation of the internal carotid artery in the guttural pouch. Equine Vet. J., 6:143, 1974.
25. Rosenblueth, A., and Bard, P.: The innervation and function of the nictitating membrane in the cat. Am. J. Physiol., 100:537, 1932.
26. Sokolovsky, V.: Achalasia and paralysis of the canine esophagus. J. Am. Vet. Med. Assoc., 160:943, 1972.
27. Thompson, J. W.: The nerve supply to the nictitaing membrane of the cat. J. Anat., 95:371, 1961.
28. Smith, J. S., and Mayhew, I. G.: Horner's syndrome in large animals. Cor. Vet., in preparation.

Chapter 7

UPPER MOTOR NEURON SYSTEM

PYRAMIDAL SYSTEM
HISTOLOGY OF THE CEREBRAL
    CORTEX
EXTRAPYRAMIDAL SYSTEM
Telencephalon
Diencephalon

Mesencephalon
Rhombencephalon
FUNCTION
CLINICAL SIGNS: UPPER MOTOR NEURON
    DISEASE
Tetany—Tremors

    The upper motor neuron (UMN) is the motor system confined to the central nervous system that is responsible for the initiation of voluntary movement, the maintenance of tone for support of the body against gravity, and the regulation of posture to provide a stable background upon which to initiate the voluntary activity. Traditionally, it is divided into pyramidal and extrapyramidal components. This separation is more significant in the primate, in whom the pyramidal system is more highly developed and has a more important function than has been observed in domestic animals.

    The pyramidal system consists of those neurons whose cell bodies are located in the motor area of the cerebral cortex, and whose axons descend through the white matter of the cerebrum and brain stem, including the pyramid on the ventral surface of the medulla. Their telodendron is in the grey matter of the spinal cord. This is an uninterrupted, monosynaptic, corticospinal pathway from the cerebrum to the spinal cord by way of the pyramids of the medulla.

    In contrast, the extrapyramidal system consists of neurons that originate in the cerebral cortex, including the motor area, and descend into the brain stem directly or by way of subcortical nuclei. Synapse occurs with additional neurons in the subcortical nuclei and brain stem nuclei. Axons course from specific brain stem nuclei caudally through the spinal cord, without traversing the pyramids of the medulla. The telodendron of the final neuron is in the grey matter of the spinal cord. This is a multineuronal, multisynaptic, corticospinal pathway. These two systems overlap anatomically and function together. They will be considered together as the upper motor neuron in clinical discussions.

PYRAMIDAL SYSTEM

    The development of the pyramidal system is related directly to the capacity of the animal to perform finely skilled movements. In primates its termination in

125

the spinal cord is most dense in the areas of the lateral portion of the ventral grey column, in which the cell bodies of the general somatic efferent lower motor neuron to muscles of the digits are located. Here it may synapse directly on the dendritic zone of the alpha motor neuron (GSE). Such development has been observed in the primate and the raccoon, two unrelated species that possess considerable manipulative ability in their thoracic limb digits.[1] This system is developed poorly in domestic animals, especially in the horse, the ox, and the sheep. In the horse this system makes a sizable contribution to the facial muscles for lip movement, suggesting that these muscles perform the most highly skilled activity of this species.

The cell body of the neuron of the pyramidal system is located in the motor area of the cerebrum, which usually is situated in the frontal lobe or adjacent parietal lobe. In primates, this mostly involves the precruciate gyrus. In carnivores, it overlaps on the sensory area and is limited to the postcruciate gyrus and rostral ectomarginal gyrus.[6, 13] In ungulates, it is located medially along the frontal lobe in the region of the precruciate gyrus.[9] Stimulation studies have shown that these motor areas can be subdivided into regions of the body that are innervated by lower motor neurons receiving impulses from the pyramidal system neurons that originate in these specific parts of the motor area. This is referred to as a somatotopic organization. The various portions of the body are represented topographically on specific areas of cerebral gyri. The homunculus drawn for the human brain depicts this phenomenon. Regions involved in more highly skilled functions have a larger representation in the motor area. Muscles with small motor units have a larger area of representation. The primary motor area of one cerebral hemisphere serves the musculature on the opposite side of the body. In the carnivore the postcruciate gyrus is related to the innervation of the appendicular musculature.[6, 11] The ectomarginal gyrus is related to the motor function of the cervical muscles and the muscles of specific areas of the head. Many of these cell bodies are large, and are referred to as giant pyramidal cells or Betz's cells. They are located in lamina V of the cerebral cortex of the gyri in the motor area.

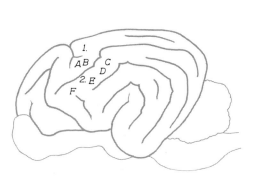

1. POSTCRUCIATE GYRUS
   A. Pelvic limb
   B. Thoracic limb
2. ROSTRAL ECTOMARGINAL GYRUS
   C. Ear
   D. Eyelid
   E. Masseter, temporal mm.
   F. Lateral cervical mm.

Figure 7–1. Topography of the cerebral motor cortex.

The axons of these cells descend through the white matter of the brain, which includes, in this order: the corona radiata of the motor cortex, the internal capsule of telencephalon and diencephalon, the crus cerebri of the mesencephalon (in which they occupy the medial two thirds), the longitudinal fibers of pons, and the pyramid of medulla. Caudal to the obex of the medulla, approximately 75 per cent or more of these axons cross in the pyramidal decussation located adjacent to the ventral median fissure, and pass through the grey matter to the dorsal part of the lateral funiculus. Here they descend as the lateral corticospinal tract medial to the ascending spinocerebellar tracts.[54] In the dog, approximately 50 per cent of these axons terminate in the cervical spinal cord grey matter, 20 per cent in the thoracic grey matter, and 30 per cent in the lumbosacral grey matter.[28] Most influence the general somatic efferent lower motor neuron by way of synapse with inter-neurons.[42, 44] The remaining 25 per cent or less descend without crossing in the ventral funiculus adjacent to the ventral median fissure as the ventral cortico-spinal tract. This tract is not as well defined as the lateral tract. The axons of the ventral corticospinal tract descend the spinal cord as far as the midthoracic level, and the majority cross at their termination. In ungulates, the entire pyramidal system is confined to the cervical spinal cord.[3] A few axons have been found caudal to the cervical segments in the horse.[8, 9]

In addition to influencing the spinal nerve lower motor neuron, this system also affects the cranial nerve lower motor neuron. This is mediated by axons that leave the descending pathway as it moves through the brain stem to synapse on or near the general somatic efferent and special visceral efferent lower motor neuron. These are called corticonuclear (corticobulbar) fibers. The pyramidal system axons are organized regionally in the central white matter. In the crus cerebri the pyramidal system is in the center, with the axons to the pelvic limb lateral, those to the thoracic limb in the middle, and those to the muscles of the head medial.

Disturbances in the pyramidal system demonstrate the different role this system plays in primates as compared to domestic animals. Lesions in the cerebral origin of this system in man cause a paralysis of contralateral voluntary muscle activity. In dogs examined a few days after experimental removal of the motor area there is no defect in the gait, but there is a deficiency in the response to postural reaction testing in the contralateral limbs.[59] Lesions in this same area in all domesticated animals present a similar clinical syndrome. Section of the canine pyramidal system in the crus cerebri or pyramid also does not affect the gait.[24]

HISTOLOGY OF THE CEREBRAL CORTEX

The cerebral cortex is made up of an elaborate organization of neural structures with innumerable interconnections that form the basis for the numerous functions allotted to it. These include consciousness, intellect, emotion, behavior, perception, and control of somatic and visceral motor functions. These are performed by the reciprocal relationship of the cortex with the rest of the central and the peripheral nervous systems.

The cerebral cortex varies from 1.5 to 4 mm in thickness, and is situated between the pia mater and the underlying white matter of the corona radiata, which it covers. It contains neuronal cell bodies of many different sizes and shapes: axons, telodendria, the processes of the dendritic zone, and neuroglial cells. The neurons in the cortex constitute a system of chains of interrelated neurons. It is a laminated structure based either on the organization of the processes, the study of which is called myeloarchitectonics, or on the arrangement of the cell bodies, the study of which is termed cytoarchitectonics. When viewed according to the organization of the cell bodies, as many as six layers can be recognized. The extent to which each of these six laminae is developed varies throughout the cerebrum. In general, the neopallium has six layers, and the archipallium and paleopallium each have less than six. Some functional significance has been attached to the variation in lamination in the different regions of the cerebrum. Various maps have been prepared showing the laminar variations that occur throughout the cerebrum. Some include over one hundred different areas based on cytoarchitectonic studies.

In general, the neuronal cell bodies are of two types. The stellate or granule cell has a round cell body and short processes, which usually are confined to the cortex. The pyramidal cell has a pyramidal-shaped cell body that varies in size and has long processes. The axon of the pyramidal cell projects from the cortex into the white matter of the corona radiata as an association axon to another cortical area in the same hemisphere, or as a commissural axon that crosses to a cortical area in the opposite hemisphere, or as a projection axon that projects to nuclear areas in the brain stem or spinal cord. The corticospinal neuron is an example of the latter type. Each cortical area receives axons from other cortical areas in the same hemisphere (association), from the opposite hemisphere (commissural), and from the brain stem, especially the thalamus (projection). The study of the arrangement of these processes in the cortex, and of the processes of the granule cells, is referred to as myeloarchitectonics.

In the neocortex, the six layers from external to internal consist of the molecular layer, external granular layer, pyramidal cell layer, internal granular layer, ganglion cell layer, and polymorphic cell layer. The processes of the molecular and external and internal granular layers are confined mostly to the cortex. Axons from the pyramidal, ganglionic, and polymorphous layers constitute the cortical efferents that form the association, commissural, and projection pathways.

EXTRAPYRAMIDAL SYSTEM

The extrapyramidal system embraces diverse, scattered groups of interconnected and functionally related structures that form a series of neurons in a multisynaptic pathway from the brain to the lower motor neuron of the brain stem and spinal cord. These pathways do not traverse the pyramids of the medulla, but function with the pyramidal system in the initiation of voluntary movement and in providing tonic mechanisms for the support of the body against gravity. These functions are performed ultimately by the influence of this system (UMN) on the alpha and gamma motor neurons (LMN) in motor nuclei in the brain stem and in the ventral grey column of the spinal cord.

The cell bodies of neurons in the extrapyramidal system are located in nuclei in all divisions of the brain. The more important of these will be described for each of the divisions, along with the course of the axons. Only the extrapyramidal nuclei in the mesencephalon and rhombencephalon have axons that descend the spinal cord to influence the activity of the lower motor neuron.

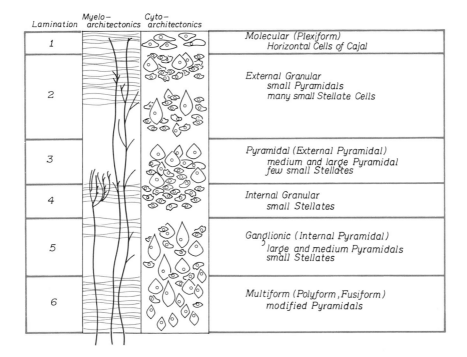

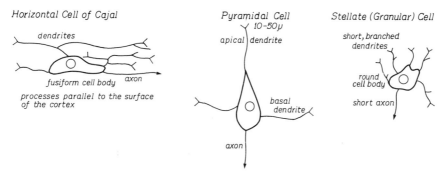

Figure 7–2. Histology of the cerebral cortex.

Telencephalon

1. Extrapyramidal neurons are located in the cerebral cortex throughout the cerebrum, but mostly in the frontal and parietal lobes, in which they occur in the cortex of the motor area and adjacent gyri. These project to basal nuclei and other extrapyramidal nuclei in the brain stem.

2. The basal nuclei are subcortical collections of neuronal cell bodies. These include the septal nuclei, amygdala and claustrum, which function in the limbic system. The caudate nucleus, putamen, and pallidum are extrapyramidal basal nuclei. The putamen and pallidum are referred to as the lentiform nucleus because of their overall shape on transverse or dorsal section. The corpus striatum refers to

all three of these extrapyramidal basal nuclei and the intervening internal capsule that is traversed by their processes.

The caudate nucleus is located primarily in the floor of the lateral ventricle, medial to the internal capsule. The large head and most of the body are rostral to the diencephalon. The body extends caudally dorsolateral to the diencephalon, medial to the internal capsule, and is continued by a small tail into the temporal lobe of the cerebrum, in which it is lateral to the internal capsule. It receives afferents from extrapyramidal neurons in the cerebral cortex and projects mostly to the adjacent pallidum.[55]

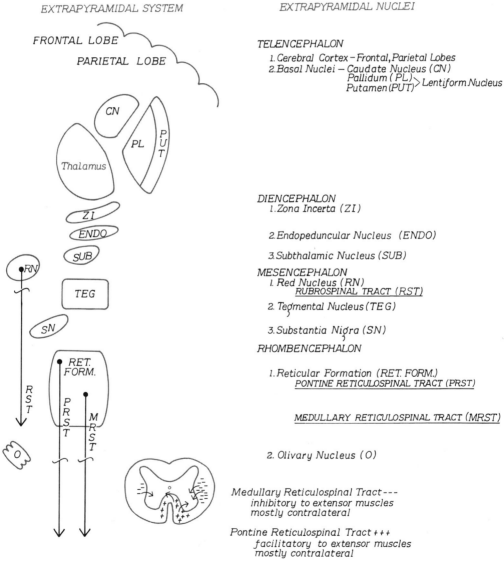

EXTRAPYRAMIDAL SYSTEM

FRONTAL LOBE

PARIETAL LOBE

CN

PL   P U T

Thalamus

ZI

ENDO

SUB

RN

TEG

SN

RET. FORM.

P R S T

M R S T

R S T

O

EXTRAPYRAMIDAL NUCLEI

TELENCEPHALON
1. Cerebral Cortex – Frontal, Parietal Lobes
2. Basal Nuclei – Caudate Nucleus (CN)
   Pallidum (PL)
   Putamen (PUT) > Lentiform Nucleus

DIENCEPHALON
1. Zona Incerta (ZI)

2. Endopeduncular Nucleus (ENDO)

3. Subthalamic Nucleus (SUB)

MESENCEPHALON
1. Red Nucleus (RN)
   RUBROSPINAL TRACT (RST)

2. Tegmental Nucleus (TEG)

3. Substantia Nigra (SN)

RHOMBENCEPHALON

1. Reticular Formation (RET. FORM.)
   PONTINE RETICULOSPINAL TRACT (PRST)

MEDULLARY RETICULOSPINAL TRACT (MRST)

2. Olivary Nucleus (O)

Medullary Reticulospinal Tract --- inhibitory to extensor muscles mostly contralateral

Pontine Reticulospinal Tract +++ facilitatory to extensor muscles mostly contralateral

Figure 7–3.   The extrapyramidal system.

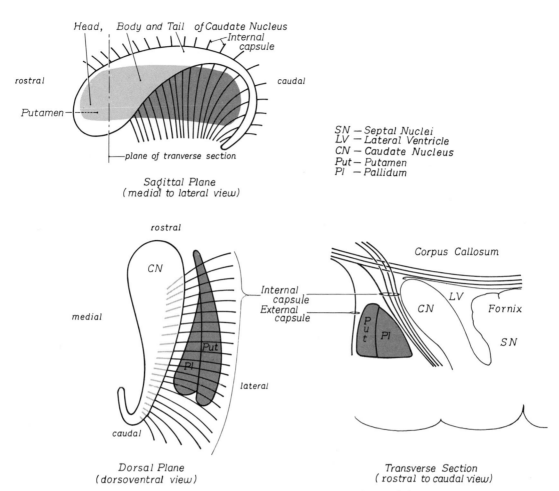

Figure 7–4. Extrapyramidal nuclei of the telencephalon.

The lentiform nucleus comprises the pallidum (globus pallidus) medially and the putamen laterally, separated by a layer of white matter. It is bounded medially by the internal capsule and laterally by the thin external capsule. This nucleus begins rostrally in the frontal lobe, in which it is separated from the head and body of the caudate nucleus by the internal capsule. It extends caudally through the parietal and into the temporal lobe to a level caudal to the amygdala in the pyriform lobe, in which the lateral ventricle and hippocampus are located. It is dorsal to the amygdaloid nucleus and lateral to the optic tract and internal capsule.

A feedback circuit is provided by a multisynaptic pathway from cortical extrapyramidal neurons to caudate nucleus, to pallidum, to ventral rostral nucleus of thalamus, to cerebral cortex. At the time of cortical initiation of voluntary movement such a circuit provides a modifying control mechanism. Certain thalamic nuclei serve to project information from the brain stem to the cerebrum. The ventral rostral thalamic nucleus is an example of such a projection nucleus for the extrapyramidal system.

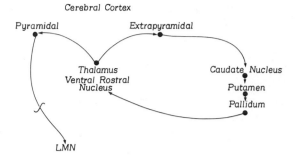

Diencephalon

The extrapyramidal nuclei are located in the ventrolateral region of the thalamus.

1. The endopeduncular nucleus is located in the rostral thalamus between the optic tract and the internal capsule medial to the lentiform nucleus. It extends caudally lateral to the hypothalamus.

2. The zona incerta is a narrow nucleus located dorsomedial to the internal capsule and lateral to the external medullary lamina of the thalamus. This nucleus extends through most of the thalamus.

3. The subthalamic nucleus is in the caudal thalamus, caudal to the endopeduncular nucleus on the dorsomedial surface of the crus cerebri.

All three of these nuclei are connected to the extrapyramidal nuclei in the telencephalon and caudal brain stem by afferent and efferent axons, but none projects directly to the spinal cord lower motor neuron.

Mesencephalon

There are three extrapyramidal nuclear areas in the midbrain.

1. The substantia nigra is so named because its cell bodies contain a melanin pigment that increases with age and is macroscopic in some species.[33] This nucleus can be found throughout the mesencephalon dorsal to the crus cerebri and ventral to the tegmentum. It is bounded rostrally by the subthalamic nucleus. Some of these neurons project rostrally to the caudate nucleus in which dopamine, synthesized in the substantia nigra neurons, is secreted as the neurotransmitter. This is referred to as the nigrostriatal pathway.

2. The tegmental nucleus is an ill-defined area in the reticular formation of the tegmentum of the mesencephalon. It extends the length of the mesencephalon. Rostrally it is dorsolateral to the red nucleus in the tegmentum.

3. The red nucleus is in the tegmentum at the level of the rostral colliculus ventrolateral to the oculomotor nucleus. It receives a group of afferent axons from the ipsilateral motor area of the cerebral cortex by way of the internal capsule and crus cerebri. Axons of the cell bodies in the red nucleus decussate at the level of the nucleus in the tegmentum, and descend as the rubrospinal tract through the ventrolateral mesencephalon, pons, medulla, and lateral funiculus of the spinal

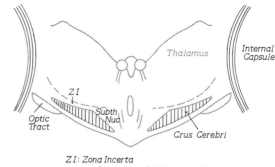

ZI: Zona Incerta
Subth Nuc: Subthalamic Nucleus

Figure 7–5. Extrapyramidal nuclei of the diencephalon.

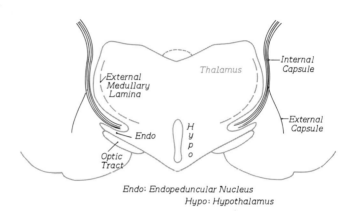

Endo: Endopeduncular Nucleus
Hypo: Hypothalamus

cord. Here the tract is associated closely with the lateral corticospinal tract deep to the superficially positioned ascending spinocerebellar tracts in the dorsal portion of the lateral funiculus. This tract descends through the entire spinal cord. Its axons terminate on interneurons in the ventral grey column of the spinal cord that influence the activity of the lower motor neuron. This corticorubrospinal system is organized somatotopically.[23, 47] The neurons in the thoracic limb area of the motor cortex project on the dorsal part of the red nucleus, whose

Figure 7–6. Extrapyramidal nuclei of the mesencephalon.

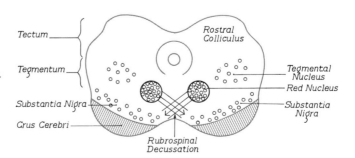

neurons project on the spinal cord grey matter that innervates the thoracic limb. Corticorubral neurons from the pelvic limb region of the motor cortex synapse in the ventral portion of the red nucleus, whose neurons descend in the rubrospinal tract to influence the pelvic limb lower motor neuron. The rubrospinal tracts are considered to be especially important in the control of somatic motor activity in the domestic animal.[25] They are predominantly facilitatory to motoneurons of flexor muscles.

Rubrobulbar neurons course with the rubrospinal neurons, and at various levels leave the rubrospinal tract as it courses through the caudal brain stem. The rubrobulbar neurons synapse in the cranial nerve nuclei for general somatic efferent and special visceral efferent function.

The red nucleus also receives a group of afferent axons from the contralateral lateral (dentate) nucleus of the cerebellum. These axons enter the mesencephalic tegmentum, and synapse on neurons in the red nucleus. These cell bodies of the red nucleus project rostrally to the ventral rostral nucleus of the thalamus, in which synapse occurs, and these thalamic neurons project to the cerebral cortex. The red nucleus in this instance is part of a cerebellorubrothalamic system that is part of a feedback circuit to the cerebral cortex. The cerebellum receives cortical projections by way of the pontine nucleus and middle cerebellar peduncle. The complete circuit involves the corticopontocerebellar and cerebellorubrothalamic pathways.

In addition, there are afferent and efferent connections of the red nucleus with the telencephalic basal nuclei.

Rhombencephalon

1. The reticular formation is located in the core of the medulla, the pons, the tegmentum of the midbrain, and the caudal diencephalon. It appears to be an ill-defined meshwork of a variety of cell types engulfed in a diffuse network of neuronal processes. Anatomic studies have defined nuclear areas belonging to the reticular formation. It receives projections primarily from the cerebellum, spinal cord, and higher levels of the brain, including extrapyramidal nuclei. The reticular formation, in turn, projects to these three areas. A large projection serves the spinal cord.[3, 4, 41]

Many functions have been attributed to the reticular formation. These include activation of the cerebral cortex (ascending reticular activating system — ARAS), control of vital functions such as respiratory and cardiac functions, control over voluntary excretion, control over vomiting and swallowing, and control over muscle tone and motor function. Some textbooks divide the reticular formation into an ascending portion that functions in the activation of the higher brain structures, and a descending portion that influences ventral grey column internuncial activity and the alpha and gamma efferent neurons affecting motor tone and motor activity. The descending portion includes its participation in the extrapyramidal system.

Studies in the cat have defined an area of the reticular formation in the pons that exerts facilitatory influence on motoneurons of extensor muscles by way of a descending reticulospinal tract.[44] This pontine reticulospinal tract courses mostly in the contralateral ventral funiculus. Similarly, an area of the medullary reticular formation has inhibitory influence on the motoneurons of extensor muscles in the spinal cord by way of a medullary reticulospinal tract that courses in the lateral funiculus in a medial intermediate position, mostly on the contralateral side. The axons that course in these two tracts cross at their place of origin in the reticular formation. A few remain ipsilateral.

2. The olivary nucleus is located ventrally in the medulla, from a level caudal to the facial nucleus to a level caudal to the obex rostral to the pyramidal decussation. It is dorsolateral to the pyramids and medial lemniscus, medial to the descending hypoglossal axons. It comprises three nuclear groups that at some levels have the appearance of fingers directed ventrolaterally. This extrapyramidal nucleus receives afferents from many of the extrapyramidal nuclei in the telencephalon, diencephalon, and mesencephalon. Its efferents project primarily to the contralateral portion of the cerebellum. This is a primary source of extrapyramidal system projection to the cerebellum. The axons cross the midline dorsal to the pyramids, intermingle with the medial lemniscus, and continue in an arc dorsolaterally to enter the caudal cerebellar peduncle, where they are distributed to the cerebellum.

A feedback circuit exists to the cerebral cortex by way of the cerebellum through this nucleus.

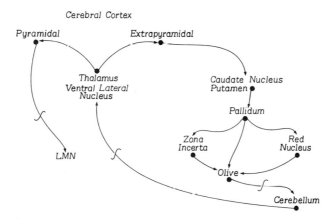

In this presentation of the extrapyramidal portion of the upper motor neuron, the final efferent pathways by which this system exerts influence over the lower motor neuron are rubrospinal, medullary, and pontine reticulospinal tracts. Other descending tracts influence motor tone and motor activity by their connections with the ventral grey column of the spinal cord. These include the vestibulospinal tract, the medial longitudinal fasciculus, and the tectospinal tract. These sometimes are included in descriptions of the extrapyramidal descending projections. In this book they are considered together with different systems that have their own anatomic components and functional attributes, separate from but interrelated with the extrapyramidal system.

A comparison of the development of the upper motor neuron tracts in the cranial cervical spinal cord of man, the cat, and the horse reveals the decrease in importance of the pyramidal system (corticospinal tract) and the increase in the contribution of the extrapyramidal system (rubrospinal tract) in the domestic animal.

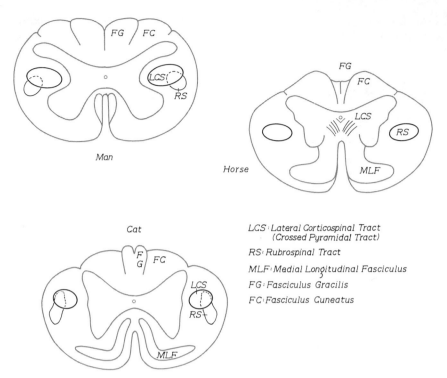

Figure 7–7. Comparison of first cervical spinal cord segment in man, the cat, and the horse.

FUNCTION

The functions of the upper motor neuron can be summarized as: (1) the initiation of voluntary activity of the motor systems, and (2) the maintenance of muscle tone to support the body against gravity and to establish the posture upon which the voluntary activity can be performed.

The extrapyramidal system exerts its functions by influencing the activity of the alpha and gamma motor neurons in the ventral grey column of the spinal cord. Its activity in modulating muscle tone involves its control over the myotatic reflex. The sensory receptor organ for this reflex is the neuromuscular spindle located in the belly of the skeletal muscles. These spindle-shaped structures are composed of intrafusal fibers, which are modified small muscle cells. The intrafusal fibers are parallel to the extrafusal fibers, which are the larger skeletal muscle cells. A connective tissue capsule encloses the group of intrafusal fibers and is attached to the endomysium of the adjacent extrafusal fibers. Within the spindle there are two types of intrafusal fibers. One type (nuclear bag) is interrupted near its middle by a nonstriated dilation containing many cell nuclei. The second type (nuclear chain) has no central dilation, although its nuclei are accumulated in the middle of the fiber. These features create for the neuromuscular spindle a central distended nuclear bag region augmented by a lymph space that envelops the middle portion of the intrafusal fibers. The poles of the spindle are tapered and contain the contractile striated portion of the intrafusal fibers.

The intrafusal fibers are innervated in the polar regions by small myelinated neurons whose cell bodies are in the ventral grey column of the spinal cord, intermingled with the larger general somatic efferent neurons. These small neurons are called gamma neurons or efferents, while the larger GSE neurons are referred to as alpha neurons or efferents.

The nuclear bag region is surrounded by the processes of a sensory neuron whose axon is large and classified as Ia. These Ia afferents, with their annulospiral endings on the nuclear bag, have their cell bodies in spinal ganglia, and the axon courses through the dorsal root and the dorsal grey column, into the ventral grey column, to synapse directly on an alpha motor neuron. Impulses are stimulated in the dendritic zone (annulospiral ending) of the Ia afferent by any action that stretches the nuclear bag region of the spindle, including passive stretch of the skeletal muscle by gravity, tapping the tendon of the muscle with a blunt instrument, or active stretch by contraction of the intrafusal fibers mediated by the gamma efferent.

Posture is maintained against the steady force of gravity by this mechanism. The force of gravity stretches extensor muscles and the nuclear bag region of the spindles. The Ia afferent is stimulated. In turn, the Ia afferent stimulates the alpha motor neuron (GSE), causing contraction of the extrafusal fibers of the extensor muscle. Collaterals of the Ia afferent stimulate interneurons in the ventral grey column that are inhibitory to the GSE neurons innervating the muscles antagonistic to the action of the extensor muscle. The activity of this myotatic reflex

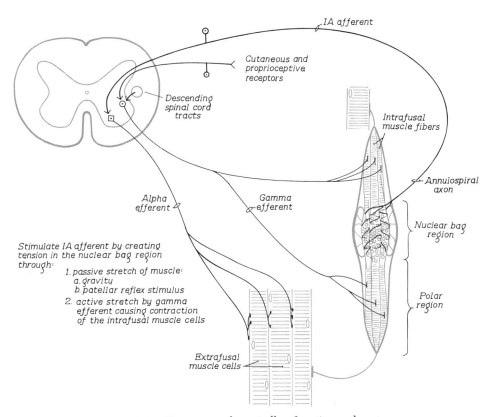

Figure 7–8. Neuromuscular spindle—function and anatomy.

maintains the constant low-level state of contraction known as muscle tone. Other collateral axons of the Ia afferent are involved in ascending proprioceptive pathways to the cerebellum and sensory cortex, providing higher centers with information on the state of muscle contraction to be used in the proper coordination of motor activity. The gamma efferent is subject to influence by descending spinal cord tracts of the extrapyramidal system.

Golgi tendon organs are the receptors (dendritic zone) of Ib sensory neurons that are located in tendons. They have a higher threshold to the stimulus of stretching muscles than Ia annulospiral afferents, and are stimulated when the tendon is stretched by contraction of the extrafusal fibers of the muscle. Within the ventral grey column of the spinal cord, the Ib afferent projects on interneurons that are inhibitory to the alpha motor neuron innervating the contracting muscle, and that are facilitatory to the alpha motor neuron innervating the antagonist of this muscle, thus lowering its threshold to stimulus. This inverse myotatic reflex provides for smooth coordination of skeletal muscle activity and protects against overstretching of tendons.

The classic example used by the physiologist to demonstrate the role of the extrapyramidal system in the control of motor tone is the phenomenon of decerebrate rigidity. When the brain stem is transected between the colliculi of the midbrain, an uninhibited extensor tonus of all the antigravity muscles is produced. The head and neck are extended markedly in a posture of opisthotonos, and all four limbs in the quadriped are extended rigidly. This is explained as a release mechanism. The tonic mechanism or myotatic reflex involving the lower motor neuron has been released from the effects of the descending inhibitory upper motor neuron pathways. The facilitatory centers in the pontomedullary reticular formation for motor tone can function autonomously (pontine reticulospinal tract). The inhibitory centers in the pontomedullary reticular formation require continual input from the cerebral cortex, basal nuclei, and cerebellum to function (medullary reticulospinal tract). This input is sacrificed by the lesion, causing the imbalance in function observed as a release phenomenon. In decerebrate rigidity there is a release of the alpha and gamma efferent neurons from the influence of the inhibitory descending upper motor neuron spinal cord tracts. The vestibulospinal tract contributes its facilitatory influence to that of the pontine reticulospinal tract.

The myotatic reflex and normal tonic mechanisms also can be influenced by disturbances in the spinal cord segments. As a result of the intoxication caused by the growth of *Clostridium tetani* in the tissues and the production of the tetanus toxin, or by the absorption of ingested strychnine, a similar release phenomenon occurs, consisting of opisthotonos and persistent rigid extension of all four limbs.[40, 56, 58] These toxins are inhibitory to the activity of interneurons in the ventral grey column of the spinal cord which are known as Renshaw cells. These interneurons normally are inhibitory to the alpha motor neuron and are stimulated by recurrent collaterals of the alpha motor neurons. They function to limit the duration, intensity, and distribution of the motor neuron discharge. These toxins cause postsynaptic inhibition at the telodendron of the Renshaw cells. The clinical signs reflect the released alpha motor neuron activity from this source of inhibition.

A recent review of the neural control of locomotion has attempted to apply a model for normal voluntary locomotor function to clinical problems in animals.[29] The basic assumption is that two systems control skeletal muscle movement. The postural control system maintains posture by controlling trunk muscles and the antigravity (extensor) muscles of the proximal limbs. The vestibulospinal and reticulospinal tracts from the medulla and pons facilitate these postural muscles and inhibit most flexor muscles. The voluntary control system initiates voluntary locomotor movement and emanates from the cerebral cortex, extrapyramidal basal nuclei, and red nuclei. It influences spinal motoneurons by way of the corticospinal and rubrospinal tracts. Their function is opposed to that of the postural system, and is facilitatory to flexor muscles and all distal limb muscles, while simultaneously inhibiting antigravity muscles.

Basic locomotor activity may involve recruitment of reflexes by these control mechanisms, alternating between the voluntary and postural systems. The voluntary system recruits flexor reflexes (muscles) to initiate the protraction phase of the gait, and the postural system recruits extensor reflexes for the supporting and propulsive phases of the gait. This hypothesis is attractive and is supported by physiologic studies, but it oversimplifies the voluntary control system. The components that are described can be absent, and other components that presumably are brain stem mechanisms can function in the voluntary initiation of locomotion.

Clinical and experimental lesions that destroy the motor cortex or lentiform and caudate nuclei in the domestic animal provide evidence that these anatomic structures are not necessary for the initiation of voluntary movement. Progressing caudally, evidence of paresis of voluntary movement only first occurs with lesions in the rostral midbrain, but experimental destruction of the red nucleus does not induce paresis. Postural reactions are deficient, possibly due to some loss of volun-

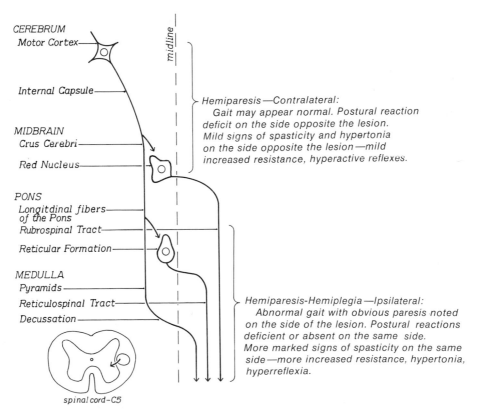

Figure 7–9.   Diagram of upper motor neuron pathways for voluntary movement.

tary facilitation of flexor muscles necessary to initiate the motor phase of most of these reactions. Whereas experimental lesions that destroy the lateral corticospinal and rubrospinal tracts do not produce a gait deficiency, clinical disease (infarction) that destroys all of the lateral funiculus but spares the other funiculi produces an ipsilateral hemiplegia. The loss of other descending motor systems in this funiculus, presumably reticulospinal, must be responsible for the inability to initiate movement. Although the voluntary initiation of locomotion in domestic animals is assumed to be a brain stem function, it has not been defined specifically in anatomic terms.

CLINICAL SIGNS: UPPER MOTOR NEURON DISEASE

Paresis. Disturbance to the mechanism for initiating voluntary motor function causes paresis (weakness) or paralysis, depending on the severity of the lesion. The severity of the paresis increases as the location of the lesion descends in the upper motor neuron to involve more of the pathways.

Unilateral lesions of the upper motor neuron rostral to the red nucleus cause contralateral hemiparesis that is so mild it may not be apparent in the gait. However, the response to postural reaction testing is deficient. This is exemplified by experimental removal of the motor area of the cerebrum or complete removal of the cortex of one hemisphere. Chronic lesions confined to one cerebrum or its internal capsule involving the upper motor neuron present a similar clinical syndrome. Lesions that involve the upper motor neuron in the motor cortex or internal capsule also involve the ascending cerebral pathway for general proprioception. The contralateral deficit that is observed in the postural reactions is designated hemiparesis, and in reality is also a reflection of this proprioceptive deficit. Unilateral lesions in the midbrain tegmentum, substantia nigra, and crus cerebri produce a contralateral hemiparesis that usually is observed as a mild deficiency in gait and in postural reactions. The degree of paresis may depend on the acuteness of the lesion. An acute destructive lesion in the rostral midbrain from the migration of a *Cuterebra* larva involved the entire right crus cerebri in a cat. This lesion was continued rostrally by a large hematoma in the right ventrolateral diencephalon. This cat had a dense hemiplegia on the left side and mild paresis on the right side.

Unilateral lesions in the pons and medulla usually produce an ipsilateral hemiparesis of the gait and a postural reaction deficiency. The gait dysfunction is more obvious if the unilateral lesion is further caudal in the medulla or cranial cervical spinal cord.

Apparently the anatomic landmark for focal lesions that produce ipsilateral hemiparesis is somewhere in the middle of the mesencephalon. When the lesion occurs rostral to this area, the hemiparesis is contralateral and less profound.

A lesion that destroys only the lateral funiculus of the cervical spinal cord causes complete paralysis of the ipsilateral limbs. This is a hemiplegia. Lesions that involve both sides of the caudal brain stem or cervical spinal cord cranial to the second thoracic spinal cord segment cause tetraparesis or tetraplegia (quadriplegia). Lesions of the spinal cord caudal to the third thoracic spinal cord segment cause loss of voluntary movement in the pelvic limbs or paraparesis if partial, paraplegia if complete.

If the lesion that disturbs the upper motor neuron pathways does not interfere with the grey matter or roots of the spinal cord in the cervical or lumbosacral intumescence, no loss of the reflex arcs occurs and no lower motor neuron clinical signs appear.

Myotatic Reflexes. The disturbance to the descending upper motor neuron pathways involved in the maintenance of muscle tone usually causes signs of myotatic reflexes released from the effects of the inhibitory UMN pathways.[31] All spinal reflexes are intact. Myotatic reflexes—patellar, biceps, triceps—may be intact, or hyperactive (hyperreflexia), or clonus may be observed. Hypertonia is manifested by increased resistance to passive manipulation of the limbs, and represents exaggerated contraction of muscles subjected to stretch due to the released myotatic reflex. Flexor reflexes may show a prolonged afterdischarge, which is observed as repetitive flexion of the limb in the absence of repeated stimuli. The crossed extensor reflex is an example of this release phenomenon when exhibited in a recumbent animal that exerts no voluntary effort to remove itself from the stimulus. In most cases of focal spinal cord lesions that disturb the descending upper motor neuron pathways, one or more of these signs of a released lower motor neuron are observed. Occasionally, hypotonia instead of hypertonia is seen. However, reflexes are still intact because of the lack of direct disturbance of the lower motor neuron. Whether this represents a greater disturbance to the descending facilitatory pathways is not known.

A naturally occurring disease syndrome in cats causes acute destruction of the cerebral portions of this upper motor neuron and demonstrates its limited effect on locomotion.

CEREBRAL VASCULAR DISEASE IN CATS. A neurologic syndrome has been recognized in cats which consists of a peracute onset of signs of a cerebral disturbance that most often are unilateral. These signs are caused by an extensive ischemic necrosis of cerebral tissue.

The disease affects adult cats of all ages and both sexes. Although it tends to occur more commonly in the summer months, a few cases have been seen in the fall and winter.

The onset is variable. Some cases show only severe depression with mild ataxia, or circling, or both. Some animals circle continuously. Others begin with seizures, and the seizure activity may be unilateral and consist of tonic or clonic activity of the muscles on one side of the head, trunk, and limbs. Changes in attitude and behavior are common, and may involve severe aggression. Pupils often are dilated, and blindness may be apparent. For the first 1 to 2 days there may be an observable hemiparesis.

These acute signs usually resolve in a few days to residual signs of a nonprogressive unilateral cerebral lesion. Destruction of the sensorimotor cortex or its cerebral pathway causes an obvious deficit in the contralateral postural reactions, but there is little interference with the gait. The loss of the visual cerebral cortex or optic radiation results in a contralateral failure to respond to a menacing gesture, but pupillary responses to light are normal. Unilateral cerebral lesions often cause an animal to pace slowly in a circle toward the side of the abnormal cerebrum. These lesions are usually in the frontal lobe, and the head turning and circling toward the diseased cerebrum sometimes are referred to as part of the adversive syndrome. The specific cause is unknown, but these are fairly reliable signs. Occasionally, a cat continues to have seizures. These may be generalized or partial motor seizures in which the seizure activity is observed in the muscles on the side of the head and body opposite to the diseased cerebrum. This shows the influence of the cerebral upper motor neuron on the lower motor neuron to the opposite side of the head and body. Involvement of limbic system structures such as the amygdala and hippocampus may be the cause of the behavioral change, which is often permanent.

Occasionally, bilateral blindness persists along with dilated unresponsive pupils, because of ischemic necrosis of the optic chiasm. Careful examination may reveal a unilateral facial hypalgesia, contralateral to the cerebral lesion. No other cranial nerve deficits have been observed. Spinal flexor reflexes are normal, as is pain perception from the limbs. There may be mild hypertonia and hyperreflexia of tendon reflexes that is more pronounced on the side on which the postural reactions are deficient.

The lesion consists of a variable degree of ischemic necrosis of the cerebral hemisphere, usually unilateral but occasionally bilateral. Most of the necrosis is entirely ischemic. Occasionally, hemorrhages occur in the parenchyma or in the leptomeninges. The necrosis may be multifocal or the infarction may involve up to two thirds of one entire cerebrum. Frequently the major infarction lesion has been in the distribution of the middle cerebral artery. In chronic cases, gross atrophy is most marked in the vicinity of this vessel on the lateral side of the infarcted cerebrum.

Vascular lesions have been found in only a few cases. These have consisted of a large thrombus in the middle cerebral artery, venous thrombosis, and vasculitis consisting of mononuclear cells in old cases and neutrophils in early cases. The case with the thrombosed middle cerebral artery had an extensive associated vasculitis with neutrophils and eosinophils. In one case autopsied 3 months after the onset, a dead nematode was found in the thalamus. Its significance remains to be proved.

Neutrophils are abundant in the degenerate tissue of an acute ischemic lesion if the blood supply remains. These soon are replaced by mononuclear cells that phagocytize the dead debris. In a few cases there is no evidence of a primary inflammatory lesion associated with the blood vessels. No lesions have been found in other organs, including the heart. Up to the present time tissue culture studies for viral isolation have been unrewarding.

Hematologic studies and urinalyses have been normal in these subjects. CSF often has a mildly elevated protein level, with little to no cell accumulation. Scintigraphy and electroencephalography sometimes have indicated the location of the lesion.

The prognosis for life is good, since this is not a progressive disorder. Only one known case has died, 12 hours after the onset of clinical signs. All others have lived; however, their behavioral changes often have interfered with their relationships with their owners. In a few instances persistent uncontrollable seizures have been a problem.

Involuntary Adventitious Movements. In primates disturbances to the extrapyramidal system in the brain sometimes result in the production of repetitive, involuntary, adventitious movements. Examples of these are postural tremor, athetosis, dystonia, ballism, chorea, and myoclonus.[15] The presence of one of these signs is not pathognomonic for any one specific disease or deficiency of any one nuclear area.

A postural tremor is produced by small, rapid, alternating contractions of opposed muscle groups. It is observed at rest and often disappears with activity. It is evident especially in the hands and fingers, and is characteristic of the patient with parkinsonism. These patients also may develop rigidity of joints from incapacitating relentless muscle hypertonia. In the past therapy for this has included surgical destruction of a specific anatomic site in the extrapyramidal system that is responsible for initiating the tremor and hypertonia. More recently, therapy has involved the replacement of a deficient neurotransmitter substance, dopamine.

Athetosis is slow, writhing movements of the extremities. Dystonia is the same phenomenon in the axial musculoskeletal system. Ballism is violent flailing of a limb. Chorea is continual but irregular jerky rapid movements of different muscle groups. Myoclonus is repetitive, rhythmic, contractions of the same group of muscles that may persist during sleep and under light anesthesia. Comparable diseases and signs in domestic animals are rare.

Experimental lesions in these extrapyramidal nuclei of dogs and cats do not produce overt signs of paresis or adventitious movements. In some instances dogs with such lesions may tend to circle or turn the head to one side. A hereditary disease occurs in Kerry blue terriers in which a bilateral symmetric degeneration occurs in the substantia nigra and caudate nucleus, along with the cerebellar cortex. The clinical signs of severe spastic dysmetric ataxia reflect the cerebellar lesion that precedes the extrapyramidal lesion.[61]

EQUINE NIGROPALLIDAL ENCEPHALOMALACIA. A disease is found in horses that causes an acute destruction of extrapyramidal nuclei, with signs of muscle rigidity. Nigropallidal encephalomalacia occurs in horses that consume a specific plant over a prolonged period.[16, 20, 37, 60] The plant usually involved is *Centaurea solstitialis*, star thistle, found mostly in California and Oregon. Signs of intoxication appear suddenly after weeks of grazing on this plant, with marked hypertonia, rigidity of the muscles of the head causing facial immobility, retraction of the lips and nose, protrusion of the tongue, and inability to prehend food, which results in death from starvation. Continual purposeless chewing movements may occur. Limb hypertonia is less evident. The patients are depressed. The major lesion is a bilateral symmetric necrosis of the substantia nigra and pallidum related to the chronic consumption of this plant. The lesion occurs suddenly, and is ischemic in nature. It is found only in horses and can be reproduced experimentally. The pathogenesis is unknown.

These signs are similar to the hypertonia and rigidity seen in some of the diseases of the extrapyramidal nuclei in man, and reflect the role of this system in the maintenance of normal muscle tone and motor activity. It is of interest that the muscles most obviously affected in the horse have the largest representation in the motor area of the cerebral cortex.

CANINE MYOCLONUS. Involuntary adventitious movements are common only in one clinical disease of domestic animals, canine myoclonus. Its pathogenesis differs from that usually observed in man. Myoclonus occurs in dogs and usually is related to a previous nonsuppurative encephalitis or myelitis caused by the canine distemper virus.[7, 34, 35, 51, 52, 57] Many synonyms for this disease exist in the literature, including canine chorea, flexor spasm, and tremor syndrome. Most veterinarians call it distemper chorea. By definition it is not chorea as it occurs in man, but myoclonus, a repetitive, rhythmic contraction of the same group of muscles, up to 60 per minute. Repetitive flexion of one limb, thoracic or pelvic, or both limbs on one side, or contractions of the muscles of mastication, are examples of the groups involved. The muscle groups involved may change as the disease progresses. There may be mild paresis of these muscles. The movements usually persist during sleep and at times under light anesthesia. These signs usually follow the overt signs of encephalitis. Occasionally, myoclonus precedes these signs or it may appear with no other signs of encephalomyelitis. The pathogenesis of the myoclonus is unknown. Experimental studies have shown that once the myoclonus has been established, the segments of the spinal cord that contain the lower motor neuron of the muscles involved in the myoclonus can be cut off from the brain by transection of the spinal cord cranial to their level, and the myoclonus still persists. It even continues following section of the dorsal roots of these spinal cord segments. Ventral root section abolishes the myoclonus. It is hypothesized that a pacemaker is established in the spinal cord motor neuron pool that causes a spontaneous depolarization and discharge of the alpha motor neuron. Lesions are not always evident in the vicinity of this motor neuron pool. There is no specific treatment, and the accompanying signs of encephalomyelitis may progress. Occasionally, the encephalitic signs regress or stabilize and the myoclonus persists. In a few cases the myoclonus has resolved spontaneously.

The following two diseases of domestic animals may represent a disturbance of the myotatic reflex mechanism. No lesions have been found in the nervous system.

"SCOTTY CRAMPS". Hyperkinetic episodes occur in Scottish terrier dogs and often are called "Scotty cramps."[38, 39] The syndrome also has been reported in Cairn terriers. The signs, which are variable with each case, commence between 6 weeks and 18 months of age, and are stimulated by exercise or excitement. Increased "stiffness" and hyperflexion followed by hyperextension of the limbs are observed. Rapid extension of the pelvic limbs may cause the animal to lose its balance. Occasionally, the pelvic limbs become resistant to flexion and act like pillars, so that the dog is unable to walk. The spasms may affect the cervical and facial musculature. These episodes are not accompanied by any disturbance in consciousness. A short period of rest usually alleviates the signs. Treatment with diazepam (Valium), a muscle relaxant that functions in the CNS, stops the signs and continual daily therapy decreases their incidence. Physiologic studies suggest that the muscle hypertonicity is the result of a spinal cord disturbance and is not due to a muscle disorder. The disturbance may involve the myotatic reflex mechanism. Pharmacologic studies have suggested that this may be a disorder of serotonergic neurons that normally inhibit motor activity.

SPASTIC SYNDROME. Spastic syndrome, crampiness, or stretches, occurs most commonly in the Holstein and Guernsey breeds, commencing between 3 and 7 years of age.[49] It becomes evident in the standing animal as episodes of marked extension of the pelvic limbs. The prolonged spasms are evident in the extensor muscles of the lumbar vertebrae. The signs often are stimulated when the animal gets up, and disappear when it lies down. In most cattle the signs are mild, with the episodes lasting from a few seconds to several minutes, or occasionally longer. These signs persist for the duration of the animal's life. The syndrome is thought to be inherited as a single recessive factor with incomplete penetrance. The pathogenesis is unknown. It may represent a primary disturbance of the myotatic reflex, or a defect in the postural reflex mechanism.

Tetany—Tremors

Because tetany and tremors represent a neuromuscular disturbance that in some instances may have its genesis in the extrapyramidal system, a differential diagnosis is described briefly here.

Tetany. Tetany is a disorder marked by intermittent tonic muscular contractions, as opposed to tetanus, which is a sustained muscular contraction usually manifested in the antigravity muscles. In some instances tetany may accompany the tetanus that occurs in the disease tetanus or in strychnine poisoning. Tetany may accompany other signs of diffuse brain disease, such as encephalitis caused by a variety of agents, polioencephalomalacia from abnormal thiamine metabolism and lead intoxication, and acute organophosphate intoxication.

Transport tetany has been described in lambs shortly after arrival at a feedlot. Ewes and cows, especially late in gestation, are susceptible to a similar syndrome of tetany following prolonged transport.[5, 27, 46] Mortality is high, with death following a period of coma. The pathogenesis is unknown beyond the obvious involvement of severe physical stress, but hypocalcemia and hypomagnesemia often accompany the tetany. A similar syndrome occasionally is seen in horses, especially in lactating mares, that have been feeding on lush pasture and suddenly become severely stressed. Hypocalcemia is a constant finding, and the response to calcium therapy may be dramatic.

Grass tetany occurs in lactating cattle that recently have been exposed to fresh lush pasture, and often is accompanied by hypomagnesemia and hypocalcemia. Calves may show tetany with an electrolyte imbalance associated with profuse diarrhea, or tetany with hypomagnesemia, hypocalcemia, and occasionally diarrhea when fed solely on a whole milk diet.

Hereford calves with hereditary neuraxial edema are unable to get up at birth.[17] When stimulated, they show tetany of the limbs and neck that lasts from 1 to 2 minutes. If supported, the limbs remain rigidly extended.

Tetany also may occur in white muscle disease of calves and lambs.

Tetany is found most commonly in dogs in association with parturition, and usually hypocalcemia and occasionally hypoglycemia are present. It also may occur in chronic kidney disease accompanied by uremia, especially when of a congenital nature. These dogs also may be hypocalcemic. Inadvertent removal of both parathyroid glands causes hypocalcemia and tetany.

Tremors. Tremors, trembling, or shaking also can occur as the only clinical sign or as one of a group of clinical signs associated with a diffuse disturbance of brain function.

LARGE ANIMALS. In animals that graze, a number of diseases of suspected mycotoxic origin have been recognized.[18, 36] Paspalum staggers or dallis grass poisoning affects cattle, sheep, and horses that graze on grasses of the genus *Paspalum,* which support the growth of the fungus *Claviceps paspali.* Tremors, hyperexcitability, and ataxia occur. Similarly, animals grazing on plants infected by various species of *Penicillium* may show a tremor that is exacerbated by forced movement or excitement. This produces a spastic ataxia which may cause them to fall, and convulsions may occur. A number of tremorgenic toxins have been isolated from these fungi.

Some plants themselves may produce a toxin at various stages of their growth that on ingestion produces tremors, staggering, and ataxia, with occasional falling. Probably the best example of this is phalaris staggers, which is seen commonly in sheep in Australia and New Zealand that graze on Harding grass (*Phalaris tuberosa*).[21, 22] Some sheep collapse suddenly and die after an acute course, whereas others show signs of a chronic neurologic disturbance consisting of tremors, ataxia, and occasionally convulsions. A tryptamine alkaloid is being investigated as the possible toxic substance that may interfere with serotonin metabolism in these animals.[30] Cobalt may be protective for the chronic neurologic form.

The outbreak of possibly similar phalaris staggers has been reported in cattle in California grazing on canary grass (*Phalaris minor*). Only the chronic signs of intoxication were seen, with a spastic (stiff-legged) ataxia accompanied by falling, trembling, difficulty in prehension, and licking movements of the tongue. All signs were exacerbated by excitement. Organophosphate poisoning could not be excluded completely from this report as a cause.

Rye grass staggers may occur in grazing sheep, cattle, and horses.[14] It is less fatal than the type caused by the phalaris grasses. Clinical signs vary in severity, from slight spasms and stiffness of the limbs after running to total tetany, causing immobility and often lateral recumbency. The signs are aggravated by excitement and forced locomotion. Recovery usually follows removal of the animal from the rye grass pasture. The toxic principle is unknown.

A toxic alcohol, tremetol, present in white snakeroot (*Eupatorium rugosum*) causes severe muscle tremors, salivation, vomiting, and dyspnea, which progress to recumbency, coma, and death.

Constant tremors also have been seen at or near birth in lambs, calves, and pigs with congenital failure of myelin formation. This has been described as hypomyelinogenesis in sheep and pigs and as an hereditary leukodysplasia in Jersey calves.[32, 50] Other breeds of cattle have been described with the same clinical signs and lesions. In border disease of sheep, abnormal myelin formation and clusters of swollen interstitial glia in the CNS have been found.[2, 26, 43] Newborn lambs with this disease quiver constantly and often have an abnormal hair coat. The name "hairy shaker disease" has been applied to this disorder. There is some evidence to support the possibility of a transmissible agent in the pathogenesis of this disease.[19] The porcine disease has been referred to as myoclonia congenita.[62] However, it is important to recognize that the myoclonus or tremor is only associated with voluntary movement. This is also true in the lambs and calves. The tremor is absent when the animal is recumbent and not moving. Both inheritance factors and viral agents have been implicated in the abnormal myelin formation in the central nervous system of affected swine. If nursed properly some of these animals will spontaneously recover from the clinical signs.

Shivering is a rare idiopathic disease in horses, primarily in those of the heavier breeds.[12] The clinical signs usually are observed when the animal first is moved, especially backward. They are most prominent in the pelvic limbs and tail, and consist of spasmodic, jerky, extension of the tail, tense, trembling pelvic limb muscles, quivering of the superficial rump and thigh muscles (shivering), and an occasional elevation and abduction of one pelvic limb, which is held in space momentarily before being returned slowly to the ground. These signs last only a few minutes and disappear with rest, but appear again on the next movement. This disease is insidiously progressive. There is no effective therapy.

SMALL ANIMALS.　In dogs, tremors are associated most often with other signs of diffuse brain disease frequently caused by an intoxication. Metaldehyde (snail bait), organophosphates, chlorinated hydrocarbons, and fluoroacetate are the most common causes of these signs. Occasionally, tremors occur with varying degrees of diffuse nonsuppurative encephalitis. Tremors also may accompany the tetany of hypocalcemia and sometimes appear in hypoglycemic animals.

In mature dogs a syndrome of unknown pathogenesis occurs characterized by a sudden onset of constant tremors all over the body, including the head and eyeballs. It is exaggerated by handling, forced locomotion, and excitement. It decreases, but does not disappear with total relaxation. The dogs are alert and responsive, and have no insufficiency in cranial nerve function. The tremors may be severe enough to cause an ataxic gait, but strength seems normal. Occasionally, one of these dogs convulses. All laboratory studies for blood cytology and chemistry, including electrolytes, are normal. CSF determinations are normal. No history or evidence of intoxication can be found. Anticonvulsant therapy with primidone, phenobarbital, diphenylhydantoin, and diazepam has not proved obviously efficacious. In some dogs the signs resolve in a few weeks, while others take months, and a few never fully recover. The signs usually do not progress. The pathogenesis of this disease is unknown.

REFERENCES

1. Amann, J. F.: The organization of spinal motoneurons and their relationship to corticospinal fibers in the racoon (Procyon lotor). Ph.D. thesis, Ithaca, N.Y., Cornell University, 1971.
2. Barlow, R. M., and Dickinson, A. G.: On the pathology and histochemistry of the central nervous system in border disease of sheep. Res. Vet. Sci., 6:230, 1965.
3. Barone, R.: Les voies descendantes dans le névraxe des Equidés. Bull. Acad. Vet. Fr., 39:137, 1966.
4. Belmusto, L., Waldring, S., and Owens, G.: Localization and patterns of potentials of the respiratory pathway in the cervical spinal cord in the dog. J. Neurosurg., 22:277, 1965.
5. Blood, D. C., and Henderson, J. A.: Veterinary Medicine. 4th ed., Baltimore, Williams & Wilkins, 1974.
6. Breazile, J. E., and Thompson, W. D.: Motor cortex of the dog. Am. J. Vet. Res., 28:1483, 1967.
7. Breazile, J. E., Blaugh, B. S., and Nail, N.: Experimental study of canine distemper myoclonus. Am. J. Vet. Res., 27:1375, 1966.
8. Breazile, J. E., Jennings, D. P., and Swafford, B. C.: Conduction velocities in the corticospinal tract of the horse. Exp. Neurol., 17:357, 1967.
9. Breazile, J. E., Swafford, B. C., and Biles, A. R.: Motor cortex of the horse. Am. J. Vet. Res., 27:1605, 1966.
10. Breazile, J. E., Swafford, B. C., and Thompson, W. D.: Study of the motor cortex of the domestic pig. Am. J. Vet. Res., 27:1369, 1966.
11. Buxton, D. F., and Goodman, D. C.: Motor function and the corticospinal tracts in the dog and racoon. J. Comp. Neurol., 129:341, 1967.
12. Catcott, E. J., and Smithcors, J. F.: Equine Medicine and Surgery. 2nd ed., Wheaton, Ill., American Veterinary Publications, Inc., 1972.
13. Chambers, W. W., and Liu, C. N.: Corticospinal tract in the cat. J. Comp. Neurol., 108:23, 1957.
14. Clegg, F. G., and Watson, W. A.: Rye grass staggers in sheep. Vet. Rec., 72:731, 1960.
15. Cooper, I. S., Samra, K., and Bergmann, L.: The thalamic lesion which abolishes tremor and rigidity of Parkinsonism. A radiologic-clinico-anatomic correlation study. J. Neurol. Sci., 8:69, 1969.
16. Cordy, D. R.: Nigropallidal encephalomalacia in horses associated with ingestion of yellow star thistle. J. Neuropathol. Exp. Neurol., 13:330, 1954.
17. Cordy, D. R., Richards, W. P. C., and Stormont, C.: Hereditary neuraxial edema in Hereford calves. Pathol. Vet., 6:487, 1969.
18. Cysewski, S. J.: Paspalum staggers and tremergen intoxication in animals. J. Am. Vet. Med. Assoc., 163:1291, 1973.
19. Dickinson, A. G., and Barlow, R. M.: The demonstration of the transmissibility of border disease of sheep. Vet. Rec., 81:114, 1967.
20. Fowler, M. E.: Nigropallidal encephalomalacia in the horse. J. Am. Vet. Med. Assoc., 147:607, 1965.
21. Gallagher, C. H., Koch, J. H., and Hoffman, H.: Diseases of sheep due to ingestion of Phalaris tuberosa. Aust. Vet. J., 42:279, 1966.
22. Gallagher, C. H., Koch, J. H., Moore, R. M., and Steel, J. D.: Toxicity of Phalaris tuberosa for sheep. Nature, 204:542, 1964.
23. Hongo, T., Jankowska, E., and Lundberg, A.: The rubrospinal tract. 1. Effects on alpha-motor neurons innervating hind limb muscles in cat. Exp. Brain Res., 7:334, 1969.
24. Hukuda, S., Jameson, H. D., and Wilson, C. B.: Experimental cervical myelopathy. III. The canine corticospinal tract. Anatomy and function. Surg. Neurol., 1:107, 1973.
25. Ingram, W. R., and Ranson, S. W.: Effects of lesions in the red nuclei in cats. Arch. Neurol. Psychiatry, 28:483, 1932.
26. Innes, J. R. M., and Saunders, L. Z.: Comparative Neuropathology. New York, Academic Press, 1962.

27. Kronfeld, D. S., and Hammel, E. P.: Differential diagnosis, treatment, and prevention of tetany in cattle. Am. Assoc. Bovine Pract. Proc., 1974.
28. Lassek, A. M., Dowd, L. W., and Weil, A.: The quantitative distribution of the pyramidal tract in the dog. J. Comp. Neurol., *51*:153, 1930.
29. Latshaw, W. K.: A model for the neural control of locomotion. J. Am. Anim. Hosp. Assoc., *10*:598, 1974.
30. Lee, H. J., Kuchel, R. E., Good, B. F., and Trowbridge, R. F.: The etiology of phalaris staggers in sheep. IV. The site of preventive action and its specificity to cobalt. Aust. J. Agri. Res., 8:502, 1957.
31. Magoun, H. N., and Rhines, R.: Spasticity, the Stretch Reflex, and Extrapyramidal Systems. Springfield, Ill., Charles C Thomas, 1948.
32. Markson, L. M., Terlicki, S., Shand, A., Sellers, K. C., and Woods, A. J.: Hypomyelinogenesis congenita in sheep. Vet. Rec., *71*:269, 1959.
33. Marsden, C. D.: The development of pigmentation and enzyme activity in the nucleus substantiae nigrae of the cat. J. Anat. (Lond.), 99:175, 1965.
34. Mason, M. M.: Rhythmic myoclonic convulsions in dogs. Vet. Rec., 58:247, 1946.
35. McGovern, V. J., Steel, J. D., Wyke, B. D., and Dobson, M. E.: Canine encephalitis causing a syndrome characterized by tremor. Aust. J. Exp. Biol. Med. Sci., 28:433, 1950.
36. Mendel, V. E., Crenshaw, D. L., Baker, N. F., and Muniz, R.: Staggers in pastured cattle. J. Am. Vet. Med. Assoc., *154*:769, 1969.
37. Mettler, F. A., and Stern, G. M.: Observations on the toxic effects of yellow star thistle. J. Neuropathol. Exp. Neurol., 22:164, 1963.
38. Meyers, K. M., Dickson, W. M., and Schaub, R. G.: Serotonin involvement in a motor disorder of Scottish terrier dogs. Life Sci., *13*:1261, 1973.
39. Meyers, K. M., Lund, J. E., Padgett, G., and Dickson, W. M.: Hyperkinetic episodes in Scottish terrier dogs. J. Am. Vet. Med. Assoc., *155*:129, 1969.
40. Muylle, E., Oyaert, W., Ooms, L., and Decraemere, H.: Treatment of tetanus in the horse by injections of tetanus antitoxin into the subarachnoid space. J. Am. Vet. Med. Assoc., *167*:47, 1975.
41. Nyberg-Hansen, R.: Sites and mode of termination of reticulospinal fibers in the cat. J. Comp. Neurol., *124*:71, 1965.
42. Nyberg-Hansen, R., and Brodal, A.: Sites of termination of corticospinal fibers in the cat. An experimental study with silver impregnation methods. J. Comp. Neurol., *120*:369, 1963.
43. Osborne, B. I., Clarke, G. L., Stewart, W. C., and Sawyer, M.: Border disease-like syndrome in lambs: Antibodies to hog cholera and bovine viral diarrhea viruses. J. Am. Vet. Med. Assoc., *163*:1165, 1973.
44. Petras, J. M.: Afferent fibers to the spinal cord. The terminal distribution of dorsal root and encephalospinal axons. Med. Serv. J. Can., 22:668, 1966.
45. Petras, J. M.: Cortical, tectal, and tegmental fiber connections in the spinal cord of the cat. Brain Res., 6:275, 1967.
46. Pierson, R. E., and Jensen, R.: Transport tetany of feedlot lambs. J. Am. Vet. Med. Assoc., *166*:260, 1975.
47. Pompeiano, O., and Brodal, A.: Experimental demonstration of a somatotopical origin of rubrospinal fibers in the cat. J. Comp. Neurol., *108*:225, 1957.
48. Rinvick, E., and Walberg, F.: Demonstration of a somatotopically arranged corticorubral projection in the cat. An experimental study with silver methods. J. Comp. Neurol., *120*:393, 1963.
49. Roberts, S. J.: Hereditary spastic disease affecting cattle in New York State. Cor. Vet., 55:637, 1965.
50. Saunders, L. Z., Sweet, J. D., Martin, S. M., Fox, F. H., and Fincher, M. G.: Hereditary congenital ataxia in Jersey calves. Cor. Vet., *42*:559, 1952.
51. Turbes, C.: Studies on involuntary movements at rest in the dog. Anat. Rec., *118*:362, 1954.
52. Turbes, C. C., Abreau, B., and Richards, A.: Experimental studies of involuntary motor activity. Neurology, *13*:351, 1963.
53. Udall, D. H.: The Practice of Veterinary Medicine. Ithaca, N.Y., 1954.
54. Verhaart, W. J. C.: The pyramidal tract—its structure and function in man and animals. World Neurol., 3:43, 1962.
55. Webster, K. E.: The cortico-striatal projection in the cat. J. Anat., 99:329, 1965.
56. Weinstein, L.: Tetanus—current concepts. N. Engl. J. Med., 289:1293, 1973.
57. Whittier, J. R.: Flexor spasm syndrome in the carnivore. Am. J. Vet. Res., *17*:720, 1956.
58. Wilson, V. J.: Inhibition in the central nervous system. Sci. Am., *214*:102, 1966.
59. Woosley, C. N.: Postural relations of the frontal and motor cortex of the dog. Brain, 56:353, 1933.
60. Young, S., Brown, W. W., and Klinger, H.: Nigropallidal encephalomalacia in horses caused by ingestion of weeds of the genus *Centaurea*. J. Am. Vet. Med. Assoc., *157*:1602, 1970.
61. de Lahunta, A., and Averill, D. R., Jr.: Hereditary cerebellar cortical and extrapyramidal nuclear abiotrophy in Kerry Blue Terriers. J. Am. Vet. Med. Assoc., *168*:1119, 1976.
62. Fletcher, T. F.: Ablation and histopathologic studies on myoclonia congenita in swine. Am. J. Vet. Res., *29*:2255, 1968.

Chapter 8

GENERAL PROPRIOCEPTION SYSTEM — GP

SENSORY SYSTEMS
GENERAL PROPRIOCEPTION
SPINAL NERVES
Proprioceptive Pathway for Reflex Activity and
  Cerebellar Transmission
Cerebellar Pathway
Proprioceptive Pathway to the Somesthetic
  Cortex for Conscious Perception

Lateral Cervical Nucleus
CRANIAL NERVES
Reflex
Conscious Perception
CLINICAL SIGNS
DISEASES

SENSORY SYSTEMS

Sensory systems are characterized by a peripheral afferent neuron with a dendritic zone (modified in many neurons to form a receptor organ), an axon that courses into the grey matter of the central nervous system, a cell body in a ganglion of the peripheral nervous system, and centrally located relay nuclei and tracts primarily passing to a specific thalamic projection nucleus, which relays to a sensory area of the cerebral cortex. Each type of sensation is known as a modality, a form of energy converted by the receptor organ into a neuronal impulse. These include touch, temperature, movement, light, sound, chemicals, and pressure, and they inform the nervous system of the features of the external and internal environments of the body. In some instances there is a specific neuroanatomic structural pathway for certain modalities. Most receptor organs have a low threshold for a certain modality, but still can be stimulated by other modalities. This form of energy to which a receptor organ is most sensitive is referred to as the adequate stimulus. Anatomically, there are encapsulated and nonencapsulated receptor organs. The neuronal terminal of the encapsulated receptor (dendritic zone) is associated with a well-developed connective tissue capsule, of which there are many varieties. In the nonencapsulated forms there is no connective tissue modification of the dendritic zone. Although the connective tissue modification of the encapsulated endings may provide the structural features necessary for that receptor to be sensitive to one specific modality or energy form, the sensitivity is not limited necessarily to that one modality. Several forms of energy may excite that receptor. Even without obvious connective tissue modification, the nonencapsulated receptors exhibit low thresholds of sensitivity to one specific modality. The histologic characteristics of the receptor do not necessarily restrict the receptor to sensitivity to one specific modality. Nevertheless, they are classified as thermoreceptors, mechanoreceptors, chemoreceptors, and photoreceptors, based on their adequate stimulus.

Receptors have been classified according to their location in the body. Exteroceptors are located on the surface of the body, and are sensitive to changes in the external environment affecting the body surface. These include general somatic afferent (GSA) neurons for touch, temperature, pressure, and noxious stimuli, and special somatic afferent (SSA) neurons for light and sound. Proprioceptors are sensitive to movement, and are located in the internal mass of the body in muscles, tendons, and joints (general proprioception—GP), and in the labyrinth of the inner ear (special proprioception—SP). Interoceptors are located within the body viscera, and are sensitive to changes in the internal environment. These include general visceral afferent (GVA) neurons for body temperature, blood pressure, gas concentration, pressure and movement in viscera, and special visceral afferent (SVA) neurons for chemical energy (smell and taste).

The sensation of pain is a cerebral interpretation, a subjective response to the stimulation of various receptors called nociceptors. This group of receptors is nonselective in the form of energy that elicits its maximal response, but the stimulus threshold for these modalities is high. The intensity of stimulation necessary to evoke an impulse from these receptors is at a level that is potentially destructive to tissue; for example, high-intensity excitation by mechanical, electrical, thermal, or chemical stimuli.

GENERAL PROPRIOCEPTION—GP

General proprioceptive neurons constitute a sensory system to detect the state of position or movement in muscles, tendons, and joints. Two basic pathways will be described for this system. One involves the pathway for segmental reflex activity and for transmitting proprioceptive information to the cerebellum. The other involves the transmission of proprioceptive information to the sensory somesthetic cerebral cortex. These pathways will be considered separately for spinal nerves and cranial nerves.

SPINAL NERVES

The general proprioceptive (GP) afferent has its dendritic zone (receptor organ) in a muscle, a tendon, or a joint. The Ia afferent in neuromuscular spindles and the Golgi tendon organs are examples of such receptors. The axons course proximally in peripheral nerves to the spinal nerve and through the spinal ganglion associated with the dorsal root of that spinal nerve. The cell body of the GP afferent is in the segmental spinal ganglion. The axon continues in the dorsal root and enters the spinal cord along the dorsolateral sulcus.

Proprioceptive Pathway for Reflex Activity and Cerebellar Transmission

REFLEX. The axons enter the dorsal grey column of the spinal cord. Some axons (Ia) synapse directly on alpha motor neurons (general somatic efferent) in the ventral grey column to complete a reflex arc. Others (Golgi tendon organ) indirectly influence an alpha motor neuron and complete the reflex arc by synapsing on an interneuron. Activity of some interneurons influences alpha motor neurons in other segments of the spinal cord by passing cranial and caudal in the fasciculus proprius of the lateral funiculus, which is the white matter immediately adjacent to the grey matter. This also is referred to as the propriospinal fiber system, which connects adjoining and distant segments of the spinal cord. This provides a means of interrelating neural activity within the spinal cord.

Cerebellar Pathway

FROM TRUNK AND PELVIC LIMBS

Dorsal Spinocerebellar Tract. The GP axon enters the dorsal grey column and synapses on a cell body medially at the base of the dorsal grey column. This is in the nucleus thoracicus (Clarke's nucleus).[5] The axon of this cell body enters the lateral funiculus of the same side and passes cranially on the surface of the dorsal portion of the lateral funiculus in the dorsal spinocerebellar tract. Here it is lateral to the lateral corticospinal and rubrospinal tracts. The nucleus thoracicus extends from approximately C8 to L4 in the cat. Pelvic limb GP afferents must course cranially to the cranial lumbar segments to synapse in this nucleus. The dorsal spinocerebellar tract passes cranially through the entire spinal cord and joins the caudal cerebellar peduncle by way of the superficial arcuate fibers on the surface of the medulla.[4, 10] It is distributed primarily to the cerebellar cortex of the vermal and paravermal lobules.

Ventral Spinocerebellar Tract. The GP axon enters the dorsal grey column and synapses on cell bodies near its base laterally.[6, 12] These form a continuous column from the cranial thoracic segments caudally throughout the lumbar and sacral segments. Most axons of these cell bodies cross to the opposite lateral

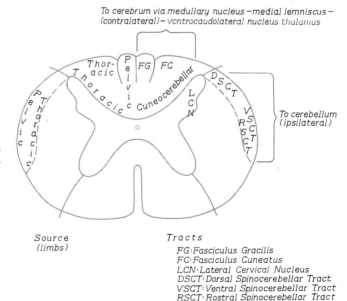

Figure 8–1. General proprioceptive pathways at the second cervical segment.

To cerebrum via medullary nucleus —medial lemniscus — (contralateral)—ventrocaudolateral nucleus thalamus

To cerebellum (ipsilateral)

Source
(limbs)

Tracts

FG: Fasciculus Gracilis
FC: Fasciculus Cuneatus
LCN: Lateral Cervical Nucleus
DSCT: Dorsal Spinocerebellar Tract
VSCT: Ventral Spinocerebellar Tract
RSCT: Rostral Spinocerebellar Tract

funiculus by way of the ventral white commissure. In the contralateral lateral funiculus they form the ventral spinocerebellar tract on the surface of the lateral funiculus ventral to the dorsal spinocerebellar tract.

This tract courses cranially throughout the spinal cord, through the medulla and pons on the lateral side to reach the rostral cerebellar peduncle, which it joins, and then courses caudally into the cerebellum, mostly to the vermal and paravermal lobules of the contralateral side.[4, 10] Many of these ventral spinocerebellar tract axons recross in the cerebellum before terminating, thus influencing the cerebellum on the same side on which the axons were stimulated.

From Cervical Region and Thoracic Limbs

Cuneocerebellar Pathway. This thoracic limb pathway is homologous to the dorsal spinocerebellar tract from the pelvic limbs.[11, 18] The GP axons pass dorsal to the dorsal grey column and enter the lateral portion of the dorsal funiculus, which is the fasciculus cuneatus. They pass cranially in the fasciculus cuneatus to the caudal medulla, in which they terminate in the lateral cuneate nucleus. This nucleus is located dorsally in the medulla, dorsolateral to the parasympathetic nucleus of the vagus, ventromedial to the caudal cerebellar peduncle, rostral to the obex and medial cuneate nucleus, and caudal to the spinal vestibular nucleus. It contains afferents from the dorsal roots of spinal nerves C1 to T8.

Axons of the cell bodies in the lateral cuneate nucleus enter the adjacent caudal cerebellar peduncle and pass into the cerebellum.

Cranial (Rostral) Spinocerebellar Tract. This thoracic limb pathway is homologous to the ventral spinocerebellar tract from the trunk and pelvic limbs. The GP axons enter the dorsal grey column and synapse on cell bodies near its base. The axons of these cell bodies enter the ipsilateral lateral funiculus and course cranially medial and ventral to the ventral spinocerebellar tract. They enter the cerebellum through both the caudal and rostral cerebellar peduncles.

In summary, these spinocerebellar pathways provide the cerebellum, predominantly ipsilaterally, with information about where the trunk and limbs are in space, both during movement and during a fixed posture. This information aids the cerebellum in its role of regulating posture, tone, locomotion, and equilibrium.[24]

Proprioceptive Pathway to the Somesthetic Cortex for Conscious Perception

FASCICULUS GRACILIS AND FASCICULUS CUNEATUS. The GP axon in the dorsal root enters the spinal cord at the dorsolateral sulcus, passes dorsal to the dorsal grey column, and enters the dorsal funiculus and courses cranially. GP axons from the pelvic limbs and caudal trunk (caudal to T6) course in the medial portion of the dorsal funiculus in the fasciculus gracilis.[8] Cranial to T6 the GP axons are situated more laterally in the fasciculus cuneatus. The dorsal funiculus is organized somatotopically so that the GP axons from the more caudal levels are situated medially in the dorsal funiculus. As the funiculus passes cranially, the GP axons are contributed to the lateral aspect. Thus cervical GP axons are the most lateral in the funiculus. Some axons may terminate in the spinal cord grey matter of the segments cranial to their origin.

NUCLEUS GRACILIS AND MEDIAL CUNEATE NUCLEUS. The GP axons in the fasciculus gracilis terminate in the nucleus gracilis in the dorsal part of the caudal medulla. This nucleus begins in the fasciculus gracilis caudal to the obex at the

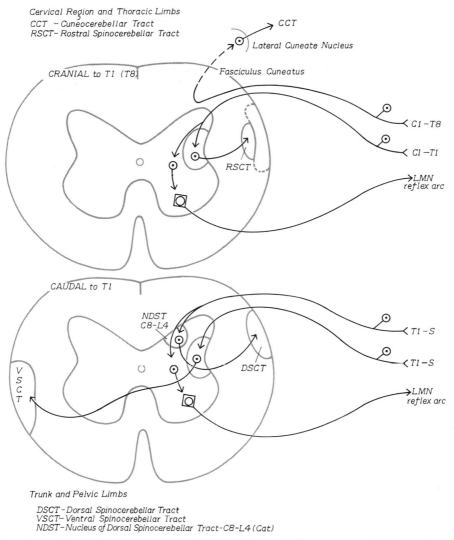

Figure 8–2.   General proprioceptive pathways to the cerebellum — spinocerebellar pathways.

level of the pyramidal decussation. It is lateral to the dorsal median sulcus and extends rostrally to the level of the obex, where it is dorsal to the parasympathetic nucleus of the vagus and medial to the medial cuneate nucleus.

The GP axons in the fasciculus cuneatus (exclusive of those in the cuneocerebellar pathway) terminate in the medial cuneate nucleus in the dorsal part of the caudal medulla. This nucleus extends caudally in the fasciculus cuneatus to the level of the pyramidal decussation. It is lateral to the nucleus gracilis and extends rostrally proximal to the obex. Its rostral portion is medial to the caudal portion of the lateral cuneate nucleus (cuneocerebellar pathway).

MEDIAL LEMNISCUS — VENTRAL CAUDAL LATERAL NUCLEUS, THALAMUS. Axons from the nucleus gracilis and medial cuneate nucleus course ventrally and transversally through the medulla as the deep arcuate fibers to the opposite side

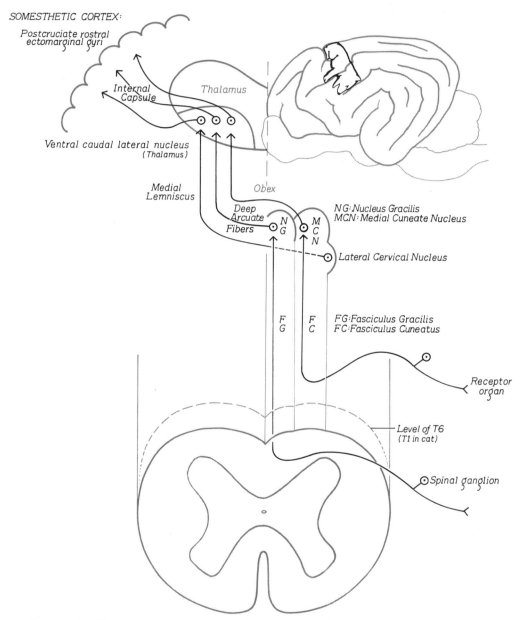

Figure 8–3.   General proprioception, spinal nerve, conscious pathway to somesthetic cortex.

of the midline. Here they form the medial lemniscus dorsal to the contralateral pyramid and ventromedial to the olive.[17]

The medial lemniscus, oriented in a dorsal plane, courses rostrally through the medulla dorsal to the pyramid. As it passes through the dorsal part of the trapezoid body, it is medial to the dorsal nucleus of the trapezoid body. In the pons it is located dorsal to the longitudinal fibers. In the mesencephalon it is ventral in the caudal tegmentum, dorsal to the substantia nigra, and shifts laterally as it courses through the tegmentum of the rostral mesencephalon and into the caudal diencephalon. The medial lemniscus terminates in a specific projection nucleus of the thalamus, the ventral caudal lateral nucleus. This nucleus is ill defined; it is located ventral in the thalamus, dorsal to its external medullary lamina. The axons of this nucleus project to the sensory, somesthetic cortex of the cerebrum by way of the internal capsule.

The somesthetic cortex is described classically as located in the parietal lobe of the cerebrum caudal to the cruciate sulcus.[1, 2] In the dog it overlaps with the motor cortex, being located in the caudal part of the postcruciate gyrus and the rostral ectomarginal gyrus. There is a somatotopic organization of the medial lemniscus, the ventral caudal lateral nucleus of the thalamus, and the somesthetic cortex.[13]

All sensory systems project to localized regions of the cerebral cortex called primary sensory areas. Five of these are well established: auditory, visual, olfactory, gustatory, and somesthetic. The somatotopic organization of the somesthetic cerebral cortex reflects the density of receptor organs in the different regions of the body. For example, the prehensile organs of an animal (the lips of a pig, a horse, and a dog, and the forepaws or hands of a raccoon, a cat, a monkey, and a man) have an abundance of receptor organs for this function, and a correspondingly large representation in the somesthetic cortex.[1, 2, 14, 22, 23]

Lateral Cervical Nucleus. An additional somesthetic pathway for general proprioception occurs by way of the lateral cervical nucleus.[3, 7, 19, 21] This nucleus projects from the lateral side of the dorsal grey column in the first two or three cervical spinal cord segments. It receives afferents from the spinocervical tract in the ipsilateral lateral funiculus. The cell bodies of this tract are located in the nucleus proprius of the dorsal grey column along the entire spinal cord.[25]

The axons of the cell bodies in the lateral cervical nucleus flow cranially and cross to the opposite side of the caudal medulla to join the contralateral medial lemniscus. Their course in the medial lemniscus to the ventral caudal lateral nucleus of the thalamus and the somesthetic cortex is similar to that of the deep arcuate fibers that make up the medial lemniscus. There is some evidence to support the finding that this nucleus also projects axons to the cerebellum. In the dog and cat this nucleus serves mainly as a relay for tactile sensation.

CRANIAL NERVES

The majority of the GP axons in the head are considered to course from the receptor organ in muscles of mastication, facial and extraocular muscles, and the temporomandibular joint in the nerve branches from the trigeminal nerve (cranial nerve V). These GP axons in the ophthalmic, maxillary, and mandibular nerves course through the trigeminal ganglion and enter the pons with the trigeminal nerve. The axons course rostrally along the lateral border of the central grey substance of the fourth ventricle and mesencephalic aqueduct in the mesencephalic tract of the trigeminal nerve.

Level of Metencephalon–Mesencephalon

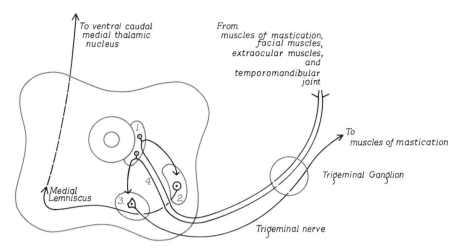

Figure 8–4. Trigeminal proprioceptive pathways. *1:* Nucleus of the mesencephalic tract of the trigeminal nerve; *2:* pontine sensory nucleus of the trigeminal nerve; *3:* motor nucleus of the trigeminal nerve; *4:* mesencephalic tract of the trigeminal nerve.

Although cell bodies of peripheral afferent neurons normally are located in ganglia of the peripheral nervous system, the cell bodies of these neurons are an exception to this rule. The cell bodies of these GP axons are located in the nucleus of the mesencephalic tract of the trigeminal nerve in a narrow band on the lateral border of the central grey substance throughout the mesencephalon.

Reflex. For reflex function the axons may pass directly to the adjacent general somatic efferent and special visceral efferent nuclei of cranial nerves to synapse on the alpha motor neuron. These alpha motor neurons may be in-

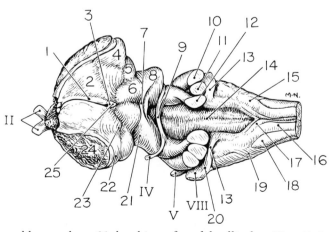

Figure 8–5. Dorsal view of brain stem. *1:* Stria habenularis thalami; *2:* dorsal aspect of thalamus; *3:* habenular commissure; *4:* lateral geniculate nucleus; *5:* medial geniculate nucleus; *6:* rostral colliculus; *7:* commissure of caudal colliculi; *8:* caudal colliculus; *9:* crossing of trochlear nerve fibers in rostral medullary velum; *10:* middle cerebellar peduncle; *11:* caudal cerebellar peduncle; *12:* rostral cerebellar peduncle; *13:* dorsal cochlear nucleus; *14:* dorsal median sulcus in fourth ventricle; *15:* lateral cuneate nucleus; *16:* fasciculus cuneatus; *17:* nucleus gracilis; *18:* spinal tract of trigeminal nerve; *19:* superficial arcuate fibers; *20:* left ventral cochlear nucleus; *21:* brachium of caudal colliculus; *22:* optic tract; *23:* brachium of rostral colliculus; *24:* cut surface between cerebrum and brain stem; *25:* pineal body or epiphysis; *II:* optic nerves; *IV:* trochlear nerve; *V:* trigeminal nerve; *VIII:* vestibulocochlear nerve.

fluenced indirectly by interneurons in the pontine sensory nucleus of the trigeminal nerve, which are stimulated by the GP axons of the mesencephalic tract.

Conscious Perception. The GP axons in the mesencephalic tract course caudolaterally to terminate in the pontine sensory nucleus of the trigeminal nerve. This nucleus is located in the caudal pons and rostral medulla, where it is situated between the entrance of the trigeminal nerve and its motor nucleus, ventromedial to the middle and rostral cerebellar peduncles. The axons of these cell bodies cross through the ventral reticular formation to the opposite side to form the trigeminal lemniscus (quintothalamic tract), which joins the medial lemniscus and courses rostrally to the caudal thalamus in this lemniscus. They terminate in the ventral caudal medial nucleus of the thalamus adjacent to the ventral caudal lateral nucleus. Axons of these cell bodies course through the internal capsule to the somesthetic cortex.

CLINICAL SIGNS

Ataxia (incoordination) is the principal sign observed with lesions in the general proprioceptive system. This sometimes is referred to as sensory ataxia as opposed to motor ataxia of cerebellar cortical disease. Ataxia is a result of lack of kinesthesia, a lack of the sense of motion or of the position of the body or limbs in space.

The animal may show a standing posture with the distal portion of the extremities placed more lateral than normal, a basewide stance. On moving, the limbs may swing to the side and circumduct or abduct more than normal, or cross beneath the trunk, or adduct more than normal, sometimes interfering with the opposite limb. There may be a delay in initiating protraction of the limb on getting up or on walking, causing a longer stride than normal and a tendency for the hindquarters to appear slightly lower (crouched) than usual. This may contribute to the wobbly appearance of the pelvic limb gait. The animal may walk on the dorsal surface of its distal extremity, or "knuckle over." Occasionally, a degree of overresponse is seen during flexion of the limb when the animal is in movement. The uninhibited flexion causes the limb to be lifted higher than usual. This may be combined with excessive abduction. The excessive flexion is often called hypermetria, and also occurs in a more severe form in cerebellar disease.

This hypermetria with general proprioceptive deficit may be explained by the lack of spinocerebellar input to the cerebellar cortex. Spinocerebellar neurons terminate in the cerebellar cortex, in which Purkinje neurons are activated. These are inhibitory neurons that indirectly affect brain stem neurons through their effect on neurons in the cerebellar nuclei. Thus spinocerebellar activation of the cerebellar cortex typically results in inhibition of the brain stem mechanism that induces voluntary locomotion, so that once limb flexion is induced for the protraction phase of locomotion, it is inhibited in turn in time for the appropriate extensor support phase to occur. A deficiency in this inhibition induced by the spinocerebellar deficit results in a prolonged flexor phase of the gait observed as hyperflexion or hypermetria.[9, 16]

Defects may be observed in the response of the patient to testing postural reactions such as placing, hopping, proprioceptive positioning, and the tonic neck test. In mild lesions subtle dysfunctions may become apparent in the pelvic limbs by forcing the animal to hop slowly on each limb, and in the thoracic limbs by forcing the animal to wheelbarrow with its head and neck extended. An occasional tendency to "knuckle over" is a sign of deficit.

With unilateral lesions in the spinocerebellar system the signs of proprioceptive deficit are ipsilateral, and asymmetry is obvious in the response to postural reaction testing.

Lesions in the thalamus, internal capsule, or somesthetic cortex on one side cause an abnormal response to postural reactions on the contralateral side. Part of the explanation for the asymmetric postural reactions may be related to the disruption of the thalamocortical pathway of the GP system, in addition to the disruption of the telencephalic portion of the upper motor neuron.

It may be difficult to separate paresis from proprioceptive deficiency on clinical examination of the patient, but this usually does not interfere with the interpretation of the gross location of the lesion. The upper motor neuron and GP systems accompany each other through most of the neuraxis. Mild compression of the spinal cord at the thirteenth thoracic segment causes paraparesis and ataxia in the pelvic limbs because of interference with the upper motor neuron in the ventral and lateral funiculi and the GP system in the lateral (and dorsal) funiculi. Thoracic limb function is normal.

A unilateral midcervical spinal cord lesion produces a profound upper motor neuron and GP deficit in the gait and postural reactions in the ipsilateral thoracic and pelvic limbs, with only a mild dysfunction in postural reactions in the contralateral pelvic limb.

Clinicopathologic and experimental studies indicate that lesions of the spinocerebellar system have a more profound influence on gait than do lesions of the dorsal columns.[15] Experimental section of the dorsal column bilaterally at C4 in the dog initially produced a high stepping gait in the thoracic limbs, but after 2 to 3 weeks it was nearly completely compensated.[20] The same results have been found in cats and monkeys.

DISEASES

Clinical diseases that affect the spinal nerve component of this system have been discussed in conjunction with the lower motor neuron in Chapter 4. Although most of the deficit resulting from peripheral nerve injury is described as caused by the general somatic efferent lower motor neuron loss, some may be due to loss of the general proprioception system. If the peroneal nerves are compressed for a prolonged period of time by ropes placed just above the tarsus to tie the dog to a surgery table, a transient neurologic deficit may be observed after recovery from anesthesia. At this level the nerve is compromised distal to its muscle innervation to the flexors of the tarsus and extensors of the digits. Nevertheless, the dog can stand and walk on the dorsum of the paw. There is no evidence of paresis. The dysfunction is presumably due to the loss of function of the GP and general somatic afferent neurons present in the nerve at the site of the compression. Hypalgesia or analgesia may accompany the proprioceptive deficit.

Spinal cord diseases are described in Chapter 10. No clinical signs have been associated with diseases that affect the cranial nerve component of this system.

REFERENCES

1. Adrian, E. D.: Afferent areas in brain of ungulates. Brain, 66:89, 1943.
2. Adrian, E. D.: The somatic receiving area in the brain of the Shetland pony. Brain, 69:1, 1946.
3. Brodal, A., and Rexed, B.: Spinal afferents to the lateral cervical nucleus in the cat. An experimental study. J. Comp. Neurol., 98:179, 1953.
4. Grant, G.: Spinal course and somatotopically localized termination of the spinocerebellar tracts. An experimental study in the cat. Acta Physiol. Scand., 56 Suppl., 193, 1962.
5. Grant, G., and Rexed, B.: Dorsal spinal root afferents to Clarke's column. Brain, 81:567, 1958.
6. Ha, H., and Liu, C.-N.: Cell origin of the ventral spinocerebellar tract. J. Comp. Neurol., 133:185, 1968.
7. Ha, H., and Liu, C.-N.: Organization of the spino-cervico-thalamic system. J. Comp. Neurol., 127:445, 1966.
8. Hand, P. J.: Lumbosacral dorsal root terminations in the nucleus gracilis of the cat. Some observations on the terminal degeneration in other medullary sensory nuclei. J. Comp. Neurol., 126: 137, 1966.
9. Hartley, W. J., and Palmer, A. C.: Ataxia in Jack Russell terriers. Acta Neuropathol., 26:71, 1973.
10. Holmquist, B., and Oscarsson, O.: Location, course, and characteristics of uncrossed and crossed ascending spinal tracts in the cat. Acta Physiol. Scand., 58:57, 1963.
11. Holmquist, B., Oscarsson, O., and Rosen, I.: Functional organization of the cuneocerebellar tract in the cat. Acta Physiol. Scand., 58:216, 1963.
12. Hubbard, J. I., and Oscarsson, O.: Localization of the cell bodies of the ventral spinocerebellar tract in lumbar segments of the cat. J. Comp. Neurol., 118:199, 1962.
13. Johnson, J. I., Jr., Welker, W. I., and Pubols, B. H., Jr.: Somatotopic organization of raccoon dorsal column nuclei. J. Comp. Neurol., 132:1, 1968.
14. Landgren, S., and Silfvenius, H.: Projection to cerebral cortex of group I and muscle afferents from the cat's hindlimb. J. Physiol., 200:353, 1969.
15. Lassek, A. M.: Motor deficits produced by posterior rhizotomy versus section of the dorsal funiculus. Neurology, 4:120, 1954.
16. Latshaw, W. K.: A model for the neural control of locomotion. J. Am. Anim. Hosp. Assoc., 10:598, 1974.
17. Matzke, H. A.: The course of the fibers arising from the nucleus gracilis and nucleus cuneatus of the cat. J. Comp. Neurol., 94:439, 1951.
18. Oscarsson, O.: Functional organization of the spino- and cuneocerebellar tracts. Physiol. Rev., 45:495, 1965.
19. Rexed, B., and Brodal, A.: The nucleus cervicalis lateralis—a spinocerebellar relay nucleus. J. Neurophysiol., 14:399, 1951.
20. Reynolds, P. J., Talbott, R. E., and Brookhart, J. M.: Control of postural reactions in the dog: The role of the dorsal column feedback pathway. Brain Res., 40:159, 1972.
21. Truex, R. C., Taylor, M. J., Smyth, M. Q., and Glidenberg, P. L.: The lateral cervical nucleus of cat, dog and man. J. Comp. Neurol., 139:93, 1970.
22. Welker, W. I., and Campos, G. B.: Physiological significance of sulci in somatic sensory cerebral cortex in mammals of the family Procyonidae. J. Comp. Neurol., 120:19, 1963.
23. Welker, W. I., and Seidenstein, S.: Somatic sensory representation in the cerebral cortex of the raccoon (Procyon lotor). J. Comp. Neurol., 111:469, 1959.
24. Petras, J. M., and Cummings, J. F.: The origin of spinocerebellar pathways. II. The nucleus centrobasalis of the cervical enlargement and the nucleus dorsalis of the thoracolumbar spinal cord. J. Comp. Neurol., in press.
25. Craig, A. D.: Spinocervical tract cells in cat and dog, labeled by the retrograde transport of horseradish peroxidase. Neurosci. Let., 3:173, 1976.

Chapter 9

GENERAL SOMATIC AFFERENT SYSTEM—GSA

SPINAL NERVE
Reflex GSA Pathway
GSA Pathway for Conscious Perception—Pain
  Pathway

CRANIAL NERVE
Reflex GSA Pathway
GSA Pathway for Conscious Projection
CLINICAL SIGNS
DISEASES

The general somatic afferent system is referred to as the "pain, temperature, touch" system. The receptor organs, both encapsulated and nonencapsulated, are classified as exteroceptors, being stimulated by physical contact with the external environment. These exteroceptors are classified further physiologically as mechanoreceptors, thermoreceptors, and nociceptors on the basis of the form of energy that is their adequate stimulus.

SPINAL NERVE

The axons course from the receptor organ on the surface of the body through peripheral nerves, spinal nerves, and through the segmental spinal ganglion related to the dorsal root. These GSA neurons are unipolar, and the cell body is in the spinal ganglion. The axon continues proximally through the dorsal rootlet to the dorsolateral sulcus, where it enters the spinal cord. The axon branches dorsal to the dorsal grey column and courses cranially and caudally through the adjacent two or three segments. The pathway formed by these axons at the apex of the dorsal grey column is referred to as the dorsolateral fasciculus (Lissauer's tract). Collaterals of these axonal branches enter the dorsal grey column all along the segments that are traversed. They pass into the middle of the dorsal grey column, giving off collaterals to interneurons located at the apex of the dorsal grey column in an area called substantia gelatinosa.

Reflex GSA Pathway. The GSA axons synapse on interneurons in the grey matter of the spinal cord, which in turn influence the alpha motor neurons. Interneurons with axons passing in the fasciculus proprius can influence the alpha motor neurons of adjacent segments to stimulate the complete general somatic efferent system of the lower motor neuron of the reflex arc. This is the reflex path-

160

way for the flexor reflex, limb withdrawal phenomenon. It only requires the peripheral nerves to the area stimulated, the muscles that contract, and the segments of the spinal cord from which the peripheral nerves originate.

The surface of the body can be mapped according to the distribution of general somatic afferent receptor organs either associated with peripheral nerves, or associated with specific dorsal roots (dermatomes).[5, 9] The latter is referred to as dermatomal mapping, and represents the distribution of a dorsal root's axons (receptor organs) over the body surface. This demonstrates the embryonic fate of the dorsal root axons that innervated the dermatomal portion of the somite. As the dermatome contributed to the body surface, its dorsal root innervation extended with it by way of branches of spinal or peripheral nerves.

Studies in the dog have shown that each dermatome of the trunk extends from the dorsal to the ventral midline, and there is a craniocaudal overlap of up to three dorsal roots in the lumbosacral region.[5]

Sensory deficit, like motor deficit, is more obvious with disrupted peripheral nerves than with a disrupted spinal nerve or its roots.

A noxious stimulus (a pin or forceps) applied to the skin of the medial side of the antebrachium causes withdrawal of the limb by flexion of the shoulder, elbow, carpus, and digits. The axons of the nociceptors course proximally in the medial cutaneous antebrachial nerve, the musculocutaneous nerve, and the sixth, seventh, and eighth cervical spinal nerves and their dorsal rootlets. Collaterals of these axons terminate on interneurons in the grey matter of these and the adjacent spinal cord segments. These interneurons synapse on alpha motor neurons of the same segments and those caudal to this site that have axons coursing to the flexor muscles of the shoulder (spinal roots and nerves C7, C8, T1 and the axillary and radial nerves), the flexors of the elbow (spinal roots and nerves C6, C7, C8 and the musculocutaneous nerve), the flexors of the carpus (spinal roots and nerves C8, T1, T2 and the median nerve), and the flexors of the digits (spinal roots and nerves C8, T1, T2 and the median and ulnar nerves).

The flexor withdrawal response may be part of an animal's conscious perception of pain, but this requires additional central pathways not needed for the segmental reflex arc. The two responses must be distinguished from each other. Ascertaining cerebral response to noxious stimuli is especially important in evaluating spinal cord disease.

GSA Pathway for Conscious Perception—"Pain Pathway."   General somatic afferent axons that enter the dorsal grey column through the substantia gelatinosa synapse on cell bodies at the base of the dorsal grey column.[12, 14] The axons of these dorsal grey column neurons cross to the opposite ventral portion of the lateral funiculus medial to the ventral spinocerebellar tract and form the lateral spinothalamic tract. In primates this is essentially an entirely crossed system, and the spinothalamic tract is composed of axons that are uninterrupted from their place of origin at a cell body in the dorsal grey column to their termination in a thalamic nucleus. In domestic animals the axons leaving cell bodies in one dorsal grey column enter the lateral funiculus of both sides of the spinal cord. The spinothalamic pathway in the lateral funiculus is dorsal in the cat and ventral in the pig.[1, 2, 3, 4, 8] There is evidence that the pathway is interrupted frequently by axons leaving the path, entering the grey matter to synapse on another neuron whose axon rejoins the spinothalamic pathway of the same or opposite side. Thus, in contrast to man, animals have a diffuse, bilaterally represented multisynaptic pathway for the conduction of impulses stimulated by noxious stimuli.

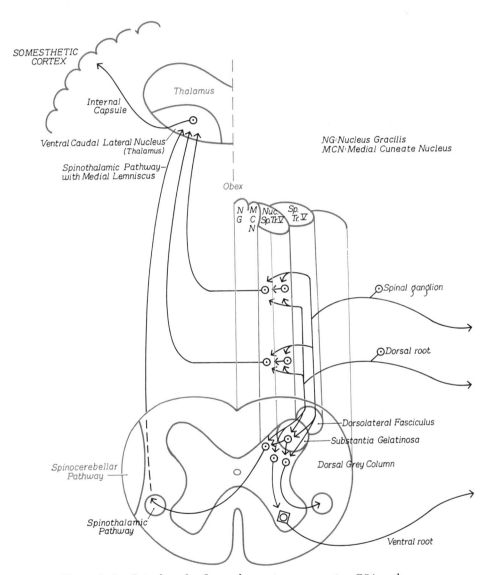

Figure 9–1. Spinal cord reflex and conscious perception GSA pathways.

In primates hemisection of the spinal cord causes ipsilateral motor deficit (upper motor neuron) and contralateral sensory deficit (general sensory afferent) caudal to the lesion. This syndrome, called Brown-Séquard, is explained by the level of crossing being at the origin of these systems, which is the brain stem for the upper motor neuron and approximate site of entrance to the spinal cord for the general somatic afferent system. The contralateral hypalgesia is not as evident in the domestic animal because of the bilateral spinal cord pathways for the GSA system. Nevertheless, clinical experience with a few unilateral lesions in the spinal cord and rostral brain stem occasionally has demonstrated a contralateral hypalgesia. This would suggest that a contralateral pathway may predominate.

Experimental evidence indicates that in addition to the spinothalamic pathway, other tracts in the lateral funiculus, such as spinoreticular and fasciculus proprius pathways, also may conduct the modality of "pain."

In the standard description of the conscious pathway for the general somatic afferent system, the axons in the spinothalamic tract pass cranially through the entire spinal cord, and through the medulla, pons, and midbrain associated with the lateral aspect of the medial lemniscus. In the caudal thalamus these axons synapse in the specific projection nucleus for the general somatic afferent system in spinal nerves, the ventral caudal lateral nucleus of the thalamus. Axons of these

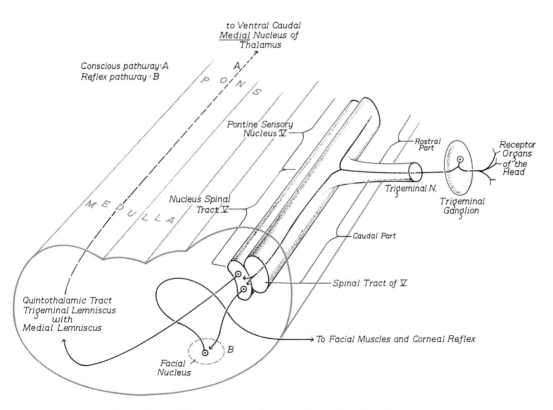

Figure 9–2. Trigeminal nerve, general somatic afferent pathways.

cell bodies enter the internal capsule and are distributed to the somesthetic cortex.[7] Conscious perception of pain may occur at both the thalamic and cortical levels of this pathway.

As these spinothalamic axons traverse the brain stem, collaterals terminate in the reticular formation in its ascending division. These are afferents to the ascending reticular activating system (ARAS) concerned with the arousal of the cerebral cortex, the maintenance of the state of consciousness.

There is evidence that considerable modulation of pain occurs at the termination of primary afferents in the dorsal grey column. Neurons in the substantia gelatinosa are inhibitory to the neurons that project into the spinothalamic 'pain' pathway. Most nociceptive afferents are small axons that terminate mostly on the spinothalamic projection neurons. Large diameter non-nociceptive axons terminate on other projection neurons in the dorsal grey column and on large numbers of substantia gelatinosa neurons. By this mechanism these inhibit the 'pain' pathway by modulating the activity of the nociceptive afferents.

CRANIAL NERVE

The general somatic afferent axons course from the receptor organ on the surface of the head through the branches of the ophthalmic, maxillary, and mandibular nerves, and the trigeminal nerve and ganglion. The cell bodies of these unipolar GSA neurons are in the trigeminal ganglion, which is located in the canal for the trigeminal nerve in the rostral part of the petrosal bone. The trigeminal nerve enters the pons through the caudolateral portion of the transverse fibers of the pons as they form the middle cerebellar peduncle. This is rostral to the origin of the facial and vestibulocochlear nerves.

The GSA axons of the trigeminal nerve course caudally on the lateral side of the medulla in the spinal tract of the trigeminal nerve. This tract is shaped like a quarter circle, with the concave surface medial. As it passes from rostral to caudal, it is medial to the cochlear nuclei in the vestibulocochlear nerve, and to the dorsal spinocerebellar tract as it enters the caudal cerebellar peduncle in the superficial arcuate fibers. At the obex it becomes superficial on the lateral side of the medulla between the fasciculus cuneatus dorsally and the dorsal spinocerebellar tract ventrally. The tract continues caudally into the first cervical spinal cord segment, in which it is continued by the dorsolateral fasciculus (Lissauer's tract). Throughout this course a nuclear column is located medial to this tract. In the pons, it is the pontine sensory nucleus of the trigeminal nerve. Throughout the medulla and into the first cervical segment, it is the nucleus of the spinal tract of the trigeminal nerve. This nuclear column is similar in shape to the spinal tract of the trigeminal nerve. In the cervical spinal cord it is continuous with the substantia gelatinosa. General somatic afferent axons in the spinal tract of the trigeminal nerve terminate in the nuclear column medial to it, the pontine sensory nucleus and nucleus of the spinal tract of the trigeminal nerve.

Reflex GSA Pathway. Axons of the cell bodies in this nuclear column project to the lower motor neuron nuclei of cranial nerves to complete reflex arcs. The closure of the eyelids on stimulation of the cornea (ophthalmic nerve) and the eyelids (ophthalmic and maxillary nerves) is evidence of the termination of these trigeminal neurons on cell bodies in the pontine and spinal tract nuclei whose axons terminate on the special visceral efferent neurons of the facial nucleus. These are the corneal and palpebral reflexes.

   GSA Pathway for Conscious Projection.   Other axons from cell bodies in the pontine sensory nucleus and nucleus of the spinal tract of the trigeminal nerve predominantly cross to the opposite side, become associated with the medial lemniscus, and course rostrally with this bundle. These are sometimes referred to as the trigeminal lemniscus or the quintothalamic tract. In the caudal thalamus these axons synapse in the specific projection nucleus of the thalamus for the GSA system in cranial nerves, the ventral caudal medial nucleus. Axons of these cell bodies enter the internal capsule and are distributed to the head region of the somesthetic cortex.

CLINICAL SIGNS

   In the neurologic examination of animals, the most reliable modality for testing the GSA system is that of nociception—pain. Analgesia means complete absence of pain perception. Hypalgesia means decreased pain perception.

   Pain is not just an exteroceptive modality, but is the subjective interpretation of nerve impulses produced peripherally by a stimulus that is actually or potentially harmful to tissue. This interpretation of pain varies with each individual.[2, 10, 11] The interpretation of these impulses is modified and conditioned by past experiences and memories, by an understanding of the cause of the impulses, and by the consequence expected. The degree of attention and emotional state of the individual also modifies the response. The response often is related more to the significance of an injury than to its size. Even in animals a considerable variation occurs in the cerebral response to stimuli considered by the investigator to be noxious or painful. This often makes interpretation of dysfunction of the spinothalamic pathway difficult. A stimulus that elicits a "pain" response in the normal small animal in most cases is the application of pressure to the base of the toenails with forceps. Response to pin pricking is often unreliable, because many normal patients show no cerebral response. In large animals for whom a pin or forceps may not be adequate, an electric prod may be used. The horse often responds well to a pin or closed forceps. The area most sensitive to a noxious stimulus in the head of domestic animals is the nasal mucosa. If an area of hypalgesia or analgesia is suspected, this region should be tested.

   Interpretation of an intact or interrupted spinothalamic pathway is most important in the evaluation of the degree of nervous tissue damage following injury. Injuries to the spinal cord that cause complete motor paralysis and complete analgesia or lack of sensation to noxious stimuli caudal to the lesion have a poor prognosis and require prompt surgical intervention if it is warranted. Patients with complete motor paralysis but with hypalgesia or depressed response to noxious stimuli caudal to the lesion have a better prognosis. The presence of a cerebral response to noxious stimuli indicates that some pathways in the spinal cord are intact at the site of the lesion. With peripheral nerve lesions, the same signs of paralysis but accompanied by hypalgesia in the area of distribution of the involved peripheral nerves indicate that the nerve is still intact, and the prognosis is not as grave as it would be with paralysis and analgesia.

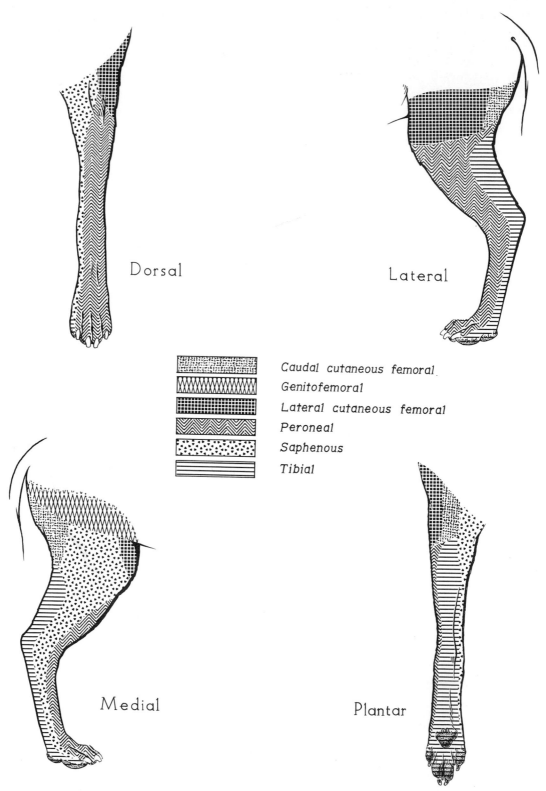

Caudal cutaneous femoral
Genitofemoral
Lateral cutaneous femoral
Peroneal
Saphenous
Tibial

Figure 9–3. Peripheral nerve innervation of skin of left pelvic limb. (From Evans, H. E., and de Lahunta, A.: Miller's Guide to the Dissection of the Dog. Philadelphia, W. B. Saunders Co., 1971.)

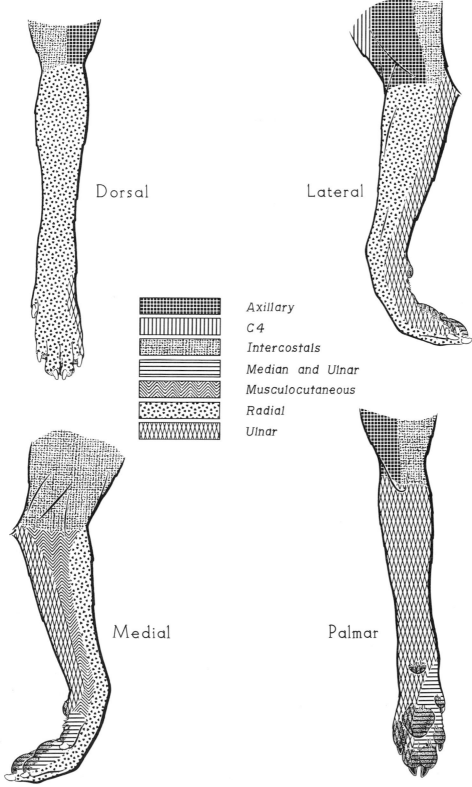

Dorsal

Lateral

Axillary
C 4
Intercostals
Median and Ulnar
Musculocutaneous
Radial
Ulnar

Medial

Palmar

Figure 9–4. Peripheral nerve innervation of skin of left thoracic limb. (From Evans, H. E., and de Lahunta, A.: Miller's Guide to the Dissection of the Dog. Philadelphia, W. B. Saunders Co., 1971.)

DISEASES

Clinical diseases that affect the spinal and peripheral nerve components of this system were considered in conjunction with the lower motor neuron in Chapter 4. Spinal cord diseases will be discussed in Chapter 10.

Hypalgesia or analgesia of the face is caused by lesions that interfere with the trigeminal nerve, its ganglion, or its tract in the pons and medulla. The most common causes are injuries, neoplasms, and granulomas. The presence of facial analgesia in an animal with intracranial injury is a poor prognostic sign, because it suggests contusion of the caudal brain stem. Facial hypalgesia (cranial nerve V) on the same side as a facial muscle paresis (cranial nerve VII) and vestibular ataxia (cranial nerve VIII) suggest an intracranial and usually medullary location of the lesion and a more cautious prognosis. Otitis media-interna can affect only cranial nerves VII and VIII, not V. The bilateral nonsuppurative trigeminal neuritis that causes paralysis of the muscles of mastication also may produce a hypalgesia, but it is difficult to detect.

When the eyeball is denervated of its sensory nerves (trigeminal-ophthalmic nerve), degenerative changes occur in the cornea.[13] This is referred to as neurotrophic keratitis, and consists of edema and erosion of epithelial cells. The relationship of the cellular metabolism of the cornea to its sensory nerve supply is not clearly understood.

Lesions that destroy the ventral caudal medial thalamic nucleus or its projection pathway in the internal capsule or the somesthetic cortex may produce a subtle hypalgesia of the contralateral face. This may best be determined by palpation of the nasal mucosa with a blunt instrument.

REFERENCES

1. Anderson, F. D., and Berry, C. M.: Degeneration studies of long ascending fiber systems in the cat brain stem. J. Comp. Neurol., *111*:195, 1959.
2. Breazile, J. E., and Kitchell, R. L.: Pain perception in animals. Fed. Proc., *28*:1379, 1969.
3. Breazile, J. E., and Kitchell, R. L.: A study of fiber systems within the spinal cord of the domestic pig that subserve pain. J. Comp. Neurol., *133*:373, 1968.
4. Breazile, J. E., and Kitchell, R. L.: Ventrolateral spinal cord afferents to the brain stem in the domestic pig. J. Comp. Neurol., *133*:363, 1968.
5. Fletcher, T. F., and Kitchell, R. L.: The lumbar, sacral and coccygeal tactile dermatomes of the dog. J. Comp. Neurol., *128*:171, 1966.
6. Halliwell, R. E. W.: Pathogenesis and treatment of pruritus. J. Am. Vet. Med. Assoc., *164*:793, 1974.
7. Hamey, T., Bromley, R. B., and Woosley, C. N.: Somatic afferent area I and II of dog's cerebral cortex. J. Neurophysiol., *19*:485, 1956.
8. Kennard, M. A.: The course of ascending fibers in the spinal cord of the cat essential to the recognition of painful stimuli. J. Comp. Neurol., *100*:511, 1954.
9. Kirk, E. J.: The dermatomes of the sheep. J. Comp. Neurol., *134*:353, 1968.
10. Melzack, R.: The perception of pain. Sci. Am., *204*:41, 1961.
11. Melzack, R., and Wall, P. D.: Pain mechanisms: A new theory. Science, *150*:971, 1965.
12. Ralston, H. J.: The organization of the substantia gelatinosa Rolandi in the cat lumbosacral spinal cord. Z. Zellforsch. Mikrosk. Anat., *67*:1, 1965.
13. Scott, D. W., and Bistner, S. I.: Neurotrophic keratitis in a dog. Vet. Med. Small Anim. Clin., *68*:1120, 1973.
14. Szentágothai, J.: Neuronal and synaptic arrangement in the substantia gelatinosa Rolandi. J. Comp. Neurol., *122*:219, 1964.
15. Kerr, F. W. L.: Pain—A central inhibitory balance theory. Mayo Clinic Proc., *50*:685, 1975.

Chapter 10

SPINAL CORD DISEASE

NEUROLOGIC EXAMINATION
GAIT
POSTURAL REACTIONS
SPINAL REFLEXES
CRANIAL NERVES
SUMMARY OF SIGNS WITH LESIONS AT SPECIFIC LOCATIONS IN THE SPINAL CORD
Lumbosacral: Fourth Lumbar to Fifth Caudal Segment
Thoracolumbar: Third Thoracic to Third Lumbar Segment
Caudal Cervical: Fifth Cervical to Second Thoracic Segment
Cranial Cervical: First Cervical to Fifth Cervical Segment
SPINAL CORD DISEASE IN SMALL ANIMALS
LUMBOSACRAL SPINAL CORD DISEASE (L4–Cd)
Trauma
Inflammation
Degeneration
Neoplasia
Malformation
THORACOLUMBAR SPINAL CORD DISEASE (T3–L3)

Trauma
Inflammation
Degeneration
Neoplasia—Intramedullary
Malformation
CERVICAL SPINAL CORD DISEASE (C1–C5)
Trauma
Inflammation
Degeneration
Neoplasia—Intramedullary
Malformation
CERVICAL INTUMESCENCE SPINAL CORD DISEASE (C6–T2)
Trauma
Inflammation
Degeneration
Neoplasia
Malformation
SPINAL CORD DISEASE IN LARGE ANIMALS
Trauma
Inflammation
Degeneration
Neoplasia—Intramedullary
Malformation

The objective of this chapter is first to review the method and interpretation of the neurologic examination, which determines the location of the lesion in the spinal cord. Following that, the different kinds of lesions that affect the spinal cord are discussed on a regional basis in general and according to species.

NEUROLOGIC EXAMINATION

There are four parts to the neurologic examination: examination of gait, postural reactions, spinal reflexes, and cranial nerves. All are necessary to determine whether a lesion is confined to the spinal cord, and at what level. As indicated in Chapter 4, spinal reflexes only require specific peripheral nerves and the spinal cord segments with which they connect. The spinal reflex response should not be confused with the perception of pain. In addition to the sensory component of the peripheral nerves and their spinal cord segments, the pain pathway requires the ascending spinothalamic system in the lateral funiculus of the spinal cord, and the brain stem, and the related thalamocortical system. These all must be intact and functional for the normal perception of pain. A dog with a transverse spinal cord lesion at T13 has normal or hyperactive reflexes, but no perception of pain from the pelvic limbs or trunk caudal to the lesion.

A postural reaction depends on the same components as the reflex, in addition to the ascending pathways through the white matter of the spinal cord and brain stem to the cerebellum and somesthetic cortex of the cerebrum, and the descending upper motor neuron pathways that return from the cerebrum and the brain stem and comprise spinal cord white matter (lateral and ventral funiculi).

GAIT

In most spinal cord disease the abnormality of the gait and the postural reactions reflect the degree of involvement of the ascending general proprioceptive tracts (ataxia) and the descending upper motor neuron tracts (paresis). Determination of the degree and site of hypalgesia or analgesia helps to localize the lesion and to indicate its severity.

The degree of paresis is shown by the ability of the patient to stand, support itself, and walk. Be aware that an animal with severe upper motor neuron paresis with spasticity may be unable to stand, but if placed in a supporting position may extend its limbs and support its weight in a reflex response, although it is unable to move voluntarily. This reflex extensor thrust does not indicate voluntary movement and strength. Ataxia is manifested by a tendency to cross the limbs so that they interfere with one another, to walk on the dorsal surface of the paw, to have a longer stride with a prolonged supporting phase before protraction, to abduct the limb, especially on turns, or to appear mildly hypermetric.

The gait should be examined in a place in which the patient can move freely, unleashed, and the ground surface is not slippery. The floor of many examining rooms is too slippery for adequate evaluation of gait. In some cases of vertebral column injury with spinal cord contusion resulting in paresis and ataxia, moving the patient on a slippery floor may cause it to fall, and further injury may result.

The degree of functional deficit dictates the need for further examination of the animal's strength and coordination. In a patient that is severely tetraparetic, is recumbent and unable to support its weight or move its limbs when weight is borne on them, there is no need for further tests to be performed for postural reactions. A paraplegic patient does not have to be examined for postural reactions in the pelvic limbs, but the thoracic limbs should be examined carefully. Occasionally, a patient with progressive myelitis may present as paraplegic because of an extensive thoracolumbar spinal cord location of the lesion, and also may have an asymmetric thoracic limb gait because of a less severe focus of the lesion in the cervical spinal cord. An early sign in dogs with ascending myelomalacia associated with an acute intervertebral disk extrusion may be a hesitant, stumbling, awkward gait in the thoracic limbs. The severity of pelvic limb weakness is evaluated best by holding the patient suspended at the base of the tail and observing its gait. The degree of pelvic limb dysfunction from thoracolumbar spinal cord lesions may be graded according to the following scheme.[136]

Grade	Sign
0	Absence of purposeful movement—paraplegia
1	Unable to stand to support; slight movement when supported by the tail—severe paraparesis
2	Unable to stand to support; when assisted moves limbs readily but stumbles and falls frequently—moderate paraparesis and ataxia
3	Can stand to support but frequently stumbles and falls—mild paraparesis and ataxia
4	Can stand to support; minimal paraparesis and ataxia
5	Normal strength and coordination

POSTURAL REACTIONS

Following observation of the gait for strength and coordination the postural reactions can be tested, especially to determine if there are less obvious deficiencies in strength and coordination when the gait appears to be normal.

Wheelbarrowing. The thoracic limbs may be tested by supporting the patient under the abdomen so that the pelvic limbs are off the ground surface, and forcing the patient to walk on its thoracic limbs. The normal animal walks with symmetric movements of both thoracic limbs and the head extended in normal position. Patients with lesions of the peripheral nerves of the thoracic limbs, cervical spinal cord, or brain stem may have asymmetric movements, with stumbling or knuckling over on the dorsum of the paw of the affected limb. Hypermetria occasionally is observed. With more severe lesions in this area that involve the central nervous system, there is a tendency to carry the head flexed with the nose close to and occasionally reaching the ground surface for support. If no deficit is observed, extend the neck while the animal is wheelbarrowed. This sometimes reveals a mild deficit, a tendency to knuckle over on the dorsum of the paw, which was not observed before. This is often helpful in confirming a cervical spinal cord lesion in Great Danes or Doberman pinschers that have a cervical vertebral malformation and show mild pelvic limb paresis and ataxia, but no overt thoracic limb signs.

Hopping—Thoracic Limb. While still supporting the pelvic limbs, hop the animal laterally on one thoracic limb while holding the other off the ground surface so that the entire weight of the body is supported by the limb to be tested. Move the dog forward and to each side but especially laterally, and observe the strength and coordination of the limb. Repeat this on the other thoracic limb and compare the response. Asymmetry occurs with paresis or ataxia. Hypermetria may occur with general proprioceptive or cerebellar deficits. This is an effective way of determining minor deficits when the gait appears to be normal, as is the case with contralateral cerebral sensorimotor cortex lesions.

If a dog presents with a grade 0 to 1 spastic paraplegia and a mild asymmetry in the hopping reaction of the thoracic limbs with no other abnormality of their function, this justifies the diagnosis of a multifocal lesion with a major lesion between T3 and L4 and a minor lesion cranial to C5. Canine distemper myelitis is a common cause of this kind of syndrome.

Extensor Postural Thrust. The same sequence of tests can be done on the pelvic limbs. The extensor postural thrust reaction is performed by holding the patient off the ground surface by supporting it caudal to the scapulae and lowering it to the ground surface, and observing the patient extend its pelvic limbs to support its weight. Moving the patient forward and backward in this position tests the symmetry of pelvic limb function, their strength and coordination.

Hopping—Pelvic Limb. Continuing to support the patient by the thorax so that the thoracic limbs are not in contact with the ground surface, one pelvic limb can be held up and the patient forced to hop laterally on the supporting limb. Both pelvic limbs should be tested in this way and the response compared.

Hemistanding and Hemiwalking. The patient's ability to stand and walk on the thoracic and pelvic limbs on one side can be tested by holding the opposite thoracic and pelvic limbs off the ground surface and forcing the patient to walk forward or to the side. These are referred to as the hemistanding and hemiwalking reactions.

A patient with a unilateral lesion of the sensorimotor cortex or internal capsule may have a normal gait, but show deficits in its postural reactions on the side opposite the lesion. Attempts to hemiwalk on the contralateral side are exaggerated (hypermetric) and spastic, and stumbling may occur. With unilateral cervical spinal cord lesions the limbs on the same side as the lesion show a deficiency in the gait, are unresponsive on postural reaction testing, and unable to support the animal in the hemiwalking reaction.

Placing. Other postural reactions that can be tested include placing with the thoracic limbs. The patient is supported off the ground surface, and its thoracic limbs are brought to the edge of a table or similar surface so that the dorsal surface of the paws makes contact. This test should be performed on both thoracic limbs simultaneously and individually, with and without blindfolding the patient. Vision can compensate for the lack of sense of position when the general proprioceptive system is abnormal.

Tonic Neck Reaction. The tonic neck reaction involves extension of the head and neck so that the nose is directed dorsally. The normal patient responds by extension of all the joints of both thoracic limbs. A patient with disease of the general proprioceptive system in the cervical spinal nerves, cervical spinal cord, or medulla fails to extend its carpus, or digits, or both, and these joints flex passively so that the weight is borne on the dorsal surface of the paw. The same response may occur if a patient is paretic either as a result of disease of the motor neurons that innervate the thoracic limb, or disease of the white matter of the spinal cord that influences these motor neurons.

Proprioceptive Positioning. Proprioceptive positioning tests this afferent system by determining the patient's ability to recognize when a paw has been flexed so that the weight is borne on its dorsal surface. The normal animal returns the paw to its usual position. In patients with severe paresis, response to this test may be deficient.

SPINAL REFLEXES

Muscle tone and spinal reflexes are evaluated best when the patient is in lateral recumbency and is as relaxed as possible. It is important to test muscle tone, tendon reflexes, and the flexor reflex to noxious stimuli in that order so as to maintain the cooperation of the patient.

Muscle Tone. Muscle tone is evaluated by passive manipulation of each limb individually. The degree of resistance is determined to be less than normal (hypotonic), normal, or greater than normal (hypertonic). The latter condition may be referred to as spasticity. The degree of spasticity varies from a mild increased resistance to passive manipulation to a marked increase that may be "clasp knife" in character. It is referred to as "clasp knife" because as attempts are made to flex a limb, the degree of extension of the limb increases, until suddenly it gives way to complete flexion of the limb without resistance.

Hypotonia usually occurs with lower motor neuron disease, whereas upper motor neuron disease is characterized by hypertonia or spasticity. The functional integrity of the lower motor neuron is necessary to cause muscle cell contraction and to maintain muscle tone. It is also necessary to maintain the normal health of the muscle cell it innervates. When denervated, these cells degenerate. This is observed clinically as neurogenic atrophy, and can be detected electromyographically by the production of abnormal potentials in resting muscle. The upper motor neuron influences the activity of the lower motor neuron to produce voluntary motor activity and to maintain muscle tone for support of the body against gravity. Although the upper motor neuron includes both facilitatory and inhibitory functions on the activity of the lower motor neuron, when the upper motor neuron is diseased the result usually seen is a release of the lower motor neuron to antigravity muscles from inhibition and overactivity of the facilitatory mechanism. This release is observed as hypertonia or spasticity.

Extensor Thrust. With the animal in a nonsupporting position of lateral recumbency, place the palm of the hand against the ventral surface of the paw and exert a sudden mild pressure against the paw. This is a reflex response that evaluates muscle tone, and the function of the femoral nerve and L4–L5 spinal cord segments. The normal animal extends the limb mildly against the hand of the examiner. In some cases of upper motor neuron disease it is extended vigorously against the hand. In cases of lower motor neuron disease there is no response.

Patellar Reflexes. The most reliable tendon reflex is the patellar reflex. It is obtained by lightly tapping the patellar tendon when the patient is in lateral recumbency and is as relaxed as possible for proper evaluation. A neurologic hammer used in pediatric examinations is the most useful instrument, but any hard object such as scissor handles can be used. The reflex can be elicited in all normal dogs, and is mediated by the femoral nerve through the fourth to fifth lumbar spinal cord segments. The degree of normal response varies with the breed. Large breeds of dogs have a brisker reflex than the short-legged breeds such as the dachshund. The response should be evaluated as absent (0), hyporeflexic (plus 1), normal (plus 2), hyperreflexic (plus 3), or clonic (plus 4). An absent reflex or hyporeflexia occurs when a portion of the reflex arc is diseased. Hyperreflexia or clonus often is present in upper motor neuron disease.

The localizing value of this reflex can be demonstrated by the following example. Examination of an acutely paraplegic dachshund that had normal perineal and flexor reflexes but hypotonia and no patellar reflex suggested an L4, L5 spinal cord lesion and possible midlumbar (L3–L4) location of an intervertebral disk extrusion.

Biceps and Triceps Reflex. In the thoracic limb the biceps and triceps reflexes can be elicited in most dogs that are relaxed and in lateral recumbency. Lightly tapping the tendon of insertion of the triceps proximal to the olecranon elicits a slight extension of the elbow. The reflex is mediated by the radial nerve through the seventh and eighth cervical and first and second thoracic spinal cord segments. The biceps reflex is elicited by placing a finger on the distal ends of the biceps and brachialis muscles at the level of the elbow. Tapping this finger with the hammer elicits a slight flexion of the elbow. The muscle contraction can be palpated in some instances when no movement of the joint is seen. The musculocutaneous nerve mediates this reflex through the sixth, seventh, and eighth cervical spinal cord segments. The normal patient has a mild reflex response to these stimuli. In a few normal patients response is difficult to elicit and appears absent. These reflexes also are absent when there is disease in some portion of the reflex arc, and they may be hyperactive in some cases with disease of the upper motor neuron.

Flexor Reflex—Pelvic Limb. The flexor reflexes to painful stimuli determine the integrity of the reflex arc, as well as the pathway in the central nervous system that is concerned with the patient's response to painful stimuli. The most reliable stimulus is pressure exerted on the base of the toenail with hemostats. Many animals do not respond to the stimulus of a pin. In the pelvic limb, the flexor reflex is mediated by the sciatic nerve through the sixth and seventh lumbar spinal cord segments and the first sacral segment. Abnormality of the motor portion of the sciatic nerve distal to the pelvis causes paralysis, hypotonia, and atrophy of the flexors of the stifle, tarsus, and digits, as well as of the extensors of the tarsus and digits. There is no resistance to flexion or extension of the paw. On walking with a sciatic nerve paralysis, the tarsus will be lower on the affected side and the paw may be placed on its dorsal surface; however, the limb is able to support weight as long as the femoral nerve is intact.

Sensory branches of the peroneal nerves supply the dorsal surface of the paw. The plantar surface is supplied by sensory branches of the tibial nerve. The medial side of the paw is supplied by the saphenous nerve, a branch of the femoral nerve at the femoral triangle. This enters the spinal cord through the fourth to fifth lumbar segments. A patient may have a contused sciatic nerve from a pelvic fracture and have no function of the muscles innervated by this nerve, and analgesia of the lateral, dorsal, and plantar surfaces of the paw. However, the intact saphenous nerve provides sensation to the medial surface of the paw. If this area is stimulated, the patient will flex the hip with the intact innervation of the iliopsoas muscle, but the stifle, tarsus, and digits will fail to flex. For this reason, both the medial and lateral surfaces of the paw should be tested for reflex response as well as for pain perception.

Pain Perception. The patient shows signs of pain when the impulses generated by a noxious stimulus have entered the spinal cord over the peripheral nerves and dorsal roots and are relayed to tracts in the lateral funiculi of the spinal cord bilaterally. These tracts ascend the spinal cord in the lateral funiculi, and continue through the medulla, pons, and mesencephalon to specific nuclei in the thalamus for relay to the somatic sensory cerebral cortex. Pain may be evidenced when the impulses reach the thalamus or cerebrum.

Flexor Reflex—Thoracic Limb. In the thoracic limb the thoracodorsal, axillary, musculocutaneous, radial, median, and ulnar nerves primarily are responsible for flexion of the shoulder, elbow, carpus, and digits when a painful stimulus is applied to the paw. These arise from the sixth cervical to the second thoracic spinal cord segments. The specific sensory nerve stimulated depends on the location of the stimulus. The median and ulnar nerves innervate the skin of the palmar surface of the paw; the radial nerve supplies the dorsal surface. In the forearm the radial nerve supplies the skin on the cranial and lateral surfaces. The ulnar nerve supplies the caudal surface and the musculocutaneous nerve innervates the medial surface.

Crossed Extensor Reflex. In patients with upper motor neuron disease and release of the lower motor neuron, a crossed extensor reflex may be elicited in the recumbent animal when the flexor reflex is stimulated. This occurs in the limb opposite the one being tested for a flexor reflex. To avoid voluntary extension of the contralateral limb as a response to pain, the flexor reflex first should be elicited with a mild stimulus, and the opposite limb should be observed for extension. This reflex often is difficult to interpret in a patient that still has some voluntary movement of the limbs. It is an abnormal reflex, indicative of upper motor neuron disease when it is elicited in a patient in lateral recumbency. It has not proved useful in determining the prognosis of spinal cord lesions.

Perineal Reflex. The perineal reflex is elicited by stimulating the anus with a mild noxious stimulus, and observing contraction of the anal sphincter and flexion of the tail. It is mediated by branches of the sacral and caudal nerves through the sacral and caudal segments of the spinal cord.

CRANIAL NERVES

In evaluating spinal cord disease, the examination of cranial nerves is useful to exclude or implicate diffuse or multifocal lesions in an animal that presents with the signs of spinal cord disease. On examining the eyes, signs of a sympathetic paralysis (Horner's syndrome) may correlate directly with the location of a spinal cord lesion in the first three thoracic spinal cord segments, or with an unusually acute severe cervical spinal cord lesion that interferes with the lateral tectotegmentospinal system.

SUMMARY OF SIGNS WITH LESIONS AT SPECIFIC LOCATIONS IN THE SPINAL CORD

Lumbosacral: Fourth Lumbar to Fifth Caudal Segment

Complete malacia from fourth lumbar through fifth caudal segments:
Flaccid paraplegia: no support, gait, or movement of pelvic limbs and tail. Normal thoracic limbs.
No postural reactions in pelvic limbs.
Areflexia: flexor, patellar, perineal reflexes.
Atonia: soft muscles, no resistance to manipulation of pelvic limbs or tail.
Neurogenic atrophy: in chronic lesions.
Dilated anus.
Analgesia from pelvic limbs, tail, and perineum.
Partial malacia of gray and white matter between the fourth lumbar and fifth caudal segments:
Flaccid paraparesis and ataxia of pelvic limbs with normal thoracic limbs.
Postural reactions of pelvic limbs attempted, but poorly accomplished.
Hyporeflexia or areflexia: flexor and patellar reflexes.
Hypotonia: normal or weak resistance to manipulation of pelvic limbs.
Slight neurogenic atrophy: in chronic lesions.
Normal or depressed pain perception (hypalgesia) from pelvic limbs, tail, and perineum.

Thoracolumbar: Third Thoracic to Third Lumbar Segment

Complete malacia—focal site between third thoracic and third lumbar segments:

Spastic paraplegia: no voluntary support, gait, or movement of pelvic limbs. Normal thoracic limbs. With acute lesions the thoracic limbs may be spastic (Schiff-Sherrington syndrome).

No postural reactions in pelvic limbs.

Reflexes normal or hyperactive: flexor and patellar.

Crossed extensor reflex may occur.

Muscle tone normal or hypertonic.

Analgesia from area caudal to the lesion.

Partial malacia—focal site between third thoracic and third lumbar segments:

Spastic paraparesis and ataxia of pelvic limbs with normal thoracic limbs.

All postural reactions poorly performed in pelvic limbs.

Reflexes normal or hyperactive: flexor and patellar.

Crossed extensor reflex may occur.

Muscle tone normal or hypertonic.

Pain perception normal or depressed from area caudal to the lesion.

Caudal Cervical: Fifth Cervical to Second Thoracic Segment

Partial malacia of gray and white matter between fifth cervical and second thoracic segments:

Tetraparesis and ataxia of all four limbs, with the thoracic limb deficit worse than that of the pelvic limb, or tetraplegia, with the patient in lateral recumbency.

Thoracic limbs: hyporeflexic or areflexic; normal tone or hypotonic; neurogenic atrophy if a chronic lesion.

Pelvic limbs: normal reflexes or hyperreflexic; normal tone or hypertonic; no atrophy.

Pain perception normal or depressed from all four limbs, or depressed from thoracic limbs only.

All postural reactions poorly performed with the thoracic limb function worse than that of the pelvic limb.

Miosis, protruded third eyelid, ptosis, and enophthalmos (T1–T3 lesion).

Cranial Cervical: First Cervical to Fifth Cervical Segment

Partial malacia—focal site between first and fifth cervical segments:

Spastic tetraplegia with patient in lateral recumbency: (1) No postural reactions present. (2) Reflexes normal or hyperactive in all four limbs. (3) Crossed extensor reflexes may occur. (4) Muscle tone normal or hypertonic. (5) Hypalgesia from area caudal to the lesion.

Spastic tetraparesis and ataxia of all four limbs. The deficit in the pelvic limbs is often worse than in the thoracic limbs. Occasionally, the opposite is found. (1) Postural reactions poorly performed. (2) Reflexes normal or hyperactive. (3) Crossed extensor reflexes may occur. (4) Muscle tone normal or hypertonic. (5) Pain perception normal or depressed from area caudal to the lesion.

Bladder dysfunction often accompanies severe spinal cord disease. Total lower motor neuron paralysis occurs with sacral spinal cord lesions. Severe or total focal thoracolumbar spinal cord lesions produce an upper motor neuron type of paralysis. Paralysis is less common with cervical spinal cord lesions, unless the lesion is severe. With both LMN and UMN paralysis, retention of urine occurs. Overflow takes place with both, but is more constant with lower motor neuron disease. It is less frequent in UMN disease because greater intraluminal pressure is required to overcome the tone in the striated urethral muscle. If the integrity of the bladder wall is retained, reflex urination may follow within a variable period of time. Reflex urination is more efficient in upper motor neuron disease, utilizing the intact peripheral nerves and sacral spinal cord segments. In lower motor neuron disease this must be mediated within the wall of the bladder.

SPINAL CORD DISEASE IN SMALL ANIMALS

LUMBOSACRAL SPINAL CORD DISEASE (L4–Cd)

Some examples of lumbosacral spinal cord disease already have been considered in Chapter 4 on lower motor neuron disease.

Trauma

External Injury. Fracture with displacement of L7 is a common injury which usually produces total paralysis of the tail, anus, perineum, bladder, and rectum. The degree of pelvic limb paresis and ataxia depends on the degree of involvement of the lumbar roots and nerves. If both the L6 and L7 spinal nerves are compromised on the cranial and caudal aspects of the fractured vertebra, in addition to the S1 roots coursing through the L7 vertebral foramen, there is a complete sciatic nerve paralysis, unilateral or bilateral. The flexor reflex is absent from the stifle, tarsus, and digits, but hip flexion and the patellar reflex are preserved. There is analgesia of the dorsal, lateral, and plantar surfaces of the hind paw, but not of the medial surface (femoral, saphenous nerves, L4–L5 roots).

If the trauma from the accident is severe, hemorrhage and necrosis may occur in the spinal cord segments cranial to the site of the fracture and produce paraplegia with atonia, areflexia, and analgesia of the pelvic limbs, perineum, anus, and tail.

There is a better prognosis for direct injury to the spinal roots and nerves than for injury to spinal cord segments. Spinal roots are more resistant to injury because of their structure, they tend to recover more often following contusion, and even can regenerate if necessary. For these reasons, although vertebral canal displacement may be severe with an L7 fracture and luxation, the prospect for recovery is not hopeless.

Internal Injury. Intervertebral disk extrusions in the middle and caudal lumbar vertebral column are not common but do occur. Their location is predicted by the nature of the lower motor neuron signs they produce and by the paresis, ataxia, or paralysis of the gait. An L3–L4 extrusion often produces a loss of the patellar reflex because of involvement of the adjacent L4 and L5 spinal cord segments. If L6 and L7 are spared, the flexor reflex is preserved. An L4–L5 or L5–L6 extrusion produces loss of the flexor reflex. At the L4–L5 articulation, the spinal cord segments L6, L7, and S1 are vulnerable. At the L5–L6 articulation the roots of these segments are vulnerable. Decreased or absent anal and tail tone and perineal reflex, along with lower motor neuron bladder paralysis, accompany extrusions at or caudal to the L5–L6 articulation.

Similarly, other forms of space-occupying lesions can be located in this region of the spinal cord. The following case report is a typical example.

Signalment. An 8-year-old male Weimaraner.

Chief Complaint. The patient had lumbar pain and pelvic limb dysfunction.

History. Two and one-half weeks prior to referral, this dog was presented to a veterinarian with the complaint of an arched back and soreness in this area. The signs persisted without a definite diagnosis. One week prior to referral, soreness during examination was noticed in the right pelvic limb. Neurologic signs were first evident to the owner 3 days before presentation, and consisted of paresis, ataxia, or both, of the right pelvic limb. These signs had progressed by the time of the referral examination.

Physical Examination. The dog was an alert, aggressive patient with normal thoracic limb function. The pelvic limbs were paretic and ataxic, especially the right one. It frequently was placed on its dorsal surface, crossed under the body, or abducted widely. When bearing weight, the right tarsus was closer to the floor than the left tarsus. Occasionally, the limbs only partially supported the caudal trunk. If weight was added to the pelvis by manual pressure, the pelvic limbs could not support the body due to paresis.

Postural reactions were most deficient in the right pelvic limb. Hopping and proprioceptive positioning were performed poorly on the right and showed a fair but not normal response on the left. Muscle tone was moderately hypotonic in the right pelvic limb, and slightly hypotonic to normal in the left pelvic limb. The tail was hypotonic. The anus showed only equivocal hypotonia. Atrophy was evident in the right caudal thigh muscles and all the right leg muscles. The right pelvic limb flexor reflex was depressed markedly. Pain was perceived and the hip flexed, but stifle, tarsal, and digital flexion were absent. On striking the patellar tendon some contraction was observed in the quadriceps muscle, but the only action seen was hip flexion. In the left pelvic limb the patellar reflex was plus 1 to 2. The flexor reflex was intact but slightly depressed. Pain perception was normal. Pressure applied to the spines of the vertebrae elicited pain from the caudal lumbar and sacral vertebrae. Brisk extension of the tail elicited pain.

Anatomic Diagnosis. The lesion involved the spinal cord segments or roots L6, L7, S1–S3, and caudal primarily on the right side. The site of pain on vertebral manipulation suggested a root lesion.

Laboratory Findings: CSF. Cisternal CSF examination revealed 93 mg of protein per dl and no WBC. Plain radiography showed no lesion.

Myelography. It was not possible to enter the subarachnoid space between L5 and L6. Radiopaque dye was introduced between L4 and L5. The dye column caudal to the injection site stopped abruptly over the caudal end of the body of L5. CSF from the L4–L5 tapping site contained 430 mg of protein per dl and no WBC.

Surgery. A laminectomy at L5, L6, and L7 revealed an elongate mass in the epidural space beween the laminae on the right side and the spinal cord, which was compressed dorsolaterally to the left. The right roots and spinal nerves from L5 caudally were compressed ventrally. The mass was dissected free of the neural structures and removed. It was not attached to the meninges of the spinal cord or the roots. It was diagnosed as a fibrosarcoma.

Outcome. The dog improved mildly in a few weeks, then remained stable for about 8 months, when the same signs appeared again. Euthanasia then was performed.

Inflammation (see Chapter 4)

Polioencephalomyelitis in pigs.
Rabies encephalomyelitis in all species.

Canine distemper myelitis.
Toxoplasma myelitis.
Equine protozoal myelitis.

Degeneration (see Chapter 4)

Ischemic myelopathy: fibrocartilaginous emboli.
Diffuse myelomalacia.
Hereditary abiotrophy: Swedish Lapland dog.

Neoplasia

Intramedullary.   Spinal cord gliomas or metastases to the parenchyma are uncommon. Diagnosis requires myelography.

Extramedullary.   See trauma and case report in the preceding section.

Malformation (see Chapter 2)

Myelodysplasia and meningomyelocele commonly are associated with spina bifida of the caudal lumbar or sacral vertebrae. Segmental hypoplasia may isolate sacral and caudal segments, producing analgesia. As a rule, the malformation does not interfere enough with grey matter morphology to cause lower motor neuron signs. The pelvic limb gait may be ataxic and weak. Although all individuals are susceptible, this malformation is found more commonly in Manx cats and English bulldogs.

THORACOLUMBAR SPINAL CORD DISEASE (T3–L3)

Trauma

External Injury.   External injuries most often are caused by automobiles, gunshot wounds, and wounds acquired while fighting. Characteristically, such spinal cord trauma is sudden in onset, usually immediately related to the time of the accident, but occasionally it may follow the accident by a few hours. It generally is nonprogressive; however, it may progress within the first 24 hours posttrauma, and only in the second 24 hours posttrauma if there is continual bleeding or excessive movement at the site of the vertebral column injury with continued trauma to the spinal cord. Following this, the signs remain stable or improve.

Most fractures in this region occur at the thoracolumbar junction, but they can occur at any level. They vary in type and degree of subluxation. Be aware that the radiograph can determine only the degree of subluxation present at that time. It may have been far worse at the time of the injury, but immediately returned to a normal position. Always examine the radiograph for the size of the intervertebral disks. They often are extruded with external injury, and their normal location is reduced in size. In fact, a narrow space between two vertebrae may be the only evidence of an external injury, and be diagnostic for an acutely extruded intervertebral disk. In rare cases the external injury causes spinal cord contusion without vertebral column injury.

Sudden complete compression of the thoracolumbar spinal cord causes paralysis of all the muscles caudal to the lesion and analgesia of the skin. Unlike incomplete, subacute, or chronic spinal cord lesions in this region, a specific syndrome of muscle tone and reflexes accompanies the paraplegia observed in these acute complete lesions. This is referred to as the Schiff-Sherrington syndrome. Although the lesion is caudal to T2, there is rigid extension of the thoracic limbs. However, they still function normally in the postural reactions and all efforts of voluntary movement. Despite the fact that the paralysis is caused by direct interference with the upper motor neuron, there is remarkable hypotonia of the pelvic limbs. However, all spinal reflexes caudal to the lesion are normal. The level of the lesion can be determined best by locating a line of analgesia, or the level of detection of the panniculus reflex, or both. This line usually is caudal to the spinal cord lesion by one to two spinal cord segments because of the caudal distribution of the cutaneous branches of the spinal nerves after they emerge from the intervertebral foramina.

The term Schiff-Sherrington syndrome has been applied to the phenomenon of thoracic limb extensor hypertonia associated with paraplegia from acute thoracolumbar spinal cord lesions.[115, 116] It is explained by the fact that there are neurons located in the lumbar spinal cord that are responsible for the tonic inhibition of extensor muscle alpha motoneurons in the cervical intumescence. These are called "border cells," and their cell bodies are located on the dorsolateral border of the ventral grey column from L1 through L7, with a maximal population from L2 through L4.[125] Their axons cross to the contralateral fasciculus proprius of the lateral funiculus, where they ascend to their termination in the cervical intumescence. Acute severe lesions cranial to these "border cell" neurons and caudal to the cervical intumescence that suddenly deprive the cervical intumescence neurons of this source of tonic inhibition cause a "release" of these latter neurons, which results in the extensor hypertonia observed in the thoracic limbs. There is no compromise of the descending upper motor neuron system to the cervical intumescence and therefore the thoracic limbs can function normally in the gait and postural reactions, except for the hypertonia.

In primates such acute spinal cord lesions cause spinal cord shock caudal to the lesion. This is a physiologic phenomenon that severely depresses lower motor neuron function of all the spinal cord segments caudal to the site of the morphologic lesion. It results in complete atonia and areflexia caudal to the lesion, which persists for 2 to 3 weeks. This phenomenon may result from the functional disturbance caused by the sudden widespread disorganization that occurs on the dendritic zone and cell body of the general somatic efferent motor neuron.[58] This is produced by the degeneration of telodendria of the efferent spinal cord neurons that were interrupted by the lesion.

Spinal shock in domestic animals is of much less magnitude and is of no clinical significance. Spinal reflexes always are present caudal to the lesion by the time the veterinarian observes the injured patient. Possibly, the hypotonia in the pelvic limbs is attributable to spinal shock, but the degree of lower motor neuron depression is not sufficient to interfere with the spinal reflexes. This species difference in the phenomenon of spinal shock may be due to the fact that fewer spinal cord efferent neurons synapse directly on the GSE motoneuron in domestic animals, and thus less direct synaptic disorganization occurs. Pelvic limb hypotonia and thoracic limb hypertonia usually disappear in 10 to 14 days after the onset of neurologic signs. Normal to increased tone appears in the pelvic limbs, along with hyperreflexia.

Although the Schiff-Sherrington syndrome indicates severe spinal cord dysfunction and a cautious prognosis, it does not infer that no recovery can occur. It does not signify the degree of morphologic disturbance at the site of the spinal cord injury. Some recovery may follow the resolution of spinal cord hemorrhage and edema, and remyelination of intact axons.

Whenever the possibility exists that a patient has a vertebral column injury, the area should not be handled more than necessary. As a rule, the location of these injuries can be found with minimal manipulation of the patient. The entire examination can be performed with the animal in lateral recumbency. To determine whether the thoracic limb hypertonia represents the Schiff-Sherrington phenomenon or is due to a cervical spinal cord injury, minimal stimulation of the forepaws with a pin or mild pressure with forceps readily determines if pain and voluntary movement are present. In the Schiff-Sherrington syndrome they are present in the thoracic limbs but absent in the pelvic limbs. With cervical spinal cord injuries, there is more equal tone and deficit in pain and voluntary movement in all four limbs.

Therapy should be prompt and vigorous (see Chapter 19).[164] Corticosteroids and the hypertonic solution, mannitol, are used to reduce spinal cord edema. Recent studies suggest that dimethyl sulfoxide (40 per cent intravenous 1 gm per kg) may be effective in treating these injuries. Surgery usually involves decompression, reduction, and immobilization. There may be a discrepancy between the degree of vertebral column and spinal cord injuries. In most instances it is not possible to judge the severity of the spinal cord injury by the degree of displacement of the vertebrae, and it is dangerous to give a prognosis based solely on the degree of subluxation observed on radiographs. Some cases that appeared hopeless radiographically have made some recovery.

Currently extensive research is being performed on the pathophysiology of spinal cord injury.[89,158] A posttraumatic progressive hemorrhagic necrosis has been recognized that is related to local hypoxia from direct vascular injury, or the accumulation of toxic amounts of neurotransmitter amines that cause further vasoconstriction and tissue damage, or both. Surgical and medical treatments for this condition are being studied.

Internal Injury. Numerous lesions can slowly or suddenly occupy space in the vertebral canal and injure the spinal cord by compression. These are referred to as internal injuries, and usually are not associated with any source of external trauma.

INTERVERTEBRAL DISK DISEASE.[34,47,51,104,136] Intervertebral disk protrusion-extrusion occurs in all breeds of dogs. It is most common in the chondrodystrophic breeds (dachshund, Pekingese, French bulldog), and it can occur in these breeds at a young age. This is releated to the early spontaneous degeneration of the intervertebral disks that takes place in these breeds. The occurrence of this neurologic syndrome at 3 years of age is not uncommon, and occasionally it appears at 2 years. If the dog is less than 1 year old with thoracolumbar signs, look for another cause. The incidence is also high in miniature poodles, beagles, and cocker spaniels. It is found occasionally in other breeds (nonchondrodystrophic) associated with aging, and therefore generally is not observed before about 5 years of age.

Studies have shown that about 80 per cent of intervertebral disk protrusions occur between T11 and L3. On radiographs these may be evident on the floor of the vertebral canal if they are calcified, or their protrusion may be indicated by the narrowing of the intervertebral disk space that prolapsed its nuclear contents. It may be necessary to use myelography to demonstrate the lesion.[84]

These protrusions or extrusions produce varying degrees of an ischemic myelopathy in the spinal cord by interfering with the circulation of blood through the parenchyma. Most slow or mild compressions result in some degree of demyelination and axonal degeneration. Sudden large extrusions may produce focal hemorrhage and myelomalacia in the grey and white matter. There is no evidence of a myelitis other than the normal vascular response to the tissue damage.

The signs caused by the extrusion vary from pain without neurologic deficit, to mild paraparesis and ataxia, to severe paraparesis and ataxia, to paraplegia with pain response intact, to paraplegia with pain response absent. The pain associated with these intervertebral disk lesions may not represent direct meningeal involvement, but could result from the disruption of the periosteum and annulus fibrosis associated with the protrusion or extrusion. These structures are innervated by general somatic afferent neurons.

In mild cases it may be impossible to distinguish between paresis and ataxia, but this is not important in establishing the location of the lesion and providing a prognosis. In all cases spinal reflexes are intact. In most cases they are hyperactive, and hypertonia is evident on manipulation of the limbs. These are the classic signs of upper motor neuron disease. Occasionally, hypotonia occurs without other signs of lower motor neuron disease. Pain sensation (general somatic afferent—spinothalamic pathway) is almost always intact in paraparetic cases. Paraplegic animals with pain sensation have a better prognosis than those in whom there is no cerebral response to an unequivocally noxious stimulus, such as forceps pressed on the base of the toenail. In the latter cases, it is helpful to establish the line of analgesia by pinching the skin with forceps along the ventral abdomen and along the dorsum of the vertebral column. Keep in mind the caudoventral course of the caudal thoracic and lumbar nerves across the abdomen. The dorsal branches of the thoracolumbar spinal nerves also course caudally, which accounts for the line of analgesia being caudal to the site of the lesion by one to two segments. The level of detection of the panniculus reflex may be interpreted similarly.

It is the responsibility of the examiner to establish the degree of paresis, spinal reflex function, and cerebral response to pain in order to establish a prognosis and select a course of therapy.

In some instances lumbar intervertebral disk extrusions cause a necrosis in a number of segments without developing into progressive myelomalacia. When the examiner can establish from indications of loss of lower motor neuron function that extensive grey matter necrosis has occurred, the prognosis is poor and surgery usually is not warranted.

The degree of paraparesis and ataxia should be graded according to a scheme such as the one described in the examination portion of this chapter. This permits the clinician to follow the course of the patient to greater advantage.

Therapeutic procedures are varied and include rest with and without administration of corticosteroids, fenestration, which is the surgical removal of degenerate nucleus pulposus, and a procedure for removal of the vertebral arches to decompress the spinal cord with removal of the extruded intervertebral disk material. The latter is called a dorsal decompressive laminectomy or hemilaminectomy. The therapeutic procedure selected depends on the duration and extent of the clinical signs, the past medical and surgical history of the patient, and the experience and expertise of the examining clinician.[35, 133] Decompressive laminectomy is indicated in the paraplegic patient. The shorter the duration of signs before surgery, the better is the prognosis. If pain sensation is still intact in the paraplegic patient, the prognosis is better. However, in some cases improvement has occurred following delayed decompression of dogs with paraplegia and analgesia. There are numerous descriptions of the surgical procedures applicable to this disease.[36, 37, 38, 39, 70, 137, 138] Each surgeon has established guidelines for the selection of the form of therapy, if any, to be employed. Considerable variation exists in these guidelines, although in many cases the experimental work of Tarlov has served as a basis.[133]

The following case description exemplifies the value of a thorough neurologic evaluation of the patient prior to the recommendation of therapy.

Signalment. A 4-year-old female dachshund.

History. Four days prior to admission, the owner noticed that the dog's gait in the hind limbs was stiff and the dog appeared to be in pain. One day later, the patient became paralyzed completely in the hind limbs. Hyperesthesia was evident over the caudal thoracic vertebrae.

Physical Examination. On the day of examination the animal was alert and responsive. The patient lay in lateral recumbency and attempted to bite anyone that handled it. It seemed to be in severe pain. When placed on the ground, it showed no voluntary movement of the pelvic limbs. It readily wheelbarrowed, but the gait with the thoracic limbs was asymmetric. There was some awkwardness in the use of the thoracic limbs, there was a short stride in the left forelimb, and occasionally the dog had difficulty keeping the head elevated and the nose dropped toward the floor.

Spinal Reflexes. The flexor, patellar, and perineal reflexes all were intact. The patellar reflex was hyperactive (plus 3). There was a slightly increased resistance to passive manipulation of the pelvic limbs. No atrophy was evident. No pain was elicited when the digits were compressed.

The thoracic limbs evidenced marked increased resistance to manipulation. Flexor reflexes were intact and pain was perceived.

Postural Reactions. No postural reactions were present in the pelvic limbs. There was a variable response in the thoracic limbs, but often abnormal, to placing, hopping, and the tonic neck tests.

The abdominal muscles were completely flaccid. No intercostal muscle activity was evident. Respirations were predominantly diaphragmatic. Analgesia was apparent in the pelvic limbs, abdomen, and thorax up to the thoracic inlet. In the thoracic limbs and cranial to the thoracic inlet, pain was perceived. There was no panniculus reflex or local mass reflex along the thoracic and lumbar epaxial region.

Cranial Nerves. Cranial nerve examination was unremarkable except for the pupils. Considering the excited state of the dog, they both seemed smaller than normal. The third eyelids were prominent but not fully protruded.

Ancillary Procedures. Radiographs demonstrated a narrow intervertebral disk between segments T12 and T13. Cerebrospinal fluid from the cerebellomedullary cistern contained 60 mg of protein per dl, many neutrophils, and some mononuclear cells and erythrocytes.

Diagnosis. Diffuse myelomalacia from the cranial lumbar segments to the cranial thoracic segments. In this instance, the progressive myelomalacia spared the lumbosacral intumescence.

The abnormal gait and postural reactions in the thoracic limbs suggested a lesion of a mild nature in the cervical spinal cord. The partial bilateral Horner's syndrome indicated involvement of the cranial thoracic segments. The line of analgesia in the cranial thoracic area pointed to a severe spinal cord lesion at that level that also could account for the paraplegia. The lack of intercostal muscle activity and obvious diaphragmatic respirations suggested that these muscles were denervated by a diffuse thoracic spinal cord grey matter lesion, leaving only the phrenic nerves (cervical spinal cord segments 5, 6, and 7) for the control of respirations. The abdominal muscle atonia indicated denervation of these muscles by a caudal thoracic and cranial lumbar spinal cord grey matter lesion. The denervation of intercostal and abdominal muscles thus suggested a diffuse lower motor neuron lesion in the thoracic spinal cord which could be explained by a myelomalacia. The upper motor neuron signs in the paralyzed pelvic limbs indicated that the myelomalacia did not descend caudal to the L3 segment.

There is no therapy available for a spinal cord lesion of this nature as extensive as these signs suggest.[48] Euthanasia was recommended.

Necropsy. At necropsy there was extrusion of the T12–T13 intervertebral disk. The spinal cord was discolored grossly and soft from L3 to C8. On transverse section, total malacia of the segments from L3 to T3 was found, with partial sparing of the first two thoracic and caudal cervical segments. The segments caudal to L3 were normal.

NEOPLASIA.   Extradural and intradural extramedullary neoplasms compress the spinal cord and produce an ischemic myelopathy.[17,53,97,143] An intradural extramedullary neoplasm is one that is contained within the dura, but is primarily outside the spinal cord parenchyma. In this position it usually displaces and compresses the spinal cord parenchyma, and only occasionally does it infiltrate the spinal cord.

In dogs neurofibromas commonly are intradural, but occasionally they are found in the epidural space. Meningiomas and metastatic choroid plexus carcinomas usually are intradural. A neuroepithelioma occurs intradurally in young dogs. In cats of all ages the most common spinal cord neoplasm is lymphosarcoma.[159] It usually is extradural in the epidural space. Occasionally, it is found intradural. The same neoplasm occurs extradurally in dogs, but is much less common. Meningiomas also occur intradurally in cats. Most metastatic neoplasms are extradural.

These extramedullary neoplasms typically produce a progressive neurologic disability. Although usually slow in onset and progression, it is not unusual for the clinical signs to come on fairly suddenly and progress rapidly. From retrospective study of necropsied cases it would appear that some of these masses may grow slowly for a considerable period of time, with the spinal cord adapting to the compression. The onset of neurologic signs may represent the critical point when the compression interferes with the spinal cord circulation, resulting in lesions and clinical signs. It is astounding to observe at necropsy how severe a compression there is in an animal that was still ambulatory. The adaptation of the spinal cord to compression that is produced slowly appears to be phenomenal, whereas sudden compression produces a devastating effect on spinal cord structure and function. Neoplasms often are located laterally, and therefore it is common for the neurologic signs to be asymmetric, at least at the onset of the observed disability. The paresis and ataxia are more pronounced on the side of the lesion.

Plain radiographs are normal, unless the neoplasm has invaded or originated from a vertebra. A myelogram usually demonstrates the location of the neoplasm, and careful comparison of ventrodorsal and lateral views should differentiate extradural from intradural lesions.[14, 43, 129]

A thorough physical examination and thoracic radiographs should be made to diagnose metastatic neoplasia.

Canine Neuroepithelioma.   An intradural mostly extramedullary neoplasm occurs in the thoracolumbar region of young dogs.[121, 134] Between 1970 and 1975, seven cases were observed. The ages at the time of examination for neurologic deficit ranged from 6 months to 3 years and 2 months. The patients were four females and three males. There were four German shepherds, one mastiff, one beagle, and one Old English sheepdog. All neoplasms were solitary and were located between T10 and L2 spinal cord segments in the leptomeninges. Five were on the left and two on the right. The signs often were fairly rapid in onset and progression. Occasionally, temporary improvement was observed with steroid therapy, but this was followed by continued progression of signs. At examination three dogs were grade 0 paraplegics, and four were about grade 3 paraparetics. Myelography is necessary for diagnosis. In one case surgical removal was followed by improvement, which has not deteriorated over a period of 8 months.

Examination of the neoplasm microscopically by numerous pathologists has resulted in mixed opinions. The general consensus is that this may represent a neuroepithelioma arising on the spinal cord surface from undifferentiated neuroepithelial cells. The clinician must be aware of this disease when examining young dogs with signs of progressive thoracolumbar spinal cord disease. There is some indication that it is more common in the German shepherd.

Canine Multiple Cartilaginous Exostoses. Although not a neoplastic disease, multiple cartilaginous exostoses occur in young dogs and may invade the vertebral canal as a space-occupying lesion.[10, 16, 42, 45] These exostoses represent a benign proliferation of cartilage and bone associated with an epiphyseal plate in bones, and grow by endochondral formation. These growths are covered by hyalin cartilage and undergo normal endochondral ossification similar to that at the epiphyseal plate. They are common in long bones, ribs, and vertebrae. They form large, easily palpable masses at these sites. Those that grow from a vertebral arch into the canal cause extradural spinal cord compression and progressive neurologic signs. Most occur in the thoracic or lumbar vertebrae. These growths cease spontaneously when normal bone growth stops at the epiphyseal plates under the control of the endocrine system. There is no sex or breed predilection, but a familial basis is suspected. It is considered an hereditary disease in man. The onset of neurologic signs occurs prior to 1 year of age unless the compression is caused by subsequent development of a neoplasm from multiple cartilaginous exostoses. Surgical excision is necessary only for cosmetic purposes, if abrasions occur over a mass, or if signs of spinal cord compression occur.

Vertebral osteomas may occur in young dogs and produce excessive pain with or without signs of spinal cord compression. The pain is similar to that observed with osteomyelitis but leukocytosis, fever, and response to antibiotics do not occur.

VERTEBRAL MALFORMATION. Vertebral column malformation should be considered in young dogs less than 1 year old that have signs of a progressive thoracolumbar spinal cord lesion, usually beginning between 3 and 9 months of age.[8, 43] The disease is *not* restricted to the brachycephalic breeds. Careful physical examination usually discloses the malformation because of the deviation of the vertebral column. There may be an associated line of hypalgesia. The neurologic deficit usually is symmetric.

Radiographs generally reveal a marked dorsal deviation of the thoracic vertebral column, kyphosis, with one or more wedge-shaped vertebral bodies and ventrally deviated spines at the most dorsal point of the kyphosis. At this point the vertebral canal is smaller than normal. A myelogram shows compression of the subarachnoid space by a symmetric decrease in diameter of the vertebral canal over one or more of the wedge-shaped vertebral bodies.

These dogs are born with this vertebral column malformation, which often is referred to as "hemivertebra" because of the wedge-shaped appearance of one or more of the vertebrae at the dorsal aspect of the kyphosis. Hemivertebra is a misnomer, however, because more than one half of the vertebra is formed, and it is fallacious to propose that this resulted from a failure of the two vertebral body ossification centers to develop and fuse. There is only one such ossification center in the normal dog.

Since there is no spinal cord malformation, neurologic signs do not appear until the spinal cord is compressed. Presumably, the onset of neurologic signs, that is, spinal cord compression, is delayed for one of two reasons, or both. Either the kyphosis is progressive as the dog grows, ultimately resulting in compression, or as the dog grows the vertebral canal at the site of the malformation does not grow sufficiently by resorption and remodeling to accommodate the growth of the spinal cord, and compression results.

If surgical decompression is to be performed, be aware that the vertebral column may be quite unstable at the site of the malformation and some immobilization should be performed prior to completion of the laminectomy.

VERTEBRAL OSTEOMYELITIS — DISKOSPONDYLITIS. Diskospondylitis is an inflammation of the vertebral bodies and associated intervertebral disk.[39, 55] It is usually a septic condition from a hematogenous source, but occasionally is associated with an adjacent tissue infection. *Staphylococcus aureus, Corynebacterium diphtheroides, Streptococcus canis, Brucella canis,* and *Nocardia* have been cultured from these lesions. Cultures frequently are negative and even biopsy may not reveal sepsis.

The most diagnostic clinical sign is severe vertebral column pain associated with a progressive paraparesis and ataxia. The neurologic deficit results from the bone proliferation associated with the lesion that encroaches on the vertebral canal and compresses the spinal cord. Fever and hematologic abnormalities may not be present. Some cases have a history of previous vertebral column trauma.

Radiographs reveal an irregular bone proliferation of the vertebral bodies adjacent to an intervertebral disk which is usually narrow. Lytic lesions often are present in the vertebrae at this site. The reactive bone proliferation extends outward in all directions. The part that invades the vertebral canal causes extradural spinal cord compression.

Treatment should include long-term antibiotic therapy specific for the organism that is cultured, spinal cord decompression, and vertebral immobilization to allow arthrodesis of the involved vertebrae.[39]

SPONDYLOSIS DEFORMANS AND DURAL OSSIFICATION. Although spondylosis deformans and dural ossification frequently are incriminated as causes of spinal cord compression, they rarely cause this condition. The proliferative bone lesion of spondylosis deformans produces ventral and lateral exostosis on the vertebral bodies, but rarely enters the vertebral canal to compress the spinal cord.[81, 82] A myelogram is required to confirm whether this bone lesion actually has compressed the spinal cord.

Dural ossification, erroneously called pachymeningitis, is a common finding, especially in the larger breeds of dogs.[83, 117, 140] It occurs at an early age (1 to 2 years), but its development is more extensive in the older dog. Although it can occur at all levels of the spinal cord dura mater, it is found most commonly ventrally in the cranial and caudal cervical areas and the lumbar area. It also may occur laterally and dorsally, and almost surround the spinal cord at some levels. Despite the massive development of this condition, associated spinal cord lesions are rare.

Inflammation

Canine Distemper Myelitis. Dogs of any age are susceptible to the canine distemper virus. Its effect on the nervous system is variable, and may be dependent on the strain or properties of the virus. Some dogs with this disease present with signs caused by the predominant action of this virus on the spinal cord, with or without a history of previous systemic illness. If the nonsuppurative myelitis that occurs is most developed between segments T3 and L3, there are signs of a spastic paraparesis and ataxia that is often asymmetric, or spastic paraplegia.

This disease is especially suspect in dogs that are less than 1 year old. The history should indicate that the neurologic signs have been progressive.

Clinical information that contributes to this etiologic diagnosis is the finding of other neurologic deficits that cannot be explained by a focal thoracolumbar spinal cord lesion alone. Mild thoracic limb deficit in a paraplegic dog can be explained only by two lesions—one mild cervical spinal cord lesion and one severe thoracolumbar lesion. A head tilt, abnormal nystagmus, and/or head tremor suggest cerebellovestibular dysfunction. Visual deficit in a dog with normal eyeballs suggests central visual pathway disease. Typically, the inflammatory demyelinating lesion in this disease is most prominent in the white matter of the optic tracts, cerebellar peduncles, and the spinal cord, although no part of the brain is immune to it. The diffuse distribution of lesions, as well as their progressive nature, should suggest an inflammatory disease.

A mild increase in mononuclear cells, or protein, or both in the cerebrospinal fluid may be observed in cases of canine distemper encephalomyelitis. The presence of lesions of chorioretinitis observed with the ophthalmoscope also suggest exposure to this virus.

To date, there is no specific therapy for this central nervous system viral disease, and the prognosis is poor. In most cases the lesions continue to progress. In a few instances they have ceased spontaneously and some improvement has occurred, either as a result of compensatory mechanisms, or possibly owing to relief of the inflammation and remyelination of intact axons.

Toxoplasmosis. *Toxoplasma gondii,* the protozoan that causes toxoplasmosis, may affect the CNS of dogs and cats, but is much less common than canine distemper. It may be focal or diffuse in distribution, and usually alters the CSF more remarkably than the canine distemper virus. In some instances neutrophils may appear in the CSF.[161]

Cryptococcosis. *Cryptococcus neoformans* produces a severe diffuse meningitis with ependymitis and some associated encephalomyelitis in dogs and cats. Although pelvic limb paresis and ataxia may be the most obvious clinical signs, the diffuse nature of the lesion usually causes signs of cervical spinal cord and brain involvement as well. The CSF generally contains large complements of inflammatory cells and protein, and consistently contains the organism, which can be identified readily. Both toxoplasmosis and cryptococcosis may produce a characteristic granulomatous chorioretinitis that can be observed with the ophthalmoscope.

Suppurative Myelitis. Bacterial-induced suppurative myelitis usually is associated with encephalitis and meningitis. Clinical signs mostly are referable to the meningitis, and consist of hyperesthesia, a stiff neck and gait, and severe pain induced by any manipulation of the patient. It often is accompanied by fever, anorexia, increased white blood cell count on hematologic study, and neutrophils in the CSF. The degree of CSF pleocytosis and protein elevation is variable. The response to antibiotic therapy is variable. Relapses are frequent and may be thwarted only by prolonged therapy.

Degeneration

Degenerative Myelopathy in German Shepherds.   A degenerative myelopathy occurs predominantly in the aging German shepherd, and is characterized by a slowly progressive paraparesis and ataxia of the pelvic limbs.[6, 49, 50] Most patients are over 5 years old. A history of a progressive course over 5 to 6 months is common. Its onset is insidious, and loss of position sense is often the first indication of the disease. Paw-dragging, crossing the limbs, and incomplete extension of the limb for full support usually is accompanied by increased or abnormal reflexes in the pelvic limbs. Occasionally, hypotonia and hyporeflexia have been observed. The signs may be asymmetric. There often occurs a general wasting (disuse atrophy) of the muscles in the caudal thoracic and lumbosacral region. Postural reactions often are poorly performed in the pelvic limbs, especially the response to proprioceptive positioning. Although the dog eventually may be unable to get up on the pelvic limbs, grade 0 paraplegia or analgesia have not been observed. Thoracic limb function appears normal.

Although radiographs often may demonstrate dural ossification or spondylosis deformans in a dog of this age, these lesions rarely affect the spinal cord. Significant geriatric intervertebral disk protrusion can be eliminated by plain radiography as well as by myelography. Small prominences of the annulus fibrosis are common and may compress the spinal cord, but do not produce lesions or clinical signs. In degenerative myelopathy, myelograms demonstrate a normal subarachnoid space not compromised by a space-occupying mass (neoplasm), or excessive dural ossification, or the rare encroachment of spondylosis deformans in the vertebral canal. CSF usually shows no abnormality unless the protein level is increased slightly.

The lesion consists of a diffuse degeneration of white matter in both the ascending and descending spinal cord tracts in all funiculi in all the segments of the spinal cord. It is referred to as a multisystem degeneration. The lesion is most extensive in the thoracic region. This is a degeneration of individual neurons and not groups of neurons in specific regions of these funiculi. Both the myelin sheaths and the axons degenerate. The lesion also may involve peripheral nerves, which accounts for the occasional case with some lower motor neuron signs. A typical case report follows.

Signalment.   The patient was an 8-year-old male German shepherd.

History.   Four months prior to admission, the owner noticed a slight ataxia in the hind limbs. In time, weakness became obvious and the ataxia more pronounced, and both progressed slowly until the animal became severely paraparetic 10 to 12 weeks following the onset of the signs.

Physical Examination.   On admission the dog was alert and responsive. The animal was unable to use the pelvic limbs unaided. When wheelbarrowed, the head was held erect and the gait of the thoracic limbs was normal. When supported, a very slight swinging motion of the pelvic limbs was evident (grade 1 paraparesis).

Spinal Reflexes.   The flexor, patellar, and perineal reflexes were intact. The patellar reflex was of normal amplitude (plus 2). Muscle tone was normal, and there was moderate increased resistance to passive manipulation of the pelvic limbs. Pain was perceived when the digits were compressed. All reflexes, tone, and resistance were normal in the thoracic limbs.

Postural Reactions. No postural reactions were present in the pelvic limbs. They were normal in the thoracic limbs.

Cranial Nerves. There were no abnormalities noticed.

Ancillary Procedures. Radiographs revealed minor spurring of the vertebral bodies ventrally, indicative of spondylosis. There was no lesion seen involving the vertebral canal. A myelogram also did not reveal any significant lesion within the vertebral canal. Cerebrospinal fluid contained 1 white blood cell per cmm and 30 mg of protein per dl.

Leukodystrophy in Afghan Hounds. A primary myelin degeneration occurs in young Afghan hounds of both sexes, starting usually between 3 and 13 months of age, and progressing in 2 to 3 weeks from mild paraparesis and pelvic limb ataxia to paraplegia.[18] As the disease progresses, the thoracic limbs often are affected and tetraplegia may ensue. As the paraparesis worsens, paresis of the axial musculature of the middle to caudal trunk is evident.

Dogs that have caudal thoracic or cranial lumbar spinal cord lesions producing paraplegia can support their trunks fairly well when the pelvic limbs are supported only by holding the dog up by the tail and allowing it to walk on the thoracic limbs. If there is a focal lesion in the middle or cranial thoracic spinal cord, or a diffuse thoracic spinal cord lesion, as in this disease, because of the loss of the upper motor neuron to the motoneurons of the axial muscles of a larger portion of the trunk, the dog is unable to support the trunk in this maneuver. It will fall to either side unless both the trunk and the tail are supported by the examiner.

Initially, pelvic and thoracic limb reflexes are preserved, but in time these may be compromised as the lesion extends into the adjacent ventral grey columns of the lumbosacral and cervical intumescence.

The lesion is an extensive symmetric demyelination of large portions of the lateral and ventral funiculi and occasionally the dorsal funiculi, primarily in the thoracic spinal cord segments. There may be no CSF abnormality, despite the extensive necrosis. Breeding studies have indicated an hereditary basis for this disease. An autosomal recessive inheritance is proposed.

Demyelinating Myelopathy in Miniature Poodles. An idiopathic demyelination of the brain stem and spinal cord has been reported in miniature poodle puppies, with the onset of signs usually between 2 and 4 months of age.[25] The signs are those of progressive, diffuse spinal cord white matter disease. Spastic paraparesis is followed rapidly by paraplegia and tetraplegia. Hypertonia and hyperreflexia are marked. When tetraplegic, the patient lies in lateral recumbency with the thoracic limbs rigidly extended. The patient remains alert and responsive, and has no demonstrable cranial nerve deficit. Pain perception is retained. The lesion is restricted to white matter, in which the destruction is extensive. In general, the axons are spared. The myelin degeneration occurs symmetrically in all funiculi of all segments of the spinal cord, especially in the cervical segments, and may affect the reticular formation of the medulla and cerebellar peduncles in a patchy or diffuse manner. The pathogenesis is unknown, but a familial (hereditary) basis is suspect.

Ischemic Myelopathy. Ischemic myelopathy caused by vascular emboli presumed to be fibrocartilage can occur at any level of the spinal cord. If it occurs in the thoracolumbar region, a *sudden* spastic paraparesis with ataxia or paraplegia results. The signs are ipsilateral or bilateral, with or without symmetry, depending on the location and degree of ischemic myelopathy. These lesions usually do not produce pain on vertebral manipulation. Radiographs are normal.

A myelogram may suggest slight spinal cord swelling at the site of the lesion. CSF may contain more protein than normal.

Recovery may be spontaneous if the ischemic episode is mild. Some evidence of improvement should be apparent during the first week of the disease. If the ischemia is severe, an infarct or focal myelomalacia results, with permanent neurologic deficit. See Chapter 4 for further discussion of this disease.[156, 157]

Neoplasia — Intramedullary

Intramedullary neoplasia of the spinal cord is less common than the extramedullary form. Gliomas are the most common form of intramedullary neoplasia. There is no clear clinical feature that differentiates these two forms of neoplasia. Parenchymal destruction may be greater with the intramedullary form, and clinical signs appear earlier and are more severe when comparing neoplasms of similar size. Much depends on the rate of growth of the neoplasm.

Diagnosis can be confirmed only by myelography, and in some cases exploratory laminectomy may be necessary to distinguish the intramedullary from extramedullary form of neoplasia. Intramedullary neoplasms are much less amenable to surgical removal because of their intimate relationship with the parenchyma that has been infiltrated with the neoplastic cells.

Malformation

Canine Myelodysplasia. The myelodysplasia referred to as spinal dysraphism usually produces symmetric pelvic limb ataxia that can be observed by 4 to 6 weeks of age.[26, 79] It was described in Chapter 2, and is the most common congenital malformation in the dog.

The disease is most prevalent in the Weimaraner breed, in which it is considered to be inherited as a codominant gene. It has been reported in many other breeds. Breeding clinically affected Weimaraners to normal German shepherds or Norwegian elkhounds produces some clinically affected puppies. Breeding the normal offspring of these matings also produces some affected puppies.

The classic clinical sign observed is a symmetric use of the pelvic limbs, referred to as "bunny hopping." This is associated with a variable degree of proprioceptive deficit, with a tendency to overextend a limb on getting up or walking and standing or walking on the dorsal surface of the paw. Paresis is observed only occasionally. Patellar reflexes are normal. The pelvic limb flexor reflex stimulated in one limb usually elicits a simultaneous flexion of both limbs. Postural reactions are performed poorly in these limbs.

In dogs that are affected severely by the spinal cord malformation, there also may be abnormalities of the musculoskeletal system accompanied by scoliosis, spondylosis, koilosternia, kinked tails, and decreased pelvic muscle mass. In litters with affected offspring, some pups may be born dead or die shortly after birth.

Occasionally, a remarkable abnormality of vestibular system function is observed for a few weeks in dogs with clinical signs of the spinal cord malformation. This consists of a severe head tilt and a tendency to drift or fall to the same side. The pathogenesis of this disturbance has not been found, and it may resolve spontaneously or be compensated.

Spinal cord lesions are described in Chapter 2. It should be remembered that any clinical signs related to these lesions are present at birth and do not progress.

Signs of progressive pelvic limb ataxia in Weimaraners that were born with normal gait and posture are caused by some other acquired disease.

Other Malformations. Be aware of the association between vertebral column and spinal cord malformations. They can occur at any level, but more often are caudal thoracic and lumbar. Scoliosis or kyphosis may be associated with spinal cord aplasia, hypoplasia or a myelodysplasia with syringomyelia, hydromyelia, central canal abnormalities or hyperplasia of spinal cord tissue, or both. Neurologic signs are present at birth but usually are not apparent until 4 to 6 weeks of age in puppies and kittens, when they first become ambulatory. Ataxia most commonly accompanies the myelodysplasia, whereas paresis is more evident in hypoplasia, and paraplegia in cases of aplasia. The signs are nonprogressive. The cause of these isolated cases is unknown.

CERVICAL SPINAL CORD DISEASE (C1–C5)

Trauma

External Injury. Fractures of cranial cervical vertebrae may produce considerable displacement, yet present with remarkably few signs of neurologic deficit. The attitude, posture, and gait all depict the severe neck pain that is present. This is especially true for fractures of the cranial aspect of the body of C2.[136] Following anesthesia for radiography or surgery, the instability is exacerbated and the dog is often worse, with obvious neurologic signs of cervical spinal cord compression.

Spinal cord concussion or contusion can occur with or without fractures of the cervical vertebrae and intervertebral disk extrusion.

The principles described for external injury of the thoracolumbar spinal cord also apply to the cervical spinal cord. Unlike the Schiff-Sherrington syndrome, the thoracic limb hypertonia in cervical spinal cord injury usually is associated with pelvic limb hypertonia and severe paresis of voluntary function of all the limbs.

The following case report exemplifies unilateral cervical spinal cord injury.

Signalment. A 10-year-old male mongrel.

History. On the morning of examination, the patient was found with about 4 inches of skin torn over the midthoracic vertebral spines, and having difficulty with its gait. The animal had been normal when put outdoors the night before.

Physical Examination. The patient was a stoic but responsive and cooperative dog that walked with an obvious asymmetry to its gait. The toes of both the right thoracic and right pelvic limbs were dragged along the floor. This was not noted on the left side. Weight was supported more by the left limbs than the right, but occasionally the dog swayed slightly on the left limbs. The limbs were not noticeably abducted.

Spinal Reflexes. All flexor reflexes were normal. Crossed extension occurred in the right thoracic and pelvic limbs. Pain perception was normal from all limbs. The patellar reflex was hyperactive (plus 3) on the left side and a prolonged clonus (plus 5) was elicited on the right side. The perineal reflex was normal.

Passive manipulation of the limbs elicited a mild increased resistance on the left side and marked resistance on the right side. Clonus could be elicited in the right pelvic limb merely by putting pressure on the plantar surface of the paw.

Postural Reactions. All these tests demonstrated a deficit on the right side. The left limbs responded normally to the tonic neck and eye test, proprioceptive positioning, placing, hopping, and extensor postural thrust. The right limbs responded poorly if at all to these tests. If the right limbs were held up, the patient could support itself and walk on the left limbs. If the left limbs were held up, the dog could support itself only momentarily on the right limbs before collapsing. Normal gait was not possible on the right limbs alone.

Diagnosis. These clinical signs indicated a lesion on the right side of the cervical spinal cord cranial to C6. The sudden onset suggested trauma or a vascular disturbance as the mechanism for the lesion.

Radiography. Many lead pellets were found in the cervical region. One was located in the vertebral canal on the right side at C2.

While surgery was under consideration for removal of this foreign body, the dog suddenly expired from a venous embolus that arose from an area of the femoral vein injured by the same gunshot accident. This embolus had occluded the conus arteriosus and pulmonic valve.

Internal Injury

INTERVERTEBRAL DISK EXTRUSION.[90,162] Cervical pain is the sign most commonly associated with cervical intervertebral disk extrusion. Although any of the disks can be affected, the C2–C3 articulation has the highest incidence. If the spinal cord is compressed, signs of neurologic deficit appear, involving all four limbs. Pelvic limb paresis and ataxia usually exceed that of the thoracic limbs, but occasionally the reverse occurs, with marked hypertonia and loss of voluntary function of the thoracic limbs. Hypertonia and hyperreflexia are observed in all four limbs.

In those cases with more severe thoracic limb deficit, the extrusion has been largest on the midline, compressing more of the central portion of the spinal cord. Perhaps this involves more of the upper motor neuron to these limbs, since they course more medially to reach the grey matter in which they terminate. Occasionally, more caudally located cervical intervertebral disk extrusions also cause more severe thoracic limb deficit. Pain on manipulation of the cervical vertebrae does not always accompany the neurologic signs. Sometimes the neurologic signs are asymmetric and an ipsilateral spastic hemiparesis occurs.

In some cases there are continual irregular contractions or spasms of the cervical muscles usually associated with neck pain, with or without mild signs of ataxia and paresis.

NEOPLASIA—EXTRAMEDULLARY. Primary or metastatic neoplasms of the vertebral column, epidural space, or meninges can cause extramedullary compression of the cervical spinal cord. The kinds of neoplasms have been discussed in the section on thoracolumbar lesions. Meningiomas have been seen more commonly at the C1 or C2 levels in the dog. They cause varying degrees of progressive spastic tetraparesis and ultimately recumbency, but rarely tetraplegia. If the lesion is unilateral, the signs may be asymmetric at their onset. Plain radiographs are normal unless there is a vertebral column neoplasm. Usually a myelogram is necessary to demonstrate the space-occupying lesion. Neurofibromas usually produce an ipsilateral spastic hemiparesis initially.

VERTEBRAL MALFORMATION—MALARTICULATION

Atlantoaxial Subluxation. Atlantoaxial subluxation occurs in miniature or toy breeds of dogs as a result of fracture, degeneration, or malformation of the dens.[43, 44, 65, 98] A fracture with subluxation is not limited to these small breeds. The pathogenesis of the absence of the dens in these small breeds is unknown. A degenerative process is suspected, causing dissolution of the bone and leaving only a remnant on the cranial articular surface of the axis. There is speculation that the mechanism is similar to the femoral head necrosis observed in Legg-Perthes disease, and possibly is related to the early development of the sex hormones in these breeds.[73] The main portion of the dens and the cranial articular surface of the axis (centrum 1) have an ossification center that is seen first at 3 weeks, and that fuses with the intercentrum 2 (cranial epiphysis) of the axis at 7 to 9 months of age. The apex of the dens (proatlas) has an inconstant ossification center that fuses to the dens at 3 to 4 months.[147]

Luxation is found most commonly in the young dog 6 to 18 months old, but it is not limited by age. The loss of the dens may precede the subluxation by a considerable period of time if the dense connective tissue between the dorsal arch of the atlas and the spine of the axis resists the instability between the body of the axis and body of the atlas. Normally, the transverse ligament of the atlas helps maintain the dorsoventral alignment of the atlas and axis by holding the dens in the caudal articular fovea of the atlas.

Without a dens this supporting mechanism is lost, and the cranial aspect of the body of the axis rotates dorsally into the vertebral canal. When subluxation has occurred, the transverse ligament of the atlas may be forced cranially into a vertical position.

Radiographs demonstrate a narrowed vertebral canal over the cranial aspect of the body of the axis, where it has pivoted dorsally into the canal. The space between the arch of the atlas and the spine of the axis is widened. Usually, there is no dens evident on the axis. In a few cases a remnant may be apparent on the ventral aspect of the canal over the body of the atlas.

The clinical signs vary from reluctance to have the head patted, to severe neck pain, to varying degrees of spastic tetraparesis, and occasionally recumbency. Often the thoracic limb paresis is more profound than the pelvic limb paresis. The dogs can stand and walk with their thoracic limbs positioned caudally under the thorax. They walk with a short, stiff stride and often place one paw in front of the other. Spasticity is severe in these limbs. The thoracic limb deficit may reflect the more pronounced midline rather than lateral spinal cord compression.

These patients should be handled with extreme care. The atlantoaxial region should not be manipulated. The signs may worsen after forced exercise. If the ataxia and paresis cause the dog to fall, the subluxation may be exacerbated, along with the spinal cord deficit. In one instance this was known to produce severe medullary edema leading to the death of the animal. Under anesthesia there is no muscle tone to support the alignment, and the danger of further subluxation is even more critical.

Surgery may be successful if spinal cord and medullary edema are prevented. The procedure is to wire the arch of the atlas to the spine of the axis. This requires passing a needle with wire beneath the arch of the atlas. Because the dura usually adheres to this arch in C1, the needle passes through the dura as well. Extreme care must be taken so as not to injure the spinal cord. It must be remembered that by the time these dogs are presented with clinical signs, there already has been extensive damage to the spinal cord. Any further insult from the surgical procedure may readily precipitate signs of medullary edema with respiratory and cardiac arrest.

C5, C6, and C7: Great Danes, Doberman Pinschers. Cervical spinal cord compression caused by caudal cervical vertebral malformation-malarticulation occurs primarily in Great Danes and Doberman pinschers, producing clinical signs referred to as the wobbler syndrome.[22, 43, 100, 101, 123, 143]

The onset of clinical signs in the Great Dane usually occurs prior to 1 year of age, often by 2 years of age, and occasionally later than 2 years. It has even been known to occur at 7 years. More Doberman pinschers are affected clinically after 2 years of age, but a few show signs before 1 year, like the Great Dane. There is no sex predilection. The condition often affects the most rapidly growing Great Dane puppy.

The owner generally only recognizes an abnormality of the pelvic limbs, which is ataxia. The onset usually is insidious, with the owner assuming that the ataxia is normal for the rapid growth of the dog. In some cases the onset is sudden. The signs normally are progressive, and often the thoracic limbs are abnormal by the time the dog is presented for examination.

Upon examination, there is obvious bilateral paresis and ataxia of the pelvic limbs and occasionally of the thoracic limbs. When the signs are mild, they may be most evident as the animal gets up. It may be unsteady and tend to overextend a pelvic limb. During walking and especially on turning, the pelvic limbs may cross each other, abduct widely, or, in more severe cases, tend to collapse. The pelvic limb stride may be longer than usual and asymmetric, causing an awkward swaying movement of the hindquarters. Periodically, the animal may drag its toes or step with the dorsal surface of its paw on the ground. This often has caused the toenails to be worn dorsally. The signs are less obvious when the patient is gaited at faster speeds over a straight course. Abrupt change in speed or direction often exacerbates the deficit and frequently causes pelvic limb collapse. The animal gives the impression of not knowing where its limbs are because of a proprioceptive deficit.

Thoracic limb signs, when present, are similar but usually less remarkable than in the pelvic limbs. These include occasional stumbling with flexion of the carpus, so that the dorsal surface of the paw strikes the ground surface. The limbs may cross each other. In some instances, the thoracic limbs have a restricted motion, appearing rigid. This spastic gait with limited joint flexion may give the appearance that the thoracic limbs tend to "float" on protraction before striking the ground. This may appear as hypermetria. The Doberman pinschers show this spastic thoracic limb dysfunction more often than the Great Danes.

The response to testing postural reactions usually is abnormal, especially in the more paretic and ataxic animals. Hopping and proprioceptive positioning demonstrate the greatest deficits. If there are signs of thoracic limb abnormality, the animal may flex the carpus and rest the dorsal surface of the paw on the ground, or collapse when the head and neck are extended fully. If the patient is forced to walk on its thoracic limbs with the pelvic limbs held off the ground, and the head and neck in full extension, it may drag its paws on their dorsal surfaces. This proprioceptive deficit sometimes has been the only sign of abnormality in the thoracic limb function. Manipulation of the neck usually does not elicit pain.

These signs suggest a cervical spinal cord white matter lesion involving ascending proprioceptive tracts and descending motor tracts. Laboratory studies of blood, urine, and cerebrospinal fluid have revealed no abnormalities, except for an occasional mild elevation in protein content of the cerebrospinal fluid.

In studying the gait disorder that occurs in this disease, it first must be determined that this is a neurologic disorder and not an abnormal gait caused by one or more of the several skeletal diseases that occur in the young, rapidly growing dogs of the giant breeds.

Coxofemoral dysplasia, osteochondrosis dessicans, hypertrophic osteodystrophy, and genu valgum are some of these diseases. On observing the gait, the examiner must keep in mind the question of whether the patient is unwilling to perform a function because of pain from skeletal disease, or is unable to perform it due to neurologic dysfunction. In the skeletal diseases the stride usually is shortened, and the gait may appear choppy. There may be an asymmetric posture or function of the limbs, or both. In all instances, however, in the absence of neurologic disease the patient knows the position of its limbs at all times. The limbs are not crossed, or abducted excessively, nor do they appear to be positioned widely apart. If the patient responds to postural testing there is no failure to perform the tests. Careful palpation of the joints may reveal a lesion or cause pain. In some instances, the animal may have both a neurologic and a skeletal disease, but careful testing should reveal the neurologic deficit. The examiner must decide whether the dog will not or can not carry out a function. The former indicates skeletal disease, the latter neurologic disease. The ataxic dog with a cervical spinal cord lesion does not have control over the position of its limbs. This accounts for the wide-based, abducted gait with stumbling and flexing of the digits so that the dorsal surface of the paw is placed on the ground surface.

The signs described indicate a focal cervical spinal cord lesion. The spastic paresis is caused by the interference with the descending upper motor neuron tracts, and the ataxia is due to the lesion in the ascending proprioceptive tracts, especially the spinocerebellar tracts. Typically, pelvic limb signs are worse than those in the thoracic limbs. This may reflect the more superficial position of the pelvic limb spinocerebellar tracts in the spinal cord at the site of the injury, or the further distance of the pelvic limbs from the center of gravity of the animal, or both. The occasional mild scapular muscle atrophy reflects the chronicity of the lesion, with neuronal loss from the grey matter of the C6 and C7 segments. An electromyogram may reveal denervation potentials in these muscles.

In the young dog the primary neurologic disease to differentiate is canine distemper myelitis. Careful neurologic examination of the patient with cervical spinal cord myelitis from canine distemper usually reveals other abnormalities that cannot be explained by a lesion that is localized solely in the cervical spinal cord. The distemper lesion in the nervous system usually is disseminated, and most of the time signs reflect the site of greatest damage. Paraplegia with mild thoracic limb deficit requires two lesions of different severity, one cervical and one thoracolumbar. Head tilts or tremor and abnormal nystagmus depend on a cerebellovestibular lesion. It is not unusual for a dog with encephalomyelitis caused by the canine distemper virus to present with signs of spinal cord disease. The cerebrospinal fluid is often abnormal. Further, this disease is most prevalent in dogs of the same age as those affected most frequently by the cervical vertebral malformation.

Focal cervical spinal cord neoplasms are not common at this young age, but they cannot be excluded. Neurofibroma, meningioma, and neuroepithelioma have been seen in young animals, and require myelography for diagnosis.

Intervertebral disk extrusions, not associated with caudal cervical vertebral malformation-malarticulation, usually occur in older dogs and most often can be identified readily by plain radiographs. Cervical pain, not usually observed in dogs with cervical vertebral malformation-malarticulation, is often the prominent sign in cervical disk disease.

Radiographs of the caudal cervical vertebrae of the normally extended and fully flexed neck in lateral view are the most helpful. In a few cases the ventrodorsal view has revealed asymmetry of vertebral structures. The following observations may reflect the source of the spinal cord contusion:

1. Malarticulation: One of the caudal cervical vertebrae may be malarticulated so that the craniodorsal aspect of its vertebral body is displaced into the vertebral

canal. This may be stable and be evident on both flexed and extended neck views. It may be unstable and only be apparent on the flexed neck view. This unstable malarticulation is referred to as spondylolisthesis (spondylo = vertebra, listhesis = slipping).

2. Malformation: These changes may reflect the response of the vertebrae and adjacent soft tissues to the abnormal forces associated with or resulting in the malarticulation. The cranial orifice of the vertebral foramen may be stenotic, with or without deformity of the craniodorsal or cranioventral aspects of the vertebral body. Exostoses may occur, especially at the cranioventral aspect of the vertebral body. There may be degenerative changes in the associated intervertebral disks, which may culminate in complete collapse of the disk and ankylosis of the adjacent vertebrae. Degenerative periarticular arthritis may be apparent at the synovial joints.

Most dogs have a combination of malarticulation and malformation. A few dogs have demonstrated the typical physical and neurologic signs, but no radiographic abnormality can be seen on plain radiographs. A myelogram may reveal soft tissue changes associated with the caudal cervical vertebrae. Proliferation of the interarcuate ligament (yellow ligament) or protrusion-extrusion of the intervertebral disk may be identified.

In a few instances, surgery has revealed extensive proliferation of the cranial articular processes in a ventromedial direction encroaching on the vertebral foramen and the spinal cord. Asymmetry in these processes may be evident on a ventrodorsal radiograph.

At necropsy, disarticulation of cervical vertebrae often reveals a compressed spinal cord segment at the cranial orifice of one or more of the caudal cervical vertebrae. The vertebral foramen is often funnel-shaped, with the smaller orifice at the cranial end. Occasionally, an enlarged interarcuate ligament rests on the dorsal surface of the compressed spinal cord at the entrance to a vertebral foramen.

Microscopy has revealed a focal spinal cord injury usually limited to the sixth and/or seventh cervical spinal cord segments. Occasionally, the fifth segment was involved. There was a variable degree of degeneration of the grey and white matter in these segments, involving almost all of the funiculi. Myelin degeneration was the most pronounced lesion in the white matter. Axonal degeneration was less prominent.

Sometimes there is a focal area of necrosis in one or more of the funiculi. At the site of the focal spinal cord lesion, there often is a paucity of neurons in the grey matter with an abundance of hypertrophied astrocytes.

In the spinal cord segments cranial to this focal lesion, the white matter degeneration is limited primarily to the ascending tracts in the dorsal funiculi and the superficial portions of the dorsolateral funiculi. Caudal to the focal lesion, the white matter degeneration is limited to the descending spinal cord tracts in the ventral funiculi and deep portions of the lateral funiculi. This pattern of noninflammatory degeneration of ascending neurons cranial to the injury and descending neurons caudal to the injury is explained by a Wallerian-type of degeneration of the axon and its myelin that occurs in the segment of the neuron which is separated from its cell body. In this disease, the neurons are destroyed at the site of the injury, usually the sixth, or seventh, or both cervical spinal cord segments.[57, 141, 142]

The prognosis for spontaneous recovery is poor. A few young dogs have been

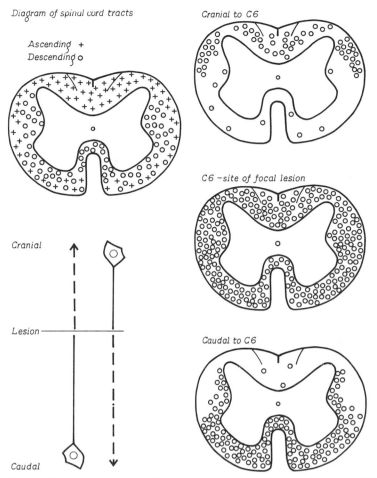

Figure 10–1.   Pattern of spinal cord degeneration following a focal segmental lesion.

found to improve following rest in a confined place. Most cases either remain static or slowly progress until the animal may become unable to get up.

Surgery is advocated as the best therapy for this disease.[28, 41, 107, 130, 131] The procedure employed depends on the type of malarticulation-malformation that is present, and the experience of the surgeon. Three procedures are advocated.

Dorsal decompressive laminectomy (DDL) alone is advocated for a stenotic cranial orifice of a vertebral foramen, or a stable malarticulation. A DDL with arthrodesis of the articular processes is advocated for the unstable malarticulation without a deformity of the craniodorsal aspect of the vertebral body. Malarticulations with a prominent craniodorsal projection of the vertebral body should have a ventral decompression with excision of this projection and fusion of the vertebral bodies.

The cause of this disease is unknown. A study on overnutrition in Great Dane dogs indicated a possible role of excess dietary calcium, hypercalcemia, and hypercalcitonism in this disease.[54] The inhibitory effect of calcitonin on bone resorption and remodeling may contribute to the stenosis of the vertebral foramen. Many affected animals have a history of excessive feeding and supplementation. Genetics may play a role in the predisposition for this disease.[123] Closely related affected animals from different litters have been observed, and it has been found that breeding affected animals resulted in a high incidence of this disease in the progeny.

C3: Basset Hound.   A possible hereditary malformation of the third cervical vertebra has been observed in male basset hounds under 6 months old.[93] Spinal cord compression occurs at either the C2–C3 or C3–C4 articulation.

OSTEOMYELITIS—ABSCESS (see discussion of Thoracolumbar Spinal Cord Disease, p. 186).   In the cervical vertebrae this disease occurs more frequently in the caudal vertebrae. In areas of the country in which the parasite *Spirocerca lupi* exists, it may be the cause of such a caudal cervical lesion.

Spondylosis Deformans—Dural Ossification (see discussion of Thoracolumbar Spinal Cord Disease.

Inflammation

The discussion of these diseases under the thoracolumbar spinal cord is referable to the cervical area, only the clinical signs indicate cervical spinal cord disease (see p. 187).

Degeneration

Ischemic Myelopathy—Fibrocartilaginous Emboli.   Ischemic myelopathy from vascular emboli presumed to be fibrocartilage may occur in the cervical spinal cord and produce bilateral or unilateral clinical signs. Most cases have been unilateral, producing ipsilateral spastic hemiparesis or hemiplegia. The signs usually are sudden in onset, with full development in less than 6 hours. In one case that was an exception it took at least 48 hours for the complete development of the hemiplegia. In this patient a rapidly developing myelopathy associated with a neoplasm was considered, but the density of the paralysis was unusual and more characteristic of an infarct. In such cases varying degrees of Horner's syndrome have been observed ipsilaterally, presumably from the sudden complete interruption of the lateral tectotegmentospinal system.

The CSF often has a mild elevation of its protein content, and for the first 24 hours or so may have an increased neutrophil population. A myelogram may reveal a swollen spinal cord at the site of the ischemic lesion.

Spontaneous recovery often has been observed, especially if some voluntary movement has been retained in the thoracic limb. Signs of improvement usually are evident during the first week after the onset of the signs. This improvement may be accounted for by the resolution of edema and hemorrhage, and collateral circulation to areas that were ischemic but not yet necrotic. In time, the dog may compensate for the permanent loss of a portion of its spinal cord parenchyma, and this also may contribute to its continued improvement.

At necropsy, the lesion usually is limited to the lateral funiculus and adjacent grey matter on one side. A few hemorrhages may be present in the soft necrotic tissue.

In one case the patient showed a remarkable tendency to force itself toward

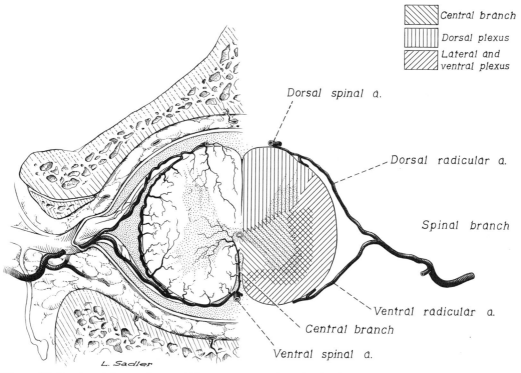

Figure 10–2. Arterial vasculature of the canine spinal cord. The lesion distribution following fibro-cartilaginous emboli reflects multiple vascular occlusion. (From J. Am. Anim. Hosp. Assoc., *12*:37, 1976.)

the paralyzed side. The dog would not lie on its normal side, but immediately rolled to its paralyzed side. No neck or head disorientation was evident, and no abnormal nystagmus. This dog recovered, and it was assumed that the unilateral cervical spinal cord lesion involved the ventral funiculus with its vestibulospinal tract, which accounted for the torsion of the dog's trunk.

The following is a case report of a dog with this lesion in the right lateral funiculus of the cervical spinal cord.

Signalment. A 4-year-old female sheltie.

Chief Complaint. The patient was unable to get up.

History. Four days prior to examination, the patient was playing outside with another dog when it lay down and was unable to get up.

Physical Examination. The dog was reluctant to stand and walk. If supported, it moved the left limbs well but not the right limbs. Both right limbs were severely paretic, and hypertonic with no atrophy. The right patellar reflex was brisk. Flexor reflexes were intact and when elicited in the left limbs, crossed extension occurred in the right limbs. Postural reactions were absent in the right limbs. Most were performed adequately in the left limbs but the patient fell easily if pushed when hemiwalking on the left side. No neck pain was elicited.

Ancillary Procedures. Radiographs were normal.

CSF contained 23 RBC and 12 mononuclear cells per cmm, and 44 mg of protein per dl.

Diagnosis. The lesion was on the right side of the spinal cord, probably cranial to the C6 segment. The sudden onset, nonprogression of signs, lack of pain, normal radiographs, and elevated protein levels in the CSF with a few mononuclear cells suggest ischemic myelopathy.

Outcome. Over a period of 10 days in the hospital with no treatment, the dog slowly improved. At discharge, it could just stand and walk. After 3 months, the only residual deficit the owner noted was a slight tendency for the right thoracic limb to slide out on the slippery kitchen floor when the dog lowered its head to eat. Its gait was normal.

Demyelinating Myelopathy: Miniature Poodles

Leukodystrophy: Afghan Hounds. In these suspected familial diseases, pelvic limb deficits are the first to be observed. As the disease progresses, the cervical spinal cord and thoracic limb function become involved. (See discussion under thoracolumbar spinal cord disease, p. 189.)

Neoplasia—Intramedullary (see Thoracolumbar Spinal Cord Disease, p. 190.)

Malformation

Myelodysplasia. Myelodysplasia usually is restricted to the thoracolumbar spinal cord. Cervical spinal cord malformations are rare but produce signs present at birth that are static and do not progress in severity.

Swimmer Syndrome in Puppies. This is not a disorder of the cervical spinal cord, but is discussed here because of its consideration in a differential diagnosis of malformations.

Occasionally one or more of a litter of puppies is found with its limbs too abducted to stand and walk at a time when it normally should. These puppies make swimming motions with their abducted limbs in their attempts to move. There may be associated severe dorsoventral compression of the thorax. They are alert, responsive, and strong. There is no detectable neurologic deficit. In time, permanent secondary joint deformities and ankylosis may occur in the limbs. The condition seems to represent a musculoskeletal growth abnormality. The pathogenesis is not well understood. There may be two mechanisms for this disease.

1. The disease has been reported in English bulldogs, Sealyham terriers, and Pekingese dogs with achondroplasia or osteochondrodystrophy. This may be a metabolic or endocrine disease causing imperfect ossification of the long bones at the epiphyses, which may contribute to the development of the swimmer syndrome.

2. The disease also occurs in puppies of breeds with no detectable underlying skeletal disease. German shepherds, black and tan coonhounds, and miniature poodles have been involved. In these animals poor management may contribute to the syndrome. Puppies raised on a hard, slippery surface are unable to adduct their limbs to support themselves and walk, and the pressure of the body on the hard surface contributes to the deformity of the thorax.

In most necropsies of these dogs no discernible abnormality has been found in the nervous or musculoskeletal systems.

If the condition is recognized early, it may be reversed by management procedures. These include hobbling the puppies by tieing their limbs in an adducted position and bedding them on deep, soft material such as a box of crumpled newspaper or on thick padding or blankets. Owners that have the most success attend these puppies continually.

CERVICAL INTUMESCENCE SPINAL CORD DISEASE (C6–T2)

Lesions in this location produce signs of lower motor neuron paresis in the thoracic limbs and upper motor neuron paresis in the pelvic limbs. The thoracic limb paresis is sometimes more profound than that in the pelvic limb. Involvement of the dorsal grey column results in more profound thoracic limb hypalgesia. T1–T3 lesions produce ipsilateral Horner's syndrome.

Trauma

External Injury. External injury causing vertebral fractures or intervertebral disk extrusions may contuse the cervical intumescence. These are more often cranial thoracic than caudal cervical.

External injury that causes avulsion of roots of the brachial plexus may contuse the associated spinal cord and produce spastic paresis and ataxia of the ipsilateral pelvic limb.

Internal Injury

INTERVERTEBRAL DISK EXTRUSION. Protrusion or extrusion of a caudal cervical intervertebral disk may contuse the cervical intumescence. Neck pain often is present. Radiographs are usually diagnostic. Sometimes myelography is necessary. Always obtain cerebrospinal fluid prior to taking the myelogram. It is usually normal with intervertebral disk extrusions, or protein levels may be elevated slightly. A marked elevation of protein and mononuclear cells suggests an inflammatory lesion in the spinal cord and not intervertebral disk extrusion, even if the plain radiographs indicate the latter.

NEOPLASM—EXTRAMEDULLARY. The most common neoplasm that is found at this location in the dog is a neurofibroma of a spinal nerve or root that compresses the spinal cord at the intumescence.[163]

The signs vary with the rate of growth of the lesion and the awareness of the owner. Generally, it presents as a "lameness" in one thoracic limb with no radiographically demonstrable lesion. The "lameness" becomes a paresis and may be associated with diffuse muscle atrophy in the affected thoracic limb. As the paresis progresses in that limb, the ipsilateral pelvic limb develops a spastic paresis and ataxia caused by the compression of the spinal cord by the neoplasm growing through the intervertebral foramen and along the roots to the spinal cord. Continual spinal cord compression causes tetraparesis. Thoracic limb paresis is usually more conspicuous than the pelvic limb paresis.

In some cases of this disease, the unilateral thoracic limb atrophy is severe and associated with pain and lameness in that limb. Nevertheless, the limb is still functional. The only indication that the spinal cord is affected may be a slight tendency for the ipsilateral pelvic limb to slide out to the side on a slippery floor, and its postural reactions may be slightly slower.

When this lesion begins in a single spinal nerve or its roots, neurologic signs are not observed in the gait. Only when it applies pressure to the adjacent cervical intumescence is the neurologic deficit observed in the gait. If the lesion begins at the T1 or T2 spinal nerve and compresses the adjacent spinal cord and subsequently the intumescence, the ipsilateral upper motor neuron pelvic limb deficit may precede the lower motor neuron thoracic limb signs. Such a lesion may produce paraplegia and mild lower motor neuron thoracic limb signs.

Usually this neoplasm is intradural but extramedullary, and compresses the spinal cord at the site of origin of the rootlets. It is amenable to surgical removal, but the involved roots must be sacrificed. In some instances, it may not be possible to separate the mass from the adjacent spinal cord tissue. In this disease the spinal cord compression may be severe and yet the patient is still ambulatory. In a few cases the lesion is extradural to the spinal cord.

The following two cases are examples of this lesion at the cervical intumescence.

Signalment.   A 7-year-old German shepherd.

History.   Two weeks prior to examination, the owner first noticed some difficulty with the use of the left forelimb. During the next 10 days, the same difficulty involved the left hind limb as well.

Physical Examination.   The patient was in good physical condition, alert, and responsive. When standing, the left forepaw often was placed knuckled on its dorsal surface. When walking, the left forelimb was thrown forward more than the right so that it landed on the palmar surface of the paw. Otherwise it knuckled over on the dorsal surface of the paw. The left hind paw frequently was knuckled over on its dorsal surface. Atrophy was evident in the left supraspinatus, infraspinatus, and triceps muscles.

Spinal Reflexes.   The flexor reflex of the left forelimb was weak compared to the right. The triceps reflex was present bilaterally and was symmetric. The flexor reflexes in the hind limbs were intact and symmetric. Pain was perceived from all the limbs. The left patellar reflex was hyperactive, with transient clonus present (plus 4). The right patellar reflex was normal (plus 2). Increased resistance was noted in the left hind limb on manipulation.

Postural Reactions.   On tonic neck and eye testing, the left forelimb did not support weight properly and often knuckled. Pain was evident on neck manipulation. Proprioceptive positioning was performed poorly in the left forelimb, fairly in the left hind limb, and normally on the right side. Hopping and placing were abnormal on the right side. On extensor thrust the left hind limb was extended more than normal when compared to the right. When held by both left limbs, the patient supported its weight well on the right limbs and could walk on them. When held by the right limbs the left limbs could not support the weight of the dog.

Radiography and Myelography.   Plain radiographs revealed no lesion. A myelogram revealed a block to the flow of the dye at C6. Euthanasia was requested.

Necropsy.   The left C6 rootlets were enlarged by a mass that pushed the spinal cord parenchyma to the right. It was diagnosed as a neurofibroma.

Signalment.   A 10-year-old male springer spaniel.

Chief Complaint.   The patient had neck pain and weakness.

History.   Two weeks prior to admission, the dog suddenly developed cervical pain and the body was curved to the left (concave left). The pain persisted, and the dog became reluctant to move, or developed weakness that prevented normal freedom of movement. The gait difficulty progressed.

Physical Examination.   The dog was mildly depressed and apprehensive. Paresis was pronounced in both thoracic limbs, with frequent collapse onto the carpus of the right limb. The pelvic limbs were paretic, but less so than the thoracic limbs. Postural reactions demonstrated that the right thoracic limb was more paretic than the left pelvic limb. Manipulation of the base of the neck occasionally elicited pain. The dog also continually moaned on being urged to move, as if the effort to walk caused pain. Muscle atrophy was pronounced in the thoracic limbs. The thoracic limbs were hypotonic and spinal reflexes were depressed markedly. Pain response was normal. The pelvic limbs were hypertonic and hyperreflexic (plus 3 patellar bilaterally). These signs progressed over a 7-day period of observation, and the thoracic limb atrophy increased. This atrophy occurred in all the muscles, but was pronounced in the scapular musculature.

Anatomic Diagnosis. A lesion involving the spinal cord grey matter or the associated roots that contribute to the brachial plexus and the white matter, with descending tracts to the lumbosacral segments.

Radiography. Intervertebral disks C5–C6 and C6–C7 were calcified markedly without obvious protrusion.

Radiopaque dye injected into the subarachnoid space at the L5–L6 level slowed to a narrow point at the level of the caudal end of the body of C5. There was no indentation of the dye column at the site of the intervertebral disks. Normal cervical myelograms showed dye flowing freely through this area.

Laboratory Findings. Examination of CSF revealed no abnormality.

Surgery. Dorsal laminectomy was performed at C5 and C6. No epidural lesion was seen. The dura was opened longitudinally and a mass was found invading the parenchyma on the right side. Because it was not amenable to removal, euthanasia was performed.

Necropsy. There was a mass in the right sixth cervical spinal nerve and its roots, which invaded the spinal cord at the origin of these roots. Both to the naked eye and microscopically, the mass had the characteristics of a neurofibroma.

Inflammation

Canine distemper myelitis occasionally affects grey matter in a multifocal distribution. The sporozoan *Toxoplasma gondii* frequently affects grey matter. If a portion of the lesion is in the C6 to T1 segments of the spinal cord, clinical signs referable to this area are seen. As a rule, clinical signs also are found in these two diseases that are indicative of the multifocal nature of the lesion. The granulomatous myelitis form of reticulosis also must be considered.[31, 63] CSF studies are helpful in confirming these diagnoses.

Degeneration

Ischemic myelopathy from vascular emboli presumed to be fibrocartilage commonly produces unilateral lesions in the cervical intumescence. The disease usually results in an acute onset of a very severe neurologic deficit. Usually, the severer the degree of lower motor neuron deficit in the thoracic limb, the poorer are the chances for the patient's spontaneous improvement.

The following two case reports are concerned with this disease at this location.

Signalment. A 6-year-old male border collie.

Chief Complaint. The dog was unable to stand.

History. Five days prior to examination, in the evening, the dog suddenly was noted to have difficulty using the right thoracic limb. By the following morning, it could not use the right pelvic limb.

Physical Examination. The dog was alert and responsive. It could not stand up, but when given assistance readily moved the left limbs but not the right limbs. The right pelvic limb was hypertonic and supported weight in a reflex response. The left pelvic limb was not normal in its use, but was much better than the right pelvic limb. The right thoracic limb was atonic and could not support weight. The left thoracic limb was normal.

The right pupil was smaller than normal. The right third eyelid protruded, and the palpebral fissure was reduced slightly in size.

There was essentially no response to postural reaction testing in the right limbs. Occasionally, a slight attempt at hopping occurred in the right pelvic limb. The left pelvic limb was slow on hopping and proprioceptive positioning was abnormal. Hemiwalking was slightly weak on the left side, and the left thoracic limb occasionally knuckled when walking with the neck extended.

Muscle tone was reduced markedly in the right thoracic limb, and increased mildly in both pelvic limbs. There was a slight indication of atrophy in the right scapular muscles. Patellar reflexes were brisk bilaterally. The biceps and triceps reflexes were brisk in the left thoracic limb and absent in the right limb. The flexor reflexes were normal, except in the right thoracic limb, in which the reflex was absent. There was marked hypalgesia over most of the right thoracic limb distal to the elbow.

Radiography.   Plain and contrast radiographs were normal.

Laboratory Findings.   CSF contained 187 RBC and 4 mononuclear cells per cmm, and 57 mg of protein per dl.

Diagnosis.   The signs indicate a focal cervical spinal cord lesion on the right side of the C6 to T3 segments. The grey matter lesion at this site accounts for the lower motor neuron paralysis and dense hypalgesia in the right thoracic limb. The lateral funicular lesion accounts for the upper motor neuron paralysis of the right pelvic limb.

The sudden onset without a history of trauma, the lack of progression, lack of neck pain, normal radiographs, and abnormal CSF suggest that ischemic myelopathy is the kind of lesion present.

Outcome.   No improvement occurred after 10 days of hospitalization. Euthanasia was performed.

Necropsy.   There was ischemic and hemorrhagic infarction of the right side of the spinal cord from C6 to C8 in the dorsal and lateral funiculi and the grey matter on the right side. The ventral funiculus was spared. Fibrocartilaginous emboli were found in small arteries and veins associated with the parenchymal lesion.

The lack of lesion in the cranial thoracic segments indicated that the Horner's syndrome was caused by the destruction of the lateral tectotegmentospinal tract by the lateral funicular lesion.

Signalment.   A 3-year-old male schnauzer.

Chief Complaint.   The dog was unable to get up.

History.   Four days prior to the referral examination, the owner noticed early in the morning that the dog was unable to use its right pelvic limb. By the time it was presented to the referring veterinarian later that morning, it could not use either right limb. These signs did not change in the interval prior to examination. There was no obvious source of injury, and no pain was associated with the problem.

Physical Examination.   The dog was alert and responsive. There was no evidence of cerebral or cranial nerve involvement, but the right pupil and palpebral fissure were smaller than the left, and the right third eyelid was protruded.

The dog was in right lateral recumbency. Any attempt to put it in left lateral recumbency was met with strenuous resistance. The pelvic limbs extended caudally, and flailed along with the left thoracic limb until the dog righted itself to a sternal or right lateral recumbent position. The neck and head were well oriented, but the trunk frequently was curved. The disorientation stimulated on placing the dog in left lateral recumbency only seemed to involve the limbs and trunk caudal to the neck. On the animal's struggling to move out of left lateral recumbency, the body flexed, with the concavity to the right side. When in sternal recumbency the body often was twisted, mostly with the concavity to the right side. The left limbs seemed to be pushing the dog over to the right side during these periods of disorientation.

The dog could not stand to walk. If held up, the left limbs moved but were stiff or hypertonic. The right limbs did not move, except for an occasional attempt with the right thoracic limb. It was difficult to hold the dog straight to test this because of the tendency of the trunk to twist and fall to the right.

Postural reactions were intact on the left, but very brisk and spastic (hypertonic). The right thoracic limb made small, essentially useless attempts to hop; the right pelvic limb did not move. Placing, proprioceptive positioning, and hemiwalking were absent on the right side.

The pelvic limbs showed hypertonia, especially the right limb. The left thoracic limb was hypertonic, but the right thoracic limb was hypotonic. Patellar reflexes were brisk on the left, and the dog was too tense to adequately grade the reflex on the right. Flexor reflexes were intact except for the right thoracic limb, in which the reflex was depressed. There was a mild hypalgesia on the right side of the body from the thoracic limb caudally. This seemed slightly more evident in the right thoracic limb.

Radiography. Plain radiographs were normal.

Laboratory Findings. CSF contained 9 RBC and 8 mononuclear cells per cmm, and 30 mg of protein per dl.

Diagnosis. These signs suggest a lesion of the caudal cervical and cranial thoracic spinal cord on the right side. The grey matter lesion accounts for the hypotonia and hyporeflexia of the right thoracic limb and Horner's syndrome, if the T1 through T3 segments were involved. The white matter lesion accounts for the spastic paralysis of the right pelvic limb and also possibly Horner's syndrome, by its interference with the descending lateral tecto-tegmentospinal tract in the lateral funiculus.

The tendency to lean, fall, and roll right with the trunk but without head, neck, or eye abnormalities suggests an ipsilateral (right) ventral funiculus lesion with loss of the vestibulospinal tract on that side.

The sudden onset, without a history of trauma, and the lack of progression, lack of neck pain, normal radiographs, and abnormal CSF suggest ischemic myelopathy for the lesion.

Outcome. The dog improved over a period of 7 days hospitalization. It could stand and walk at discharge. Five months later, examination only showed abnormality in proprioception of the right pelvic limb. It stood, walked, and ran freely without obvious abnormality.

Neoplasia

Intramedullary neoplasms are not common but could locate at this site.

Malformation

Malformations that are restricted to this location have not been observed.

SPINAL CORD DISEASE IN LARGE ANIMALS

A differential diagnosis for the entire spinal cord will be described according to the various kinds of lesions that occur. Those that are limited to a specific segment of the spinal cord will be indicated. If the assessment of the clinical signs and of the location of the lesion is accurate, then the consideration of the differential diagnosis can be more selective.

Trauma

External Injury. In fractures and subluxation, the clinical signs reflect a focal spinal cord contusion related to the site of the vertebral column injury. Horses are prone to sacral fractures on falling while backing off transport vans. Cattle are susceptible to caudal, sacral, or lumbar fractures from breeding accidents. The bones of foals or calves with calcium deficiency may be more susceptible to fracture. These are usually thoracic or lumbar vertebral fractures. Vertebral body abscesses often result in a pathologic fracture and occur more commonly in cattle, sheep, and pigs.

The Schiff-Sherrington syndrome has not been observed in these species.

As a rule, the signs are sudden in onset and either remain static or improve. In one instance, an 11-month-old Appaloosa did not become recumbent for 48 hours following a fracture of the lamina of L5. When presented with a large animal that is recumbent and unable to get up, it often is necessary to sling the animal in order to evaluate the degree of function retained in the thoracic limbs and help locate the lesion to a cervical or thoracolumbar site. If a fracture is present, gentle palpation of the area may cause excessive pain to the patient.

An animal that is recumbent as a result of a caudal cervical spinal cord lesion usually still can flex the neck laterally on each side. The more cranial the location of the cervical spinal cord lesion, the less able is the animal to do this.

Sometimes in cattle a line of hypalgesia or analgesia can be determined only by using an electric prod. A pin or forceps is usually sufficient in horses. It is especially important to locate the site of the spinal cord lesion accurately if radiography is to be performed.

Internal Injury

MALFORMATION-MALARTICULATION C1–C7: THE WOBBLER SYNDROME. Although many of the equine spinal cord and some brain lesions that do not produce recumbency cause the animal to wobble, the term "wobbler syndrome" has been used most often to refer to a specific disease syndrome. In this syndrome the cervical spinal cord is contused by a malarticulation or malformation between C1 and C7.[20, 24, 33, 60, 64, 79, 87, 105, 109, 111, 112, 113, 119, 120, 122, 128]

Synonyms for this syndrome include wobbles, and equine sensory ataxia. The latter refers to the pronounced signs of ataxia caused by the interference of the cervical spinal cord lesion with the general proprioception pathways. However, paresis also occurs and becomes evident as the deeper upper motor neuron pathways are interfered with.

Horses often develop a wobbly gait, and because this "wobbler syndrome" has been recognized widely and published in the literature, it has been assumed that most wobbly horses have this syndrome of a focal cervical spinal cord contusion from a vertebral abnormality. Unfortunately, most of these horses have not been studied carefully at necropsy. When such a study is carried out, it is found that there are a significant number of these horses that do not have the expected lesions. Instead, primary degenerative spinal cord lesions and inflammatory lesions often are found.

Cervical vertebral malarticulation-malformation causes cervical spinal cord compression in many breeds of horses, usually within the first year or two of life. Onset is most prevalent in the weanling or yearling periods. It may be gradual and insidious, or sudden and associated with some form of trauma. Typically, the signs of pelvic limb ataxia are the most pronounced. These are more evident at a slow walk or while turning in circles. The pelvic limb stride may be asymmetric, with one limb having a longer stride than the other. Occasionally, both pelvic limb strides are prolonged. In a few cases the stride is shortened and the hoof stabs sharply into the ground. One or both limbs may scuff the ground during the protraction phase of the gait. If the pelvis is pushed gently or the tail pulled as the horse walks, the ataxic-paretic horse may be pulled easily to the side, may stumble, cross one limb in front of the other, or step on itself. This is called the sway response.

When the horse walks in a wide or small circle, the outside pelvic limb often swings wide and high on protraction. This is referred to as abduction, circumduction, or hypermetria, and is assumed to be a sign of a proprioceptive deficit. Swinging the horse in a tight circle may cause it to pivot for a prolonged period on the inside pelvic limb, whereas the normal animal steps around briskly. This is a sign of a spinal cord lesion, but it has not been determined if it is a sign of general proprioception or upper motor neuron deficit. The latter is suspected.

Thoracic limb signs usually are less evident and may require careful observation to determine. In some animals there is quite remarkable spasticity, causing a stiff gait with less flexion of the joints on protraction. This may cause the limbs to appear to float before the supporting phase begins. Occasionally, a thoracic limb hoof scuffs on protraction. This may be elicited or accentuated by walking the horse with the neck extended and head held as high as possible. When signs are more severe, the horse often stumbles on the thoracic limbs and crosses one in front of the other. The stumbling may be exacerbated by moving the horse in a tight circle. During circling it may tend to pivot on the most affected thoracic limb, similar to the response of the pelvic limbs in this action.

The standing sway test with the thoracic or pelvic limbs is performed by gently pushing or pulling the horse by the withers or pelvic region, respectively. The normal horse resists this movement or steps sharply around. The ataxic, paretic horse may delay on protraction and then step on the opposite limb or abduct the opposite limb excessively.

Paresis may be detected by squeezing firmly so as to apply a downward pressure to the loin and withers regions separately. The horse may respond by extending its vertebral column, and if it is weak the thoracic or pelvic limbs, respectively, tend to flex and buckle. It is possible to cast the very weak horse in this manner.

On backing these horses, the severely affected horse may tend to collapse in the pelvic limbs, or be very slow to protract the limbs backward and sink toward the ground as this delay is prolonged. The mildly affected horse may back readily, but be slightly awkward (ataxic) in the placement of its hooves.

Blindfolding these horses only slightly accentuates the ataxia at best. Most horses with this disease show little change in their signs on walking blindfolded on smooth ground.

If a slope is available, gaiting the horse in a straight line and in circles on the slope may augment subtle signs of neurologic deficit. It is not unusual for the gait to appear more normal when the horse is trotted in a straight line on a flat surface. However, if a horse is turned loose in a paddock and observed as it changes speeds and makes sudden turns, the signs may be observed more readily.

The disparity in signs between the pelvic and thoracic limbs may reflect the greater distance of the pelvic limbs from the center of gravity of the horse, the more superficial position of the pelvic limb spinocerebellar tracts in the lateral funiculus, where they are contused readily, or possibly the greater percentage of upper motor neuron synapses in the grey matter of the cervical intumescence.

As a rule, the clinical signs are fairly symmetric, reflecting disturbance of the ascending general proprioception pathways (ataxia) and descending upper motor neuron pathways (paresis). Rarely are there unequivocal signs of disturbance of the ascending general somatic afferent pathway (pain).

The course of the disease is variable. In most animals, the signs remain static or slowly progress. Occasionally, they improve, but reports of spontaneous recovery are rare. There is no practical therapy for the condition.

CSF seldom is altered by the condition.

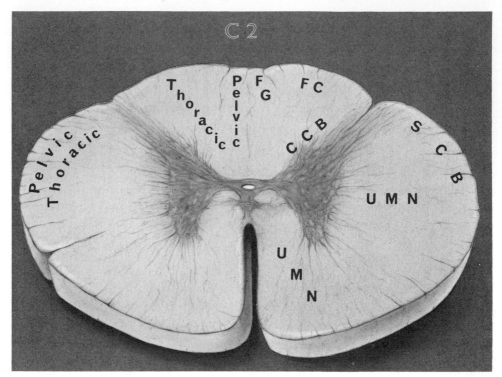

Figure 10–3.   Transverse section of cervical spinal cord. The more superficial location of pelvic limb spinocerebellar tracts may explain the more profound signs of ataxia in these limbs.

Radiographs require careful evaluation. There is considerable dorsal displacement of the vertebral bodies at their intervertebral articulations in normal horses when the normally extended and flexed views are compared. In a few cases the malarticulation is flagrant. In most cases the malarticulation is subtle but careful measurement of the cranial and caudal orifices of each vertebral foramen usually will reveal stenosis of one or more of these openings. Myelography and vertebral venography will often show compression of the subarachnoid space and venous plexus, respectively, where the foramina are stenotic or malarticulation is obvious. Cisternal myelograms in normal horses usually show a narrow ventral line at the intervertebral articulations in lateral radiographs of the flexed neck. If both the dorsal and ventral dye lines are narrowed at a flexed intervertebral articulation, this usually indicates abnormal stretching of the spinal cord at that site. Focal spinal cord lesions have been correlated with this radiographic observation at the C3–C4 articulation.

Cervical venography is performed with the neck in full flexion. A 4.5 inch 10-gauge needle with a grip handle is inserted into the marrow cavity of the axis. Forty cc of 80 per cent sodium iothalamate (Angio-Conray) are injected by an automatic injection unit set at 90 pounds per square inch of pressure. A 5-second delay is allowed before exposure of the radiographs. This outlines the cervical vertebral ventral internal venous plexus and vertebral veins. At the site of the spinal cord compression the plexus also may be compressed and the dye will not be visible.

The malarticulation-malformation of the cervical vertebrae has been classified previously in this syndrome.[112] Type 1 is a fusion in flexion of the axis and C3, and occurs in weanlings. In type 2 there is a symmetric overgrowth of the cranial articular processes of C4 related to excessive motion at this joint. This excess movement sometimes is referred to as spondylolisthesis. It is most common in yearlings. The type 3 malformation is an asymmetric overgrowth of one of the cranial articular processes, usually at C5, C6, or C7. These malformations produce varying degrees of abnormality in movement and compromise the vertebral canal, which directly compresses the spinal cord or interferes with its venous drainage, causing white matter degeneration. In some instances, the cranial or caudal orifice of the vertebral foramina of C3 or C4 has been found to be smaller than normal, causing compression of the spinal cord. The focal spinal cord lesion may be only 1 to 2 cm long, and shows a remarkable demyelination in most all funiculi, with some evidence of axonal degeneration. In some the dorsal funiculi are spared. In the severe lesion some cavitation may occur in the white matter, and neurons may be depleted from the grey matter and replaced by hypertrophied astrocytes. Secondary degeneration occurs in the ascending pathways cranial to this focal lesion and in the descending pathways caudal to the focal lesion.

The specific cause of the various cervical vertebral abnormalities is unknown. They may result from a number of factors. Although inheritance has often been incriminated, a recent study of Thoroughbreds does not support a genetic basis.[170] A rapid rate of growth causing imbalance between muscle and skeletal structures has been implicated. The syndrome often is seen in young, large, rapidly growing horses with long necks in whom a disparity in growth of the vertebral column and spinal cord may account for the focal stretching of the latter. In addition, nutritional factors may be implicated, as in the canine syndrome.

Horses that develop exostosis of their cervical vertebral articular processes may suffer spinal cord compression and signs similar to those described for the wobbler syndrome. These vertebral lesions occur more frequently in the older horse and less frequently in the age range of the more typical animal with the wobbler syndrome. How these articular lesions relate to the overall pathogenesis of the vertebral abnormalities that occur in the wobbler syndrome is unknown.

ATLANTO-OCCIPITAL MALFORMATION OF ARABIAN HORSES. Arabian horses of either sex may be born with an atlanto-occipital malformation that may seriously compromise the spinal cord at birth or shortly after. In most there is no discernible atlanto-occipital joint, with complete fusion of the atlas with the occipital bone. If the joint is present it is malformed, and the vertebral foramen of the atlas is extremely narrow cranially. The axis may be displaced ventrally, with the dens articulating ventral to the malformed body of the atlas. In some, the dens may be hypoplastic. Despite this deformity in the vertebral canal between the atlas and the axis, the spinal cord compression has occurred within the foramen of the atlas, which is reduced markedly in size.

The signs of cranial cervical spinal cord compression may be present at birth and cause inability to stand or severe symmetric ataxia and paresis if the foal can stand. Extending the neck to nurse may be difficult and cause the foal to fall. In one case there was an audible click at the site of the malformation when the head was moved. Some foals are born with no clinical neurologic signs and develop them in the first few weeks or months. This suggests that at birth the vertebral foramen of the atlas was large enough for the size of the spinal cord, but as the foal grew it failed to remodel and enlarge simultaneous with the growing spinal cord, which became progressively more compressed at this site. Once the neurologic signs are apparent, they progress at a moderate rate. In most of the animals examined the gait has a remarkable spastic quality, especially in the thoracic limbs. They may stumble and fall to either side or backward. Their signs usually are more pronounced than those of most horses with the wobbler syndrome.

An important diagnostic feature is the posture of the neck. It is more extended than normal, and appears stiff due to the lack of mobility at the atlanto-occipital joint. Palpation reveals the abnormality of the joint. The transverse process (wing) of the atlas usually is reduced in size, and if the jugular process of the occipital bone is palpable, the normal space between the jugular process and wing of the atlas may not be felt. They either will be immovable, or there will be limitied motion between them.

Radiographs confirm this diagnosis and reveal the degree of deformity. A myelogram shows the site of spinal cord compression.

This disease is suspected to be genetic in origin. All known cases have been observed in Arabian horses.[67] In one instance two affected offspring were produced from the same consecutive matings. This malformation represents a disturbance in the normal development of the caudal occipital and cranial cervical sclerotomes.

A similar condition has been reported in a Holstein-Friesian calf.[69]

NEOPLASIA

Lymphosarcoma. In cattle lymphosarcoma often may develop in the epidural space at any level of the spinal cord and produce clinical signs referable to the area of the spinal cord that is compressed. This usually affects adult cattle, but can occur in animals that are under 1 year of age. Finding evidence of this lesion in other sites in the body and in the blood helps confirm the suspicion, but it can occur at this site without involvement of any other organ and no evidence of leukemia on the hemogram.

In one instance of a cow with this lesion in the vertebral foramen of C4, before persistent signs of ataxia and paresis occurred, the animal occasionally would collapse after lowering its head to eat from the floor.

Neurofibroma. Neurofibromas are found most often in cattle of all ages. A neurofibroma was observed in a 2-month-old calf with signs of a thoracolumbar focal spinal cord lesion. These frequently are seen in various peripheral nerves in cattle at slaughter houses, with no evidence of having produced neurologic signs.

Extramedullary neoplasms are rare in horses. An intradural extramedullary lymphoreticular neoplasm was observed compressing and infiltrating the C8 and T1 segments of a 1 and one-half-year-old quarter horse. The signs appeared quite suddenly, and the horse was unable to get up 24 hours later. The signs suggested a caudal cervical lesion.

The thoracic limbs were more paretic than the pelvic limbs. The pelvic limbs were severely hypertonic, had normal flexor and plus 3 patellar reflexes, and pain was perceived readily. The thoracic limbs were hypotonic, hyporeflexic, and hypalgesic. The neck could readily be flexed laterally.

EPIDURAL ABSCESS. Abscesses frequently occur in the extradural space of cattle, sheep, and pigs. They may involve the adjacent bone or be restricted to the epidural space. The adjacent spinal cord becomes compressed. The temperature, pulse, and respiration may be normal, but chronic abscesses often are associated with an elevated plasma protein level because of the increased globulin fraction. *Corynebacterium pyogenes, Streptococcus* species, or *Staphylococcus* species are isolated most frequently. Only in exceptional cases does the abscess invade the dura and break into the leptomeninges. Since the abscess is restricted to the epidural space, there are usually no inflammatory cells in the CSF. This is a rare lesion in horses.

Inflammation

Protozoal Myelitis. Horses are susceptible to a protozoal myelitis and encephalitis.[11, 12, 19, 27, 114] The identity and life cycle of the protozoan remain unknown. The organism has many similarities to *Toxoplasma gondii*, but some significant differences. It can produce a focal or diffuse myelitis at any level of the spinal cord in horses of any age. Mostly young mature horses are affected. It is more common in standard breeds. The focal nature of the lesion has been referred to as segmental myelitis.

The clinical signs are variable in onset. Often the recognition of neurologic signs is preceded by a variable period of lameness that defies accurate diagnosis. There may be a history of repeated unsuccessful therapy for musculoskeletal disease.

The neurologic signs are often asymmetric, with one limb much more affected than the other. The lesion affects grey matter as readily as white matter, and if this involves the intumescence, there may be clinical signs of grey matter disease. These include neurogenic atrophy, hypotonia and hyporeflexia for the ventral grey column, and hypalgesia for the dorsal grey column.[110] A caudal cervical spinal cord lesion first may produce an ipsilateral thoracic limb deficit, followed by an ipsilateral hemiparesis, followed by tetraparesis and ataxia. A thoracolumbar lesion may cause an inability to back up, and the horse may collapse on its pelvic limbs and sit like a dog. The signs usually are progressive, but the rate varies. Some may collapse within a few days, while others remain static for weeks. Improvement or recovery has not been observed.

CSF studies in many cases have been remarkably unrewarding. In a few instances, an increase in mononuclear cells and protein levels has been noted. This has been found mostly in lumbosacral CSF from horses with lumbosacral lesions.

CSF enzymes are being evaluated in this disease at present. Toxoplasma serum antibodies usually are absent.

The lesion consists of a proliferative inflammation of grey matter and white matter, with a variable degree of necrosis of myelin, and axonal degeneration. Hemorrhage occurs occasionally. The inflammatory cells are mostly mononuclear and include lymphocytes, plasma cells, and macrophages, usually in a perivascular arrangement. The macrophages also may be free in the tissues. Eosinophils often are present, as well as multinucleated giant cells. Frequently, a similar nonsuppurative meningitis accompanies this parenchymal lesion. Glial cells may proliferate. Neuronal degeneration occurs on the edge of necrotic lesions. In a few cases protozoal organisms are abundant. They mostly are contained in macrophage cytoplasm. A few form rosettes in neuronal cytoplasm or free in the tissues. In many cases, these are difficult to find.

Indications for this diagnosis include signs of a moderately progressive lesion in a mature horse, asymmetry of signs, signs of grey matter disease, signs of severe ataxia and paresis, and involvement of only a single animal on a farm.

This same disease can occur in the brain stem, cerebellum or cerebrum, or both, and produce clinical signs referable to that area. These are considered with the appropriate neuroanatomic system.

There is no specific therapy for this disease. There is some indication that steroids enhance its progress. Therapy and control must await specific identification of the protozoan and its life cycle.

Equine Herpes I Virus—Myeloencephalopathy and Vasculitis. Equine herpes virus type I rhinopneumonitis, may produce a diffuse multifocal ischemic or hemorrhagic myelopathy and encephalopathy with leptomeningeal vasculitis.[13, 21, 30, 32, 59, 71, 85, 118, 126, 135, 145, 146] The equine rhinopneumonitis virus causes mild upper respiratory disease in horses of all ages and abortion in pregnant mares. Occasionally, neurologic signs have accompanied outbreaks of abortion and respiratory disease caused by this virus. The neurologic syndrome also may occur as the only illness on a farm.

The neurologic signs usually are sudden in onset, but vary in severity from mild ataxia to severe paralysis. After a few days the signs generally do not progress significantly. Mild ataxia may be transient and be followed by complete recovery, or progress to tetraparesis and lateral recumbency in a 2- to 3-day period. Some horses become recumbent in 24 hours. Some cases with mild ataxia may improve, but retain some permanent gait abnormality. Despite the severity of the signs, bladder paralysis commonly occurs in early stages, and the animal may dribble urine constantly from an enlarged bladder. The tail is often hypotonic. Most often the signs are symmetric in the pelvic limbs. Occasionally, the signs are asymmetric. Even a severe hemiparesis may result. Sometimes the onset of neurologic signs is preceded or accompanied by a fever. In a few instances the signs that are sudden in onset are referable to a diffuse cerebral or brain stem lesion.

CSF may be xanthochromic and contain a significant elevation of protein, with the normal number of leukocytes or only a slight pleocytosis.

The spinal cord lesion usually is a diffuse myelopathy consisting of foci of myelin degeneration and axonal swelling in the white matter of one or more funiculi that are often linear and oriented along the route of a penetrating blood vessel. Sometimes a portion of the grey matter is involved. Occasionally, a few lipid-filled macrophages are present in the lesion, but the general lack of inflammatory cells in the necrotic lesion is remarkable. Sometimes there is hemorrhage associated with this degenerative lesion. Careful study of the leptomeningeal blood vessels often reveals a vasculitis, especially of small arteries. A mare with hemiplegia had a large infarct in the lateral funiculus of the midcervical spinal cord. Similar lesions may be found in the brain. Ischemic or hemorrhagic infarcts may occur in the brain stem or cerebrum, along with a vasculitis of leptomeningeal or cerebrocortical blood vessels.

It is assumed that the parenchymal lesions are caused by interruption of the blood supply related to the vasculitis that is present. This produces the disseminated focal areas of degeneration or necrosis. The vasculitis may be associated with an antigen-antibody reaction. Inclusion bodies have not been found.

The virus has been isolated from the diseased nervous tissue of horses.[118, 135, 145, 146] The same disease and lesions have been reproduced by inoculating experimental horses with the recovered virus.[135]

This diagnosis should be suspected when a neurologic disease is sudden in onset with little change after 2 to 3 days, involves more than one horse on a farm, is associated with recent abortions or upper respiratory disease on the farm, causes disturbance of bladder function, and is reflected in abnormal CSF determinations. Demonstration of a rising serum neutralization titer to the equine herpesvirus I also helps confirm the diagnosis.

Because of the nature of the lesion, prompt therapy with high levels of corticosteroids may be beneficial. Spontaneous recovery often occurs in mildly ataxic and paretic animals. Most recover in a 1- to 4-week period. A few require months. Recumbent animals have been reported to get up after 4 to 21 days.[145, 146]

Although most clinical signs are referable to the spinal cord, occasionally the brain stem and cerebral lesions also produce clinical signs referable to the area of destruction.

Equine Nonsuppurative Myelitis. Occasionally, a mature horse is presented with moderately progressive signs of a fairly symmetric ataxia and paresis, and a mild diffuse nonsuppurative myelitis is found at necropsy. No obvious microbial agents have been found. Whether this condition is related to the protozoal disease or is a separate entity is not known at this time.

Viral Leukoencephalomyelitis of Goats. A viral leukoencephalomyelitis occurs in kids usually 2 to 4 months old.[166-169] Signs begin in one or both pelvic limbs and progress rapidly, with varying degrees of paraparesis or tetraparesis reflecting the multifocal distribution of the lesion. If the primary lesion is limited to the thoracolumbar spinal cord, only paraparesis and pelvic limb ataxia occur. Cervical lesions usually produce tetraparesis followed by recumbency. Signs usually reflect the predominant white matter distribution of the lesion, and spasticity and hyperreflexia are evident.

Cerebrospinal fluid usually contains a remarkable mononuclear pleocytosis of between 100 and 1000 leukocytes per cmm and a variable protein elevation.

The lesion consists of a severe proliferative granulomatous nonsuppurative leukoencephalomyelitis with varying degrees of necrosis of myelin and axons. Lymphoreticular cells predominate in the inflammatory reaction. The lesion is widely disseminated through the central nervous system but is more severe in the spinal cord. An interstitial pneumonia may also occur.

The disease has been transmitted in goats by inoculation of filtered diseased tissue but no virus has been isolated. Epidemiologic observations suggest infection occurs in utero or shortly after birth. No treatment has been recognized.

Parasitic Myelitis — Cerebrospinal Nematodiasis

Parelaphostrongylus tenuis, — GOATS AND SHEEP. In goats and sheep the migration of the adult nematode, *Parelaphostrongylus tenuis,* through the spinal cord and brain can produce a variety of clinical signs, depending on where the greatest damage occurs.[4, 5, 62, 77, 139] This parasite is the meningeal worm of white-tailed deer, and has a neurotrophic life cycle in that species without producing clinical signs.[2, 3] In goats and sheep, most of the clinical signs are referable to the spinal cord lesion and consist of lameness, paresis, and ataxia of one or both pelvic limbs, paraplegia, hemiparesis, tetraparesis and ataxia, and tetraplegia. Mild vestibular signs and blindness also have been caused by the migration of the parasite in the brain. Death may occur. The signs are often progressive, and change as the migratory route changes; they may remain static or even improve spontaneously.

The CSF frequently has a pleocytosis greater than 200 WBC per cmm and consisting of mononuclear cells and eosinophils. There is often hemorrhage in the CSF from the lesion, and protein levels usually are increased moderately to higher than 100 mg per dl. The presence of eosinophils is particularly helpful in making a differential diagnosis. These rarely occur in CSF without parasitism.

This diagnosis should be considered whenever more than one animal in a flock is affected with a neurologic syndrome, and yet they do not all show the same clinical signs, suggesting the multifocal nature of the lesion.[7, 87]

A number of anthelmintics have been tried for the treatment and prophylaxis of this disease.[124] These include diethylcarbamazine (Caricide) with dexamethasone (Azium), levamisol (Ripercol), and thiabendazole. None has been tested adequately for its efficacy. For the patient with neurologic disease, diethylcarbamazine with dexamethasone is recommended. For the prophylactic treatment of a flock, levamisol is recommended.

Strongylus vulgaris—HORSES. In horses, migration of the larval form of *Strongylus vulgaris* may produce signs of spinal cord disease.[72, 106, 127, 132, 160] This is an abnormal route for this species of equine parasite. More often the migration is in the brain, but spinal cord lesions do occur. The clinical signs depend on the location of the lesion. They are usually sudden in onset. In theory, this is a progressive disease, and the signs progress and change as the larva migrates. However, this is dependent on the continual migration of the larva. CSF studies should reflect the destruction produced and the reaction to the parasite, as was noted in the goats with cerebrospinal nematodiasis.

Degeneration

Degenerative Myeloencephalopathy in Horses. A slowly progressive symmetric ataxia and paresis have been observed in young horses and zebras that have a diffuse degenerative myeloencephalopathy.[76, 80] The age at onset may vary from birth to 2 years, but it appears most often in the first few months of life. The signs are progressive and may begin in the pelvic limbs, but soon involve the thoracic limbs. In most cases the thoracic limb deficit is as pronounced as the pelvic limb deficit. In addition to the ataxia and paresis, there is often marked spasticity in the gait.

The neurologic signs indicate a symmetric cervical spinal cord white matter lesion—abnormal positioning, decreased strength, and spasticity of limbs. There is no hypalgesia, hypotonia, hyporeflexia, or muscle atrophy, and no sign of brain disease.

Laboratory studies on blood and CSF are all normal. Plain and contrast radiographs as well as myelograms and vertebral venograms are normal.

There are no gross lesions in the central nervous system. On examination with the microscope, a diffuse degeneration of neurons in the white matter of all spinal cord funiculi is seen. It is more pronounced in the thoracic segments and in the dorsal spinocerebellar tract. It is least evident in the dorsal funiculi. Myelin degeneration is the most strongly marked lesion, with a variable degree of astrocytosis. Swollen eosinophilic (dystrophic) axons are present mostly in the grey matter, and are especially prominent in the nucleus thoracicus, in the thoracic segments, and in the gracilis and cuneate nuclei of the medulla. Neuronal degeneration also occurs variably in the olivary, vestibular, oculomotor, pretectal, and thalamic nuclei. Therefore this is a multisystem degenerative disease of the nervous system.

This disease should be suspected in young horses with progressive pelvic and thoracic limb ataxia and paresis, especially if the signs begin in the first few months. As a rule, the signs are slightly more pronounced than in horses with the malarticulation-malformation syndrome from C2 to C7 (wobbler syndrome). Typically, spasticity is prominent. Neck palpation is normal in this disease. It is often not possible to distinguish this disease clearly from the wobbler syndrome on physical and neurologic examination.

The cause of the disease is unknown. The lesions are similar to some of the heredodegenerative diseases of man,[46, 148] sheep,[149] and cats.[150] The disease has been recognized in a family of zebras, suggesting an inheritance factor.[80] However, in horses it has been recognized in several breeds. Some similar clinical signs and lesions have been observed in nutritional deficiency diseases in sheep[152] and rats,[153, 154] in an ataxic condition of unknown cause in the red deer,[155] and in a plant poisoning in cattle.[151] Further studies are needed to define the cause, prevention, and treatment of this disease.

Haloxon Neurotoxicity in Sheep. Sheep exposed to the organophosphate anthelmintic haloxon may develop a neurotoxic response.[9, 74, 165] Acute intoxications are rare, but occasionally a delayed response occurs about 3 to 5 weeks after treatment with this compound.[85] Experimental studies suggest that older sheep are more susceptible. Clinical experience has not supported this.

The clinical signs are fairly rapid in onset, and usually remain static. Over a period of 3 to 4 months of observation the signs neither progress nor improve. Signs are all in the pelvic limbs, and consist of a symmetric spastic paraparesis and ataxia. The sheep are alert, responsive, and strong in the thoracic limbs. They run around with their pelvic limbs in a partially flexed, crouched position, and often with the dorsal surface of the hoof on the ground. There is still voluntary function in the limbs, but the strength and coordination are reduced. The limbs are hypertonic, and reflexes are normal to hyperactive. There is no atrophy and no obvious loss of pain sensation.

The lesions are unremarkable. Swollen axons have been found in the sciatic nerve and lumbar spinal cord.

Resistance of some sheep to this intoxication was found to be related to the amount of an esterase present in their plasma.[9] This enzyme was gene-determined, and when present in sufficient amounts protected the sheep against haloxon. Cholinesterase levels are not depressed significantly when the first neurologic signs appear.

Myelin Disorder of Charolais Cattle. In Charolais cattle a progressive symmetric gait disorder begins at about 1 year of age.[91] The gait is stiff and stumbling, and worse in the pelvic limbs. The animals may become recumbent and have extreme difficulty getting up. Except for an occasional head bob, there are no other signs of intracranial disease. Multiple plaques of abnormal myelin are present in the brain and spinal cord white matter. The pathogenesis is unknown, but this disease may have a familial basis.

Neoplasia — Intramedullary

Intramedullary neoplasms are rare in large animals. They present clinically similar to extramedullary neoplasma, and are difficult to differentiate. Myelography is needed for the differential diagnosis.

Malformation

Myelodysplasia in Calves. Calves born with moderate to severe ataxia and spastic paraparesis that is nonprogressive often have a focal or diffuse myelodysplasia. Spinal dysraphism, diplomyelia, and segmental hypoplasia have been observed mostly in the lumbar or sacral spinal cord. In severe cases the calf is too ataxic to stand. A vertebral column lesion such as scoliosis may accompany the spinal cord malformation. Arthrogryposis and cleft palate have been reported, along with cervical spinal cord dysraphism in Charolais calves.[68]

REFERENCES

1. Alden, C., Woodson, F., Mohan, R., and Miller, S.: Cerebrospinal nematodiasis in sheep. J. Am. Vet. Med. Assoc., 166:784, 1975.
2. Anderson, R. C.: The development of *Pneumostrongylus tenuis* in the central nervous system of white-tailed deer. Pathol. Vet., 2:360, 1965.
3. Anderson, R. C., Lankester, M. W., and Strelive, U. R.: Further experimental studies of *Pneumostrongylus tenuis* in cervids. Can. J. Zool., 44:851, 1966.
4. Anderson, R. C., and Strelive, U. R.: The effect of *Pneumostrongylus tenuis* (Nematoda: Metastrongyloidea) in kids. Can. J. Comp. Med., 33:280, 1969.
5. Anderson, R. C., and Strelive, U. R.: Experimental cerebrospinal nematodiasis *(Pneumostrongylus tenuis)* in sheep. Can. J. Zool., 44:889, 1966.
6. Averill, D. R., Jr.: Degenerative myelopathy in the aging German shepherd dog: Clinical and pathologic findings. J. Am. Vet. Med. Assoc., 162:1045, 1973.
7. Baharsefat, M., Amjadi, A. R., Yamin, B., and Ahoura, P.: The first report of lumbar paralysis in sheep due to nematode larvae infestation in Iran. Cor. Vet., 63:81, 1972.
8. Bailey, C. S.: An embryological approach to the clinical significance of congenital vertebral and spinal cord abnormalities. J. Am. Anim. Hosp. Assoc., 11:426, 1975.
9. Baker, N. F., Tucker, E. M., Stormont, C., and Fisk, R. A.: Neurotoxicity of haloxon and its relationship to blood esterases of sheep. Am. J. Vet. Res., 31:865, 1970.
10. Banks, W. C., and Bridges, C. H.: Multiple cartilaginous exostosis in a dog. J. Am. Vet. Med. Assoc., 129:131, 1956.
11. Beech, J.: Equine protozoan encephalomyelitis. Vet. Med. Sm. Anim. Clin., 69:1562, 1974.
12. Beech, J., and Dodd, D. C.: Toxoplasma-like encephalomyelitis in the horse. Vet. Pathol., 11:87, 1974.
13. Bitsch, V., and Dam, A.: Nervous disturbances in horses in relation to injection with equine rhinopneumonitis virus. Acta Vet. Scand., 12:134, 1971.
14. Bullock, L. P., and Zook, B. C.: Myelography in dogs using water-soluble contrast mediums. J. Am. Vet. Med. Assoc., 151:321, 1967.
15. Butler, H. C.: An investigation into the relationship of an aortic embolus to posterior paralysis in the cat. J. Sm. Anim. Pract., 12:141, 1971.
16. Chester, D. K.: Multiple cartilaginous exostoses in two generations of dogs. J. Am. Vet. Med. Assoc., 159:895, 1971.
17. Chrisman, C. L.: Electromyography in the localization of spinal cord and nerve root neoplasia in dogs and cats. J. Am. Vet. Med. Assoc., 166:1074, 1975.
18. Cockrell, B. Y., Herigstad, R. R., Flo, G. L., and Legendre, A. M.: Myelomalacia in Afghan hounds. J. Am. Vet. Med. Assoc., 162:362, 1973.
19. Cusick, P. K., Sell, D. M., Hamilton, D. P., and Hardenbrok, H. J.: Toxoplasmosis in two horses. J. Am. Vet. Med. Assoc., 164:77, 1974.
20. Dahme, E., and Schebitz, H.: Zur Pathogenese der spinalen Ataxie des Pferdes unter Zugrundelegung neurer Befunde. Zbl. Veterinaermed., 17:120, 1970.
21. Dalsgaard, H.: Enzootic paresis in horses as a consequence of outbreaks of rhinopneumonitis (virus abortion). Medlemsbl. Danske Dyrlaegeforen, 3:71, 1970.
22. de Lahunta, A.: Progressive cervical spinal cord compression in Great Dane and Doberman pinscher dogs (a wobbler syndrome). *In* Kirk, R. W., ed., Current Veterinary Therapy, V. Small Animal Practice. Philadelphia, W. B. Saunders, 1974, 674–675.
23. de La Torre, J. C., Johnson, C. M., Goode, D. J., and Mullan, S.: Pharmacologic treatment and evaluation of permanent experimental spinal cord trauma. Neurology, 25:508, 1975.
24. Dimock, W. W., and Errington, B. J.: Incoordination of equidae: Wobblers. J. Am. Vet. Med. Assoc., 95:261, 1939.
25. Douglas, S. W., and Palmer, A. C.: Idiopathic demyelination of brain stem and cord in a miniature poodle puppy. J. Pathol. Bacteriol., 82:67, 1961.
26. Draper, D. D., Kluge, J. P., and Miller, W. J.: Clinical and pathological aspects of spinal dysraphism in dogs. Proceedings of the 20th World Veterinary Congress, Thessaloniki, Greece, 1975.
27. Dubey, J. P., Davis, G. W., Loestner, A., and Kiryu, K.: Equine encephalomyelitis due to a protozoan parasite resembling *Toxoplasma gondii*. J. Am. Vet. Med. Assoc., 165:249, 1974.
28. Dueland, R., Furneau, R. W., and Kaye, M. M.: Spinal fusion and dorsal laminectomy for midcervical spondylolisthesis in a dog. J. Am. Vet. Med. Assoc., 162:366, 1973.

29. English, P. B.: Clinical communication: A case of hyperostosis due to hypervitaminosis A in a cat. J. Sm. Anim. Pract., 10:207, 1969.
30. Fankhauser, R.: Entzündliche Gefässveränderungen als Grundlage von Rückenmarksläsionen beim Pferd. Schweiz. Arch. Tierheilk., 110:171, 1968.
31. Fankhauser, R., Fatzer, R., Luginbuhl, H., and McGrath, J. T.: Reticulosis of the central nervous system in dogs. Adv. Vet. Sci. Comp. Med., 16:35, 1972.
32. Fankhauser, R., and Gerber, H.: Zerebrale Vaskulitis beim Pferd. Arch. Exp. Vet. Med., 24:61, 1970.
33. Fraser, H., and Palmer, A. C.: Equine incoordination and wobbler disease of young horses. Vet. Rec., 80:338, 1967.
34. Funkquist, B.: Thoraco-lumbar disc protrusion with severe spinal cord compression in the dog. I. Clinical and patho-anatomic observations with special reference to the rate of development of symptoms of motor loss. Acta Vet. Scand., 3:256, 1962.
35. Funkquist, B.: Thoraco-lumbar disc protrusion with severe spinal cord compression in the dog. II. Clinical observations with special reference to the prognosis in conservative therapy. Acta Vet. Scand., 3:317, 1962.
36. Funkquist, B.: Thoraco-lumbar disc protrusion with severe spinal cord compression in the dog. III. Treatment by decompressive laminectomy. Acta Vet. Scand., 3:344, 1962.
37. Funkquist, B.: Decompressive laminectomy in thoracolumbar disc protrusion with paraplegia in the dog. J. Sm. Anim. Pract., 11:445, 1970.
38. Funkquist, B., and Schantz, B.: Influence of extensive laminectomy on the shape of the spinal cord. Acta Orthop. Scand. (Suppl.), 56:1, 1962.
39. Gage, E. D.: Treatment of discospondylitis in the dog. J. Am. Vet. Med. Assoc., 166:1164, 1975.
40. Gage, E. D., and Hoerlein, B. F.: Hemilaminectomy and dorsal laminectomy for relieving compressions of the spinal cord in the dog. J. Am. Vet. Med. Assoc., 152:351, 1968.
41. Gage, E.D., and Hoerlein, B. F.: Surgical repair of cervical subluxation and spondylolisthesis in the dog. J. Sm. Anim. Hosp. Assoc., 9:385, 1973.
42. Gambardella, P. C., Osborne, C. A., and Stevens, J. B.: Multiple cartilaginous exostoses in the dog. J. Am. Vet. Med. Assoc., 166:761, 1975.
43. Geary, J. C.: Canine spinal lesions not involving discs. J. Am. Vet. Med. Assoc., 155:2038, 1969.
44. Geary, J. C., Oliver, J. E., and Hoerlein, B. F.: Atlanto-axial subluxation in the canine. J. Sm. Anim. Pract., 8:577, 1967.
45. Gee, B. R., and Doige, C. E.: Multiple cartilaginous exostoses in a litter of dogs. J. Am. Vet. Med. Assoc., 156:53, 1970.
46. Greenfield, J. G.: The Spino-Cerebellar Degenerations. Oxford, England, Blackwell Scientific Publications, 1954.
47. Griffiths, I. R.: Some aspects of the pathogeneses and diagnosis of lumbar disc protrusion in the dog. J. Sm. Anim. Pract., 13:439, 1972.
48. Griffiths, I. R.: The extensive myelopathy of intervertebral disc protrusions in dogs (the ascending syndrome). J. Sm. Anim. Pract., 13:425, 1972.
49. Griffiths, I. R., and Duncan, I. D.: Chronic degenerative radiculomyelopathy in the dog. J. Sm. Anim. Pract., 16:461, 1975.
50. Griffiths, I. R., and Duncan, I. D.: Age changes in the dorsal and ventral lumbar nerve roots of dogs. Acta Neuropathol., 32:75, 1975.
51. Hansen, H. J.: A pathologic-anatomical study on disc degeneration in the dog. Acta Ortho. Scand. (Suppl.), 11, 1952.
52. Hartley, W. J., and Blakemore, W. F.: An unidentified sporozoan encephalomyelitis in sheep. Vet. Pathol., 11:1, 1974.
53. Hayes, K. C., and Schiefer, B.: Primary tumors in the CNS of carnivores. Pathol. Vet., 6:94, 1969.
54. Hedhammar, A., Wu, F.-M., Krook, L., Schryver, H. F., de Lahunta, A., Whalen, J. P., Kallfelz, F. A., Nunez, E. A., Hintz, H. F., Sheffy, B. E., and Ryan, G. R.: Overnutrition and skeletal disease; An experimental study in growing Great Dane dogs. Cor. Vet., Suppl. 5, 64::1, 1974.
55. Henderson, R. A., Hoerlein, B. F., Kramer, T. T., and Meyer, M. E.: Discospondylitis in three dogs infected with Brucella canis. J. Am. Vet. Med. Assoc., 165:451, 1974.
56. Hopkins, A., and Rudge, P.: Hyperpathia in the central cervical cord syndrome. J. Neurol. Neurosurg. Psychiatry, 36:637, 1973.
57. Hukuda, S., and Wilson, C. B.: Experimental cervical myelopathy: Effects of compression and ischemia on the canine cervical spinal cord. J. Neurosurg., 37:631, 1972.
58. Illis, L. S.: The motor neuron surface and spinal shock. Mod. Trends Neurol., 4:53, 1967.
59. Jackson, T., and Kendrick, J. W.: Paralysis of horses associated with equine herpesvirus I infection. J. Am. Vet. Med. Assoc., 158:1351, 1971.
60. Jones, T. C., Doll, E. R., and Brown, R. G.: The pathology of equine incoordination (ataxia or "wobblers" of foals). Proc. Am. Vet. Med. Assoc., 91st Annual Meeting, 1954, 139–149.
61. Joshua, J. O., and Ishmael, J.: Pain syndrome associated with spinal hemorrhage in the dog. Vet. Rec., 83:165, 1968.
62. Kennedy, P. C., Whitlock, J. H., and Roberts, S. J.: Neurofilariosis, a paralytic disease of sheep.I. Introduction, symptomatology and pathology. Cor. Vet., 42:118, 1952.
63. Koestner, A., and Zeman, W.: Primary reticuloses of the central nervous system. Am. J. Vet. Res., 23:381, 1962.

64. Krunajevic, T., and Bergsten, G.: Luxation of the cervical spinal column as a cause of wobbles in a foal. Acta Vet. Scand., 9:112, 1968.

65. Ladds, P., Guffy, M., Blauch, B., and Splitter, G.: Congenital odontoid process separation in two dogs. J. Sm. Anim. Pract., 12:463, 1970.

66. Lawson, D. D.: The diagnosis and prognosis of canine paraplegia. Vet. Rec., 89:654, 1971.

67. Leipold, H. W., Brandt, G. W., Guffy, M., and Blauch, B.: Congenital atlanto-occipital fusion in a foal. Vet. Med. Sm. Anim. Clin., 69:1312, 1974.

68. Leipold, H. W., Cates, W. F., Radostits, O. M., and Howell, W. E.: Spinal dysraphism, arthrogryposis and cleft palate in newborn Charolais calves. Can. Vet. J., 10:268, 1969.

69. Leipold, H. W., Strafuss, A. C., Blauch, B., Olson, J. R., and Guffy, M.: Congenital defect of the atlanto-occipital joint in a Holstein-Friesian calf. Cor. Vet., 62:646, 1972.

70. Leonard, E. P.: Orthopedic Surgery of the Dog and Cat. 2nd ed., Philadelphia, W. B. Saunders Co., 1971.

71. Little, P. B.: Viral involvement in equine paresis. Vet. Rec., 95:575, 1974.

72. Little, P. B.: Cerebrospinal nematodiasis of equidae. J. Am. Vet. Med. Assoc., 160:1407, 1972.

73. Ljunggren, G.: Legg-Perthes disease in the dog. Acta Orthop. Scand. (Suppl.), 95:1, 1967.

74. Malone, J. D.: Toxicity of haloxon. Res. Vet. Sci., 5:17, 1964.

75. Matthias, D., Dietz, O., and Reckenberg, R.: Zur Klinik und Pathologie der spinalen Ataxie der Fohlen. Arch. Exp. Veterinaermed., 19:43, 1965.

76. Mayhew, I. G., de Lahunta, A., Whitlock, R. H., and Geary, J. C.: Equine degenerative myeloencephalopathy. J. Am. Vet. Med. Assoc., in press.

77. Mayhew, I. G., de Lahunta, A. Georgi, J. R., and Aspros, D. G.: Naturally occurring cerebrospinal Parelaphostrongylosis. Cor. Vet., 66:56, 1976.

78. McGrath, J.: Spinal dysraphism in the dog with comments on syringomyelia. Pathol. Vet. (Suppl.), 2:1, 1965.

79. Milne, D., Gabel, A., Chrisman, C., and Fetter, A.: Diagnosis and pathology of the wobbler syndrome (spondylolisthesis): A preliminary study. Proc. Am. Assoc. Eq. Pract., 19:303, 1973.

80. Montali, R. J., Bush, M., Sauer, R. M., Gray, C. M., and Xanten, W. A., Jr.: Spinal ataxia in zebras. Vet. Pathol., 11:68, 1974.

81. Morgan, J. P.: Spondylosis deformans in the dog: Its radiographic appearance. J. Am. Vet. Radiol. Soc., 8:17, 1967.

82. Morgan, J. P.: Spondylosis deformans in the dog. Acta Orthop. Scand. (Suppl.), 96:1, 1967.

83. Morgan, J. P.: Spinal dural ossification in the dog: Incidence and distribution based on radiographic study. J. Am. Vet. Radiol. Soc., 10:43, 1969.

84. Morgan, J. P., Suter, P. F., and Holliday, T. A.: Myelography with water-soluble contrast medium radiographic interpretation of disc herniation in dogs. Acta Radiol. (Suppl.), 319:217, 1972.

85. Moyer, W., and Rooney, J. R.: An epidemic central nervous system disease in horses. Proc. Am. Assoc. Equine Pract., 19:307, 1973.

86. Nicholson, S. S.: Bovine posterior paresis due to organophosphate poisoning. J. Am. Vet. Med. Assoc., 165:280, 1974.

87. Nobel, T. A., and Olafson, P.: Spinal nematodiasis in sheep. Refuah Vet., 13:51, 1956.

88. Olafson, P.: "Wobblers" compared with ataxic ("swingback") lambs. Cor. Vet., 32:301, 1942.

89. Osterholme, J. L.: The pathophysiological response to spinal cord injury. The current status of related research. J. Neurosurg., 40:5, 1974.

90. Palmer, A. C.: Clinical and pathologic aspects of cervical disc protrusion and primary tumors of the cervical spinal cord in the dog. J. Sm. Anim. Pract., 11:63, 1970.

91. Palmer, A. C., Blakemore, W. F., Barlow, R. M., Frazer, J. A., and Ogden, A. L.: Progressive ataxia of Charolais cattle associated with a myelin disorder. Vet. Rec., 91:592, 1972.

92. Palmer, A. C., Payne, J. E., and Wallace, M. E.: Hereditary quadriplegia and amblyopia in the Irish setter. J. Sm. Anim. Pract., 14:343, 1973.

93. Palmer, A. C., and Wallace, M. E.: Deformation of cervical vertebrae in basset hounds. Vet. Rec., 80:430, 1967.

94. Parker, A. J.: Canine spinal cord disease. Diagnosis and treatment of. Scope, 18:2, 1974.

95. Parker, A. J.: Diagnosing thoracolumbar cord disease. Ill. Vet., 13:12, 1970.

96. Parker, A. J.: Diagnosing cervical cord disease. Ill. Vet., 14:12, 1971.

97. Parker, A. J., Cusick, P. K., Park, R. D., and Henry, J. D.: Reticulum cell sarcoma producing spinal cord compression in a dog. J. Am. Anim. Hosp. Assoc., 10:21, 1974.

98. Parker, A. J., and Park, R. D.: Atlanto-axial subluxation in small breeds of dogs: Diagnosis and Pathogenesis. Vet. Med., 68:1133, 1973.

99. Parker, A. J., and Park, R. D.: Occipital dysplasia in the dog. J. Sm. Anim. Hosp. Assoc., 10:520, 1974.

100. Parker, A. J., Park, R. D., Cusick, P. K., Small, E., and Jeffers, C. B.: Cervical vertebral instability in the dog. J. Am. Vet. Med. Assoc., 163:71, 1973.

101. Parker, A. J., Park, R. D., and Gendreau, C.: Cervical disk prolapse in a Doberman pinscher. J. Am. Vet. Med. Assoc., 163:75, 1973.

102. Parker, A. J., Park, R. D., and Stowater, J. L.: Cervical kyphosis in an Afghan hound. J. Am. Vet. Med. Assoc., 162:953, 1973.

103. Parker, A. J., and Smith, G. W.: Meningeal cyst in a dog. J. Am. Anim. Hosp. Assoc., 10:595, 1974.

104. Pettit, C. D.: Intervertebral Disk Protrusion in the Dog. New York, Appleton-Century-Crofts, 1966.
105. Pohlenz, J., and Schulz, L. C.: Rückenmarksveränderungen bei der spinalen Ataxie des Pferdes in iher Abhängigkeit von Ort und Grad der Veränderungen am Halswirbelskelett. Deutsch. Tieraerztl. Wschr., 73:533, 1966.
106. Pohlenz, J., Schulze, D., and Eckert, J.: Spinale Nematodosis beim Pferd, verursacht durch *Strongylus vulgaris*. Deutsch. Tieraerztl. Wschr., 72:510, 1965.
107. Prata, R. G, and Stoll, S. G.: Ventral decompression and fusion for the treatment of cervical disc disease in the dog. J. Am. Anim. Hosp. Assoc., 9:462, 1973.
108. Prata, R. G., Stoll, S. G., and Zaki, F. A.: Spinal cord compression caused by osteocartilaginous exostoses of the spine in two dogs. J. Am. Vet. Med. Assoc., 166:371, 1975.
109. Prickett, M. E.: Equine spinal ataxia. Proc. Am. Assoc. Equine Pract., 14:147, 1968.
110. Rooney, J. R.: Two cervical reflexes in the horse. J. Am. Vet. Med. Assoc., 162:117, 1973.
111. Rooney, J. R.: Biomechanics of Lameness. Baltimore, Williams & Wilkins, 1969.
112. Rooney, J. R.: Clinical Neurology of the Horse. Kennett Square, Pa., KNA Press, 1971.
113. Rooney, J. R.: Equine incoordination. I. Gross morphology. Cor. Vet., 53:411, 1963.
114. Rooney, J. R., Prickett, M. E., Delaney, F. M., and Crowe, M. W.: Focal myelitis and encephalitis in horses. Cor. Vet., 60:494, 1970.
115. Ruch, T. C.: Evidence of the nonsegmental character of spinal reflexes from an analysis of the cephalad effects of spinal transection (Schiff-Sherrington phenomenon). Am. J. Physiol., 114:457, 1936.
116. Ruch, T. C., and Watts, J. W.: Reciprocal changes in reflex activity of the forelimbs induced by post-brachial "cold block" of the spinal cord. Am. J. Physiol., 110:362, 1934.
117. Sandersleben, J. von, and el Sergany, M. A.: Ein Beitrag zur sogenannten Pachymeningitis spinalis ossificans des Hundes unter Berücksichtigung pathogenetischer und ätiologischer Gesichtspunkte. Zbl. Veterinaermed. (A), 13:526, 1966.
118. Saxegaard, F.: Isolation and identification of equine rhinopneumonitis virus (equine abortion virus) from cases of abortion and paralysis. Nord. Vet.-Med., 18:504, 1966.
119. Schebitz, H., and Schulz, L. C.: Zur Pathogenese der spinalen Ataxie beim Pferd — Spondylarthrosis, klinishe Befunde. Deutsch. Tieraerztl. Wschr., 72:496, 1965.
120. Schebitz, H., and Dahme, E.: Spinal ataxia in the horse. Proc. Am. Assoc. Equine Pract., 14:133, 1968.
121. Schiefer, B., and Dahme, E.: Primäre Geschwülste des ZNS bei Tieren. Acta Neuropathol., 2:202, 1962.
122. Schulz, L. C., Schebitz, H., Pohlenz, J., and Mechlenburg, G.: Zur Pathogenese der Spinalen Ataxie des Pferdes — Spondylarthrosis Pathologish-anatomische Untersuchungen. Deutsch. Tieraerztl. Wschr., 72:502, 1965.
123. Selcer, R. R., and Oliver, J. E., Jr.: Cervical spondylopathy–wobbler syndrome in dogs. J. Am. Anim. Hosp. Assoc., 11:175, 1975.
124. Shoho, C.: Prophylaxis and therapy in epizootic cerebrospinal nematodiasis of animals by 1-diethylcarbamyl-4-methyl-piperazine dihydrogen citrate. Report of second field trial. Vet. Med., 49:459, 1954.
125. Sprague, J. M.: Spinal "border cells" and their role in postural mechanism (Schiff-Sherrington phenomenon). J. Neurophysiol., 16:464, 1953.
126. Sprinkle, T.: Diagnosis — equine rhino. Norden News, 50:16, 1975.
127. Stavrou, D.: Zur zerebrospinalen Nematodosis der Equiden. Berl. Münch. Tierärztl. Wochenschr., 24:471, 1967.
128. Steel, J. D. Whittem, J. H., and Hutchins, D. R.: Equine sensory ataxia (wobblers), Aust. Vet. J., 35:442, 1959.
129. Suter, P. F., Morgan, J. P., Holliday, T. A., and O'Brien, T. P.: Myelography in the dog: Diagnosis of tumors of the spinal cord and vertebrae. J. Am. Radiol. Soc., 12:29, 1971.
130. Swaim, S. F.: Ventral decompression of the cervical spinal cord in the dog. J. Am. Vet. Med. Assoc., 162:276, 1973.
131. Swaim, S. F.: Ventral decompression of the cervical spinal cord in the dog. J. Am. Vet. Med. Assoc., 164:491, 1974.
132. Swanstrom, O. G., Rising, J. L., and Carlton, W. W.: Spinal nematodiasis in a horse. J. Am. Vet. Med. Assoc., 155:748, 1969.
133. Tarlov, I. M.: Spinal Cord Compression, Mechanism of Paralysis, and Treatment. Springfield, Ill.: Charles C Thomas, 1957.
134. Teuscher, E., and Cherrstrom, E. C.: Ependymoma of the spinal cord in a young dog. Schweiz. Arch. Tierheilk, 116:461, 1974.
135. Thorsen, J., and Little, P. B.: Isolation of equine herpesvirus type I from a horse with an acute paralytic disease. Can. J. Comp. Med., 39:358, 1975.
136. Trotter, E. J.: Surgical repair of fractured atlas in a dog. J. Am. Vet. Med. Assoc., 161:303, 1972.
137. Trotter, E. J.: Canine intervertebral disk disease. *In* Kirk, R. W., ed., Current Veterinary Therapy, V. Small Animal Practice. Philadelphia, W. B. Saunders Co., 1974.
138. Trotter, E. J., Brasmer, T. H., and de Lahunta, A.: Modified deep dorsal laminectomy in the dog. Cor. Vet., 65:402, 1975.

139. Whitlock, J. H.: Neurofilariosis, a paralytic disease of sheep. II. *Neurophilaria cornellensis* n.g.n. sp. (*Nematoda filaroidia*), a new nematode parasite from the spinal cord of sheep. Cor. Vet., *42*:125, 1952.

140. Wilson, J. W., Greene, H. J., and Leipold, H. W.: Osseous metaplasia of the spinal dura mater in a Great Dane. J. Am. Vet. Med. Assoc., *167*:75, 1975.

141. Wright, F., and Palmer, A. C.: Morphological changes caused by pressure on the spinal cord. Pathol. Vet., *6*:355, 1969.

142. Wright, E., Palmer, A. C., and Payne, J. E.: Pressure-induced lesions in the spinal cord of rabbits. Res. Vet. Sci., *17*:337, 1974.

143. Wright, F., Rest, J. R., and Palmer, A. C.: Ataxia of the Great Dane caused by stenosis of the cervical vertebral canal; Comparison with similar condition in the basset hound, Doberman pinscher, Ridgeback, and thoroughbred horse. Vet. Rec., *92*:1, 1973.

144. Zaki, F. A., Prata, R. G., Hurvitz, A. I., and Kay, W. J.: Primary tumors of the spinal cord and meninges in six dogs. J. Am. Vet. Med. Assoc., *166*:511, 1975.

145. Charlton, K. M., Mitchell, D., Girard, A., and Corner, A. H.: Meningoencephalomyelitis in horses associated with equine herpesvirus infection. Vet. Pathol., *13*:59, 1976.

146. Little, P. B., and Thorsen, J.: Disseminated necrotizing myeloencephalitis: A herpes associated neurological disease of horses. Vet. Pathol., *13*:161, 1976.

147. Watson, A. G., and Evans, H. E.: The development of the atlas-axis complex in the dog. Anat. Rec., *184*:558, 1976.

148. Cowen, D., and Olmstead, E. V.: Infantile neuraxonal dystrophy. J. Neuropathol. Exp. Neurol., *22*:175, 1963.

149. Cordy, D. R., Ricards, W. P. C., and Bradford, G. E.: Systemic neuraxonal dystrophy in Suffolk sheep. Acta Neuropathol., 8:133, 1967.

150. Woodard, J. C., Collins, G. H., and Hessler, J. R.: Feline hereditary neuraxonal dystrophy, Am. J. Pathol., *74*:551, 1974.

151. Hooper, P. T., Best, S. M., and Campbell, A.: Axonal dystrophy in the spinal cords of cattle consuming the Cycad palm, *Cycas media.* Aust. Vet. J., *50*:146, 1974.

152. Chalmers, G. A.: Swayback (enzootic ataxia) in Alberta Sheep lambs. Can. J. Comp. Med., *38*: 111, 1974.

153. Dipaolo, R. V., Kanfer, J. N., and Newberne, P. M.: Copper deficiency and the central nervous system. Myelination in the rat: Morphological and biochemical studies. J. Neuropathol. Exp. Neurol., *33*:226, 1974.

154. Pentschew, A., and Schwarz, K.: Systemic axonal dystrophy in Vitamin E deficient rats. Acta Neuropathol., *1*:373, 1962.

155. Barlow, R. M., Butler, E. J., and Purves, D.: An ataxic condition in red deer (*Cervus elaphus*). J. Comp. Pathol., *74*:519, 1964.

156. Zaki, F., and Prata, R. G.: Necrotizing myelopathy secondary to embolization of herniated intervertebral disk material in the dog. J. Am. Vet. Med. Assoc., *169*:222, 1976.

157. Zaki, F., Prata, R. G., and Werner, L. L.: Necrotizing myelopathy in a cat. J. Am. Vet. Assoc., *169*: 228, 1976.

158. Zivin, J. A., Doppman, J. L., Reid, J. L., Tappaz, M. L., Saavedra, J. M., Kopin, I. J., and Jacobowitz, D. M.: Biochemical and histochemical studies of biogenic amines in spinal cord trauma. Neurology, *26*:99, 1976.

159. Schappert, H. R., and Geib, L. W.: Reticuloendothelial neoplasms involving the spinal cord of cats. J. Am. Vet. Med. Assoc., *150*:753, 1967.

160. Little, P. B., Lewin, U. S., and Fretz, P.: Verminous encephalitis of horses: Experimental induction with *Strongylus vulgaris* larvae. Am. J. Vet. Res., *35*:1501, 1974.

161. Averill, D. R., Jr., and de Lahunta, A.: Toxoplasmosis of the canine nervous system: Clinicopathologic findings in four cases. J. Am. Vet. Med. Assoc., *159*:1134, 1971.

162. Russell, S. W., and Griffiths, R. C.: Recurrence of cervical disc syndrome in surgically and conservatively treated dogs. J. Am. Vet. Med. Assoc., *153*:1412, 1968.

163. Oliver, J. E., Eubank, N. J., and Geary, J. C.: Neurofibrosarcoma in a dog. J. Am. Vet. Med. Assoc., *146*:965, 1964.

164. Mendenhall, H. V., Litwak, P., Yturraspe, D. J., Ingram, J. T., and Lumb, W. V.: Aggressive pharmacologic and surgical treatment of spinal cord injuries in dogs and cats. J. Am. Vet. Med. Assoc., *168*:1036, 1976.

165. Williams, J. F., Dade, A. W., and Benne, R.: Posterior paralysis associated with anthelmintic treatment of sheep. J. Am. Vet. Med. Assoc., *1969*:1307, 1976.

166. Cork, L. C.: Differential diagnosis of viral leukoencephalomyelitis of goats. J. Am. Vet. Med. Assoc., *1969*:1303, 1976.

167. Cork, L. C., Hadlow, W. J., Crawford, T. B., Gorham, J. R., and Piper, R. C.: Infectious leukoencephalomyelitis of young goats. J. Infect. Dis., *129*:134, 1974.

168. Cork, L. C., Hadlow, W. J., Gorham, J. R., Piper, R. C., and Crawford, T. B.: Pathology of viral leukoencephalomyelitis of goats. Acta neuropathol., *29*:281, 1974.

169. Cork, L. C., and Davis, W. C.: Ultrastructural features of viral leukoencephalomyelitis of goats. Lab. Invest., *32*:359, 1975.

170. Falco, M. J., Whitwell, K., and Palmer, A. C.: An investigation into the genetics of "wobbler disease" in Thoroughbred horses in Britain. Equine Vet. J., 8:165, 1976.

Chapter 11

VESTIBULAR SYSTEM—SPECIAL PROPRIOCEPTION

ANATOMY AND PHYSIOLOGY
RECEPTOR
Crista Ampullaris
Macula
VESTIBULOCOCHLEAR NERVE—CRANIAL NERVE VIII—VESTIBULAR DIVISION
VESTIBULAR NUCLEI
SIGNS OF VESTIBULAR DISEASE
UNILATERAL DISEASE
Abnormal Posture and Ataxia

Nystagmus
Postural Reactions—Strabismus
Paradoxical Central Vestibular Disease
BILATERAL DISEASE
DISEASES OF THE VESTIBULAR SYSTEM
PERIPHERAL
CENTRAL
CONGENITAL NYSTAGMUS

The vestibular system is the primary sensory system that maintains the animal's normal orientation relative to the gravitational field of the earth. This orientation is maintained in the face of linear or rotatory acceleration and tilting of the animal. The vestibular system is responsible for maintaining the position of the eyes, trunk, and limbs in reference to the position or movement of the head at any time.

ANATOMY AND PHYSIOLOGY

RECEPTOR

The receptor for special proprioception, the vestibular system, develops in conjunction with the receptor for the auditory system (SSA). They are derived from ectoderm, but are contained in a mesodermally derived structure. Together these are the components of the inner ear. The ectodermal component arises as a proliferation of ectodermal epithelial cells on the surface of the embryo adjacent to the developing rhombencephalon. This is the otic placode, which subsequently invaginates to form an otic pit and otic vesicle (otocyst), breaking away from its attachment to the surface ectoderm. This saccular structure undergoes extensive modification of its shape, but always retains its fluid-filled lumen and surrounding thin epithelial wall as it becomes the membranous labyrinth of the inner ear. Special modification of its epithelial surface at predetermined sites forms the receptor organ for the vestibular and auditory systems.

Corresponding developmental modifications occur in the surrounding mesoderm or head mesenchyme to provide a supporting capsule for the membranous labyrinth. This fluid-filled ossified structure is the bony labyrinth, contained within the developing petrose portion of the temporal bone.

The membranous and bony labyrinths are formed adjacent to the first and second branchial arches and their corresponding first pharyngeal pouch and first branchial groove. The first branchial groove gives rise to the external ear canal; the first pharyngeal pouch forms the auditory tube and the mucosa of the middle ear cavity. The intervening tissue forms the tympanum. The ear ossicles are derived from the mesoderm of branchial arches 1 (malleus and incus) and 2 (stapes). These become components of the middle ear associated laterally with the tympanum (malleus), and medially with the vestibular window of the bony labyrinth of the inner ear (stapes).

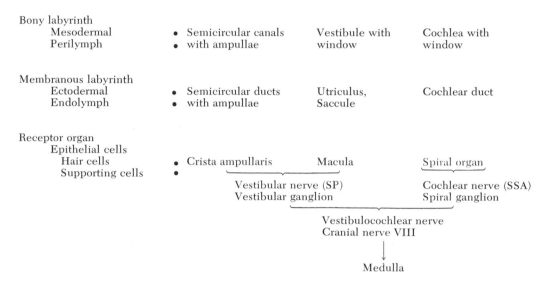

Anatomically, the bony labyrinth in the petrosal bone consists of three communicating fluid-filled portions. These are the large vestibule, and three semicircular canals and the cochlea which arise from the vestibule. These contain perilymph, a fluid similar to CSF, from which it probably is derived. There are two openings in the bony labyrinth, the vestibular and cochlear windows, which are named according to the component of the bony labyrinth in which they are located. Each is covered by a membrane, and the stapes is inserted in the membrane covering the vestibular window.

The ectodermally derived membranous labyrinth consists of four fluid-filled compartments, all of which communicate. These are contained within the components of the bony labyrinth and include the saccule and utriculus within the bony vestibule, three semicircular ducts within the bony semicircular canals, and a cochlear duct within the bony cochlea. The three semicircular ducts are the anterior (vertical), posterior (vertical), and lateral (horizontal). Each semicircular duct is oriented at right angles to the others; thus rotation of the head around any plane causes endolymph to flow within one or more of the ducts. Each semicircular duct connects at both ends with the utriculus, which in turn connects to the saccule by way of the intervening endolymphatic duct and sac. The saccule communicates with the cochlear duct by the small ductus reuniens. The endolymph

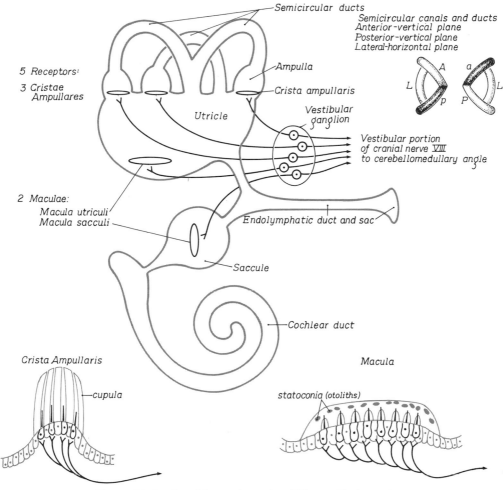

Figure 11-1. Special proprioception (SP)—vestibular system.

contained within the membranous system is thought to be derived from the blood along one wall of the cochlear duct, and is absorbed back into the blood through vessels surrounding the endolymphatic sac.

Crista Ampullaris

At one end of each membranous semicircular duct there is a dilation called the ampulla. On one side of the ampulla, a proliferation of connective tissue forms a transverse ridge called the crista. This is lined on its internal surface by columnar epithelial cells, the neuroepithelium. On the surface of the crest is a gelatinous structure that is composed of a protein-polysaccharide material called the cupula, which extends across the lumen of the ampulla. The neuroepithelium is composed of two basic cell types, hair cells and supporting cells.[1, 8, 9, 24, 30-32] The dendritic zone of the neurons of the vestibular portion of the vestibulocochlear nerve is in synaptic relationship to the hair cells. The hair cells have on their luminal surfaces 40 to 80 "hairs" or modified microvilli (stereocilia) and a single modified cilium (kinocilium). They project into the overlying cupula. Movement of fluid in the semicircular duct causes deflection of the cupula, which is oriented transversely to the direction of flow of endolymph. This bends the stereocilia and is the source of stimulus by way of the hair cell to the dendritic zone of the vestibular neuron that is in synaptic relationship with the plasmalemma of the hair cell.

There is one ampulla with its crista ampullaris in one end of each semicircular duct. Because the three semicircular ducts are all at right angles to each other, movement of the head in any plane or angular rotation stimulates a crista ampullaris and the vestibular neurons. They function in dynamic equilibrium.

The vestibular neurons are tonically active, and their activity is excited or inhibited by deflection of the cupula in different directions.[24] Each semicircular duct on one side can be paired to a semicircular duct on the opposite side by their common position in a parallel plane. These synergic pairs are the left and right lateral ducts, the left anterior and right posterior ducts, and the left posterior and right anterior ducts. While movement in the direction of one of these three planes stimulates the vestibular neurons of the crista of one duct, they are inhibited in the opposite duct of the synergic pair. For example, rotation of the head to the right causes the endolymph to flow in the right lateral duct so that the cupula is deflected toward the utriculus, and the cupula of the left lateral duct is deflected away from the utriculus. This causes increased activity of vestibular neurons on the right side and decreased activity on the left, and results in a jerk nystagmus to the right side. The anatomic orientation of stereocilia relative to the kinocilium on the surface of the crista is responsible for the difference in activity relative to the direction of the cupula deflection. Deviation of the stereocilia toward the kinocilium increases vestibular neuronal activity. These receptors are not affected by a constant velocity of movement, but respond to acceleration or deceleration.

Macula

A similar receptor is present in the utriculus and saccule located in the bony vestibule, on one surface of each of these sac-like structures. At this point the labyrinth is thickened in the shape of an oval plaque called the macula. The surface of the thickened connective tissue is covered by columnar epithelial cells. This neuroepithelium is composed of hair cells and supporting cells. Covering the neuroepithelium is a gelatinous material, the otolithic membrane, which contains calcareous crystalline bodies known as statoconia (otoliths). Similar to the hair cells of the cristae, the macular hair cells have projections of their luminal cell membrane—stereocilia and kinocilia—in the overlying otolithic membrane. Movement of the otoliths away from these cell processes is the initiating factor in stimulating an impulse in the dendritic zone of the vestibular neurons that are in synaptic relationship with the base of the hair cells. The macula in the saccule is oriented in a vertical direction (sagittal plane), while that of the utriculus is in a horizontal direction (dorsal plane); thus, gravitational forces continually affect the position of the otoliths in relationship to the hair cells. These are responsible for the sensation of the static position of the head and linear movement. They function in static equilibrium. The macula of the utriculus may be more important as a receptor for sensing changes in posture of the head, while the macula of the saccule may be more sensitive to vibrational stimuli and loud sounds.

VESTIBULOCOCHLEAR NERVE—CRANIAL NERVE VIII—
VESTIBULAR DIVISION

The dendritic zone is in synaptic relationship with the hair cells of the crista ampullaris and macula utriculi and macula sacculi. The axons course through the internal acoustic meatus with those of the cochlear division. The cell bodies of these bipolar-type neurons are inserted along the course of the axons within the petrosal bone, and form the vestibular ganglion. After leaving the petrosal bone through the internal acoustic meatus with the cochlear division of the vestibulocochlear nerve, the axons pass to the lateral surface of the rostral medulla, at the cerebellomedullary angle. This is at the level of the trapezoid body and attachment of the caudal cerebellar peduncle to the cerebellum. The vestibular neurons penetrate the medulla between the caudal cerebellar peduncle and the spinal tract of the trigeminal nerve, and terminate in telodendria at one of two sites. The majority terminate in the vestibular nuclei. A few directly enter the cerebellum by way of the caudal peduncle, and terminate in the fastigial nucleus and flocculonodular lobe. These form the direct vestibulocerebellar tract.

VESTIBULAR NUCLEI

There are four vestibular nuclei on either side of the dorsal part of the medulla adjacent to the lateral wall of the fourth ventricle.[4] From the level of the rostral and middle cerebellar peduncles, they extend caudally to the level of the lateral cuneate nucleus in the lateral wall of the caudal portion of the fourth ventricle. The four nuclei are grouped into rostral, medial, lateral, and caudal vestibular nuclei. The rostral vestibular nucleus is located ventromedial to the middle and rostral cerebellar peduncles, dorsal to the motor nucleus of the trigeminal nerve. The medial and lateral vestibular nuclei are located ventromedial to the confluence of the three cerebellar peduncles with the cerebellum. They are dorsal to the descending facial neurons. The medial nucleus continues caudally adjacent to the caudal nucleus in the dorsal medulla to the level of the lateral cuneate nucleus. The caudal cerebellar peduncle is dorsolateral to the caudal vestibular nucleus. The spinal tract of the trigeminal nerve and its nucleus are ventrolateral to the caudal vestibular nucleus in the medulla. The caudal vestibular nucleus is caudal to the lateral vestibular nucleus, which is only located at the level of the confluent cerebellar peduncles. The caudal vestibular nucleus continues caudally to the level of the lateral cuneate nucleus. These vestibular nuclei receive afferents primarily from the vestibular division of the vestibulocochlear nerve. In addition, some afferents enter from the fastigial nucleus of the cerebellum.

There are numerous projections from the vestibular nuclei.[14, 15, 20] These can be grouped into the following pathways:

Spinal Cord. The vestibulospinal tract descends in the ipsilateral ventral funiculus through the entire spinal cord, terminating in all segments on interneurons in the ventral grey column. These interneurons are facilitatory to ipsilateral alpha and gamma motor neurons to extensor muscles, inhibitory to the ipsilateral alpha motor neurons to flexor muscles, and some interneurons cross to the opposite ventral grey column and are inhibitory to the contralateral alpha and gamma motor neurons to extensor muscles. Thus the effect of stimulation of the vestibulospinal tract is an ipsilateral extensor tonus, ipsilateral facilitation of the

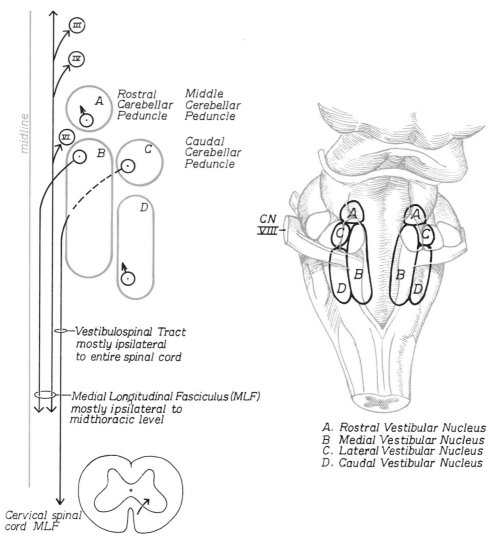

Rostral Cerebellar Peduncle

Middle Cerebellar Peduncle

Caudal Cerebellar Peduncle

Vestibulospinal Tract mostly ipsilateral to entire spinal cord

Medial Longitudinal Fasciculus (MLF) mostly ipsilateral to midthoracic level

Cervical spinal cord MLF

CN VIII

A. Rostral Vestibular Nucleus
B. Medial Vestibular Nucleus
C. Lateral Vestibular Nucleus
D. Caudal Vestibular Nucleus

Figure 11–2. Vestibular nuclei and tracts.

stretch reflex mechanism, and contralateral inhibition of this mechanism. In the cat the cell bodies of the axons in the vestibulospinal tract are in the lateral vestibular nucleus.

The medial vestibular nucleus projects axons into the medial longitudinal fasciculus, which descends in the dorsal portion of the ventral funiculus through the cervical and cranial thoracic segments, influencing the alpha and gamma motor neurons by way of interneuronal activation.

Through these spinal cord pathways the position and activity of the limbs and trunk can be coordinated with movements of the head.

Brain Stem

1. Axons course rostrally in the medial longitudinal fasciculus and reticular formation to influence the nuclei of the cranial nerves VI, IV, and III. This provides coordinated conjugate eyeball movements associated with changes in position of the head. When the brain stem is severely contused by a head injury, these pathways are interfered with and eyeball movement cannot be elicited by changing the position of the head. This is a sign that usually indicates a poor prognosis because of the severity of the associated lesion.

2. Axons project into the reticular formation. Some of these provide afferents to the vomiting center located there, which is the pathway underlying motion sickness.

3. The pathway for conscious projection of the vestibular system is not well defined. It usually is considered to be similar to the auditory system, and is mediated by way of axons that project rostrally through the midbrain to the contralateral medial geniculate nucleus of the thalamus. Synapse occurs here, and the axons of the medial geniculate neurons project by way of the internal capsule to the gyri of the temporal lobe, primarily the rostral suprasylvian gyrus.

Cerebellum. Axons of vestibular nuclear neurons project to the cerebellum through the caudal cerebellar peduncle, and terminate mostly in the flocculus of the hemisphere and the nodulus of the caudal vermis (the flocculonodular lobe),

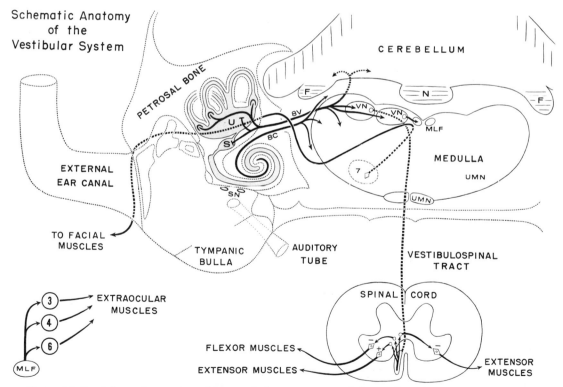

Figure 11–3. Schematic anatomy of the vestibular system. *N:* nodulus; *F:* flocculus; *UMN:* upper motor neuron; *MLF:* medial longitudinal fasciculus; *VN:* vestibular nucleus; *8V:* cranial nerve VIII, vestibular portion; *8C:* cranial nerve VIII, cochlear portion; *U:* utricle; *S:* saccule; *SN:* sympathetic neurons; *3:* oculomotor nucleus; *4:* trochlear nucleus; *6:* abducens nucleus; *7:* facial nucleus.

and the fastigial nucleus. The fastigial nucleus is the most medial of the cerebellar nuclei.

Through these pathways the vestibular system functions to coordinate the eyeballs, trunk, and limbs with movements of the head. It maintains equilibrium during active and passive movement and when the head is at rest.

SIGNS OF VESTIBULAR DISEASE

Vestibular disease produces various degrees of loss of equilibrium causing imbalance and ataxia. Strength is not interfered with, and therefore no paresis is observed. As a rule the disturbance is unilateral or asymmetric, and the signs are those of an asymmetric ataxia with preservation of strength.

UNILATERAL DISEASE

Unilateral disease of the peripheral receptor is characterized by asymmetric ataxia with preservation of strength. The same asymmetric ataxia occurs with disease of the vestibular nuclei, but usually the lesion also involves the adjacent descending upper motor neuron pathways and paresis is observed. Thus, the observation of paresis in an animal with an asymmetric vestibular ataxia is evidence that the lesion is in the medulla of the brain stem. The signs can be grouped into those that reflect disturbed tonus in axial and appendicular muscles, and those that reflect disturbance of eyeball coordination.

Abnormal Posture and Ataxia

Loss of coordination between head, trunk, and limbs is reflected in a head tilt with the more ventral ear directed toward the side of the vestibular disturbance. The trunk will tip, fall, or even roll toward the side of the lesion. The trunk may be flexed laterally, with the concavity directed toward the side of the lesion. The animal may tend to circle toward the side of the lesion. These are usually circles with short radii. It may be possible to elicit mild hypertonia and hyperreflexia in the limbs on the side of the body opposite the lesion. These signs of trunk and limb ataxia can be explained by loss of activity of the vestibulospinal tract ipsilateral to the lesion and direction of ataxia. This removes facilitation from ipsilateral extensor muscles and a source of inhibition to contralateral extensor muscles. The unopposed contralateral vestibulospinal tract causes the trunk to be forced toward the side of the lesion by excessive, unopposed extensor muscle tonus. The entire body will tip, fall, or roll toward the side of the lesion. It is not uncommon for the animal to fall when it shakes its head.

Nystagmus

Normal Vestibular Nystagmus.   The sign of disturbed vestibular input to the neurons that innervate extraocular muscles is abnormal nystagmus. Nystagmus is an involuntary rhythmic eyeball oscillation either with equal movements (pendular) or a quick and slow phase (jerk) that can occur in any plane. The direction of the jerk nystagmus is ascribed to that of the quick phase. Both eyeballs usually are affected simultaneously and in the same direction. These oscillations normally are induced by any rapid head movement. Rapid dorsoventral flexion and extension of the animal's head and neck elicits a vertical nystagmus. Similar side to side movements of the head elicit a horizontal nystagmus. The quick phase of the nystagmus is in the direction of the rotation. This can be elicited readily in most normal animals, and is called vestibular nystagmus. It is a normal reflex in which the slow component is initiated by way of the labyrinth, and the fast component results from function of a brain stem center. This reflex helps to maintain visual fixation on stationary points as the body rotates.

   Postrotatory Nystagmus.   If an animal is rotated rapidly, as it is accelerated the labyrinth moves around the fluid that deflects the cupulae of the cristae ampullaris, stimulating the vestibular nerve and thus eliciting eyeball movements. The quick phase is in the direction of the rotation. These movements cannot be observed during the stage of acceleration. In time the rotation of the endolymph reaches the speed of rotation of the labyrinth. At this constant velocity the cupulae are not deflected. Thus there is no alteration of vestibular nerve stimulus, and nystagmus does not occur. If the rotation is stopped suddenly, once again there is a disparity in the rotation of the labyrinth and the endolymph. The labyrinth is stationary, but the endolymph continues to flow for a short interval; it deflects the cupulae which stimulates the vestibular neurons, and nystagmus is elicited. Now, however, the direction of the flow is opposite to that during acceleration, and the quick phase of the nystagmus is directed opposite to the direction of the rotation. The speed and duration of this postrotatory vestibular nystagmus are variable, but should be about equal when the response to spinning is compared for both directions.

   Vestibular disease is suspected when there is a different response to spinning in one direction as compared to the other. As a rule, when the patient is rotated in a direction opposite to the side of a peripheral receptor lesion, postrotatory nystagmus is depressed. This postrotatory test stimulates both labyrinths. However, the labyrinth on the side opposite the direction of rotation is stimulated more because it is farther away from the axis of rotation. This may explain the abnormal postrotatory nystagmus that is observed with unilateral vestibular disease. On spinning away from the side of the lesion, the diseased labyrinth is farthest from the axis of rotation, cannot be stimulated properly, and a depressed postrotatory response is observed.

   Caloric Nystagmus.   The individual labyrinths can be tested separately by the caloric test. Irrigation of the external ear canal with ice cold water for 3 to 5 minutes causes the endolymph to flow in the semicircular ducts.[17] This normally induces a jerk nystagmus directed to the side opposite the one being stimulated. If the peripheral receptor on the side being tested is nonfunctional because of a disease process, no nystagmus will be observed from the caloric test. Covering the patient's eyeballs may prevent voluntary repression of the response by fixation on an object in the environment. Despite this, sometimes the animal resists this procedure and makes the test unreliable. In some normal dogs, even prolonged irrigation with cold water has failed to elicit nystagmus. Asymmetric responses suggest a deficit on the side being tested.

   Abnormal Nystagmus.   When the head is held in its normally extended position or if held flexed laterally to either side or held extended fully, no nystagmus is found. In vestibular system disease a nystagmus may be observed. If it is seen when the head is in its normal extended position, it is called a spontaneous nystagmus. If it is induced by holding the head fixed in lateral flexion or full extension, it is called a positional nystagmus.

In peripheral receptor disease the nystagmus is either horizontal or rotatory, and always in a direction (quick phase) away from the side of the lesion. The direction of rotatory nystagmus is defined by the change in the 12 o'clock position of the limbus during the quick phase. This direction does not change when the position of the head is changed. With disease of the vestibular nuclei or vestibular pathways in the cerebellum, the nystagmus may be horizontal, rotatory, or vertical, and may change in direction with changes in position of the head. Thus vertical nystagmus, or nystagmus that changes in direction on changing position of the head, is suggestive of central involvement of the vestibular system.

In some cases of severe vestibular system disturbance there is a slight head oscillation that corresponds to the rate of the spontaneous nystagmus. In addition, occasionally there is an eyelid contraction concomitant with the nystagmus. This is probably elicited reflexly.

Postural Reactions — Strabismus

Most postural reactions are intact, except for the righting response. Usually the patient experiences difficulty righting itself, with an exaggerated response toward the side of the lesion. When the head is extended in the tonic neck reaction, the eyeballs should remain in the center of the palpebral fissure in the dog and cat. This often fails to occur on the side of the vestibular disturbance, and results in a dropped or ventrally deviated eyeball.

In ruminants, it is normal for the eyeballs to deviate ventrally on neck extension. In horses there is normally a slight ventral deviation, which is more pronounced in the eyeball ipsilateral to a vestibular system lesion.

Occasionally, in vestibular disease an eyeball is noticed deviated ventrally or ventrolaterally without extension of the head and neck. This appears as a lower motor neuron strabismus, but can be corrected by moving the head into a different position or by inducing the patient to move its eyeballs to gaze in different directions. This is referred to as a vestibular strabismus. There is no paralysis of the cranial nerves that innervate the extraocular muscles. The ventrally deviated eyeball is on the side of the lesion in the vestibular system. Sometimes the opposite eyeball may appear to be deviated dorsally.

Signs of vestibular disturbance are accompanied by vomiting only occasionally.

Paradoxical Central Vestibular Disease

Some unilateral lesions in the central vestibular pathways, expecially with unilateral involvement of the cerebellar medulla and peduncles, produce a head tilt and ataxia directed toward the side opposite the lesion.[18] These are usually destructive space-occupying lesions such as gliomas, or reticulosis granulomas. No anatomic explanation has yet been offered.

Usually these lesions interfere with the general proprioceptive system afferent to the cerebellum. This produces a mild GP ataxia and postural reaction deficit, always on the same side as the lesion. This observation is the most reliable for locating the side of the lesion.

BILATERAL DISEASE

Bilateral peripheral vestibular disease with complete loss of function is characterized by symmetric ataxia with strength preserved. There is no postural asymmetry. The patient often stays crouched on the ground with its limbs spread apart. It may crawl along in this posture, occasionally staggering or falling to either side.

A characteristic jerky side to side head movement often accompanies these signs. Wide excursions of the head to either side accompany the bilateral disturbance of head orientation.

Nystagmus is not observed, and with bilateral destruction of the receptor organs no normal vestibular nystagmus can be elicited by head movement or caloric testing.

DISEASES OF THE VESTIBULAR SYSTEM

PERIPHERAL

Feline Vestibular Disease: Idiopathic-Vestibular Neuropathy.[7] This syndrome is seen in cats of all ages in the summer and early fall. It occurs suddenly as severe unilateral ataxia characterized by a head tilt and tendency to fall or roll toward the side of the head tilt. It may appear initially to the owner that the cat is unable to get up and walk. However, there is no loss of strength or ability to initiate voluntary movement. The cat is so disoriented as to its position in space that it is reluctant to move. If suddenly picked up, the cat grasps violently for a supporting surface and usually turns rapidly toward the side of the head tilt. If the cat can be supported without struggling or rolling, normal postural reactions will be elicited. These cats have no cerebral disturbance, and are extremely alert and responsive. They often stay crouched against a wall and cry distressfully.

For the first 72 hours a spontaneous nystagmus occurs in a direction opposite the head tilt. This is usually horizontal, but occasionally it is rotatory. At the onset, a head oscillation may occur simultaneous with the nystagmus. After 3 to 4 days the spontaneous nystagmus disappears, but an abnormal positional nystagmus may be elicited on altering the position of the head. The direction always remains opposite to the side of the head tilt.

As the animal becomes more willing to ambulate, it walks with a broad base and tilts to one side, with the tail often extended straight up. If it turns its head suddenly, it often staggers to the side to which it is tilted. Occasionally, it staggers to the opposite side. Sometimes the trunk sways from side to side. This is called truncal ataxia.

By 7 days the animal moves around more freely, but still with a head tilt and tendency to lean and stagger in that direction. Over the next 2 to 3 weeks the gait continues to improve. The head tilt may be the only persisting residual sign, and that may disappear.

In a cat that has recovered from or compensated for this lesion the signs may be completely absent except when the animal suddenly is stressed, and then a mild degree of asymmetric ataxia may be apparent.

Experimental labyrinthectomy in the cat produces a syndrome identical to that observed in many of the cases of feline vestibular disease.[5] The ability of these experimental cats to compensate has been determined to be dependent on functional vestibular components of the brain stem and cerebellum, particularly the fastigial nucleus of the cerebellum.

The pathogenesis of the feline disease is unknown. Although occasionally associated with a previous or concurrent upper respiratory disease, such a history is lacking in most cases. Microscopic study shows no evidence of an inflammatory lesion in the inner ear. Necropsy studies have been inadequate to determine cytologic changes in the hair cells of the receptor organs. No consistent evidence of an intoxication has been forthcoming.[6]

To date, the disease has not been found twice in the same cat. Some observers feel that bilateral signs occasionally are present. The prognosis for recovery is good. Until the pathogenesis is understood, no therapy is recommended. Many drugs have been used, including antibiotics, corticosteroids, antimotion drugs, calcium, and vitamins, but there is no concrete evidence that these increase the rate of recovery.

Canine Geriatric Vestibular Disease. A neurologic disturbance occurs in older dogs that, on careful neurologic evaluation, appears to be similar to that described for the feline vestibular disease.[3] Unfortunately, many of these cases appear to be so incapacitated at the onset of the disease that the signs are attributed mistakenly to a brain stem lesion, and the syndrome is diagnosed as "stroke." This term refers to a cerebrovascular accident that occurs in man associated with chronic vascular disease and the acute blockage of a cerebral blood vessel or its rupture and subsequent hemorrhage. Similar vascular disease in domestic animals is uncommon; however, signs indicative of cerebrovascular dysfunction occasionally do occur, and should be referable to brain stem or cerebral involvement, or both. This is not the case with these older dogs, and it is important to distinguish this fact for prognostic reasons.

The signs of the canine patient with acute vestibular disturbance all are referable to this system. They are similar to those described for the feline vestibular disease, but may be less pronounced and resolve more quickly. Vomiting may occur during the first few days of the disease. If the dog is severely affected and incapacitated by the disease, the examiner may not recognize that the signs represent a peripheral vestibular disorder until a complete neurologic examination has been performed. Normal strength and postural reactions may be masked by the ataxia and spatial disorientation.

These dogs should be handled in a manner similar to the cats. There is no specific therapy. Confinement over the period of most severe disorientation will help the patient and provide the veterinarian with the opportunity to reevaluate the patient to be sure of the diagnosis. Recurrent episodes have been observed in these dogs on the same or the opposite side.

For both the feline and canine diseases, it is important to rule out the presence of inner ear inflammation secondary to inflammation of the middle ear, otitis media and otitis interna. In most cases of the latter, the onset and severity of vestibular disturbance are not as severe as in the idiopathic disease.

Otitis Media and Otitis Interna. Vestibular signs occur in animals when the middle ear inflammation indirectly or directly affects the function of the membranous labyrinth.[22, 23] Varying degrees of unilateral vestibular disturbance appear which consist of asymmetric ataxia with strength preservation. Sometimes only a head tilt and positional nystagmus are evident. Occasionally, these signs are accompanied by an ipsilateral facial paresis to palsy, or Horner's syndrome, or both. These occur if the otitis media disturbs the function of the facial and sympathetic nerves, respectively, which course adjacent to or through the middle ear in the dog and cat.[2] Unilateral deafness may occur but is difficult to determine clinically.

Otoscopic examination of the external acoustic meatus and tympanum may reveal exudate in the middle ear. Likewise, radiographic examination may reveal the middle ear inflammation if it is extensive, filling the bulla with thick exudate, or if it affects the bone of the bulla, producing an osteitis and changing its appearance on the radiograph. Otitis media is not dependent on an associated otitis externa. The nasopharynx is also a source of infection by way of the auditory tube. Extension of the infection from the middle and inner ear locations to the meninges takes place more often in cats and pigs. Brain stem signs then accompany the peripheral vestibular signs.

The middle and inner ear inflammation may be bilateral, but if the disturbance to vestibular function is not the same the signs are asymmetric and predominate in one direction.

Occasionally, the inflammatory lesion severely affects both labyrinths, and there is complete loss of peripheral vestibular function. Signs of bilateral peripheral vestibular disease with complete loss of function prevail. Deafness often accompanies these vestibular signs, and bilateral facial palsy has been observed.

Polyneuropathy—Neuritis. Unilateral or bilateral signs of peripheral vestibular disease have been observed with facial paresis or paralysis in mature dogs without evidence of otitis media. In some instances, there has been an associated hypothyroidism and pituitary chromophobe adenoma. Response to thyroid therapy has been unsatisfactory in most cases.

A few cases have occurred with no associated endocrine disease and have resolved spontaneously.

Congenital Peripheral Vestibular Disorder. Varying degrees of peripheral vestibular disturbance have been observed in litters of German shepherd puppies and Siamese kittens. The onset of signs is usually around 3 to 4 weeks of age. The signs often regress or are compensated for by 2 to 4 months of age. A return to normal function may occur, but recurrences have been noted in the few months following recovery. Head tilt is the most salient sign. Ataxia is often mild. There is usually no abnormal nystagmus. In fact, normal vestibular nystagmus usually cannot be elicited by moving the head. In at least one Siamese cat the peripheral vestibular disorder was accompanied by deafness. Pathologic studies have revealed no inflammatory lesion, but have not been adequate to substantiate or obviate a degenerative disease or malformation. The close relationship of affected litters suggests an hereditary basis, but this remains to be proved.

A congenital, presumably vestibular system abnormality has been recognized in related litters of Burmese cats. The signs are present at or shortly after birth, when rolling is constant in the severely affected kittens. Others show a head tilt and asymmetric ataxia. The signs appear to be nonprogressive. No lesions have been seen in the brains or in inner ears that were preserved with formalin, decalcified, and serial sectioned. Viral isolation studies have been unrewarding. A familial basis is suspected for this congenital disease.

Injury. Head injuries may fracture the petrosal bone and cause bleeding from the external ear canal through a ruptured tympanum. The vestibular signs may be masked by the signs referable to an accompanying brain stem contusion. If the signs are referable primarily to disturbance of the peripheral receptor the prognosis is better, since compensation may occur if the cerebellum and brain stem are intact.

Degeneration.   Prolonged therapy with streptomycin, dihydrostreptomycin, kanamycin, and neomycin has been found to cause degeneration of the labyrinthine receptors of the vestibular system, or the auditory system, or both.[12, 26-29] The cat seems to be more susceptible than the dog. The peripheral receptor degeneration is well established. More recent investigations do not support any primary degeneration of neurons in brain stem nuclei.[11]

Neoplasia.   Neurofibroma of the vestibulocochlear nerve usually produces signs of unilateral peripheral vestibular disturbance prior to its compression of the brain stem and the additional signs that accompany such compression.

CENTRAL

Signs of vestibular system disturbance referable to disease of the vestibular nuclei or their neuronal pathways are similar to those seen in peripheral vestibular system disease.[16]

Vestibular signs usually only seen with disease of the central pathways include consistently vertical nystagmus, nystagmus that changes direction with different positions of the head, and a tendency to roll in one direction. The latter may occur to a limited degree with peripheral disease.

The lesion is localized to the central pathways mostly by the presence of signs that accompany the brain stem involvement of other functional systems. Evidence of upper motor neuron paresis and general proprioceptive ataxia is the most useful sign. Cerebellar signs, cranial nerve deficits (other than facial), and disturbances to the sensorium from lesions that involve the reticular formation (ARAS) also localize the vestibular disturbance to the brain stem pathways. Beware of the paradoxical vestibular syndrome. Cerebellar lesions that affect the vestibular system may cause a vestibular head tilt, strabismus, and ataxia on the side opposite that of the lesion. The lesion is localized by observing the side that shows the deficient postural reactions from the lesion in the general proprioceptive or upper motor neuron systems, or both.

Inflammation—Meningoencephalitis.   Canine   distemper,   toxoplasmosis, cryptococcosis, and primary reticulosis are lesions that are disseminated widely through the central nervous system, and often include the central vestibular pathways. In the granulomatous inflammatory form of primary reticulosis, a focal space-occupying lesion often occurs on one side of the cerebellar medulla. This sometimes produces the paradoxical central vestibular syndrome.

In cats, the viral agent that produces feline infectious peritonitis also affects the meninges and ependymal surfaces and the adjacent parenchyma of the CNS.[13, 21] In some cases the nervous system lesion predominates, and may be accompanied by a chronic uveitis of the eyeball. Chronic illness characterized by partial anorexia and persistent fever that are unresponsive to antibiotic therapy, accompanied by uveitis and mild signs of neurologic disturbance sometimes referable to the cerebellar vestibular systems, are typical of this disease. CSF may be remarkably altered, with a large pleocytosis of mostly mononuclear cells and a few neutrophils, and a protein content of 200 to 400 mg per dl. The gamma globulin fraction of serum protein often is increased markedly.

An aberrant parasite wandering through the central vestibular system may produce severe signs of vestibular disturbance. *Cuterebra* larvae have been found in cats and adult *Parelaphostrongylus tenuis* in goats.

In ruminants, the bacterium *Listeria monocytogenes* causes inflammation of the brain stem with signs referable to this location, including vestibular disturbance. Varying degrees of upper motor neuron paresis, head tilt, abnormal nystagmus, and facial paresis are typical of this disease.

Neoplasia. Neoplasms at the cerebellomedullary angle affect the vestibular system.[16, 18, 19] Signs of neurologic disturbance are progressive. Neoplasms at this location often are not accompanied by an increased CSF pressure at the cerebellomedullary cistern. The contents of the CSF vary. It may be normal or similar to that seen with viral inflammations, or show markedly elevated protein levels without a commensurate increase in white blood cells. Cranial nerve deficits such as facial paresis or hypalgesia are more common in small animals with neoplastic disease than with inflammatory disease at this site.

The neoplasm may be at the surface of the parenchyma, compressing it—e.g., a meningioma, neurofibroma, medulloblastoma, or choroid plexus papilloma—or it may be located within the parenchyma, infiltrating and compressing the adjacent tissue—e.g., a glioma, or a metastatic neoplasm.

Degeneration. Thiamine (vitamin B_1) deficiency occurs in cats fed all-fish diets that contain thiaminase.[10] Occasionally, it follows chronic anorexia without vitamin therapy. Terminally, there is a hemorrhagic necrosis bilaterally symmet-

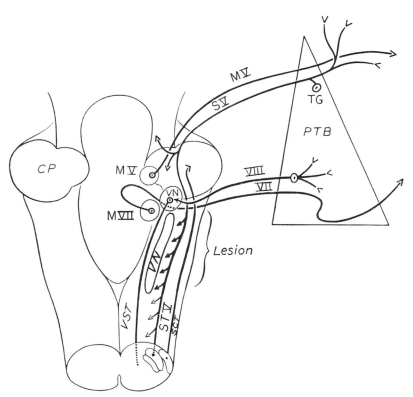

Figure 11–4. Diagram of cranial neuronal anatomy related to a granuloma that produced right-sided vestibular signs of ataxia and head tilt, complete right facial analgesia without denervation of muscles of mastication, and mild right hemiparesis and general proprioceptive ataxia in a 5-year-old pony. (From Cor. Vet., *40*:622, 1970.) *CP:* cerebellar peduncles; *MV:* motor neurons of trigeminal nerve; *MVII:* motor facial neurons; *SV:* sensory neurons of trigeminal nerve; *TG:* trigeminal ganglion; *STV:* spinal tract of trigeminal nerve; *VIII:* cranial nerve VIII, vestibular portion; *VN:* vestibular nucleus; *VST:* vestibulospinal tract; *SCT:* spinocerebellar tracts; *PTB:* petrous temporal bone.

ric in the brain stem periventricular grey matter, which includes lateral geniculate nuclei, oculomotor nuclei, caudal colliculi, and vestibular nuclei. The earliest signs of the disease are usually a mild vestibular ataxia, followed by convulsions with marked head ventroflexion. Pupils may be dilated and poorly responsive to light. Terminally, there is semicoma, continual crying, opisthotonus, and persistent extensor tonus. Prompt therapy with 1 to 2 mg of thiamine intramuscularly in the early stages of the disease results in complete remission of signs. Sometimes signs of acute vestibular disturbance accompany a prolonged period of inappetence, and complete remission of signs follows thiamine therapy.

Injury. Intracranial injury may affect the central vestibular pathways in addition to other functional systems in the brain stem. The degree of vestibular disturbance manifested depends on the degree of disturbance of the other functional system (UMN, ARAS) which would mask the vestibular disturbance. Abnormal nystagmus may be the only sign of vestibular disturbance evident in the tetraplegic, semicomatose patient.

CONGENITAL NYSTAGMUS

Congenital nystagmus occurs in man as an inherited functional abnormality, or secondary to congenital lesions in the visual system of the infant. The nystagmus is usually pendular. Congenital nystagmus was observed in a female Belgian sheepdog and three of her six offspring from one litter. The nystagmus was usually pendular with a variable frequency, but it was often very rapid. There was no obvious visual deficiency. Occasionally, the head was held tipped to one side. No ataxia was evident. Necropsy revealed a lack of development of an optic chiasm. The optic nerve fibers continued into the ipsilateral optic tract without decussation.

REFERENCES

1. Ades, H. W., and Engström, H.: Form and innervation of the vestibular epithelia. First Symposium on the Role of Vestibular Organs in Space Exploration, NASA. Scientific and Technical Information Division, Office of Technological Utilization, Washington, D.C., U.S. Government Printing Office, 1965, 23–42.
2. Blauch, B., and Strafuss, A. C.: Histologic relationships of the facial (7th) and vestibulocochlear (8th) cranial nerves within the petrous temporal bone in the dog. Am. J. Vet. Res., 35:481, 1974.
3. Blauch, B., and Martin, C. L.: A vestibular syndrome in aged dogs. J. Am. Anim. Hosp. Assoc., 10:37, 1974.
4. Brodal, A.: Anatomical aspects on functional organization of the vestibular nuclei. Second Symposium on the Role of Vestibular Organs in Space Exploration, NASA—SP115. Scientific and Technical Information Division, Office of Technological Utilization, Washington, D.C., U.S. Government Printing Office, 1966, 119–142.
5. Carpenter, M. B., Fabrega, H., and Glinsmann, W.: Physiological deficits occurring with lesions of labyrinth and fastigial nucleus. J. Neurophysiol., 22:222, 1959.
6. Coats, A. C.: Vestibular neuronitis. Trans. Am. Acad. Ophthalmol. Otolaryngol., 73:395, 1969.
7. De Lahunta, A.: Feline vestibular disease. *In* Kirk, R. W., ed., Current Veterinary Therapy, III. Philadelphia, W. B. Saunders, 1968, 466–468.
8. Engström, H.: The first-order vestibular neuron. Fourth Symposium on the Role of the Vestibular Organs in Space Exploration, NASA—SP187. Scientific and Technical Information Division, Office of Technological Utilization, Washington, D.C., U.S. Government Printing Office, 1968, 123–135.
9. Engström, H.: Form and organization of the vestibular sensory cells. *In* Stahle, J., ed., Vestibular Function on Earth and in Space. New York, Pergamon, 1970, 87–96.

10. Everett, G. M.: Observations on the behavior and neurophysiology of acute thiamine deficiency in cats. Am. J. Physiol., *141*:439, 1944.
11. Lundquist, Per-G., and Wersäll, J.: Sites of action of ototoxic antibiotics after local and general administration. *In* Stahle, J., ed., Vestibular Function on Earth and in Space. New York, Pergamon, 1970, 267–274.
12. McGee, T. M., and Olszewski, J.: Streptomycin sulfate and dihydrostreptomycin toxicity, behavioral and histopathological studies. Arch. Otolaryngol., 75:295, 1962.
13. Montali, R. J., and Strandberg, J. D.: Extraperitoneal lesions in feline infectious peritonitis. Vet. Pathol., 9:109, 1972.
14. Nyberg-Hansen, R.: Origin and termination of fibers from the vestibular nuclei descending in the medial longitudinal fasciculus. An experimental study with silver impregnation methods in the cat. J. Comp. Neurol., *122*:355, 1964.
15. Nyberg-Hansen, R., and Mascitti, T. A.: Sites and mode of termination of fibers of the vestibulospinal tract in the cat. J. Comp. Neurol., *122*:369, 1964.
16. Palmer, A. C.: Pathogenesis and pathology of the cerebellovestibular syndrome. J. Sm. Anim. Pract., *11*:167, 1970.
17. Palmer, A. C.: A test for vestibular function in sheep. Br. Vet. J., *114*:307, 1958.
18. Palmer, A. C., Malinowski, W., and Barnett, K. C.: Clinical signs including papilloedema associated with brain tumours in twenty-one dogs. J. Sm. Anim. Pract., *15*:359, 1974.
19. Pedersen, N. C., Holliday, T. A., and Cello, R. M.: Feline infectious peritonitis. Proc. Am. Anim. Hosp. Assoc., 147, 1974.
20. Petras, J. M.: Afferent fibers to the spinal cord. The terminal distribution of dorsal root and encephalospinal axons. Med. Serv. J. Can., 22:668, 1966.
21. Slausson, D. O., and Finn, J. P.: Meningoencephalitis and panophthalmitis in feline infectious peritonitis. J. Am. Vet. Med. Assoc., *160*:729, 1972.
22. Spreull, J. S. A.: Otitis media of the dog. *In* Kirk, R. W., ed., Current Veterinary Therapy, V. Philadelphia, W. B. Saunders Co., 1975, 675–683.
23. Spreull, J. S. A.: Treatment of otitis media in the dog. J. Sm. Anim. Pract., 5:107, 1964.
24. Wersäll, J., and Lundquist, Per-G.: Morphological polarization of the mechanoreceptors of the vestibular and acoustic systems. Second Symposium, Role of Vestibular Organs in Space Exploration, NASA. Scientific and Technical Information Division, Office of Technological Utilization, Washington, D.C., U.S. Government Printing Office, 1966, 57–72.
25. Wilson, V. J., Wylis, R. M., and Marco, L. A.: Projection to the spinal cord from the medial and descending vestibular nuclei of the cat. Nature, *215*:429, 1967.
26. Winston, J.: Clinical problems pertaining to neurotoxicity of streptomycin group of drugs. Arch. Otolaryngol., 58:255, 1953.
27. Winston, J., Lewey, F. H., Parenteau, A., Marden, P. A., and Cramer, F. B.: An experimental study of the toxic effects of streptomycin on the vestibular apparatus of the cat. I. Central nervous system. Ann. Otol. Rhinol. Laryngol., 57:738, 1948.
28. Winston, J., Lewey, F. H., Parenteau, A., Marden, P. A., and Cramer, F. B.: Further experimental studies of the toxic effects of streptomycin on the central vestibular apparatus of the cat. Ann. Rhinol. Laryngol., 58:988, 1949.
29. Winston, J., Lewey, F. H., Parenteau, A., Spitz, E., and Marden, P. A.: Toxic effects of dihydrostreptomycin upon the central vestibular mechanism of the cat. Ann. Otol. Rhinol. Laryngol., 62:121, 1953.
30. Engström, H., Lindeman, H. H., and Ades, H. W.: Anatomical features of the auricular sensory organs. Second Symposium on the Role of Vestibular Organs in Space Exploration, NASA-SP115. Scientific and Technical Information Division, Office of Technological Utilization, Washington, D.C., U.S. Government Printing Office, 1966, 33–46.
31. Lowenstein, O.: The functional significance of the ultrastructure of the vestibular end organs. Second Symposium on the Role of Vestibular Organs in Space Exploration, NASA-SP115. Scientific and Technical Information Division, Office of Technological Utilization, Washington, D.C., U.S. Government Printing Office, 1966, 73–90.
32. Spoendlin, H.: Some morphological and pathological aspects of the vestibular sensory epithelia. Second Symposium on the Role of Vestibular Organs in Space Exploration, NASA-SP115. Scientific and Technical Information Division, Office of Technological Utilization, Washington, D.C., U.S. Government Printing Office, 1966, 99–116.

Chapter 12

CEREBELLUM

DEVELOPMENT
ANATOMY
Cerebellar Afferents
Cerebellar Efferents
FUNCTION
SIGNS OF CEREBELLAR DISEASE
CEREBELLAR SYNDROMES
PRIMARY CEREBELLAR HYPOPLASIA AND/
    OR DEGENERATION
Cat

Dog
Cattle
Horses
Pigs
INFLAMMATION, NEOPLASIA, DIFFUSE
    DEGENERATION, AND INJURY
Inflammations
Neoplasms
Diffuse Degenerations
Injury

DEVELOPMENT

An understanding of the development of the cerebellum is pertinent to the determination of its normal microscopic characteristics and the pathogenesis of diseases that affect it.[1-5, 11, 32, 59, 68, 91, 92]

The cerebellum is the dorsal portion of the metencephalon; the ventral portion is the pons. The cerebellum develops from the alar plate region of the metencephalon. Its first sign is a dorsal bulge of the alar plate which extends the alar plate tissue dorsally and medially in the roof plate, in which the growths from each side eventually meet. This first growth is called the rhombic lip, arising from the side of the rhomboid fossa of the fourth ventricle. This rhombic lip consists of proliferating cells from the germinal zone adjacent to the fourth ventricle.

Two routes of migration issue from these germinal cells. One involves the migration of differentiating mantle layer cells into the substance of the rhombic lip. These cells no longer divide but continue to grow and mature, and give rise to the layer of Purkinje cells found throughout the cerebellar cortex and the neurons of the cerebellar nuclei located in the medulla of the cerebellum. The second migration involves actively dividing germinal cells that migrate to the surface of the rhombic lip, where they continue to be located as the folia develop in the cerebellum. This superficial layer of cells, the external germinal layer, continues mitosis, producing a zone of germinal cells composed of up to 10 to 12 layers of cells. Differentiation occurs along the inner aspect of these cells, and those cells that have stopped dividing migrate into the substance of the cerebellum to form the granule cell layer between the Purkinje cells and the white matter of the folium. The external germinal layer also contributes the few neurons (stellate cells) found in the most superficial of the three layers of the cerebellar cortex, the

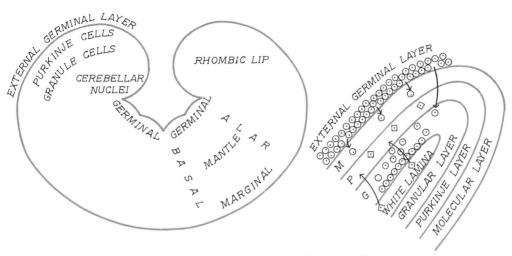

Figure 12–1. Development of the cerebellum.

molecular layer. The three layers of the definitive cerebellar cortex are from external to internal, the molecular layer, the Purkinje cell layer, and the granule cell layer. The folds produced on the surface of the cerebellum are called folia.

Purkinje cells are formed and begin differentiation early in the development of the embryo.[67, 69] The internal germinal layer adjacent to the fourth ventricle completes its activity prior to birth, leaving only a layer of ependyma to line the fourth ventricle. The external germinal layer is active late in gestation and after birth in some species. The granule cell neurons are formed from the external germinal layer later in gestation than the Purkinje cells, and their formation is not complete until the postnatal period. The degree of cerebellar development at birth correlates with the amount of motor function and coordination seen in the newborn animal.[38, 71] The foal and calf that walk at birth have a more completely developed cerebellum than the kitten, the puppy, or the human baby, who are helpless at birth. As the brain, including the cerebellum, of these latter species develops, their motor function and coordination for ambulation improve. Studies have shown a direct correlation between the development of the cerebellar cortex and mobility in the kitten.

Microscopic sections of kitten and puppy cerebellum show persistence of the external germinal layer for up to 60 to 84 days in the kitten, 75 days in the puppy, and 6 months in the calf. In the puppy, the external germinal layer is the thickest during the first 2 weeks of life. When the cells have all migrated into the molecular and granule cell layers, only the leptomeninges remain on the surface of the molecular layer. In the calf, the formation of Purkinje cells is completed at about 100 days of gestation. After that no more Purkinje cells are formed. Those that are present continue to grow and mature (differentiate) in conjunction with the continued development of the cerebellum. In the horse, ox, sheep, and pig, the external germinal layer is more active late in gestation and has mostly exhausted its germinal role prior to birth. In the calf the cerebellar primordium appears at 37 days. The external germinal layer appears at 57 days of gestation and is maximal in thickness by 183 days, when it is composed of six cell layers. Following that it slowly decreases in thickness, reaching a layer two cells thick by 2 months post-natally, and completely disappearing by 6 months postnatally.

ANATOMY

The cerebellum consists of a central median region, the vermis, named for the worm-like contortions it presents caudally, and a lateral hemisphere on each side of the vermis.[8, 9] The cerebellum is divided into two disproportionate regions: the large body of the cerebellum, and the small flocculonodular lobe. These two regions are separated by the caudolateral fissure. The flocculonodular lobe, also known as the archicerebellum or vestibular cerebellum, is confined to the ventral aspect of the cerebellum near its center. The nodulus is the most ros-tral part of the caudal vermis that is adjacent to the fourth ventricle. It connects lat-erally by a peduncle on each side to the flocculus, a small lobule on the ventral lateral aspect of the cerebellar hemisphere. The much larger body of the cerebel-lum, consisting of vermis and hemispheres, is divided into rostral and caudal lobes by the primary fissure. Within each lobe the folia are grouped into named lobules that reside in different portions of the vermis and hemispheres.

The cerebellum is attached to the brain stem by three groups of neuronal processes on each side, the cerebellar peduncles. Although arranged in a medial to lateral plane in which they attach to the cerebellum, they are named from rostral to caudal based on their connections with the brain stem. The caudal cerebellar peduncle connects the spinal cord and medulla with the cerebellum. It contains primarily afferent processes. The middle cerebellar peduncle connects the trans-verse fibers of the pons with the cerebellum, and is solely afferent to the cerebel-lum. The rostral cerebellar peduncle connects the cerebellum with the mesen-cephalon, and contains mainly efferent processes passing out of the cerebellum.

When the cerebellum is sectioned transversely or longitudinally, an exten-sive area of white matter in the center is seen. This is the cerebellar medulla that sends branches of white matter out into the overlying folia. As a group, these branches are called the arbor vitae because of their resemblance to the branches of a tree. Individually, each is the white lamina of a folium. The arbor vitae is covered by the three layers of the cerebellar cortex. In the cerebellar medulla there are situated collections of neurons that comprise the cerebellar nuclei. In domestic animals these are organized into three nuclei, from medial to lateral on each side of the median plane. They are called the fastigial, interposital, and lateral (den-tate) nuclei, respectively.

The cerebellar cortex, which is composed of three layers, forms the outer por-tion of each folium and is similar throughout the cerebellum.[70] The folial surface is covered by leptomeninges. Adjacent to this is the relatively cell-free molecular layer. This bounds the single layer of large flask-shaped neurons, the Purkinje cell layer, which in turn bounds the granule cell layer. The granule cell layer is thick and consists of numerous granule cell neurons, the cell bodies of which are small and dark-staining, giving it a characteristic cellular appearance. This layer varies in thickness and usually is thinnest in the cortex, located between folia at the depth of a sulcus.

The cerebellar cortex is uniquely organized for the distribution of afferent in-

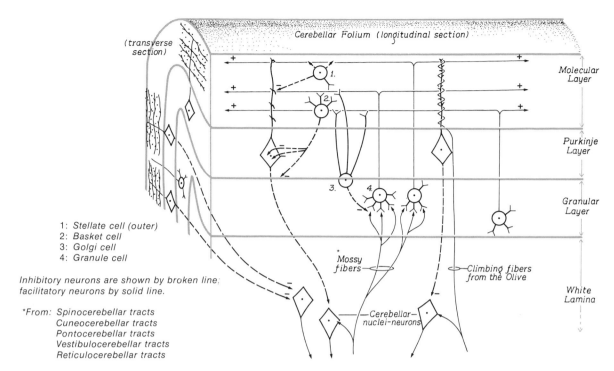

Figure 12-2. Microscopic anatomy of the cerebellum.

formation. There are two major types of afferents to the cerebellum: mossy and climbing fibers. The more abundant mossy fibers have a widespread origin in the brain stem and spinal cord. As they pass into the cerebellum, collaterals of these processes synapse in the cerebellar nuclei on neuronal cell bodies. The main process enters a folium by way of its white matter, passes into the granule cell layer, and terminates in synaptic relationship with the dendritic zone of the granule cell neurons within the granule cell layer. The axon of the granule cell courses through the Purkinje cell layer into the molecular layer, in which it branches and courses parallel to the longitudinal axis of the folium. The dendritic zone of the Purkinje cell is a maze of branched axons that is arranged in one plane in the molecular layer. This flat plane of neuronal processes is oriented transversely to the longitudinal axis of the folium. By this arrangement, the axon of the granule cell neuron traverses the dendritic zone of numerous Purkinje cells. Synapse occurs between these processes. This network can be likened to telephone wires (granule cell axons) coursing from one telephone pole (dendritic zone of a Purkinje cell) to another.

Climbing fibers are the axons of olivary neurons that enter the cerebellum through the caudal cerebellar peduncle. Collaterals synapse on neurons in the cerebellar nuclei. The main axon continues into a cerebellar folium by way of its white matter, passes through the granule cell and Purkinje cell layers into the molecular layer, and arborizes in synaptic relationship with a Purkinje cell dendritic zone.

These mossy and climbing fibers are facilitatory at their synapse with neurons of the cerebellar nuclei and the granule cells and Purkinje cells, respectively. The granule cells are facilitatory to the Purkinje cells. The stellate neurons of the molecular layer (outer and basket) are inhibitory interneurons to the Purkinje cells. The Golgi neurons of the granule layer are inhibitory interneurons to the granule cells.[39] The only axon that projects from the cerebellar cortex (an efferent axon) is that of the Purkinje cells.[37] These axons pass through the granule cell layer into the folial white matter and then to the cerebellar medulla, in which most terminate in telodendria on neurons of the cerebellar nuclei. A few Purkinje cell axons leave the cerebellum through the caudal peduncle and terminate in the vestibular nuclei. The Purkinje cell telodendria are inhibitory to the neurons in which they terminate. The efferent axons that project from the cerebellum to the brain stem are all from the neurons of the cerebellar nuclei, except for the few direct cerebellovestibular processes from Purkinje cells. It would seem that the major role of the cerebellar cortex is to modulate the continual facilitation of neurons of cerebellar nuclei by way of Purkinje cell inhibition.

In order for the cerebellum to function as a coordinator of muscular activity and regulator of muscle tone, it must receive afferent information to provide it with knowledge of where the limbs, trunk, and head are in space. Thus afferents of the general and special proprioceptive systems must project to the cerebellum. In addition, it must be apprised of the voluntary activity being induced. Thus it receives afferents from the upper motor neuron system.

Cerebellar Afferents

General Proprioception

Spinocerebellar tracts enter mostly through the caudal peduncle, with a few via the rostral cerebellar peduncle.

Cuneocerebellar tracts enter via the caudal cerebellar peduncle.

Special Proprioception

Vestibulocerebellar tracts enter directly and indirectly from the vestibular nuclei, via the caudal cerebellar peduncle.

Most of the proprioceptive neurons project to the folia of the cerebellar vermis or the adjacent paravermal folia.

Special Somatic Afferent — Visual and Auditory

Tectocerebellar processes enter by way of the rostral cerebellar peduncle and project mostly to the head of the vermis.

Upper Motor Neuron

OLIVARY NUCLEI.   Extrapyramidal nuclei of the telencephalon and brain stem project information to the cerebellum mostly through the olivary nuclei. These nuclei are located in the ventrolateral portion of the caudal medulla. They extend rostrally to just caudal to the facial nucleus, and caudally to a level just caudal to the obex. They consist of three components on each side, which vary in size throughout the length of the nuclei. Where they are most developed, they have the appearance of the three fingers oriented obliquely from dorsomedial to ventrolateral just dorsal and lateral to the pyramid and medial lemniscus. The hypoglossal axons course along their lateral border. The axons of the neurons in the olivary nuclei cross the midline and join the contralateral caudal cerebellar peduncle. These are the source of the climbing fibers to the cerebellum.

PONTINE NUCLEUS. Axons from the cerebral cortex in all areas of the hemisphere project information to the cerebellum by way of the pontine nucleus. This is the corticopontocerebellar pathway. These cerebral neurons reach this nucleus via the internal capsule, the crus cerebri, and the longitudinal fibers of the pons. Axons leave the longitudinal fibers and synapse on ipsilateral pontine neurons. The neuronal cell bodies of the pontine nucleus surround the longitudinal fibers of the pons. The axons of the cell bodies of the pontine nucleus cross the midline, forming the transverse fibers of the pons and the contralateral middle cerebellar peduncle. This peduncle projects for the most part to the cerebellar hemisphere. There is a direct relationship in the evolution of skilled motor function and the development of the motor cortex, pons, and cerebellar hemispheres. In man, the transverse fibers of the pons extend caudally over the trapezoid body, and the vermis of the cerebellum is buried by the development of the hemispheres.

RED NUCLEUS. Rubrocerebellar processes enter the cerebellum through the rostral cerebellar peduncle.

RETICULAR FORMATION. Reticulocerebellar processes enter by way of the caudal cerebellar peduncle.

Cerebellar Efferents[37]

Cerebellar Cortex. Purkinje cell axons, derived mostly from the flocculonodular lobe, project directly to the vestibular nuclei via the caudal cerebellar peduncle.

Cerebellar Nuclei

1. Fastigial nucleus neurons project to vestibular nuclei and the reticular formation by way of the caudal cerebellar peduncle.

2. Interposital nucleus neurons project to the red nucleus and the reticular formation by way of the rostral cerebellar peduncle.

3. Lateral nucleus neurons project to the red nucleus, the reticular formation, the pallidum, and the ventral lateral nucleus of the thalamus through the rostral cerebellar peduncle.

When the rostral cerebellar peduncle enters the mesencephalon, most of its efferent axons decussate in the tegmentum in the ventral tegmental decussation. This is at the level of the caudal colliculus caudal to the rubrospinal decussation. These axons cross to the opposite side to terminate in the contralateral red nucleus, the ventral lateral nucleus of the thalamus, or the pallidum.

A feedback circuit to the cerebral cortex exists by way of the direct projection of the cerebellar lateral nucleus to the contralateral ventral lateral nucleus of the thalamus, which in turn projects to the cerebrum passing through the internal capsule. An indirect route from the cerebellum to the cerebrum exists in its projection to the contralateral red nucleus and pallidum, both of which have projections to the ventral rostral nucleus of the thalamus; this in turn projects to the cerebrum.

There are essentially no efferent cerebellar axons that project in the spinal cord to directly influence the lower motor neuron. The cerebellum functions through influence over the upper motor neuron tracts that descend the spinal cord to affect lower motor neuron activity.

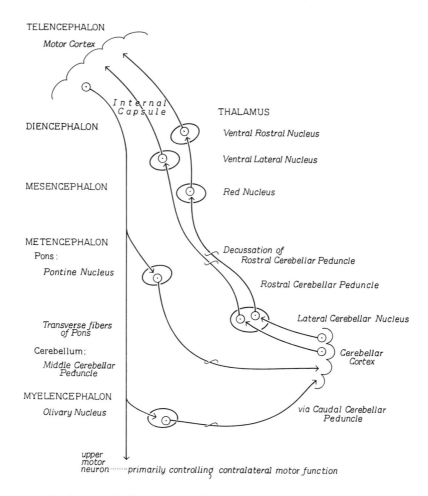

Figure 12–3. Role of the cerebellum in control of motor function: feedback circuit to cerebral cortex from the cerebellum.

FUNCTION

The cerebellum functions as a regulator, not as the primary initiator of motor activity.[36] It functions to coordinate and "smooth" movements induced by the upper motor neuron in relation to the posture of the animal to provide synergy of muscular activity. The cerebellum also functions in the maintenance of equilibrium and in the regulation of tone to preserve the normal position of the body while at rest or during motion.

In summary, the cerebellar nuclei that continually facilitate brain stem neurons in turn are regulated by the inhibitory function of the Purkinje cell neurons of the cerebellar cortex. The degree of activity of these Purkinje cell neurons depends on the afferent information reaching them directly by way of the climbing fiber afferents and indirectly via the mossy fiber afferents.

The rostral and vermal portion of the cerebellum is concerned primarily with the inhibition of lower motor neurons to extensor muscles of the neck and thoracic limbs.[21, 22] It thus participates in the overall function of the upper motor neuron to maintain support of the body against gravity.[100]

SIGNS OF CEREBELLAR DISEASE

Cerebellar disease does not cause the loss of any single function, but a general inadequacy of motor response. As a rule the cerebellum is affected diffusely by disease processes, and the patient typically presents with a bilaterally symmetric ataxia (motor ataxia) with strength preserved. With unilateral lesions, the signs of ataxia are usually ipsilateral to the lesion. Be aware of the paradoxical vestibular syndrome that occurs with unilateral cerebellar medullary and peduncle lesions that affect vestibular components of the cerebellum. With these lesions, the signs of ataxia may be contralateral to the lesion.

Cerebellar disease does not cause paresis. In severe disease the patient may be incapacitated by its ataxic condition and be unable to stand, but voluntary movements are elicited easily with normal strength. The ataxic gait is characterized by an inability to regulate the rate, range, and force of a movement, which is called dysmetria. The dysmetria usually presents as a hypermetria, an overmeasurement in the gait response observed as greater movements of the limbs than normal in all ranges of motion. Observation of the gait or postural reactions reveals a raised threshold to response. The onset of the voluntary movement is delayed, and the response, once initiated, is exaggerated. After the delay, the limb is raised too high on protraction, and then forcefully returned to the bearing surface. Inadequate Purkinje cell inhibition of the cerebellar nuclei results in the delay in cessation of a voluntary movement, and thus a hypermetric response occurs. Involvement of the flocculonodular lobe of the cerebellum may cause vestibular disturbance, a loss of equilibrium, with nystagmus, bizarre postures, and a broad-based staggering gait with jerky movements and a tendency to fall to the side or backward, especially if the thoracic limbs are elevated.

The resting posture may show a broad-based stance with the thoracic limbs, and a truncal ataxia which is a swaying of the body from side to side, forward and backward, or occasionally dorsoventrally. These may appear as gross jerky movements of the entire body. A fine head tremor is characteristic of cerebellar cortical disease, and usually is augmented by the initiation of voluntary movements such as are observed as the head reaches for food. This is an intention tremor, a form of dysmetria involving the head. In severe cerebellar abnormality the patient may be in lateral recumbency, unable to right itself to stand, with its head and neck extended in a position of opisthotonos. The rostral lobe of the cerebellum is especially inhibitory to the stretch reflex mechanism. Disease here is characterized by opisthotonos and markedly extended thoracic limbs.

Muscle tone usually is increased in domestic animals with cerebellar disease. Reflexes are normal to hyperactive. Postural reactions generally are intact, but the response may be delayed in its onset and then exaggerated. Abnormal nystagmus is observed only occasionally. The direction is variable, and may change with different positions of the head. If the head is extended and support is withdrawn suddenly, instead of returning to its normal position the head may descend ventrally further than normal. This excessive excursion is referred to as a rebound phenomenon, and is a sign of lack of cerebellar control.

It has been found that animals with significant cerebellar cortical disease fail to respond to the menace maneuver normally used to test the visual system. In the presence of normal vision and facial muscle strength, these animals fail to close their eyelids when threatened by a menacing gesture. It is known that the entire central visual pathway to the visual cortex as well as the facial neurons of cranial nerve VII must be intact for this normal response to take place. Therefore it is assumed that the pathway between the visual cortex and the facial nucleus must pass through the cerebellum. Presumably, this involves a corticopontocerebellar tract. In two instances a unilateral cerebellar lesion produced a lack of this menace response on the same side as the lesion. This would agree with the predominance of optic nerve fibers crossing through the optic chiasm to reach the contralateral visual cortex and the crossing back of corticopontocerebellar pathways at the pontine nucleus (Fig. 13–7). Varying degrees of this deficit have been observed in horses, cattle, pigs, dogs, and cats with cerebellar cortical lesions.

CEREBELLAR SYNDROMES

Primary Cerebellar Hypoplasia and/or Degeneration

Cat[72]

Feline Panleukopenia Infection.[19, 24-28, 57, 61-63, 74-76]   The feline panleukopenia virus has a predilection for the rapidly dividing cells of the cerebellar cortex of the feline fetus in utero or at the time of birth. Destruction of the actively mitotic external germinal layer results in hypoplasia of the granule layer. This has been referred to as granuloprival cerebellar hypoplasia. The action of the virus is not restricted to the external germinal layer. The nonmitotic Purkinje cells that have already differentiated also are attacked and destroyed. In a few cases necrotic lesions that presumably resulted from the inflammation caused by this virus are found in the cerebral and spinal cord white matter.

The signs are those of a mild to severe cerebellar cortical deficiency. They are observed as soon as the kitten starts to ambulate, at around 4 weeks of age. As the kitten grows and becomes more active, the signs become more obvious. However, the lesion is nonprogressive. The destruction took place in the perinatal period and no longer continues. Compensation for the cerebellar deficit is usually minimal, and the signs persist for the duration of the animal's life.

As a rule, feline panleukopenia infection in the young growing cat has no observable affect on the cerebellum. An occasional exception has been reported.

Dog[35, 93]

Viral Infections.   No in utero viral infection of the canine cerebellum has been identified. However, early postnatal infection by the canine herpes virus, which usually causes a high mortality in newborn puppies, also may affect the cerebellum.[90] If the puppy survives the infection of other organ systems, cerebellar signs may be observed caused by the destructive effect of the virus on the cerebellar tissue, which is still in its developing stage.

The signs are nonprogressive for the cerebellar destruction, which terminates when the puppy recovers from the infection.

Purkinje Cell Hypoplasia or Abiotrophy. This has been observed in a number of breeds. It usually affects more than one animal in a litter, and often more than one litter from related parents.[60] A familial basis is suspected, but often has not been verified due to lack of appropriate breeding trials. This has occurred in Laborador retrievers, Golden retrievers, cocker spaniels, Cairn terriers, and Great Danes. Sometimes the signs of diffuse cerebellar deficiency are present when the puppies start to walk. Therefore the failure to find Purkinje cells in these dogs may represent a hypoplasia. More often the puppies are normal until 8 to 12 weeks of age, and then start to develop a typical cerebellar ataxia. The signs are usually progressive, but may become static after a few weeks or continue until the animal is unable to coordinate to stand. In these cases the absence of some Purkinje cells and degenerate changes in others suggest that the disease is an abiotrophy. The Purkinje cells were formed normally, but were unable to survive due to an intrinsic defect in their metabolism. Abiotrophy refers to the lack (a-) of a vital (bios-) substance necessary for the nutritional (-trophic) life of that cell.[49, 50]

A progressive cerebellar degeneration has been described in a family of Airedales[23] and a family of Finnish harriers.[101] A cerebellar ataxia was described from birth in Bern running dogs.[48] It was associated with a loss of cerebellar Purkinje cells and a symmetric olivary nuclear degeneration. A familial basis was suspected. A severe cerebellar cortical degeneration was described in nine litters of Irish setter puppies that were unable to coordinate to stand.[83] An autosomal recessive inheritance was proposed for the cause.

An hereditary progressive ataxia with clinical signs of a cerebellar deficiency has been described in smooth-haired fox terriers.[12, 15] The onset of signs is between 10 and 16 weeks of age. The signs of cerebellar ataxia progress rapidly at first, followed by periods of slow progress and intervals of stasis. Eventually, the animals become incapacitated by the ataxia. A recessive monogenic autosomal gene with complete penetrance in the homozygous state was determined to be responsible for the disease in 23 litters with affected puppies, a total of 91 dogs. Sixty-six were normal and 25 were affected, which corresponds well to the predicted incidence of 25 per cent affected homozygous recessive puppies from a breeding of carrier parents. Pathologic studies to date have revealed only a spinal cord degeneration, mostly in the dorsospinocerebellar tracts.

Three of a litter of six Samoyed puppies were noticed to have a peculiar pelvic limb ataxia at the time the puppies became ambulatory.[53] The pelvic limbs were strong but were carried forward under the body and were markedly hypertonic and hypermetric. The animals occasionally fell to either side or backward. The thoracic limb gait appeared to be mostly normal. On hopping, the responses were slightly slow and hypermetric. No head tremor was observed, but the menace response was poor. Vision and eyelid strength were normal.

The disorder was nonprogressive over a period of 3 years of observation. The dogs were necropsied at four, 18, and 36 months. In all instances only a Purkinje cell degeneration was apparent, and this was more pronounced in the axon than in the soma. Loss of Purkinje cells was minimal.

A cerebellar hypoplasia with dysplasia and a cerebral lissencephaly occurred in two of a family of three wire-haired fox terriers. A nonprogressive symmetric dysmetric ataxia and head tremor accompanied the cerebellar malformation. Seizures began at 1 year of age and were presumed to result from the lissencephaly.

Hereditary Cerebellar Cortical and Extrapyramidal Nuclear Abiotrophy in Kerry Blue Terriers.[30, 31] From 1967 to 1970, ten Kerry blue terriers that developed a progressive cerebellar disorder were studied in a kennel in New York State. The onset was between 9 and 12 weeks of age, and both sexes were affected.

Pelvic limb stiffness and mild head tremor were the earliest signs. The gait abnormality progressed to an obvious dysmetric spastic gait and included the thoracic limbs. All movements were jerky, exaggerated, and forceful. The head tremor was exaggerated during intended movements. Strength was normal, and no involuntary adventitious movements occurred.

By 8 to 10 weeks of development of the signs the truncal ataxia became so pronounced that the side to side and to and fro oscillations of the body made linear mobility difficult. Head, trunk, and limb movements became so disorganized that leaping movements and falling backward occurred frequently.

After 20 weeks of progressive signs, the dogs often were unable to coordinate to stand without support.

There was no clinical evidence for cerebral cortical dysfunction. Cranial nerves were normal. However, there was a poor response to menacing gestures, even though there was no other evidence of facial paresis or a visual deficit.

Hematologic and CSF studies were normal.

Sequential autopsies demonstrated a progressive cerebellar cortical degeneration with ultimate loss of Purkinje cells. As the disease progressed, a bilaterally symmetric degeneration of the olivary nuclei was observed at 3 months of clinical illness. This was followed at 5 to 6 months of illness by a similar symmetric bilateral degeneration of the substantia nigra and then the caudate nuclei. The lesion was considered an abiotrophy. There was no evidence of inflammation. Viral isolation studies and intracerebral inoculation of diseased tissue into puppies and ferrets were unrewarding.

Between 1973 and 1975, three similarly affected Kerry blue terriers were recognized in California, each from a different litter. The clinical illness was first recognized in two dogs at 3 months of age and in one at 4 months. In all, the signs progressed in a fashion similar to those in the New York dogs. Necropsy of one confirmed the similar development of abiotrophy in the cerebellar cortex and extrapyramidal nuclei.

A common ancestor was found on both sides of all the pedigrees in the second and third generation of the New York litters. Similarly, a common ancestor occurred in the third and fourth generations on both sides of all the pedigrees of the affected California dogs. These two common ancestors were found to be brothers. A simple autosomal recessive inheritance is proposed for this disease.

In the New York kennel there were ten affected puppies from 23 offspring in five litters. Six affected puppies could be predicted from 24 offspring of the mating of carrier parents. The large number of observed affected animals in this study is influenced by the small total number of animals studied, and the lack of any litters without affected animals which would be expected in a larger number of matings.

In 1946, Mettler and Goss described an identical abiotrophy in a Kerry blue terrier that was about 1 year old.[79] They called it a striocerebellar degeneration. Study of a film of this dog and the microscopic slides of affected tissue confirmed that this was the same disease.

Numerous heredodegenerative diseases in man involving the cerebellum have been described and usually classified by the anatomic distribution of the lesions.[29, 54, 84] These include cerebello-olivary degeneration and olivopontocerebellar degeneration, some of which have been determined to be hereditary. More recently, cases of olivopontocerebellar degeneration have been found with degeneration of the substantia nigra and basal nuclei.[64, 66, 95]

The temporal sequence of abiotrophy in these dogs suggests a functional or anatomic relationship between these nuclear groups. In olivopontocerebellar degeneration the neuronal degeneration of the olive and pons has been described as a transsynaptic retrograde chain degeneration of neurons which synapse on neurons (Purkinje cell and granule cell) that have already degenerated. In these Kerry blue terriers the pontine nucleus did not degenerate, and the neurons of the substantia nigra and caudate nuclei that did degenerate do not synapse in the cerebellum.

The substantia nigra and caudate nuclei are anatomically and functionally connected via the dopaminergic nigrostriatal pathway.[10,20,43,44] With pharmacologic or anatomic destruction of this system, neuronal argyrophilia and depletion occur, but not the severe necrosis and "ballooning" degeneration observed in these dogs.

An alternative pathogenesis to this multisystem degeneration may be that these cellular groups have a similar biochemical characteristic or metabolic requirement that is deficient or becomes abnormal, and accounts for the pattern of degeneration observed. Although dopamine is a neurotransmitter between the substantia nigra and caudate nucleus, it does not function in the cerebellar cortex, in which gamma amino butyrate may be the inhibitory neurotransmitter.

Cattle[40, 56]

Bovine Viral Diarrhea (BVD) Virus.   This virus can destroy the developing fetal cerebellum in utero, which results in a newborn calf that is unable to coordinate to stand, or has a varying degree of cerebellar ataxia and head tremor.[16-18, 58, 78, 96] The clinical signs are nonprogressive because the cerebellar damage occurred in utero. Occasionally, some compensation may occur in the first week of life.

Affected newborn calves that have not consumed colostrum have a detectable serum antibody titer to the BVD agent. Experimental inoculation of pregnant nonimmune cows with the BVD agent at 150 days of gestation produces an acute inflammation of the cerebellum 17 days postinoculation. Severe necrosis with some hemorrhage occurs in the external germinal layer with a mononuclear, lymphocytic, and plasma cell response. Purkinje cells degenerate and edema is severe in the folial white matter. The inflammation slowly subsides over the next few weeks. At birth, only the residual scar of this acute inflammation is observed. This may be apparent grossly as a severe reduction of cerebellar tissue, and microscopically as a variable reduction or dysplasia of all the cortical layers and cavitations of the folial white matter.

From study of experimental and natural cases it has been determined that the cerebellar degeneration can result from infection between 100 and 170 days of gestation. The developing eyeball also often is affected, resulting in cataracts and retinal lesions.

Cortical Abiotrophy.   Cerebellar cortical abiotrophy that appears to be hereditary has been observed in Holsteins.[103] These calves are born and function normally until 3 to 8 months of age, when a sudden onset of ataxia occurs. The acute assault of signs peaks in a few days, then remains static or slowly progresses over the following weeks. A few become recumbent and unable to coordinate to stand in the first few days. For most calves, this takes a few weeks to occur. A few remain ambulatory.

The signs constitute a severe spastic dysmetric ataxic gait and truncal ataxia without loss of strength, affecting all four limbs and the trunk. Most are symmetric, but asymmetry has been observed. The animals stand with a basewide posture, and an intentional head tremor is obvious. The neck is held extended when standing, and opisthotonos often is observed when the calf is recumbent.

The palpebral fissure often appears widened and the ears retracted. The eyeballs may be rotated slightly so that the medial angle of the pupil is more dorsal than normal. The menace response is absent. However, vision is normal, although owners often have thought these calves were blind because they stumble into objects. Occasionally, an abnormal nystagmus has been observed. No other cranial nerve abnormality is found.

These calves are alert and responsive at all times. There is no evidence of involvement of cerebral cortical function, differentiating this brain disease from polioencephalomalacia or lead poisoning. The latter diseases profoundly affect cerebral function, causing depression, semicoma, hysteria, convulsions, and blindness. In most cases hematologic and CSF studies have been normal.

At necropsy the cerebellum is normal in size, but there is a diffuse degeneration of Purkinje cells in almost all portions of the cerebellum, and neuronal degeneration has been observed in the cerebellar nuclei.

In those calves in which pedigrees were available, one sire was found to be common in the ancestry of the parents of the affected calves. A hereditary pathogenesis is proposed for this disease.

A familial cerebellar cortical hypoplasia or abiotrophy, or both, has been reported in Hereford calves.[109]

Hereditary Hypomyelinogenesis.   Hereditary hypomyelinogenesis with primary cerebellar involvement and signs of cerebellar ataxia has been reported in Jersey, Hereford, Shorthorn, and Angus-Shorthorn breeds of cattle.[55, 94, 104] These calves usually show signs at or near birth. They generally are alert and responsive, and have a significant head tremor. The calf may be unable to coordinate to stand, or if ambulatory, walks with a spastic dysmetric gait. The absence of myelin in these cases is regarded as hypoplasia or dysmyelinogenesis. Recently this lesion was observed in a Holstein that exhibited constant tremors when trying to support itself or move voluntarily. This myoclonia was similar to that reported in lambs and pigs with myelin abnormalities.

Border Disease.   This is a congenital disturbance of newborn lambs that includes hypomyelinogenesis, abnormalities of the hair coat, and defective postnatal growth. The hypomyelinogenesis causes an ataxic gait and head or whole body tremor that resembles a cerebellar disturbance. Neurochemical studies have defined a generalized deficiency of myelin lipids with abnormal quantities of esterified cholesterol.[7, 77, 85, 87, 89] There is some evidence to support an intrauterine viral etiology for this disease.[33, 51, 80]

Horses[65]

Ataxia.   A progressive cerebellar ataxia has been observed in young Arabian horses.[6, 46, 82, 98-99, 102] The foals are usually normal at birth, and the signs begin around 3 to 4 months of age. Occasionally, signs are present at or shortly after birth. They usually consist of a remarkably spastic ataxic gait with varying degrees of dysmetria. In a few, hypermetria is severe. Strength is always normal. There is no evidence of general proprioceptive ataxia. A head tremor is almost always well developed. It is exaggerated by intended movements. A bilateral menace deficiency is apparent, although vision and facial motor function are normal. The signs of ataxia are usually only slowly progressive. In some, they remain static. Improvement has not been observed.

At necropsy, a severe diffuse absence or degeneration of Purkinje cells is found. The granule cell layer also may be partially depleted. Viral isolation studies have been unrewarding. A hereditary pathogenesis is suspected for this apparent cerebellar cortical abiotrophy.

A similar cerebellar cortical abiotrophy has been observed in the Gotland pony breed.[13, 14] Breeding studies have determined this to be a hereditary autosomal recessive disease.

Pigs

Cerebellar Degeneration. Cerebellar degeneration in utero has resulted from the vaccination of pregnant sows with live hog cholera virus.[41] The signs of cerebellar ataxia are present at birth and are nonprogressive. Congenital tremors also have occurred clinically in these pigs, and hypomyelinogenesis has been observed at necropsy.[52, 85, 86, 88]

Hypomyelinogenesis. Myoclonia congenita in newborn pigs is a clinical syndrome that has been related to a diffuse hypomyelinogenesis.[45] Although not primarily a cerebellar disease, it is included here because of the abnormal myelin formation, which may be compared with that condition recognized in calves and lambs.[85] The pathogenesis of the myoclonus is unknown. Experimental studies indicate that its genesis is in the spinal cord. Hereditary and viral etiologies have been advanced for this central nervous system disturbance.[73]

Cortical Abiotrophy. A possible hereditary cerebellar cortical abiotrophy has been noted in Yorkshire pigs,[47] in a number of litters on at least two farms.

In each instance the pigs were normal at birth and for the first 3 weeks of life. In the fourth to fifth weeks, the first indication of abnormality was an abnormal pelvic limb gait. Usually by 1 more week these signs had progressed so rapidly that the pig could not stand normally. A few remained able to stand with difficulty, and to walk with a spastic dysmetric gait. Postural reactions were slow to respond, with a marked hypertonia to the response, or no response occurred. Yet when the limbs were manipulated with the pigs in lateral recumbency, they thrashed vigorously with normal voluntary strength. Reflexes and pain perception were normal.

No head tremor was observed, but abnormal positional nystagmus often could be induced. Although the menace response was absent, vision and facial muscle strength were assessed as normal.

Cerebral function was normal at all times. These pigs remained easily excited, alert, responsive, and ate well when fed.

At necropsy at varying stages of duration of signs the only lesion observed was a Purkinje cell degeneration. This mostly involved an axonal degeneration, especially in the granule layer, with only mild degeneration of the soma of the Purkinje cells.

A hereditary pathogenesis is suspected because of the single breed involvement, closely related litters, and the finding of affected pigs in two litters from the same parents. The lesion is noninflammatory, and viral isolation studies have not been successful.

INFLAMMATION, NEOPLASIA, DIFFUSE DEGENERATION, AND INJURY

The cerebellum is subject to involvement by the same kind of lesions that affect the adjacent brain stem and other portions of the central nervous system.

Inflammations

The cerebellar white matter and cortex are affected commonly in dogs by the canine distemper virus, which causes inflammation and necrosis. *Toxoplasma gondii* and *Cryptococcus neoformans* also can affect the cerebellum in dogs and cats. The severe meningitis of the caudal fossa in cats with feline infectious peritonitis may cause cerebellar signs. The same may occur in any animal, but more commonly in calves with bacterial meningitis.

Protozoal encephalitis has been observed in the cerebellum of horses, causing asymmetric signs.

Parasitic migration may occur through the cerebellum and produce signs of a cerebellar or vestibular disturbance, or both. A *Cuterebra* larva has been observed in cats, and a *Hypoderma bovis* larva in the horse.

In all of these cases the cerebellar signs usually are accompanied by other neurologic signs suggestive of a multifocal or diffuse disease process. CSF is also usually abnormal.

The inflammatory or neoplastic form of primary reticulosis in dogs often affects the cerebellar medulla, producing asymmetric cerebellovestibular signs.

Neoplasms

Primary and metastatic neoplasms may involve the cerebellum.[105, 106] These often are unilateral at the cerebellomedullary or cerebellopontine angle, and usually produce ipsilateral signs of cerebellovestibular disturbance. They are diagnosed by the signs of adjacent brain stem involvement, including upper motor neuron paresis, general proprioceptive ataxia, ascending reticular activating system depression, and ipsilateral cranial nerve paralysis (trigeminal, facial, vestibulocochlear, glossopharyngeal, and vagal). The most common neoplasm observed at this site is the choroid plexus papilloma or carcinoma. Others include meningioma, neurofibroma, medulloblastoma, astrocytoma, and reticulosis.

Diffuse Degenerations

Cerebellar signs may accompany the signs of diffuse degenerative diseases of the CNS in cats and dogs—the leukodystrophies and lipodystrophies. These are probably most common in the Cairn and West Highland white terriers with globoid cell leukodystrophy, whose signs begin either as a mild paraparesis and pelvic limb ataxia, or as a hypermetric ataxia from cerebellar involvement.

One 4-year-old wire-haired dachshund had progressive signs of cerebellar ataxia for over 1 year. There was no clinical evidence of involvement of any other system. At necropsy there was extensive loss of Purkinje cell bodies, but the few that remained had a swollen cystoplasm containing a lipid material. Similar swollen neurons were present in numerous brain stem nuclei and the spinal cord grey matter. Cerebral cortical involvement was less. This was an unusual presentation of a lipodystrophy that has been classified as an adult case of neuronal ceroid-lipofuscinosis, based on the histochemical and ultrastructural characteristics of the cytoplasmic material.[107, 108]

Injury

Cerebellar signs may predominate following intracranial injury if this structure has received the main impact of the injury.

REFERENCES

1. Altman, J.: Postnatal development of the cerebellar cortex in the rat. I. The external germinal layer and the transitional molecular layer. J. Comp. Neurol., *145*:353, 1972.
2. Altman, J.: Postnatal development of the cerebellar cortex in the rat. II. Phases in the maturation of Purkinje cells and of the molecular layer. J. Comp. Neurol., *145*:399, 1972.
3. Altman, J.: Postnatal development of the cerebellar cortex in the rat. III. Maturation of the components of the granular layer. J. Comp. Neurol., *145*:465, 1972.
4. Altman, J., and Anderson, W.: Experimental reorganization of the cerebellar cortex. I. Morphological effects of elimination of all microneurons with prolonged x-irradiation started at birth. J. Comp. Neurol., *146*:355, 1972.
5. Altman, J., and Anderson, W.: Experimental reorganization of the cerebellar cortex. II. Effects of elimination of most microneurons with prolonged x-irradiation started at 4 days. J. Comp. Neurol., *149*:123, 1973.
6. Baird, J. D., and Mackenzie, C. D.: Cerebellar hypoplasia and degeneration in part Arab horses. Aust. Vet. J., *50*:25, 1974.
7. Barlow, R. M., and Dickinson, A. G.: On the pathology and histochemistry of the central nervous system in border disease of sheep. Res. Vet. Sci., *6*:230, 1965.
8. Barone, R., and Belkhayat, A.: La conformation et la nomenclature du cervelet des équids. Rev. Med. Vet., *121*:1013, 1970.
9. Barone, R., and Berujon, J.-B.: La morphologie du cervelet chez le Boeuf. Bull. Soc. Sci. Vet. Med. Comp., *72*:3, 1970.
10. Bedard, P.: The nigrostriatal pathway. A correlative study based on neuroanatomical and neurochemical criteria in the cat and monkey. Exp. Neurol., *25*:365, 1969.
11. Beery, F.: Untersuchungen über die Entwicklung der Motilität und die histologische Differenzierung des kleinshirns bei der Katze in den eroten Lebenswochen. Schweiz. Arch. Tierheilk., *104*:701, 1962.
12. Bjorck, G., Dyrendahl, S., and Olsson, S. E.: Hereditary ataxia in smooth haired fox terriers. Vet. Rec., *69*:871, 1957.
13. Bjorck, G., Everz, K.-E., Hansen, H.-J., and Henricson, B.: Cerebellar hypoplasia in the Gotland pony breed. Proceedings 18th World Veterinary Congress, Paris, 1967, 818.
14. Bjorck, G., Everz, K. E., Hansen, H.-J., and Henricson, B.: Congenital cerebellar ataxia in the Gotland pony breed. Zentralbl. Veterinaermed., *20*:341, 1973.
15. Bjorck, G., Mair, W., Olsson, S.-E., and Sourander, P.: Hereditary ataxia in fox terriers. Arch. Neuropathol. Suppl., *1*:45, 1962.
16. Brown, T. T.: Pathogenetic Studies of Bovine Viral Diarrhea Infection in the Bovine Fetus. Ph.D. thesis, Ithaca, N.Y., Cornell University, 1973.
17. Brown, T. T., de Lahunta, A., Bistner, S. I., Scott, F. W., and McEntee, K.: Pathogenetic studies of infection of the bovine fetus with bovine viral diarrhea virus. I. Cerebellar atrophy. Vet. Pathol., *11*:486, 1974.
18. Brown, T. T., de Lahunta, A., Scott, F. W., Kahrs, R. F., McEntee, K., and Gillespie, J. H.: Virus-induced congenital anomalies of the bovine fetus. II. Histopathology of cerebellar degeneration (hypoplasia) induced by the virus of bovine viral diarrhea-mucosal disease. Cor. Vet., *63*:561, 1973.
19. Carpenter, M. B., and Donald, H.: A study of congenital feline cerebellar malformations. J. Comp. Neurol., *105*:51, 1956.
20. Carpenter, M. B., and Peter, P.: Nigrostriatal and nigrothalamic fibers in the Rhesus monkey. J. Comp. Neurol., *144*:93, 1972.
21. Chambers, W. W., and Spraque, J. M.: Functional localization in the cerebellum. I. Organization in longitudinal corticonuclear zones and their contribution to the control of posture both extrapyramidal and pyramidal. J. Comp. Neurol., *103*:105, 1955.

22. Chambers, W. W., and Spraque, J. M.: Functional localization in the cerebellum. II. Somatotopic organization in cortex and nuclei. Arch. Neurol. Psychiatry, 74:653, 1955.

23. Cordy, D. R., and Snelbaker, H. A.: Cerebellar hypoplasia and degeneration in a family of Airedale dogs. J. Neuropathol. Exp. Neurol., 11:324, 1952.

24. Csiza, C. K.: Feline Panleukopenia Virus as an Etiological Agent of Ataxia: Pathogenesis and Immune Carrier State. Ph.D. thesis, Ithaca, N.Y., Cornell University, 1970.

25. Csiza, C. K., Scott, F. W., de Lahunta, A., and Gillespie, J. H.: Pathogenesis of feline panleukopenia virus in susceptible newborn kittens. I. Clinical signs, hematology, serology and virology. Infect. Immun., 3:833, 1971.

26. Csiza, C. K., Scott, F. W., de Lahunta, A., and Gillespie, J. H.: Pathogenesis of feline panleukopenia virus in susceptible newborn kittens. II. Pathology and Immunofluorescence. Infect. Immun., 3:838, 1971.

27. Csiza, C. K., Scott, F. W., de Lahunta, A., and Gillespie, J. H.: Respiratory signs and central nervous system lesions in cats infected with panleukopenia virus. A case report. Cor. Vet., 62:192, 1972.

28. Csiza, C. K., de Lahunta, A., Scott, F. W., and Gillespie, J. H.: Spontaneous feline ataxia. Cor. Vet., 62:300, 1972.

29. Dejerine, L., and Thomas, A.: L'atrophie olivopontocerebelleuse. Nouv. Iconogr. Salpet., 13:330, 1900.

30. de Lahunta, A.: Hereditary cerebellar cortical and extrapyramidal nuclear abiotrophy in Kerry blue terriers. Proceedings 20th World Veterinary Congress, Greece, 1975.

31. de Lahunta, A., and Averill, D. R., Jr.: Hereditary cerebellar cortical and extrapyramidal nuclear abiotrophy in Kerry blue terriers. J. Am. Vet. Med. Assoc., 168:1119, 1976.

32. Del Cerro, M. P., and Snider, R. S.: Studies on the developing cerebellum. II. The ultrastructure of the external granule layer. J. Comp. Neurol., 144:131, 1972.

33. Dickinson, A. G., and Barlow, R. N.: The demonstration of the transmissibility of border disease of sheep. Vet. Rec., 81:114, 1967.

34. Dow, R. W.: The evolution and anatomy of the cerebellum. Biol. Rev., 17:179, 1942.

35. Dow, R. W.: Partial agenesis of the cerebellum in dogs. J. Comp. Neurol., 72:569, 1940.

36. Dow, R. W., and Moruzzi, G.: The Physiology and Pathology of the Cerebellum. Minneapolis, University of Minnesota Press, 1958.

37. Eager, R. P.: Efferent corticonuclear pathways in the cerebellum of the cat. J. Comp. Neurol., 120:81, 1963.

38. Eccles, J. C.: The development of the cerebellum of vertebrates in relation to the control of movement. Naturwissenschaften, 56:525, 1969.

39. Eccles, J. C., Llinas, R., and Sasaki, K.: Golgi cell inhibition in the cerebellar cortex. Nature, 204:1265, 1964.

40. Edmonds, L., Crenshaw, D., and Selby, L. A.: Micrognathia and cerebellar hypoplasia in an Aberdeen Angus herd. J. Hered., 64:62, 1973.

41. Emerson, J. L., and Delez, A. L.: Cerebellar hypoplasia, hypomyelinogenesis, and congenital tremors of pigs associated with prenatal hog cholera vaccination of sows. J. Am. Vet. Med. Assoc., 147:47, 1965.

42. Fankhauser, R.: Cerebelläre encephalitis beim Rind. Schweiz. Arch. Tierheilk., 103:292, 1961.

43. Fibiger, H. C., McGeer, E. G., and Atmadja, S.: Axoplasmic transport of dopamine in nigrostriatal neurons. J. Neurochem., 21:373, 1973.

44. Fibiger, H. C., Pudritz, R. E., McGeer, P. O., and McGeer, E. G.: Axonal transport in nigrostriatal and nigrothalamic neurons: Effects of medial forebrain bundle lesions and 6-hydroxydopamine. J. Neurochem., 19:1697, 1972.

45. Fletcher, T. F.: Ablation and histopathologic studies on myoclonia congenita in swine. Am. J. Vet. Res., 29:2255, 1968.

46. Fraser, H.: Two dissimilar types of cerebellar disorder in the horse. Vet. Rec., 78:608, 1966.

47. Gardner, C.: Cerebellar degeneration in three pigs. Senior seminar, Flower Veterinary Library, Ithaca, N.Y., New York State College of Veterinary Medicine, 1972.

48. Good, R.: Untersuchungen uber eine Kleinhirn—rindenatrophie beim Hund. Dissertation, University of Bern, Switzerland, 1962.

49. Gowers, W. R.: A lecture on abiotrophy. Lancet, 1:1003, 1902.

50. Gowers, W. R.: The pathology of tabes dorsalis and general paralysis of the insane. Lancet, 2:1591, 1899.

51. Hamilton, A. F., and Timoney, P. J.: Bovine virus diarrhea-mucosal disease virus and border disease. Res. Vet. Sci., 15:265, 1973.

52. Harding, J. D. J., Done, J. T., Harbourne, J. F., Randall, C. J., and Gilbert, F. R.: Congenital tremor type A III in pigs, and hereditary sex-linked cerebrospinal hypomyelinogenesis. Vet. Rec., 92:527, 1973.

53. Holden, M.: Unusual ataxia in three Samoyeds. Senior seminar, Flower Veterinary Library, Ithaca, N.Y., New York State College of Veterinary Medicine, 1974.

54. Holmes, G.: A form of familial degeneration of the cerebellum. Brain, 30:466, 1907.

55. Hulland, T. J.: Cerebellar ataxia in calves. Can. J. Comp. Med. Vet. Sci., 21:72, 1957.

56. Johnson, K. R., Fourt, D. L., and Ross, R. H.: Hereditary congenital ataxia in Holstein-Friesian calves. J. Dairy Sci., *41*:1371, 1958.
57. Johnson, R. H., Margolis, G., and Kilham, L.: Identity of feline ataxia virus on the feline panleukopenia virus. Nature, *214*:175, 1967.
58. Kahrs, R. F., Scott, F. W., and de Lahunta, A.: Congenital cerebellar hypoplasia and ocular defects in calves following bovine viral diarrhea-mucosal disease infection in pregnant cattle. J. Am. Vet. Med. Assoc., *156*:1443, 1970.
59. Kaufmann, J.: Untersuchungen über die Frühentwicklung des Kleinhirns beim Rind. Schweiz. Arch. Tierheilk., *101*:49, 1959.
60. Kay, W. J., and Budzelovich, G. N.: Cerebellar hypoplasia and agenesis in the dog. J. Neuropathol. Exp. Neurol., *29*:156, 1970.
61. Kilham, L., and Margolis, G.: Viral etiology of spontaneous ataxia of cats. Am. J. Pathol., *48*:991, 1966.
62. Kilham, L., Margolis, G., and Colby, E. D.: Cerebellar ataxia and its congenital transmission in cats by feline panleukopenia virus. J. Am. Vet. Med. Assoc., *158*:888, 1971.
63. Kilham, L., Margolis, G., and Colby, E. D.: Congenital infections of cats and ferrets by feline panleukopenia virus manifested by cerebellar hypoplasia. Lab. Invest., *17*:465, 1967.
64. Klawans, H. O., and Zeitlin, Z.: L-Dopa in parkinsonism associated with cerebellar dysfunction (probable olivopontocerebellar degeneration). J. Neurol. Neurosurg. Psychiatry, *34*:14, 1971.
65. Koch, P., and Fischer, H.: Die Oldenburger Fohlenataxie als Erbkrankheit. Tierärzt Umschau., *5*:317, 1950.
66. Konigsmark, B. W., and Lipton, H. O.: Dominant olivopontocerebellar atrophy with dementia and extrapyramidal signs: A report of a family through 3 generations. J. Neuropathol. Exp. Neurol., *30*:133, 1971.
67. Lapham, L. W., Lentz, R. D., Woodward, D. J., Hoffer, B. J., and Herman, B. J.: Postnatal development of tetraploid DNA content in the Purkinje neuron of the rat: An aspect of cellular differentiation. *In* Pease, D. ed., Cellular Aspects of Neural Growth and Regulation—UCLA Forum in Medical Sciences, *14*:61, 1971.
68. Larsell, O.: The Comparative Anatomy and Histology of the Cerebellum from Monotremes Through Apes. Minneapolis, University of Minnesota Press, 1970.
69. Lentz, R. D., and Lapham, L. W.: Postnatal development of tetraploid DNA content in rat Purkinje cells: A quantitative cytochemical study. J. Neuropathol. Exp. Neurol., *29*:43, 1970.
70. Llinas, R. R.: The cortex of the cerebellum. Sci. Am., *232*:56, 1975.
71. Llinas, R. R.: Neurobiology of cerebellar evolution and development. Proceedings First International Symposium of the Institute for Biomedical Research, 1969.
72. Lockard, I., and Gillian, L. A.: Neurologic dysfunctions and their relation to congenital abnormalities of the central nervous system of cats. J. Comp. Neurol., *104*:403, 1965.
73. Mare, C. J., and Kluge, J. P.: Pseudorabies virus and myoclonia congenita in pigs. J. Am. Vet. Med. Assoc., *164*:309, 1974.
74. Margolis, G., and Kilham, L.: In pursuit of an ataxic hamster or virus-induced cerebellar hypoplasia. *In* Bailey, O. D., and Smith, D. E., eds., The Central Nervous System. Baltimore, Williams & Wilkins, 1968, 157–183.
75. Margolis, G., and Kilham, L.: Virus-induced cerebellar hypoplasia. *In* Infections of the Nervous System. Res. Publ. A.R.N.M.D., *44*:113, 1968.
76. Margolis, G., Kilham, L., and Johnson, R. H.: The parvoviruses and replicating cells: Insight into the pathogenesis of cerebellar hypoplasia. Progr. Neuropathol., *1*:168, 1971.
77. Markson, L. M., Terlecki, S., Shand, A., Sellers, K. C., and Woods, A. J.: Hypomyelinogenesis congenita in sheep. Vet. Rec., *71*:269, 1959.
78. McC. Howell, J., and Ritchie, H. E.: Cerebellar malformations in two Ayshire calves. Pathol. Vet., *3*:159, 1966.
79. Mettler, F. A., and Goss, L. J.: Canine chorea due to striocerebellar degeneration of unknown etiology. J. Am. Vet. Med. Assoc., *108*:377, 1946.
80. Osburn, B. I., Clarke, G. L., Stewart, W. C., and Sawyer, M.: Border disease-like syndrome in lambs: Antibodies to hog cholera and bovine viral diarrhea viruses. J. Am. Vet. Med. Assoc., *163*:1165, 1973.
81. Palmer, A. C.: Pathogenesis and pathology of the cerebello-vestibular syndrome. J. Sm. Anim. Pract., *11*:167, 1970.
82. Palmer, A. C., Blakemore, W. F., Cook, W. R., Platt, H., and Whitwell, K. E.: Cerebellar hypoplasia and degeneration in the young Arab horse; clinical and neuropathological features. Vet. Rec., *93*:62, 1973.
83. Palmer, A. C., Payne, J. E., and Wallace, M. E.: Hereditary quadriplegia and amblyopia in the Irish setter. J. Sm. Anim. Pract., *14*:343, 1973.
84. Parker, H. L., and Kernohan, J. W.: Parenchymatous cortical cerebellar atrophy (chronic atrophy of Purkinje cells). Brain, *56*:191, 1933.
85. Patterson, D. S. P., and Sweasey, D.: Lipid hexose: phosphorus ratio as an aid to the diagnosis of congenital myelin defects in lambs and piglets. Acta Neuropathol., *15*:318, 1970.
86. Patterson, D. S. P., Sweasey, D., and Harding, J. D. J.: Lipid deficiency in the central nervous system of Landrace piglets affected with congenital tremor A-III, a form of cerebrospinal hypomyelinogenesis. J. Neurochem., *19*:2797, 1972.

87. Patterson, D. S. P., Sweasey, D., and Hebert, C. N.: Changes occurring in the chemical composition of the CNS during fetal and postnatal development of the sheep. J. Neurochem., *18*:2027, 1971.

88. Patterson, D. S. P., Sweasey, D., Brush, P. J., and Harding, J. D. J.: Neurochemistry of the spinal cord in British saddleback piglets affected with congenital tremor type A-IV, a second form of hereditary cerebrospinal hypomyelinogenesis. J. Neurochem., *21*:397, 1973.

89. Patterson, D. S. P., Terlecki, S., Dore, J. T., Sweasey, D., and Hebert, C. N.: Neurochemistry of the spinal cord in experimental border disease (hypomyelinogenesis congenita) of lambs. J. Neurochem., *18*:883, 1971.

90. Percy, D. H., Carmichael, L. E., Albert, D. M., King, J. M., and Jonas, J. M.: Lesions in puppies surviving infection with canine herpesvirus. Vet. Pathol., *8*:37, 1971.

91. Phemister, R. D., and Young, S.: The postnatal development of the canine cerebellar cortex. J. Comp. Neurol., *134*:243, 1968.

92. Rakic, P.: Neuron-glia relationship during granule cell migration in developing cerebellar cortex. A Golgi and electronmicroscopic study in *Macacus rhesus*. J. Comp. Neurol., *141*:283, 1971.

93. Russell, J. S. E.: Defective development of the cerebellum in a puppy. Brain, *18*:523, 1895.

94. Saunders, L. Z., Sweet, J. D., Martin, S. M., Fox, F. H., and Fincher, M. G.: Hereditary congenital ataxia in Jersey calves. Cor. Vet., *42*:559, 1952.

95. Scherer, H. J.: Extrapyramidale Störungen bei der Olivopontocerebellarer Atrophie ein Beitrag zum Problem des lokalen vorzeitigen Alterns. Zentralbl. Ges. Neurol. Psychiat., *146*:406, 1933.

96. Scott, F. W., Kahrs, R. F., de Lahunta, A., Brown, T. T., McEntee, K., and Gillespie, J. H.: Virus induced congenital anomalies of the bovine fetus. I. Cerebellar degeneration (hypoplasia), ocular lesions and fetal mummification following experimental infection with bovine viral diarrhea-mucosal disease virus. Cor. Vet., *63*:536, 1973.

97. Sidman, R. L., Green, M. C., and Appel, S. H.: Catalog of the Neurological Mutants of the Mouse. Cambridge, Mass., Harvard University Press, 1965.

98. Sponseller, M. L.: Equine cerebellar hypoplasia and degeneration. J. Am. Vet. Med. Assoc., *152*:313, 1968.

99. Sponseller, M. L.: Equine cerebellar hypoplasia and degeneration. Proc. Am. Assoc. Equine Pract., *13*:123, 1967.

100. Spraque, J. M., and Chambers, W. M.: Regulation of posture in intact and decerebrate cat. I. Cerebellum reticular formation, vestibular nuclei. J. Neurophysiol., *16*:451, 1953.

101. Tontitila, P., and Lindberg, L. A.: ETT fall av cerebellar ataxi hos finsk stoväre. Svoman Elainlääkarilehti, 77:135, 1971.

102. Wheat, J. D., and Kennedy, P. C.: Cerebellar hypoplasia and its sequela in a horse. J. Am. Vet. Med. Assoc., *131*:291, 1957.

103. White, M. E., Whitlock, R. H., and de Lahunta, A.: A cerebellar abiotrophy of calves. Cor. Vet., 65:476, 1975.

104. Young, S.: Hypomyelinogenesis congenita (cerebellar ataxia) in Angus-Shorthorn calves. Cor. Vet., 52:84, 1962.

105. Zaki, F. A., Liu, S. K., and Kay, W. J.: Calcifying aponeurotic fibroma in a dog. J. Am. Vet. Med. Assoc., 106:384, 1975.

106. Zaki, F. A., and Kay, W. J.: Carcinoma of the choroid plexus in a dog. J. Am. Vet. Med. Assoc., *164*:1195, 1974.

107. Koppang, N.: Canine ceroid-lipofuscinosis—A model for human neuronal ceroid-lipofuscinosis and aging. Mech. Ageing Dev., 2:421, 1973.

108. Cummings, J. F., and de Lahunta, A.: An adult case of canine neuronal ceroid-lipofuscinosis. Acta Neuropathol. (submitted for publication).

109. Innes, I. M. R., Russell, D. S., and Wilsdon, A. J.: Familial cerebellar hypoplasia and degeneration in Hereford calves. J. Pathol. Bacteriol., *50*:455, 1940.

Chapter 13

VISUAL SYSTEM—SPECIAL SOMATIC AFFERENT SYSTEM

EMBRYOLOGY OF THE EYEBALL
HISTOLOGY OF THE PARS OPTICA
    RETINAE
Pigment Epithelium of the Retina
Photosensitive Layer (Layer of Rods and Cones)
External Limiting Membrane
External Nuclear Layer
External Plexiform Layer
Internal Nuclear Layer
Internal Plexiform Layer
Ganglion Layer
Nerve Fiber Layer
Internal Limiting Membrane
Area Centralis
CENTRAL VISUAL PATHWAY
OPTIC NERVE
OPTIC CHIASM

PATHWAY FOR CONSCIOUS PERCEPTION—
    VISUAL CORTEX
REFLEX PATHWAY
Clinical Tests
Clinical Signs
DISEASES OF THE VISUAL SYSTEM
RETINA—OPTIC NERVE
OPTIC CHIASM
OPTIC TRACTS
Bilateral
Unilateral
LATERAL GENICULATE NUCLEUS
OPTIC RADIATION—VISUAL CORTEX
Unilateral
Bilateral
Case Report

EMBRYOLOGY OF THE EYEBALL

The eyeball is derived from neuroectoderm (retina), surface ectoderm (lens, cornea), and mesoderm (cornea, sclera, and uvea).

The neuroectodermal contribution to the eyeball is induced in the open neural tube stage at its rostral end. This is in the portion of the neural tube destined to form the prosencephalon, and subsequently the diencephalon. The "optic field" neuroectoderm is induced initially by the underlying archenteron endoderm beneath the rostral ventral midline of the neural plate. This initially single primordial optic area is influenced by the adjacent rapidly infiltrating head mesenchyme. This particular portion of head mesenchyme is rostral to the notochord, and therefore is designated the prechordal mesenchyme. It helps induce the separation of the initially single optic area of neuroectoderm into two areas that first appear as depressions within the neural tube—the optic pits—in each half of the future prosencephalon. These proceed to grow laterally as evaginations from the neural tube. They are the optic vesicles. Improper separation of the optic area into two primordia by the prechordal mesenchyme leads to the development of the cyclopic malformation with a single median plane eyeball.

The optic vesicles bulge laterally from the prosencephalon and lie adjacent to the surface ectoderm, where they proliferate and induce the surface ectoderm

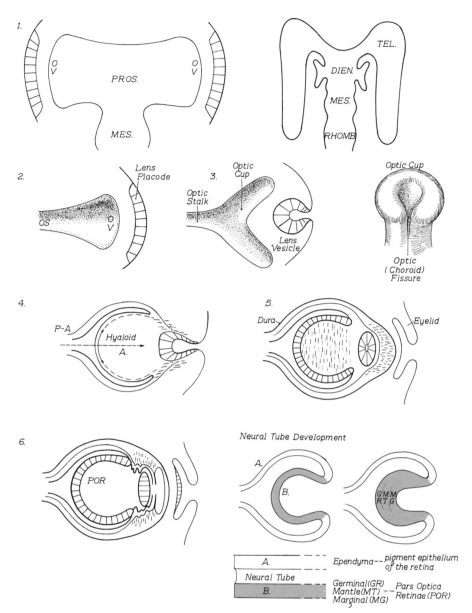

Figure 13-1. Development of the eyeball. OV: Optic vesicle, OS: Optic stalk, P-A: PIA-arachnoid.

to proliferate to form the lens placode. As the optic vesicle grows away from the prosencephalon, its connection elongates into the optic stalk. This is the precursor of the pathway of the optic nerve. The protruding lateral surface of the optic vesicle adjacent to the lens placode invaginates so that it comes to lie against the medial surface of the vesicle. This infolding forms the shape of a cup, and the structure is referred to as the optic cup. It is incomplete ventrally, where the optic or choroidal fissure develops. In time, fusion of the edges closes this fissure, except for a small notch. The infolding that produces the optic cup also involves the optic stalk, which provides a path for the optic nerve axons to enter the brain. The two layers of the optic cup differentiate into the retina.

As the optic vesicle invaginates to form the optic cup, the lens placode developing in the surface ectoderm invaginates to form the lens vesicle, which ultimately separates from the overlying surface ectoderm and remains situated at the opening to the optic cup. A fine fibrous connection remains between the inner layer of the optic cup and the posterior surface of the lens vesicle. The cavity in the lens is obliterated as the ectodermal epithelial cells that comprise it elongate and differentiate into lens fibers. Growth of the lens occurs at its equator, at which the epithelial cells at the margin of the anterior capsule proliferate, elongate, and transform into lens fibers. The characteristics of these lens fibers impart transparency to the lens.

The lens is thought to be partially responsible for the induction of the remaining ectodermal surface cells to form the surface epithelium for the cornea.

To these primordial ectodermal structures of the eyeball is added the mesodermal component. This can be considered as the addition of two layers of mesoderm corresponding to the two basic supporting mesodermal layers that are formed around the entire central nervous system, the dense protective dura and the thinner vascular pia-arachnoid.

As the loose mesoderm, mesenchyme, surrounding the brain differentiates into the vascular pia-arachnoid (leptomeninges), this process of differentiation continues along the optic stalk and over the optic cup and lens vesicle. The subarachnoid space found between the pia and arachnoid over the brain continues along the optic stalk to the optic cup. There the space is obliterated, and the mesoderm, homologous with the pia-arachnoid, differentiates into the uveal coat of the eyeball (choroid, ciliary body, and iris), and forms the endothelial layer on the internal surface of the cornea. This initially loose mesoderm completely fills the area between the lens vesicle and the corneal endothelium. A space forms in this mesoderm, leaving the mesoderm anteriorly as the corneal endothelium and posteriorly as the body of the iris and pupillary membrane. This space is the anterior chamber, which fills with aqueous. The pupillary membrane is the mesoderm situated centrally over the lens. Ultimately, it disintegrates to form the pupil. The space formed in the mesoderm between the iris and the lens is the posterior chamber, which also fills with aqueous. The uvea is the vascular tunic of the eyeball that is continuous with the pia-arachnoid, the vascular tunic of the central nervous system, at the optic stalk. The cells of these layers have some similar histologic characteristics.

The space between the fundus of the optic cup and the posterior surface of the lens is the vitreous chamber. The vitreous body that fills it is derived from secretions from the optic cup, the lens, and the enclosed mesenchyme. A blood vessel courses in the mesoderm from the base of the brain along the optic stalk in the optic fissure to supply the optic cup. A branch crosses the vitreous chamber to the posterior surface of the lens. This is the hyaloid artery, which normally disappears after birth. In cattle, a remnant of this vessel occasionally is seen emerging from the optic disk that forms at the site of the optic stalk.

As the outer layer of mesenchyme surrounding the brain differentiates into the dense pachymeninx, the dura, this process of differentiation continues along the optic stalk and optic cup. Over the optic cup this layer forms the fibrous tunic of the eyeball—the sclera. It continues anteriorly deep to the surface ectoderm to form the substance of the cornea, the substantia propria. Thus the fibrous tunic of the brain (dura) and of the eyeball (sclera) have a similar origin which reflects the initial origin of the eyeball from the neural tube.

Differentiation of the optic cup is similar to the differentiation of the neural tube, with two adjacent walls and a space between, the neural canal. The optic vesicle originally consists of proliferating neuroepithelial cells. As the lumen of the vesicle is reduced to a small space by the infolding of the lateral surface, this forms an outer and inner wall to the optic cup. The differentiation of each wall can be compared to that of the neural tube, with the formation of germinal, mantle, and marginal layers. The entire outer layer of the optic cup, which initially proliferated, later regresses to a single layer of cells. Posterior to the ciliary body, this is the pigment layer of the retina. Anterior to this it forms the outer layer of the two cell layers that cover the posterior surface of the ciliary body and iris. Thus this differentiated outer layer is homologous to the ependymal layer of the differentiated neural tube that lines the ventricular system and central canal. The inner layer of the optic cup posterior to the ciliary body differentiates into the multilayered sensory portion of the retina, the pars optica retina. Anterior to this the inner layer differentiates into a single layer of cells to form the inner layer of the two-cell layer that covers the posterior surface of the ciliary body and iris. These two layers of cells, derived from the inner and outer layers of the optic cup, are called the pars ciliaris retinae and pars iridica retinae, respectively, after the structures they cover. The rostral extent of the pars iridica retinae determines the margin of the iris. Beyond this, the mesoderm of the pupillary membrane degenerates to produce the pupillary space. Improper degeneration of this membrane leaves persistent remnants. This may be an hereditary defect in basenji dogs.[83] The outer layer of cells in the pars iridica retinae proliferates to form the smooth muscle cells of the dilator muscle of the iris. Thus, ectodermal cells are forming muscle in this site.

In the inner layer of the optic cup posterior to the ciliary body, the neuroepithelial cells proliferate as the germinal layer. With development, this layer differentiates into three layers of neurons. The outer layer of cells (toward the sclera) forms the photoreceptor neurons. These line the slit-like lumen, remnant of the neural canal, and are homologous to the ependymal layer. Two other layers of neurons differentiate, and include the layer of bipolar neurons and the ganglion cells. These are homologous to the mantle layer of the neural tube. The nerve fiber layer, a layer of axons from the ganglion cell neurons, is on the inner surface (toward the vitreous) and is homologous to the marginal layer on the surface of the neural tube. In dogs at birth, the single layer of ganglion cells is separated from an outer thick layer of undifferentiated cells which represent the primordia of the photoreceptor neurons and the bipolar cell neurons. In the first 7 days of life the definitive three layers of neurons are established.[98] The histologically mature retina is apparent by 6 weeks of age in the dog, which coincides approximately with the development of visual function.[4] The pupillary reflex is demonstrable by 3 weeks. The various media of the eyeball are not transparent until 5 to 6 weeks postnatal.[35]

The following sequence of development of the eye has been observed in the dog:[4]

Gestational day:

15—Well-developed optic vesicle and lens placode.

19—Invagination of optic vesicle to form the optic cup.

25—Lens vesicle separated from the surface ectoderm. Multicellular inner layer of optic cup differentiated into outer nuclear (mantle) and inner marginal zones. Outer layer of optic cup is a single-celled, thick layer. Retinal development progresses from central to peripheral in the optic cup inner layer as a "wave of maturation."

33—Inner neuroblastic (ganglion cell) layer separated from outer neuroblastic layer. Formation of optic nerve. Eyelid buds meet and adhere.

Birth:

Retina consists of outer neuroblastic layer, inner plexiform layer, and ganglion cell and nerve fiber layers.

Postnatal days:

7–13—Formation of inner and outer nuclear layers of retina.

16>35—Distinct inner and outer segments of rods and cones.

14—Eyelids separate.

In contrast to the dog with its short gestational period, the bovine newborn eyeball is fully developed. Studies have shown that the bovine eyeball appears well developed by the end of the second trimester of gestation.[16]

The following sequence of development has been observed in the bovine embryo-fetus.

Gestational size (mm), days (approximate):

6 mm, 25–30 days—Well-developed optic vesicle and lens placode.

10 mm, 30 days—Optic cup and lens vesicle separated from surface ectoderm. Multicellular inner layer of optic cup differentiated into outer nuclear (mantle) and inner marginal zones.

14–33 mm, 40–50 days—Separated inner and outer nuclear layers of pars optica retina.

20–40 mm, 40–50 days—Nerve fiber layer formed. Single-celled thick epithelial layer formed from a multilayered outer wall of the optic cup.

24 mm, 40 days—Well-formed optic nerve.

40 mm, 50 days—Eyelid buds meet and adhere.

410 mm, 150–180 days —All layers of the retina present.

Birth:

Eyelids are separated.

HISTOLOGY OF THE PARS OPTICA RETINAE[79, 97, 107]

Ten layers will be described, progressing from the outer (scleral) surface to the inner (vitreal) surface.

Pigment Epithelium of the Retina

This epithelium comprises a single layer of cuboidal cells, with their base on a basement membrane apposed to the choroid, and their apex facing the photosensitive layer across the potential space of the neural tube (lumen of the optic cup). Numerous processes of the apical cytoplasm and cell membrane interdigitate with the processes of the rods and cones. This close arrangement may facilitate the role of the pigment epithelium in the regeneration of rhodopsin, the visual pigment in the rods, and the removal of degenerate rod membranous lamellae by phagocytosis.[111, 114] Many melanin granules occupy the apical cytoplasm of the pigment cells throughout the retina, except over the area occupied by the

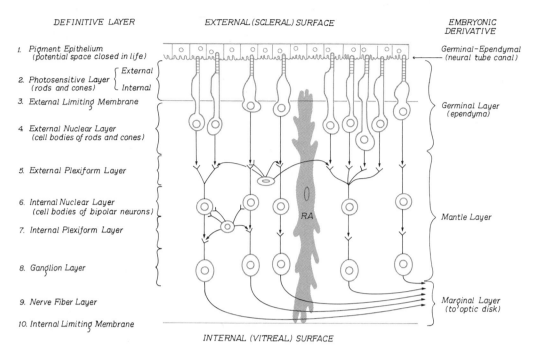

Figure 13–2. Microscopic anatomy of the pars optica retinae. HC: horizontal cell (interneuron), AC: amacrine cell (interneuron), RA: radial astrocyte (Müller's neuroglial cell).

tapetum lucidum in the choroid. The presence of these pigment granules partly accounts for the dark color of the fundus observed with the ophthalmoscope. The tapetum lucidum in the choroid is rendered more visible by the absence of melanin pigment in this epithelium.

Photosensitive Layer (Layer of Rods and Cones)

This layer, divided into two segments, represents the dendritic zone of the sensory special somatic afferent neuron, the photoreceptor cell.[97, 98] The external and internal segments of the layer are composed of modifications of the cell processes and bodies of the rod and cone cells. The external segment consists of parallel lamellae within the elongate cell processes. These are orderly stacks of flattened, double-membrane sacs in the form of disks. These membranes are oriented transversely to the axis of the cell process. The sacs are formed at the base of the external segment, migrate distally, and are cast off at the outer portion, where they are phagocytized by the pigment epithelial cells. In the rods these membranes contain the visual pigment, rhodopsin, the photoreceptor substance responsible for light absorption and the initiation of the visual stimulus. A similar substance, iodopsin, is in the cone membranous lamellae. The rod cells are sensitive to low levels of illumination (night vision). Cone cells respond to high levels of illumination (day vision), and are responsible for initiating color vision.

The external segment is connected to the internal segment by a slender stalk containing a modified cilium. The internal segment, called the ellipsoid, is elongate in rods and oval in cones, and composed mostly of endoplasmic reticulum and numerous mitochondria. It is a modification of the cell body of these photoreceptor special somatic afferent neurons.

External Limiting Membrane

This "membrane" consists of the junctional complexes between the photoreceptor cells and the supporting radial astrocytes (the cells of Müller). These latter cells surround and support all the neural elements of the retina between the basal lamina of these cells, the internal limiting membrane, and the external limiting membrane on the scleral side of the external nuclear layer.

External Nuclear Layer

This layer is composed of the cell bodies with nuclei of the photoreceptor special somatic afferent neurons. The cone nuclei are located adjacent to the external limiting membrane. The rod nuclei are smaller and constitute most of this layer. They extend in several layers toward the inner (vitreal) surface of the retina. In the dog retina, it is estimated that the ratio of the number of rod cells to cone cells is about 18 to 1. The number of cone cells increases toward the central area of the retina. Axons of the rod and cone cells course vitreally into the next layer.

External Plexiform Layer

This is a layer primarily composed of the axons and telodendria of the photoreceptor cells and the axons and dendritic zones of the bipolar neurons and their synaptic arrangements. Intermingled with these are the cell processes of the horizontal cells, an interneuron transmitting between different groups of photoreceptor cells.

Internal Nuclear Layer

This layer primarily consists of the cell bodies (nuclei) of bipolar neurons. These are the second neurons in the visual pathway, and like the photoreceptor cells, they are restricted to the retina. They connect photoreceptor neurons with ganglion cells in the visual pathway. The axon courses from the external plexiform layer, in which the dendritic zone is located, through the internal nuclear layer (cell body), into the internal plexiform layer, in which the telodendron is located. The cell body with its nucleus is situated along the course of this axon, accounting for its bipolar characteristic. On the external, scleral, surface of this internal nuclear layer the cell bodies with nuclei of the horizontal cells are located. On the opposite internal (vitreal) surface, the cell bodies of another interneuron, the amacrine cell, are located. These latter interneurons are in synaptic contact with bipolar cells, ganglion cells, and other amacrine cells. In addition, the nuclei of the radial astrocytes are located in this layer.

Whereas many rod cells are in synaptic contact with one bipolar cell, there may be only one cone cell synapsing on one bipolar cell. Thus there is a convergence of rod cell activity on the bipolar neurons.

Internal Plexiform Layer

This layer primarily is composed of the axons and telodendria of the bipolar cells and the axons and dendritic zones of the ganglion cells and their synaptic arrangements. In addition, the processes of the amacrine cells extend throughout the layer.

Ganglion Layer

This layer contains the cell bodies with nuclei of the third special somatic afferent neuron in the visual pathway. They vary in size from 6 to 35 μ in diameter. It is this neuron that transmits visually induced impulses to the brain by way of its axons in the optic nerve. These large cell bodies form an incomplete layer one to two cells thick between the internal plexiform layer and the nerve fiber layer. Nissl substance is evident in the cytoplasm of these cell bodies. There is an increased number of these cell bodies in the area centralis.[102]

Nerve Fiber Layer

This layer consists of the axons of the ganglion cells coursing on the vitreal surface of the retina to the optic disk. The axons are unmyelinated until they penetrate the sclera at the optic disk. Their myelination at this point accounts for the white color of the optic disk. The nerve fiber layer is thickest in the vicinity of the optic disk. The intermingling of scleral fibers with the ganglion cell axons at the point of origin of the optic nerve is called the lamina cribrosa. Stellate astrocytes are located in this nerve fiber layer.

Internal Limiting Membrane

This is formed by the basal cell membrane of the radial astrocyte and a basement membrane, and is the vitreal boundary of the retina.

Area Centralis

In man there is an area for most distinct vision located dorsolateral to the optic disk, and called the macula (spot), fovea, or central area. In this area the retina is composed of only cones in the photoreceptor layer, and other modifications occur to facilitate the function for most acute vision. Neuromuscular mechanisms provide that for most acute close-up vision such as reading, the light is focused on this central area in each eyeball. Domestic animals have various modifications of this area. It is difficult to identify in the dog. In the cat, it may be identified as a pale streak or oval part in the area of the tapetum lucidum dorsolateral to the optic disk in which the blood vessels (arterioles) converge.[101] The area itself is devoid of any large blood vessels. It is located dorsomedially in cattle and horses.[79] In this area centralis in the cat, there is an increase in the number of cone cells relative to rods in the photoreceptor layer. The length of the outer segments of the photoreceptor cells is increased. The bipolar and ganglion cells are increased in

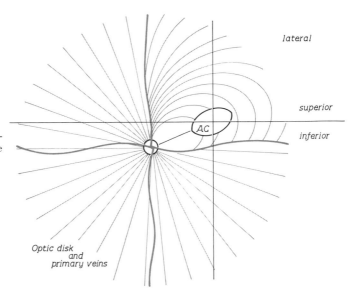

Figure 13–3. Relationship of optic disk and area centralis in the retina of the cat.

number. The axons in the nerve fiber layer form an arc as they leave the area centralis and course to the optic disk.

The optic disk, the origin of the optic nerve, varies in shape from round to oval to triangular.[1, 12, 66, 69, 108] It is usually slightly ventrolateral to the posterior pole of the eyeball and varies in its relationship to the tapetum lucidum. In toy breeds it may be in the retina entirely below the area of the tapetum lucidum. In middle-sized breeds it is usually half over the ventral area of the tapetum lucidum. In large breeds it may be entirely over the area of the tapetum lucidum.[108]

CENTRAL VISUAL PATHWAY[20, 80]

OPTIC NERVE

The growth of the ganglion cell axons through the embryonic optic stalk produces the optic nerve, cranial nerve II. The optic nerve is in fact a tract of the central nervous system based on its origin in the optic vesicle and its histologic characteristics. It is surrounded by meninges, including a subarachnoid space. It contains neuroglial cells similar to those of the brain, and has no lemnocytes. The oligodendrocytes are the source of the myelin for the axons in the optic nerve. Leptomeningeal fibers course through the nerve as septa. The optic nerves course caudally in the orbit, surrounded by their meninges and extraocular muscles. They enter the skull through the optic canals of the presphenoid bone and join on the rostroventral aspect of the brain stem, rostral to the hypophysis at the optic chiasm.

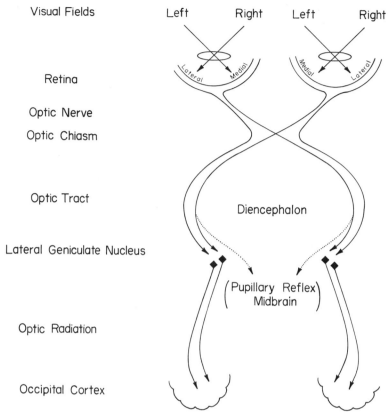

Figure 13–4. Central visual pathway for conscious perception. (From Vet. Clin. North Am., 3:491, 1973.)

OPTIC CHIASM

At the optic chiasm in domestic animals a majority of the axons in each optic nerve cross, destined to influence the contralateral cerebral hemisphere. This corresponds to the pattern that most modalities that can be localized in space (general proprioception, general somatic afferent) are represented contralaterally in the brain.

In most fish and birds, all the optic nerve axons cross in the optic chiasm. In mammals, partial decussation develops in relationship to the development of a binocular field of vision with frontal positioning of the eyeballs, and the ability to perform coordinated conjugate eyeball movements, including convergence. In primates, in whom this is most developed, the degree of decussation is slightly over 50 per cent. It is estimated that in the cat the degree of decussation is 65 per cent, in dogs 75 per cent, and in the horse and the ox 85 to 90 per cent.[22] On this basis the cat most closely resembles the primate in degree of decussation, frontal positioning of the eyeballs, and presumably conjugate movement of the eyeballs.

In general, the axons that cross in the chiasm come from ganglion cells on the medial (nasal) aspect of the retina. Axons from ganglion cells on the lateral (temporal) aspect of the retina remain ipsilateral in their course through the central visual pathway. Neuroanatomic studies in the cat have determined that this division between medial and lateral portions of the retina based on the axons that cross in the chiasm is a vertical line through the area centralis.[99, 101] Nearly 100 per cent of the axons from ganglion cells medial to this line decussate in the optic chiasm. In addition, about 25 per cent of the axons from ganglion cells lateral to this line decussate. This was determined by cutting one optic tract and studying the retrograde degeneration that occurred in the ganglion cells of the retina whose axons were severed (Fig. 13–5).

The optic tracts course caudodorsolateral over the side of the diencephalon, progressing from ventral to lateral to caudal to the internal capsule, reaching the lateral geniculate nucleus, which is the caudodorsolateral protrusion of the thalamus. Each tract contains axons mostly from the medial retina of the contralateral eyeball and the lateral retina of the ipsilateral eyeball. If the visual field is defined as the area in space observed by each eyeball when fixed at any one moment, then the lateral half of the visual field of each eyeball will stimulate the medial retina, and the medial half will stimulate the lateral retina. Thus each optic tract contains the neurons in which light generates an impulse from the same half of the visual field of each eyeball. The left optic tract contains the neurons stimulated by light from the right half of the visual field of the left and right eyeballs. Objects in the right visual fields of each eyeball therefore are represented mainly in the left central visual pathway.

When the optic tract reaches the level of the lateral geniculate nucleus, there are two courses that can be followed: a pathway for conscious perception, and a reflex pathway.

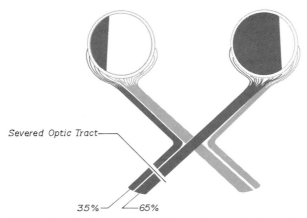

Severed Optic Tract

35%   65%

Figure 13–5. Origin in retinal ganglion cell layer of axons in the optic tract of the cat.

PATHWAY FOR CONSCIOUS PERCEPTION—VISUAL CORTEX

Approximately 80 per cent of the optic tract fibers in the cat terminate in the lateral geniculate nucleus. This nucleus contains neuronal cell bodies organized in specific laminae. There is a retinotopic anatomic relationship maintained throughout the central visual pathway.[15, 63] This is reflected in the laminations of the lateral geniculate nucleus.[22, 37, 38, 39, 42, 44, 45, 51, 57, 58, 67, 93, 103]

The axons of the neurons in the lateral geniculate nucleus project into the internal capsule and course caudally as the optic radiation in the caudal limb of the internal capsule, which forms the lateral wall of the lateral ventricle.[70] These axons terminate in the cerebral (visual) cortex on the lateral, caudal, and medial aspects of the occipital lobe.[37, 50] The gyri that comprise this area include the caudal part of the marginal and ectomarginal gyri (laterally), the occipital gyrus (caudally), and the splenial gyrus (medially). This pathway from optic tract, to lateral geniculate nucleus, to optic radiation, to visual cortex, must be intact for normal conscious visual perception to occur.

Various portions of the visual cortex have connections to the visual cortex of the opposite hemisphere, to the motor cortex of both hemispheres, to the cerebellum by way of the pons, to the tegmentum and the nuclei of cranial nerves III, IV, and VI directly or indirectly through the rostral colliculus, and to the rostral colliculus. A tectospinal tract descends from the rostral colliculus through the ventral funiculus of the cervical spinal cord to contribute to the upper motor neuron that influences the lower motor neurons in the grey matter of the spinal cord.[71] Through these pathways, responses to visual stimuli can be mediated.

Similar to the arrangement in the optic tract, the ipsilateral lateral geniculate nucleus, the optic radiation, and the visual cortex contain neurons stimulated by light from objects in the contralateral half of the visual field of each eyeball. This is a retinotopic pathway in that specific anatomic portions of the retina are represented in specific anatomic portions of the optic tract, the lateral geniculate nucleus, the optic radiation, and the visual cortex. These retinal areas have a specific representation in the visual field of each eyeball.

In primates the visual cerebral cortex is divided into functional areas. Area 17 is for stationary object vision. Areas 18 and 19 function in panoramic vision for movement, spatial relationship, and depth perception. For normal object vision interaction is required between the visual cortex and the rostral colliculus. For normal panoramic vision interaction is required between the visual cortex and the mesencephalic tegmentum. Removal of the rostral colliculus on one side produces hemianopsia in the contralateral visual field for object vision. Bilateral rostral collicular lesions produce complete blindness for still objects. Visual perception of movement and spatial orientation are lost with lesions in the mesencephalic tegmentum. Unilateral lesions of the tegmentum produce a contralateral deficit and cause severe torsion of the head so that it tilts more than 90 degrees to the side opposite the lesion. Blindfolding corrects this postural dystonia, indicating its visual basis.[112, 113]

REFLEX PATHWAY[46]

Approximately 20 per cent of the optic tract axons in the cat pass over the lateral geniculate nucleus to terminate in the pretectal area or rostral colliculus.[67] The pretectal area functions in the pupillary reflex pathway. The axons that course into the rostral colliculus follow the brachium of the rostral colliculus, which lies between the rostral colliculus and the lateral geniculate nucleus. The rostral colliculus is also a laminated structure, and in addition to the optic tract axons it receives axons from the cerebral cortex (especially the visual cortex) and the spinal cord (spinotectal tract). Axons of cell bodies in the rostral colliculus project to the tegmentum to influence nuclei of cranial nerves III, IV, and VII (tectobulbar fibers), to the spinal cord to influence ventral grey column general somatic efferent neurons (tectospinal tract), and to the cerebellum.[71] These pathways function in the coordination of head, neck, and eyeball movements in response to visual stimuli.

Clinical Tests[24, 82]

Vision can be tested by watching the patient walk in a strange environment or through a maze of obstacles.

The menace test consists of making a menacing gesture with the hand directed at each eyeball, while the other eyeball is covered. With a cooperative patient the medial and lateral aspects of each eyeball (retina) can be tested. Care must be taken not to touch any of the facial hairs or to create too much air turbulence. In the stoic patient it may be necessary to strike the eye being tested, so that the animal is aware of the test. The entire peripheral and central visual pathway must be intact for a response to occur.

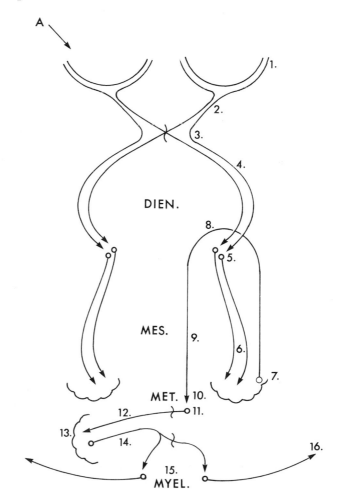

Figure 13–6. Anatomic pathway of the menace response: *1*, Retina; *2*, optic nerve; *3*, optic chiasm; *4*, optic tract; *5*, lateral geniculate nucleus; *6*, optic radiation; *7*, visual cortex; *8*, internal capsule; *9*, crus cerebri; *10*, longitudinal fibers of pons; *11*, pontine nucleus; *12*, transverse fibers of pons and middle cerebellar peduncle; *13*, cerebellar cortex; *14*, efferent cerebellar pathway; *15*, facial nuclei; *16*, facial muscles — orbicularis oculi. ʃ indicates axons crossing the midline of the brain. A lesion in the left cerebellar hemisphere would prevent a menace response directed at the left eyeball from its lateral field (*A*), because 65 to 90 per cent of the optic nerve axons cross in the chiasm.

The response observed is closure of the palpebral fissure and sometimes retraction of the eyeball or head away from the gesture. The facial nucleus and nerve must be intact for palpebral closure to occur.

In all domestic animals it has been observed that diffuse cerebellar cortical degenerative lesions cause a failure of the menace response bilaterally, with no visual deficit and normal facial nerve function. It is assumed therefore that the pathway that mediates this response from the visual cortex to the facial nucleus must pass through the cerebellum. This is probably part of the cerebropontocerebellar projection. In the horse and dog, a unilateral menace response deficit with normal vision has been observed to accompany large unilateral cerebellar lesions on the same side as the deficit. This is explained by the crossing that occurs from the cerebrum to the cerebellum at the pontine nucleus.

The pupillary light reflex response was described in Chapter 6. This tests the peripheral visual pathway and central pathway to the level of the thalamus and pretectum only. The oculomotor nucleus and nerve mediate the motor response. Loss of the pupillary response due to lesions in the afferent visual pathway usually occurs only with a severe lesion.

Clinical Signs[24]

The degree of visual deficit depends on the location and extent of the lesion in the visual pathway.

Lesions that destroy the retina or optic nerve in one eye cause blindness and a partially dilated pupil in that eyeball. This does not usually cause any disorientation of the gait, nor any head tilt or neck curvature. There is no palpebral closure in response to a menacing gesture in the affected eyeball. Light directed into the blind eyeball produces no response in either eyeball. Light directed into the normal eyeball causes both pupils to constrict. In the pupillary reflex pathway, the afferents cross both in the optic chiasm and in the pretectum to influence both oculomotor nuclei. It is through this pathway that the environmental light causes partial constriction of the pupil of the blind eyeball.

Bilateral retinal or optic nerve disease that is total causes complete blindness, with both pupils widely dilated and unresponsive to light directed into either eyeball. Optic neuritis is the most common cause of this kind of deficit.

Unilateral lesions in the optic tract, lateral geniculate nucleus, optic radiation, or visual cortex result in a visual deficit in the contralateral visual field of each eyeball. Because of the degree of decussation, the visual deficit can be appreciated only in the contralateral eyeball. This is referred to as a hemianopsia because there is a visual deficit in 50 per cent of the total visual field. In the dog, this represents about a 25 per cent retinal dysfunction in the ipsilateral eyeball and a 75 per cent retinal dysfunction in the contralateral eyeball.

In the dog and cat the visual deficit may be difficult to detect as the animal moves in its surroundings. Occasionally, an object may be bumped on the side opposite the lesion, but often there is no evidence of visual deficit. Unilateral blindfolding and maze testing of the animal may help demonstrate the deficit. In the horse and ruminants with 80 to 90 per cent crossing of optic nerve axons there is a greater tendency to walk into objects on the side of the visual deficit, contralateral to the lesion.

In all domestic animals there is a poor or absent palpebral closure response to menacing gestures to the eyeball contralateral to the lesion. If the examiner is careful, this test can be performed reliably without using a transparent barrier between the hand and the eyeball to prevent air currents and direct contact with the facial hairs.

It is important to cover the eyeball not being tested, and to menace the other eyeball from both its medial and lateral sides. The deficit will be more pronounced from the lateral side (visual field) when there are contralateral lesions in the central visual pathway.

In all unilateral lesions caudal to the optic chiasm the pupillary light reflex responses are usually normal, because of the crossing at the chiasm and pretectal area. The light always should be directed toward the lateral retina in which the area centralis is located. This occasionally may turn a slow response into a normal one.

Bilateral lesions in the optic radiations, or the visual cortex, or both, cause complete blindness with normal pupillary light reflexes.

Bilateral lesions in the optic tracts and area of the lateral geniculate nucleus, if complete, produce total blindness and dilated pupils unresponsive to light. More often the lesions are partial and clinical signs are difficult to determine. Canine distemper encephalitis often produces extensive lesions in the optic tracts without obvious clinical deficit of vision or pupillary function.

TABLE 13–1. CLINICAL SIGNS OF VISUAL DEFICIT

	Lesions				
Test	Right Optic Nerve	Right Cranial Nerve III	Right Postorbital	Right Optic Tract	Right Visual Cortex
Left eye (OS)					
Pupil	Normal size	Normal size	Normal size	Normal size	Normal size
	Light in OS	Light in OS	Light in OS	Light in OS	Light in OS
	Both constrict	Only OS constricts	Only OS constricts	Both constrict	Both constrict
Menace	Present	Present	Present	Mostly absent	Mostly absent
Right eye (OD)					
Pupil	Partial dilation	Complete dilation	Complete dilation	Normal size	Normal size
	Light in OD	Light in OD	Light in OD	Light in OD	Light in OD
	Neither constrict	Only OS constricts	Neither constricts	Both constrict	Both constrict
Menace	Absent	Present	Absent	Mostly present	Mostly present

DISEASES OF THE VISUAL SYSTEM[53, 85]

RETINA—OPTIC NERVE[17, 23, 29, 32, 64, 68, 84, 89, 90, 100]

1. There are many examples in veterinary medicine of hereditary retinal degenerations, called progressive retinal atrophy (PRA), which slowly produce blindness over a period of many months to years. Some have been shown to be hereditary in Gordon and Irish setters, miniature and toy poodles, Norwegian elkhounds, malamutes, and others.[2, 3, 7, 8, 9, 10, 11, 21, 74, 75, 76, 77] In this disease there is a slowly progressive degeneration of the photoreceptor cells. In some breeds in the early stages this may be restricted to only one type of photoreceptor cell—the rod cells in Norwegian elkhounds (night blindness), and cone cells in Alaskan

malamutes (hemeralopia or day blindness).[60, 86, 87, 88] Terminally in these diseases pupils are dilated and unresponsive to light.

2. Malformation of parts of the eyeball occurs as an hereditary disease in collie dogs. In its more severe manifestation it may produce blindness because of disruption of the retina, or optic nerve, or both.[27, 28, 91, 105, 109, 110] This is referred to as the collie eye syndrome, and may include scleral ectasia, or chorioretinal dysplasia, or both. It is a nonprogressive disease. The primary defect may relate to abnormal closure of the choroidal fissure and abnormal pigment epithelium of the retina, retarding development of the retina and choroid.

3. Eyeball hypoplasia and anophthalmia have been observed in kittens born from mothers treated for a prolonged period during gestation with *griseofulvin,* an oral treatment for fungus infections. Other malformations attributed to this teratogen include hydrocephalus, cleft palate, cranium bifidum and exencephaly, spina bifida, and cyclopian malformation.

4. Bilateral hypoplasia of the optic nerve has been observed in the cat, dog, and horse.[13, 36, 104] The optic disk is markedly diminished in size as are the optic nerve, chiasm, and tracts. The patients are blind from birth, with dilated, unresponsive pupils. Whether these cases are all hypoplasia or some are perinatal degenerations is not known.

5. Night blindness has been observed in the Appaloosa breed. They often stumble and fall while being ridden during and after dusk. They are reluctant to move in the dark. A rod cell photoreceptor deficit is assumed, but this remains to be proved.

6. Injury to the optic disk or nerve can occur associated with head trauma. Fundic examination should be performed along with the neurologic evaluation of a blind patient with brain injury before attributing the visual deficit to cerebral contusion and edema. In these latter cases dilated pupils may accompany the brain stem or oculomotor nerve compression or contusion, and be misleading as to the cause of the blindness.

7. Optic neuritis occurs in dogs as a fairly sudden onset of total blindness, usually bilateral with dilated unresponsive pupils, with or without visible abnormalities associated with the optic disk. It is a nonsuppurative inflammatory lesion with necrosis of myelin and axons, or may be a reticulosis. It is sometimes responsive to strenuous corticosteroid therapy. Any relationship of this disease to the canine distemper virus has yet to be determined.[33]

Although the onset of blindness as recognized by the owner appears to be sudden, unilateral or partial visual deficit produced as the lesion progressed may have been overlooked. Careful examination may reveal mild signs of general proprioceptive ataxia or vestibular system deficits referable to lesions in the spinal cord and cerebellar medullary region. The distribution of lesions often is similar to that in neuromyelitis optica (Devic's syndrome) in man. This human disease is thought to be immunopathologic, associated with a prior systemic viral infection.

8. Neoplasia of the presphenoid bone or meninges ventral to the brain with infiltration of the optic nerves produces bilateral blindness with dilated unresponsive pupils in the dog.

OPTIC CHIASM[14]

In domestic animals, unlike man, most pituitary neoplasms grow into the hypothalamus. The normal canine pituitary gland projects caudally away from the optic chiasm. Therefore, enlargement of this gland usually does not affect the chiasm.[25]

In one dog, a meningioma developed between the optic chiasm and pituitary gland, causing compression of both. Bilateral blindness with dilated unresponsive pupils occurred. The clinical signs were improved temporarily with corticosteroid therapy.

Occasionally, the cerebral infarction syndrome in cats (see Chapter 7) causes ischemic necrosis of the optic chiasm, resulting in blindness and dilated unresponsive pupils.

OPTIC TRACTS

Bilateral

1. Incomplete bilateral lesions may produce partial bilateral visual deficit with variable pupillary response. This is typical of the inflammation and necrosis caused by the canine distemper virus, which has a predilection for this system. Often no clinical visual deficit is observed.

2. In man, pituitary neoplasia commonly causes compression of the optic chiasm and tracts because of the rostral location of the pituitary directly ventral to the chiasm, and the lack of a meningeal barrier. In domestic animals involvement of the optic chiasm is uncommon because of the caudal position of the pituitary gland and the restrictive dural diaphragma sellae in the ruminant. Occasionally, canine pituitary neoplasms affect the optic tracts as the hypothalamus is invaded or compressed by the neoplasm. In a horse with a large pars intermedia neoplasm, sudden blindness followed ischemic necrosis of the adjacent optic tracts. Pupils were dilated and unresponsive to light.[25]

Unilateral

1. Unilateral neoplasms in the hypothalamus and thalamus often encroach upon one optic tract, resulting in a visual deficit in the contralateral eyeball with normal pupillary responses to light.

Because of the close approximation of the internal capsule and rostral crus cerebri to the optic tract, space-occupying lesions in the lateral hypothalamus, or thalamus, or both, that affect the optic tract usually also affect the internal capsule and rostral crus cerebri. This results in signs designated as a mild hemiparesis, often not evident in the gait but demonstrable by asymmetry in the response to postural testing. The deficit is contralateral to the lesion.

2. Traumatic lesions that cause necrosis of these tissues on one side of the diencephalon can result in the same residual neurologic signs—contralateral visual deficit and postural reaction deficit ("hemiparesis").

LATERAL GENICULATE NUCLEUS

Destruction of this nucleus produces signs similar to those observed with optic tract lesions.

An abnormality in the retinogeniculate projections and the neuronal organization in this nucleus has been observed in Siamese cats and white Persian tiger cats. In some, this has been associated with a congenital bilateral medial strabismus.[40, 41, 52, 56, 94]

OPTIC RADIATION—VISUAL CORTEX

Unilateral

Unilateral lesions produce hemianopsia recognized in the contralateral eyeball, as previously discussed. Pupillary size and response to light are normal.

1. Neoplastic lesions produce progressive signs of neurologic deficit. Convulsions or changes in behavior may accompany the visual deficit. Frequently, the cerebrospinal fluid pressure is elevated.[25, 31]

2. Traumatic lesions that cause necrosis of these tissues may leave a residual neurologic deficit limited to a contralateral visual deficit. If the entire hemisphere is involved, a contralateral postural reaction deficiency may be seen on neurologic examination. Immediately following the injury the neurologic signs may be more extensive, suggestive of diffuse cerebral disturbance. As the hemorrhage and edema subside, the residual neurologic deficits relate to the areas of tissue necrosis.

3. Cerebral infarction most commonly seen in cats (see Chapter 7) may destroy the optic radiation, or visual cortex, or both in one hemisphere. When the signs of the acute cerebral disturbance resolve after the first few days, it is usual to find a contralateral menace deficit from the visual pathway lesion and a contralateral postural reaction deficit from the lesion in the cerebral pathway for the upper motor neuron and general proprioceptive systems. Neither disturbance may be reflected in the routine activities of the cat. CSF may contain an increased amount of protein (20 to 100 mg per dl) and normal or slightly higher numbers of leukocytes.

4. Unilateral cerebral abscess in the horse caused by *Streptococcus equi* may directly affect the optic radiation and cause a contralateral visual deficit with normal pupils. Expansion of this lesion with accompanying cerebral edema may increase intracranial pressure and cause the occipital lobes to herniate ventral to the tentorium cerebelli. This further compromises the function of the visual cortex bilaterally, and causes total blindness if both sides are affected.[25]

Similar signs may occur in ruminants with a *Corynebacterium pyogenes* abscess.

5. In encephalitis caused by *Toxoplasma gondii*, a space-occupying granuloma may be produced in the vicinity of the optic radiation and cause a contralateral visual deficit. CSF should contain inflammatory cells, often with neutrophils and increased amounts of protein.

6. Occasionally, the focal encephalitis produced in horses by an unidentified protozoan is severe enough in one hemisphere to cause swelling and necrosis and a contralateral visual deficit.

Bilateral

Total blindness with normal pupils is characteristic of bilateral visual cortex lesions.

1. The same explanation of tentorial herniation for bilateral signs of visual deficit can be offered for any space-occupying cerebral lesion or when the brain swells following injury. Head injury that causes progressive cerebral edema causes blindness. The pupillary activity varies with the degree of brain stem involvement.

2. A malformation, hypoplasia of the prosencephalon, has been observed in calves. The lack of cerebral tissue causes the visual deficit, despite a functional brain stem.

3. Obstructive hydrocephalus compromises the optic radiation in the internal capsule, in which it forms the lateral wall of the dilated lateral ventricle. Bilateral visual deficit is a common sign of this lesion.

4. In the recovery phase of diffuse ischemic necrosis of the cerebrum caused by an overdose of anesthetic and a prolonged apnea and cardiac arrest, the only residual deficit may be that of blindness with intact pupils. In this situation the cerebral cortex has been compromised.[43, 72]

5. Polioencephalomalacia in cattle and sheep is characterized by severe cerebral disturbance, including blindness in most cases.[65] The visual deficit is due to the necrosis of cerebral cortical tissue in the visual cortex. The pathogenesis of this disease involves an abnormality in thiamine (vitamin B_1) metabolism. Lead intoxication causes a similar acute necrosis of the cerebral cortex and an associated blindness.[19] Similarly, severe water intoxication with cerebral disturbance may lead to blindness.[48]

6. Intoxication by wheat seed fungicide containing mercury causes a chronic degeneration of neurons in the cerebral cortex and their replacement by astrocytes. Convulsions and blindness may appear in the chronic stage of the disease.[55]

7. Chronic inflammation of the cerebral white matter caused by the canine distemper virus may result in a demyelination and astrocytosis of the centrum semiovale, including the optic radiation. This is a sclerosing encephalitis which may produce a unilateral or bilateral visual deficit with normal pupillary function.

8. Infarction of the cerebral white matter by septic emboli occurs in thromboembolic meningoencephalitis in cattle caused by *Hemophilus somnus*. Visual deficits may result.

Similar bilateral disseminated cerebral infarcts occurred in a pony associated with the release of a *Strongylus vulgaris* larva from the wall of the brachiocephalic trunk. Bilateral central visual deficit accompanied other signs of the acute diffuse cerebral lesion.

9. *Leukodystrophy—lipodystrophy:* Inherited metabolic disorders of the nervous system occur in dogs and cats, and are models of comparable diseases in man.[5] All are progressive, degenerative disorders of the nervous system. The onset is usually some time after weaning. Signs represent the diffuse involvement of the nervous system, but often begin with pelvic limb ataxia and paresis. In the advanced stages of the disease, blindness is a common sign. In all these diseases there is an absence or severe deficiency of a specific degradative enzyme, which leads to an abnormal accumulation of the biochemical substrate normally hydrolyzed by that enzyme. In those diseases for which a mode of inheritance has been established, a recessive gene has been implicated that is expressed in the homozygous individual. These metabolic disorders may be expressed in neurons by the accumulation of the complex lipids in neuronal cytoplasm—lipodystrophy—or in the myelin by demyelination and accumulation of complex lipids in macrophages—leukodystrophy.

Leukodystrophy involves an abnormal metabolism of myelin, and its subsequent degeneration. This white matter disease is inherited as a recessive trait in Cairn and West Highland white terriers.[34] Signs of paraparesis and ataxia begin between 3 and 6 months of age. In some cases, cerebellar signs predominate early. The signs are progressive, with diffuse involvement of the central nervous system, and include cerebellar ataxia and visual deficit. Death usually occurs prior to 1 year of age. This disease, a cerebrosidosis caused by a beta galactosidase deficiency, resembles Krabbe's disease in children. It has been reported in two related short-haired domestic cats with predominant signs of cerebellar degeneration beginning at 5 to 6 weeks of age and progressing rapidly.[47, 54]

Lipodystrophy is an abnormal neuronal metabolism associated with accumulations of complex lipids in neurons and their subsequent degeneration. This grey matter disease is inherited in German short-haired pointers and English setters. The onset of signs, including ataxia and visual deficit, is between 6 and 12 months of age. The signs progress to mental disturbance, "dummy" attitude, convulsions occasionally, and death by 2 years of age. This disease in German short-haired pointers is a GM_2 gangliosidosis, which resembles Tay-Sachs disease in man.[59] It may be due to a hexosaminidase deficiency. The English setter lipodystrophy is classified as a neuronal ceroid lipofuscinosis.[61,62]

A lipid storage disease has been reported in a Siamese cat. Neurologic disturbance, predominantly cerebellar, began at 4 months of age. The neurologic deterioration progressed, along with retarded growth and emaciation, and terminated in death at 9 months of age.[18] The disease, a sphingomyelin lipidosis, resembled Niemann-Pick disease in man. A GM_1 gangliosidosis caused by a beta galactosidase deficiency also has been reported in a Siamese cat. Signs of progressive paresis and ataxia began in the pelvic limbs at 4 months of age and progressed to tetraplegia by 6 months of age.[6, 78, 95]

Similar metabolic disorders have been reported in cattle affecting myelin or neurons, and in swine affecting neurons.[26, 49, 73, 81, 92, 106]

Case Report

Signalment.   The patient was a 7 and $1/2$-year-old male boxer.

History.   Four months prior to admission, the owner noticed that the right thoracic limb seemed to bother the dog. Occasionally, it would slide out laterally, and when standing the dog seemed to favor it by treading continually on it, as if it could not get the limb into a comfortable position. Each time the paw was placed it immediately would be retracted and replaced. One month later, the owner noticed that the right pelvic limb occasionally slid out laterally, especially on slippery floors. In the month before admission the dog showed some difficulty and caution when climbing stairs. The dog ran well on firm footing, without indicating any abnormality to the owner.

Examination.   The patient was in good physical condition, alert and responsive. No muscle atrophy was evident. While standing, the right thoracic limb frequently was treaded on the floor, as if the dog either could not find a comfortable position for it or it would not support its weight well in certain positions, and therefore kept moving it to a more satisfactory position. The right pelvic limb frequently slid out laterally on a slippery floor, and was replaced continually. When the dog walked on firm footing little deficit was seen, but on a slippery floor either or both of the right limbs often would slide out laterally on the floor. The patient ran well on a surface that was not slippery.

Spinal Reflexes.   All flexor reflexes were normal. The patellar reflex on the right side was hyperactive (plus 3), and on the left side was normal (plus 2). Muscle tone was normal. When the dog relaxed, increased resistance often could be induced by manipulating the right pelvic limb. It was not evident in the left pelvic limb or in either thoracic limb. Pain perception was intact from all limbs.

Postural Reactions.   The hopping response best demonstrated a left-right side difference. The response with the left limbs was normal, but with the right limbs the response was exaggerated, almost hypermetric in action. The extensor thrust response with the pelvic limbs was slightly asymmetric. Proprioceptive positioning was slow in the right pelvic limb. Placing was usually normal. On tonic neck and eye testing, the right forepaw occasionally knuckled onto its dorsal surface.

Cranial Nerves.   Cranial nerve examination was normal except for the visual pathway. The menace response in the right eye was deficient. When the patient was blindfolded unilaterally and walked through a maze, only a minimal difference between the two sides could be seen. There was only a suggestion that the animal had more difficulty with the left eye blindfolded. Pupillary response was normal in both eyes, direct and indirect. No fundic abnormalities were noted.

Radiographs of the cervical vertebrae and skull were normal. Cerebrospinal fluid pressure was 410 mm (normal is <170). It was clear and contained 20 mg of protein per dl and <10 cells per mm.[3]

Diagnosis. These signs indicated that the lesion was affecting the left central visual pathway caudal to the chiasm and the left cerebral upper motor neuron and general proprioceptive pathways. The progressive nature of the lesion with increased intracranial pressure indicated a space-occupying lesion, presumably a neoplasm. The dog was treated with corticosteroids and lived for about 3 months before neurologic signs worsened and euthanasia was performed. At necropsy, an astrocytoma was found in the left cerebral internal capsule and the optic radiation.

TABLE 13–2. NEURO-OPHTHALMOLOGY: REVIEW OF CLINICAL SIGNS

Extraocular:
  Size of palpebral fissure—musculus levator palpebrae (III):
    Narrow: oculomotor nerve paralysis (ptosis) with strabismus and mydriasis; sympathetic paralysis—Horner's syndrome; and facial paralysis in large animals.
    Wide: Facial paralysis in small animals.
  Protrusion of the third eyelid: sympathetic paralysis—Horner's syndrome; tetanus—when stimulated; facial paralysis—when the eye is menaced; severe depression in cats; and hyperplasia of the gland of the third eyelid.
  Strabismus: Vestibular system disturbance—ventrolateral, inconstant; oculomotor nerve paralysis—ventrolateral, constant; abducens nerve paralysis—medial, constant; and trochlear nerve paralysis—dorsal deviation of medial angle-constant.
  Nystagmus—vestibular system disturbance: peripheral disease—nystagmus to opposite side; congenital blindness—pendular; and congenital nystagmus—pendular.
  Sensory perception—trigeminal nerve: ophthalmic nerve to eyeball (cornea)—neurotrophic keratitis; maxillary nerve to eyelids laterally; and ophthalmic nerve to eyelids medially.

Intraocular:
  Size of pupil:
    Mydriasis: oculomotor nerve paralysis (ptosis) with strabismus; optic nerve paralysis with total blindness; glaucoma; iris atrophy; and retinal disease.
    Miosis: sympathetic paralysis—Horner's syndrome; acute intracerebral disease—released oculomotor nuclear function; ocular pain—oculopupillary reflex; and iritis.
  Examination: menace (vision), and pupillary light reflex.

REFERENCES

1. Ammann, K., and Müller, A.: Das Bild des normalen Augenhintergrundes beim Pferd. Berl. Münch. Tieraerztl. Wochenschr., *81*:370, 1968.
2. Aquirre, G. D., and Rubin, L. F.: Progressive retinal atrophy in the miniature poodle: An electrophysiologic study. J. Am. Vet. Med. Assoc., *160*:191, 1972.
3. Aquirre, G. D., and Rubin, L. F.: Rod-cone dysplasia (progressive retinal atrophy) in Irish setters. J. Am. Vet. Med. Assoc., *166*:157, 1975.
4. Aquirre, G. D., Rubin, L. F., and Bistner, S. I.: Development of the canine eye. Am. J. Vet. Res., *33*:2399, 1972.
5. Baker, H. J.: Inherited metabolic disorders of the nervous system in dogs and cats. *In* Kirk, R. W., ed., Current Veterinary Therapy, V. Small Animal Practice. Philadelphia, W. B. Saunders Co., 700–702.
6. Baker, H. J., Jr., Lindsey, J. R., McKhann, G. M., and Farrell, D. F.: Neuronal GM$_1$ gangliosidosis in a Siamese cat with beta galactosidase deficiency. Science, *174*:838, 1971.
7. Barnett, K. C.: Canine retinopathies. I. History and review of literature. J. Sm. Anim. Pract., *6*:41, 1965.

8. Barnett, K. C.: Canine retinopathies. II. The miniature and toy poodle. J. Sm. Anim. Pract., 6:93, 1965.
9. Barnett, K. C.: Canine retinopathies. III. The other breeds. J. Sm. Anim. Pract., 6:185, 1965.
10. Barnett, K. C.: Canine retinopathies. IV. Causes of retinal atrophy. J. Sm. Anim. Pract., 6:229, 1965.
11. Barnett, K. C.: Primary retinal dystrophies in the dog. J. Am. Vet. Med. Assoc., 154:804, 1969.
12. Barnett, K. C.: Variations of the normal ocular fundus of the dog. Am. Anim. Hosp. Assoc. Proc., 39:1, 1972.
13. Barnett, K. C., and Grimes, T. D.: Bilateral aplasia of the optic nerve in a cat. Br. J. Ophthalmol., 58:663, 1974.
14. Barnett, K. C., Kelly, D. F., and Singleton, W. B.: Retrobulbar and chiasmal meningioma in a dog. J. Sm. Anim. Pract., 8:391, 1967.
15. Bishop, G. H., and Clare, M. C.: Organization and distribution of fibers in the optic tract of the cat. J. Comp. Neurol., 103:269, 1955.
16. Bistner, S. I., Rubin, L. F., and Aquirre, G. D.: Development of the bovine eye. Am. J. Vet. Res., 34:7, 1973.
17. Bistner, S. I., Rubin, L. F., and Saunders, L. Z.: The ocular lesions of bovine viral diarrhea-mucosal disease. Pathol. Vet., 7:275, 1970.
18. Chrisp, C. E., Ringler, D. H., Abrams, G. D., Radin, N. S., and Brenkert, A.: Lipid storage disease in a Siamese cat. J. Am. Vet. Med. Assoc., 156:616, 1970.
19. Christian, R. G., and Tryphonas, L.: Lead poisoning in cattle: Brain lesions and hematologic changes. Am. J. Vet. Res., 32:203, 1971.
20. Cogan, D. G.: Neurology of the Visual System. Springfield, Ill., Charles C Thomas, 1966.
21. Cogan, D. G., and Kuwabara, T.: Photoreceptive abiotrophy of the retina in the elkhound. Pathol. Vet., 2:101, 1965.
22. Cummings, J. F., and de Lahunta, A.: An experimental study of the retinal projections in the horse and sheep. Ann. N.Y. Acad. Sci., 167:293, 1969.
23. Davis, T. E.: Bone Resorption in Hypovitaminosis A. Ph.D. thesis, Ithaca, N.Y., Cornell University, 1968.
24. de Lahunta, A.: Small animal neuro-ophthalmology. Vet. Clin. North Am., 3:491, 1973.
25. de Lahunta, A., and Cummings, J. F.: Neuro-ophthalmologic lesions as a cause of visual deficit in dogs and horses. J. Am. Vet. Med. Assoc., 150:994, 1967.
26. Donnelly, W. J. C., Sheahan, B. J., and Rogers, T. A.: GM$_1$ gangliosidosis in Friesian calves. J. Pathol., 111:173, 1973.
27. Donovan, E. F., and Wyman, M.: Ocular fundus anomaly in the collie. J. Am. Vet. Med. Assoc., 147:1465, 1965.
28. Donovan, R. H., Carpenter, R. L., Schepens, C. L., and Tolentino, F. I.: Histology of the normal collie eye. I. Topography, cornea, sclera, and filtration angle. Ann. Ophthalmol., 6:257, 1974.
29. Evans, H. E., Ingalls, T. N., and Binns, W.: Teratogenesis of craniofacial malformations in animals. III. Natural and experimental cephalic deformities in sheep. Arch. Environ. Health, 13:706, 1966.
30. Fagan, R. H.: Canine congenital nystagmus. Seminar, Flower Veterinary Library, Ithaca, N.Y., New York State College of Veterinary Medicine, 1974.
31. Finn, J. P., and Tennant, B. C.: A cerebral and ocular tumor of reticular tissue in a horse. Vet. Pathol., 8:458, 1971.
32. Fischer, C. A.: Intraocular cryptococcosis in two cats. J. Am. Vet. Med. Assoc., 158:191, 1971.
33. Fischer, C. A., and Jones, G. T.: Optic neuritis in dogs. J. Am. Vet. Med. Assoc., 160:68, 1972.
34. Fletcher, T. F., Kurtz, H. J., and Low, D. G.: Globoid cell leukodystrophy (Krabbe type) in the dog. J. Am. Vet. Med. Assoc., 149:165, 1966.
35. Fox, M. W.: Postnatal ontogeny of the canine eye. J. Am. Vet. Med. Assoc., 143:968, 1963.
36. Gelatt, K. N., Leipold, H. W., and Coffman, J. R.: Bilateral optic nerve hypoplasia in a colt. J. Am. Vet. Med. Assoc., 155:627, 1969.
37. Glickenstein, M., King, R. A., Miller, J., and Berkley, M.: Cortical projections from the dorsal lateral geniculate nucleus of the cat. J. Comp. Neurol., 130:55, 1967.
38. Guillery, R. W.: The laminar distribution of retinal fibers in the dorsal lateral geniculate nucleus of the cat: A new interpretation. J. Comp. Neurol., 138:339, 1970.
39. Guillery, R. W.: The organization of synaptic interconnections in the laminae of the dorsal lateral geniculate nucleus of the cat. Z. Zellforsch. Mikrosk. Anat., 96:1, 1969.
40. Guillery, R. W., and Kaas, J. H.: Genetic abnormality of the visual pathways in a "white" tiger. Science, 180:1287, 1973.
41. Guillery, R. W., and Kaas, J. H.: A study of normal and congenitally abnormal retinogeniculate projections in cats. J. Comp. Neurol., 143:73, 1971.
42. Guillery, R. W., and Stelzner, D. J.: The differential effects of unilateral lid closure upon the monocular and binocular segments of the dorsal lateral geniculate nucleus in the cat. J. Comp. Neurol., 139:413, 1970.
43. Hartley, W. J.: Polioencephalomalacia in dogs. Acta Neuropathol., 2:271, 1963.
44. Hayhow, W. R.: The cytoarchitecture of the lateral geniculate body in the cat in relation to the distribution of crossed and uncrossed optic fibers. J. Comp. Neurol., 110:1, 1958.

45. Hayhow, W. R.: Experimental degeneration of optic axons in lateral geniculate body of the cat. Acta Anat., 37:281, 1958.
46. Hayhow, W. R.: An experimental study of the accessory optic fiber system in the cat. J. Comp. Neurol., 113:281, 1959.
47. Hegreberg, G. A., Thuline, H. C., and Francis, B. H.: Morphologic changes in feline leukodystrophy. Fed. Proc., 30:341, 1971.
48. Heslink, P.: Water intoxication in a calf. Senior seminar, Flower Veterinary Library, Ithaca, N.Y., New York State College of Veterinary Medicine, 1975.
49. Hocking, J. D., Jolly, R. D., and Batt, R. D.: Deficiency of alpha mannosidase in Angus cattle. Biochem. J., 128:69, 1972.
50. Howard, D. R., and Braezile, J. E.: Normal visual cortical-evoked response in the dog. Am. J. Vet. Res., 33:2155, 1972.
51. Howard, D. R., and Braezile, J. E.: Optic fiber projections to dorsal lateral geniculate nucleus in the dog. Am. J. Vet. Res., 34:419, 1973.
52. Hubel, D. H., and Wiesel, T. N.: Aberrant visual projections in the Siamese cat. J. Physiol., 218:33, 1971.
53. Jensen, H. E.: Stereoscopic Atlas of Clinical Ophthalmology of Domestic Animals. St. Louis, C. V. Mosby, 1971.
54. Johnson, K. H.: Globoid cell leukodystrophy in the cat. J. Am. Vet. Med. Assoc., 157:2057, 1970.
55. Kahrs, R. F.: Chronic mercurial poisoning in swine. A case report of an outbreak with some epidemiological characteristics of hog cholera. Cor. Vet., 58:67, 1968.
56. Kalil, R. E., Jhaveri, S. R., and Richards, W.: Anomalous retinal pathways in the Siamese cat. An inadequate substrate for normal binocular vision. Science, 174:302, 1971.
57. Karamanlidis, A. N., and Magras, J.: Retinal projections in domestic ungulates. I. The retinal projections in the sheep and the pig. Brain Res., 44:27, 1972.
58. Karamanlidis, A. N., and Magras, J.: Retinal projections in domestic ungulates. II. The retinal projections in the horse and ox. Brain Res., 6:209, 1974.
59. Karbe, E., and Schiefer, B.: Familial amaurotic idiocy in male German shorthair pointers. Pathol. Vet., 4:223, 1967.
60. Koch, S. A., and Rubin, L. F.: Distribution of cones in the hemeralopic dog. J. Am. Vet. Med. Assoc., 159:1257, 1971.
61. Koppang, N.: Canine ceroid lipofuscinosis: A model for human neuronal ceroid lipofuscinosis and aging. Mech. Aging Develop., 2:421, 1973–74.
62. Koppang, N.: Neuronal ceroid lipofuscinosis in English setters. Juvenile amaurotic familial idiocy in English setters. J. Sm. Anim. Pract., 10:639, 1970.
63. Laties, A. M., and Sprague, J. M.: The projection of optic fibers to the visual centers in the cat. J. Comp. Neurol., 127:35, 1966.
64. Leipold, H. W., and Huston, K.: Congenital syndrome of anophthalmia-microphthalmia with associated defects in cattle. Pathol. Vet., 5:407, 1968.
65. Little, P. B., and Sorenson, D. K.: Bovine polioencephalomalacia, infectious embolic meningoencephalitis and acute lead poisoning in feedlot cattle. J. Am. Vet. Med. Assoc., 155:1892, 1969.
66. McCormack, J. E.: Variations of the ocular fundus of the bovine species. Vet. Scope, 18:21, 1974.
67. Meikle, T. H., Jr., and Sprague, J. M.: The neural organization of the visual pathways in the cat. Int. Rev. Neurobiol., 6:150, 1964.
68. Morris, M. L., Jr.: Feline degenerative retinopathy. Cor. Vet., 55:295, 1965.
69. Müller, A.: Das Bild des normalen Augenhintergrundes beim Rind. Berl. Münch. Tieraertzl. Wochenschr., 82:181, 1969.
70. Niimi, K., and Sprague, J. M.: Thalamo-cortical organization of the visual system in the cat. J. Comp. Neurol., 138:219, 1970.
71. Nyberg-Hansen, R.: The location and termination of tectospinal fibers in the cat. Exp. Neurol., 9:212, 1964.
72. Palmer, A. C.: Cardiac arrest and cerebrocortical necrosis. Vet. Rec., 80:390, 1967.
73. Palmer, A. C., Blakemore, W. F., Barlow, R. M., Fraser, J. A., and Ogden, A. L.: Progressive ataxia of Charolais cattle associated with a myelin disorder. Vet. Rec., 91:592, 1972.
74. Parry, H. B.: Degenerations of the dog retina. I. Structure and development of the retina of the normal dog. Br. J. Ophthalmol., 37:385, 1953.
75. Parry. H. B.: Degenerations of the dog retina. II. Generalized progressive atrophy of hereditary origin. Br. J. Ophthalmol., 37:487, 1953.
76. Parry, H. B.: Degenerations of the dog retina. VII. Central nonprogressive degeneration due to an anomaly of the ganglion cells and their axons. Br. J. Ophthalmol., 39:29, 1955.
77. Parry, H. B.., Tansley, K., and Thomson, L. C.: Electroretinogram during development of hereditary retinal degeneration in the dog. Br. J. Ophthalmol., 39:349, 1955.
78. Percy, D. H., and Jortner, B. S.: Feline lipidosis. Arch. Pathol., 92:136, 1971.
79. Prince, J. H., Diesem, C. D., Eglitis, I., and Ruskell, G. L.: Anatomy and Histology of the Eye and Orbit in Domestic Animals. Springfield, Ill., Charles C Thomas, 1960.
80. Rademaker, G. G. J., and Ter Braak, J. W. G.: On the central mechanisms of some optic reactions. Brain, 71:48, 1948.

81. Read, W. K., and Bridges, C. H.: Cerebrospinal lipodystrophy in swine. A new disease model in comparative pathology. Pathol. Vet., 5:67, 1968.
82. Roberts, S. R.: A system of testing vision in animals. J. Am. Vet. Med. Assoc., 128:544, 1956.
83. Roberts, S. R., and Bistner, S. I.: Persistent pupillary membrane in basenji dogs. J. Am. Vet. Med., Assoc., 153:533, 1968.
84. Rogers, K. T.: Experimental production of perfect cyclopia by removal of telencephalon and reversal of bilateralization in somite stage chicks. Am. J. Anat., 115:487, 1964.
85. Rubin, L. F.: Atlas of Veterinary Ophthalmoscopy. Philadelphia, Lea & Febiger, 1974.
86. Rubin, L. F.: Clinical features of hemeralopia in the adult Alaskan malamute. J. Am. Vet. Med. Assoc., 158:1696, 1971.
87. Rubin, L. F.: Hemeralopia in Alaskan malamute pups. J. Am. Vet. Med. Assoc., 158:1699, 1971.
88. Rubin, L. F.: Heredity of hemeralopia in Alaskan malamutes. Am. J. Vet. Res., 28:355, 1967.
89. Rubin, L. F., and Craig, P. H.: Intraocular cryptococcosis in a dog. J. Am. Vet. Med. Assoc., 147:27, 1965.
90. Rubin, L. F., and Lipton, D. E.: Retinal degeneration in kittens. J. Am. Vet. Med. Assoc., 162:467, 1973.
91. Saunders, L. Z.: Congenital optic nerve hypoplasia in collie dogs. Cor. Vet., 42:67, 1952.
92. Sanderson, A. T., and Anderson, L. J.: Histiocytosis in two pigs and a cow. Conditions resembling lipid storage disorders in man. J. Pathol., 100:207, 1970.
93. Sanderson, K. J.: The projection of the visual field to the lateral geniculate and medial interlaminar nuclei in the cat. J. Comp. Neurol., 143:101, 1971.
94. Sanderson, K. J., Guillery, R. W., and Shackelford, R. M.: Congenitally abnormal visual pathways in mink (*Mustela vison*) with reduced retinal pigment. J. Comp. Neurol., 154:225, 1974.
95. Sandstrom, B.: Glycogenosis of the central nervous system in the cat. Acta. Neuropathol., 14:194, 1969.
96. Scott, F. W., de Lahunta, A., Schultz, R. D., Bistner, S. I., and Riis, R. C.: Teratogenesis in cats associated with griseofulvin therapy. Teratology, 11:79, 1974.
97. Shively, J., Epling, G., and Jensen, R.: Fine structure of the canine eye: retina. Am. J. Vet. Res., 31:1339, 1970.
98. Shively, J. N., Epling, G. P., and Jensen, R.: Fine structure of the postnatal development of the canine retina. Am. J. Vet. Res., 32:383, 1971.
99. Singleton, M. C., and Peele, T. L.: Distribution of optic fibers in the cat. J. Comp. Neurol., 125:303, 1965.
100. Spratling, F. R., Bridge, P. S., Barnett, K. C., Abrams, J. T., Palmer, A. C., and Sharman, I. M.: Experimental hypovitaminosis A in calves. Vet. Rec., 77:532, 1965.
101. Stone, J.: The naso-temporal division of the cat's retina. J. Comp. Neurol., 126:585, 1966.
102. Stone, J.: A quantitative analysis of the distribution of ganglion cells in the cat's retina. J. Comp. Neurol., 124:337, 1965.
103. Stone, J., and Hansen, S. M.: The projection of the cat's retina in the lateral geniculate nucleus. J. Comp. Neurol., 126:601, 1966.
104. Weisse, I., and Stötzer, H.: Hypoplasie des Nervus opticus und Kolobom der Papille bei einem jungen Beagle. Berl. Münch. Tieraertzl. Wochenschr., 86:1, 1973.
105. Weisse, I., Stötzer, H., and Seitz, R.: Die neuroepitheliale Invagination, eine Form der Netzhaut-Dysplasie beim Beagle-Hund. Zentralbl. Veterinaermed., 20A:89, 1973.
106. Whittem, J. H., and Walker, D.: Neuronopathy and pseudolipidosis in Aberdeen-Angus calves. J. Pathol. Bacteriol., 74:281, 1957.
107. Wolff, E.: Anatomy of the Eye and Orbit. Philadelphia, W. B. Saunders Co., 1968.
108. Wyman, M., and Donovan, E. F.: The ocular fundus of the normal dog. J. Am. Vet. Med. Assoc., 147:17, 1965.
109. Yakely, W. L.: Collie eye anomaly: Decreased prevalence through selective breeding. J. Am. Vet. Med. Assoc., 160:1103, 1972.
110. Yakely, W. L., Wyman, M., Donovan, E. F., and Fechheimer, N. S.: Genetic transmission of an ocular fundus anomaly in collies. J. Am. Vet. Med. Assoc., 152:457, 1968.
111. Young, R. W., and Bok, D.: Participation of the retinal pigment epithelium in the rod outer segment renewal process. J. Cell. Biol., 42:392, 1969.
112. Denny-Brown, D., and Chambers, R. A.: Physiological aspects of visual perception. I. Functional aspects of visual cortex. Arch. Neurol., 33:219, 1976.
113. Denny-Brown, D., and Fischer, E. G.: Physiological aspects of visual perception. II. The subcortical visual direction of behavior. Arch. Neurol., 33:228, 1976.
114. LaVail, M. M.: Rod outer segment disk shedding in rat retina: Relationship to cyclic lighting. Science, 194:1071, 1976.

Chapter 14

AUDITORY SYSTEM—SPECIAL SOMATIC AFFERENT SYSTEM

ANATOMY
RECEPTOR
CRANIAL NERVE VIII—
    VESTIBULOCOCHLEAR NERVE—
    COCHLEAR DIVISION

BRAIN STEM NUCLEI AND TRACTS
THALAMOCORTICAL PATHWAY
DEAFNESS
Conduction Deafness and Nerve Deafness

ANATOMY

RECEPTOR[6, 21]

The development of the receptor for the auditory system was described with the development of the vestibular system. The cochlea, the coiled portion of the bony labyrinth, is a passageway in the petrosal bone that contains perilymph. The degree of coiling varies with the different species of animal. There are 3.25 turns in the dog cochlea compared to 2.5 in man. The portion of bone that forms the center or axis of the cochlea is the modiolus. At the base of the modiolus, the cochlea communicates with the vestibule. A shelf of bone projects into the cochlea from the modiolus. This is the spiral lamina that partially divides the cochlea into two portions, and is absent at the apex or most distal extent of the cochlea (Fig. 14–1).

The cochlear duct is the coiled portion of the membranous labyrinth that is located inside the cochlea and contains endolymph. It is a tubular structure that is situated between the spiral lamina on the medial wall of the cochlea (adjacent to the modiolus) and the opposite lateral wall of the cochlea. This completes the partitioning of the cochlea into two portions, each filled with perilymph: the scala vestibuli and scala tympani. The scala vestibuli is situated dorsal to the cochlear duct and communicates proximally with the vestibule and distally at the apex of the cochlear duct with the scala tympani. Because the cochlear duct does not reach the apex of the cochlea, this communication is possible. The site of communication is the helicotrema. The scala tympani is located ventral to the cochlear duct. It communicates distally at the helicotrema with the scala vestibuli. Proximally at the base of the coiled cochlea, it terminates at the cochlear window, which is covered by a membrane. On the other side of the cochlear window is the air-filled cavity of the middle ear in the tympanic bulla. Perilymph fills the scala vestibuli and scala tympani. At the level of the origin of the cochlea from

281

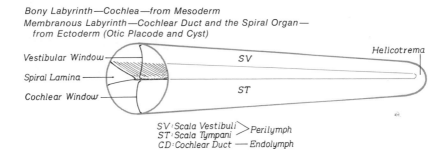

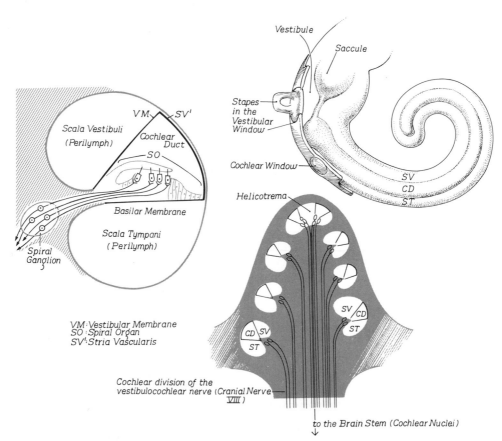

Figure 14–1.   Receptor of special somatic afferent system—auditory (SSA).

the vestibule, the cochlear duct communicates with the saccule by way of the ductus reuniens.

The cochlear duct is triangular in shape with its base, the stria vascularis and spiral prominence, situated along the outer lateral wall of the cochlea. A thin layer of tissue forms the dorsal border of the cochlear duct, the vestibular membrane. This borders the scala vestibuli and extends from the outer wall (dorsolaterally) to the middle of the medial wall, at the position of the spiral lamina. The basilar membrane, a highly organized layer of collagen-like fibers, extends from the spiral lamina (medially) to the middle of the lateral wall of the cochlea. The spiral organ (organ of Corti) is the sensory epithelium that rests on the basilar membrane, and is composed of several types of supporting cells and hair cells.[6] The hair cells have modified microvilli on their luminal surface, "hairs" or stereocilia. The tips of these cell processes (hairs) are embedded in a proteinaceous membrane, the tectorial membrane, which covers the hair cells and is attached medially along the cochlear duct. The dendritic zone of the cochlear portion of the eighth cranial nerve is in synaptic relationship with the base of the hair cells. Sound waves are transmitted from the air medium of the external ear canal to the solid medium of the tympanum and chain of three ear ossicles, which extend to the vestibular window, to the fluid medium of the perilymph in the scala vestibuli. Wave flow through the scala vestibuli is reflected to the basilar membrane by way of the endolymph of the cochlear duct or the scala tympani through its communication at the helicotrema. Movement of the highly organized basilar membrane causes the hair cells of the overlying spiral organ to move, and their stereocilia embedded in the tectorial membrane to bend. This action causes an impulse to be generated in the cochlear neurons. The basilar membrane acts like a resonator, and different portions respond maximally to specific frequencies of the sound waves. Low frequencies cause maximal vibration of the basilar membrane at the apex of the cochlear duct. High frequencies affect the proximal portion of the basilar membrane maximally.

CRANIAL NERVE VIII—VESTIBULOCOCHLEAR NERVE—COCHLEAR DIVISION

The dendritic zone of the cochlear division of the eighth cranial nerve is in synaptic relationship with the base of the hair cells in the spiral organ. The axons course medially into the modiolus. The cell bodies of these bipolar neurons are located in the modiolus at the origin of the spiral lamina, where they form the spiral ganglion. The axons course through the center or axis of the modiolus to the internal acoustic meatus, in which they join the vestibular division of the eighth cranial nerve. In the vestibulocochlear nerve the axons flow to the region of the cerebellomedullary angle at the junction of the medulla and pons, caudal to the transverse fibers of the pons. They terminate in telodendria on cell bodies located on the lateral side of the medulla, where the nerve enters. These cell bodies form the cochlear nuclei (dorsal and ventral) which bulge from the lateral side of the medulla, where they appear to be in the vestibulocochlear nerve.

BRAIN STEM NUCLEI AND TRACTS

The axons of the cell bodies in the cochlear nuclei pass into the medulla by two main pathways—ventrally through the trapezoid body, and dorsally over the caudal cerebellar peduncle by way of the acoustic stria.[8] Numerous pathways involving a variable number of synapses are available for the auditory system for reflex activity and conscious projection.

Reflexes are mediated by direct influence of neurons of the cochlear nuclei on the brain stem lower motor neuron, or indirectly by transmission through the neurons of the caudal colliculus or other auditory nuclei. Reflex regulation of sound wave frequency occurs by way of the afferent neurons of the cochlear division of the eighth cranial nerve and the cochlear nuclei, the efferent neurons of the motor nucleus of the trigeminal nerve in the pons that innervates the tensor tympani muscle, and the facial neurons that innervate the stapedius muscle.

Other neurons that belong to the auditory system and function in reflex and conscious perception pathways include the dorsal and ventral nuclei of the trapezoid body, the nucleus of the lateral lemniscus, and the caudal colliculus. The neurons of the ventral nucleus of the trapezoid body are scattered without specific arrangement throughout the trapezoid fibers. The dorsal nucleus of the trapezoid body forms a distinctly encapsulated nucleus ventrally in the rostral medulla, dorsal to the trapezoid body and dorsolateral to the pyramid, from the level of the facial nucleus in the medulla to the motor nucleus of the trigeminal nerve in the pons.[14] The lateral lemniscus is composed mostly of ascending axons in the auditory system, coursing from the rostral medulla through the pons to the caudal mesencephalon on the lateral surface of the brain stem.[9] It contains auditory axons from the cochlear nuclei or the various nuclei of the trapezoid body on the same or opposite sides. The lateral lemniscus is formed medial to the middle cerebellar peduncle, and is exposed on the lateral surface of the caudal mesencephalon rostral to the transverse fibers of the pons that form the middle cerebellar peduncle. Embedded along the ventromedial aspect of this lemniscus is the nucleus of the lateral lemniscus. The lateral lemniscus terminates at the caudal colliculus.

The caudal colliculus consists of cell bodies of neurons and axonal processes organized in laminae.[20] It is a reflex center for the auditory system. Efferent axons project to brain stem lower motor neurons by way of the tectobulbar pathways and to the cervical spinal cord through the tectospinal pathway in the ventral funiculus, which arises from the rostral colliculus.

THALAMOCORTICAL PATHWAY

Axons in the conscious projection pathway arise primarily from cell bodies in the caudal colliculus, and project in the brachium of the caudal colliculus located on the lateral side of the mesencephalon coursing rostrally to the medial geniculate nucleus of the thalamus.[25] This nucleus extends caudally beside the mesencephalon. It is the specific thalamic projection nucleus for the auditory system and projects axons by way of the internal capsule to the cerebral cortex of the temporal lobe. The auditory sensory cortex is located mostly in the sylvian and ectosylvian gyri. Studies in the dog have localized the auditory conscious projection pathway to the ectosylvian gyrus, in which the various frequencies can be arranged from rostral (high frequency) to caudal (low frequency).[27, 28, 29]

The ascending auditory pathway is characterized by diffuseness and a bilateral distribution. Despite this, at the cortical level there is a predominance of contralateral representation of each cochlear duct. Thus impulses stimulated

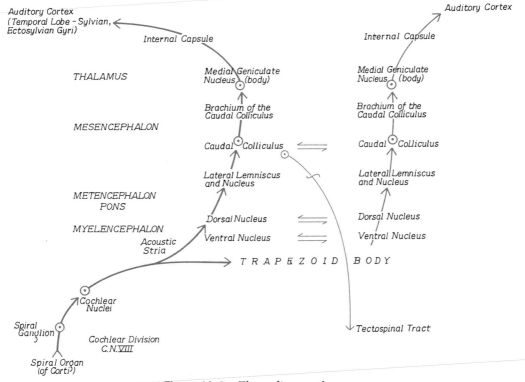

Figure 14–2.   The auditory pathway.

primarily in one cochlear duct are conducted primarily to the opposite temporal lobe. Crossing occurs at the level of the trapezoid body, between the nuclei of the lateral lemniscus and at the commissure of the caudal colliculus.

DEAFNESS[26]

Partial loss of hearing and even unilateral complete loss of hearing are difficult to establish on clinical examination of domestic animals. Complete bilateral deafness usually is caused by direct or indirect interference with the function of the receptor organ. For central lesions to produce deafness, there must be extensive damage to both cerebral hemispheres or to the pathways on both sides of the brain stem. Such lesions most likely would produce severe neurologic deficit referable to the interference with the other systems adjacent to the auditory pathways. Because of the multitude of brain stem pathways available for the auditory system, there is a large margin of safety for this function. Therefore, when presented with a deaf animal attention should be directed to those diseases that affect the receptor portion of this system. The best test for total deafness is to confront the sleeping patient with a loud noise. Inability to arouse the patient in this manner is the best evidence of total inability to hear. Less obvious degrees of deafness are difficult to evaluate, and the careful observations of the patient in its own environment by the owner may be the most reliable.

More sophisticated procedures have been developed, and include a technique of monitoring changes in respirations in response to hearing sounds, as well as recording electroencephalographic responses to auditory stimuli.[5]

Conduction Deafness and Nerve Deafness

There are two kinds of peripheral deafness, conduction and nerve deafness. Conduction deafness involves an abnormality in the gaseous or solid media that transmit the sound waves to the perilymph of the cochlea. The receptor is functional, and responds to vibrations induced in the petrosal bone by a tuning fork, but does not respond to sound waves that are unable to reach the receptor. Diseases that obliterate the external ear canal, rupture the tympanum, or interfere with the function of the ear ossicles in the middle ear produce conduction deafness.

Nerve deafness involves an abnormality in the receptor organ itself.[2, 15, 16, 23] Congenital deafness has been reported in dogs and cats caused by a lesion—degeneration, hypoplasia, or aplasia—of the spiral organ.[1, 12, 18] Frequently, the affected animals have a white hair coat.[3, 4, 11, 21, 30] There is a high incidence of congenital deafness in white cats with blue irises in which the white color is dependent on a dominant autosomal gene that has complete penetrance for white fur and incomplete penetrance for the production of a blue iris and deafness.

Congenital deafness has been observed frequently in Old English sheepdogs. It often is accompanied by a failure of pigmentation of the iris and retina and choroid. A familial trend has been observed, but the form of inheritance has not been proved. These cats and dogs with pigmentary disorders and deafness can be compared to children with similar anomalies, referred to as the Waardenburg syndrome.[7] Individuals representing many breeds of dogs have been observed with this condition. The deficit is present from birth and is permanent. An hereditary pattern has been suggested for cocker spaniels, Dalmatians, and bull terriers.[13]

Signs suggestive of a congenital bilateral vestibular disturbance have been observed in beagle puppies that have been born deaf. These include ataxia, abnormal head orientation with occasional continuous bobbing or rotatory movements, and a lack of ability to produce nystagmus. Genetic data suggest a recessive inheritance of an abnormality of development of both the vestibular and auditory receptors in the membranous labyrinth.

Ototoxicity occurs following the prolonged use of certain antibiotics.[10, 13, 17, 19] Streptomycin, neomycin, and kanamycin are drugs known to produce degeneration of the hair cells of the receptors of the vestibular system, or auditory system, or both. The specific effect depends on the chemical form of the antibiotic, the dose, and the species receiving it.

Inflammatory disease of the middle ear and inner ear that destroys the receptor of the auditory system produces deafness. This is most obvious in the animal affected bilaterally.[24]

The geriatric patient that is progressively losing its ability to hear probably has a progressive degeneration of the receptor organ or the chain of ossicles in the middle ear.

REFERENCES

1. Adams, E. W.: Hereditary deafness in a family of foxhounds. J. Am. Vet. Med. Assoc., *128*:302, 1956.
2. Altmann, F.: Histologic picture of inherited nerve deafness in man and animals. Arch. Oto-laryngol., *51*:852, 1950.
3. Bergsma, D. R., and Brown, K. S.: White fur, blue eyes, and deafness in the domestic cat. J. Hered., *62*:171, 1971.
4. Bosher, S. K., and Hallpike, C. S.: Observations on the histologic features, development, and pathogenesis of the inner ear degeneration of the deaf white cat. Proc. R. Soc. [Biol.] Series B, *162*:147, 1965.
5. Bradford, Z. J., McKinley, J. H., Rousey, C. L., and Klein, D. E.: Measurement of hearing in dogs by respiration audiometry. Am. J. Vet. Res., *34*:1183, 1973.
6. Engström, H., and Ades, H. W.: The ultrastructure of the organ of Corti. *In* Friedmann, I., ed., The Ultrastructure of Sensory Organs. Amsterdam, North Holland Publishing Co., 1973, 83–151.
7. Faith, R. E., and Woodard, J. C.: Animal models of human disease: Waardenburg's syndrome. Comp. Pathol. Bull., *5*:3, 1973.
8. Fernandez, C., and Karapas, F.: The course and termination of the striae of Monakow and Held in the cat. J. Comp. Neurol., *131*:371, 1967.
9. Goldberg, J. M., and Moore, R. Y.: Ascending projections of the lateral lemniscus in the cat and monkey. J. Comp. Neurol., *129*:143, 1967.
10. Hawkins, J. R., and Lurie, M. H.: The ototoxicity of dihydrostreptomycin and neomycin in the cat. Ann. Otol. Rhinol. Laryngol., *62*:1128, 1953.
11. Howe, H. A.: The reaction of the cochlear nerve to destruction of its end organ: A study of deaf albino cats. J. Comp. Neurol., *62*:72, 1935.
12. Igarashi, M., Alford, B. R., Cohn, A. M., Saito, R., and Watanabe, T.: Inner ear anomalies in dogs. Ann. Otol. Rhinol. Laryngol., *81*:249, 1972.
13. Innes, J. R. M., and Saunders, L. Z.: Comparative Neuropathology. New York, Academic Press, 1962.
14. Irving, R., and Harrison, J. M.: The superior olivary complex and audition: A comparative study. J. Comp. Neurol., *130*:77, 1967.
15. Johnsson, L.-G., and Hawkins, J. E.: Symposium on basic ear research. II. Strial atrophy in clinical and experimental deafness. Laryngoscope, *81*:1105, 1972.
16. Johnsson, L.-G., and Hawkins, J. E.: A direct approach to cochlear anatomy and pathology in man. Arch. Otolaryngol., *85*:43, 1967.
17. Kohonen, A.: Affect of some ototoxic drugs upon the pattern and innervation of cochlear sensory cells in the guinea pig. Acta Otolaryngol. (Stockholm) Suppl., *208*:1, 1965.
18. Lurie, M. H.: The membranous labyrinth in the congenitally deaf collie and Dalmatian dog. Laryngoscope, *58*:279, 1948.
19. McGee, T. M., and Olszewski, J.: Streptomycin sulfate and dihydrostreptomycin toxicity; behavioral and histopathologic studies. Arch. Otolaryngol., *75*:295, 1962.
20. Merzenich, M. M., and Reid, M. D.: Representation of the cochlea within the inferior colliculus of the cat. Brain Res., *77*:397, 1974.
21. Pujol, R., and Marty, R.: Postnatal maturation in the cochlea of the cat. J. Comp. Neurol., *139*:115, 1970.
22. Roberts, S.: Color dilution and hereditary defects in collie dogs. Am. J. Ophthalmol., *63*:1762, 1967.
23. Saunders, L. Z.: The histopathology of hereditary congenital deafness in white mink. Pathol. Vet., *2*:256, 1965.
24. Spreull, J. S. A.: Treatment of otitis media in the dog. J. Sm. Anim. Pract., *5*:107, 1964.
25. Strominger, N. L., and Oesterreich, R. E.: Localization of sound after section of the brachium of the inferior colliculus. J. Comp. Neurol., *138*:1, 1970.
26. Torok, N.: A review of neuro-otology pathogenesis of neuro-otological diseases. Am. J. Med. Sci., *246*:154, 1963.
27. Tunturi, A. R.: Audio frequency localization in the acoustic cortex of the dog. Am. J. Physiol., *141*:397, 1944.
28. Tunturi, A. R.: Classification of neurons in the ectosylvian auditory cortex of the dog. J. Comp. Neurol., *142*:153, 1971.
29. Tunturi, A. R.: The pathway from the medial geniculate body to the ectosylvian auditory cortex in the dog. J. Comp. Neurol., *138*:131, 1970.
30. Wolff, D.: Three generations of deaf white cats. J. Hered., *33*:39, 1942.

Chapter 15

VISCERAL AFFERENT SYSTEMS

GENERAL VISCERAL AFFERENT
  SYSTEM
ANATOMY
Receptor—Peripheral Nerves
Brain Stem Nuclei and Tracts

FUNCTIONAL CONCEPTS
SPECIAL VISCERAL AFFERENT
  SYSTEM—TASTE
SPECIAL VISCERAL AFFERENT
  SYSTEM—SMELL

GENERAL VISCERAL AFFERENT SYSTEM

ANATOMY

Receptor—Peripheral Nerves

The receptors of the general visceral afferent system are located throughout the viscera of the body, in which they are stimulated by a number of different modalities.[5, 15] Stretch, distention, or pressure on or in a viscus are the most common modalities. Some receptors are sensitive to chemical changes in the environment. Free endings and a variety of encapsulated ones are found at the dendritic zone of the neurons in this system. The axons course over the peripheral nerves most available to the viscus. In the head these are the facial nerve to the middle ear and blood vessels of the head, the glossopharyngeal nerve to the caudal tongue, pharynx, and carotid body and sinus, and the vagus nerve to the pharynx and larynx. In the thoracic and abdominal cavities these are the vagus nerve and the peripheral branches of the sympathetic trunk, the splanchnic nerves. Here in the body cavities the general visceral afferent (GVA) axons course toward the central nervous system in nerves that contain neurons of the parasympathetic and sympathetic portions of the general visceral efferent system. Visceral afferent axons from the peripheral blood vessels course through peripheral nerves to the segmental spinal nerves.

The cell bodies of these GVA neurons are located in the geniculate ganglion of the facial nerve, the distal ganglia of the glossopharyngeal and vagus nerves, and the spinal ganglia of the involved spinal nerves.[3, 14]

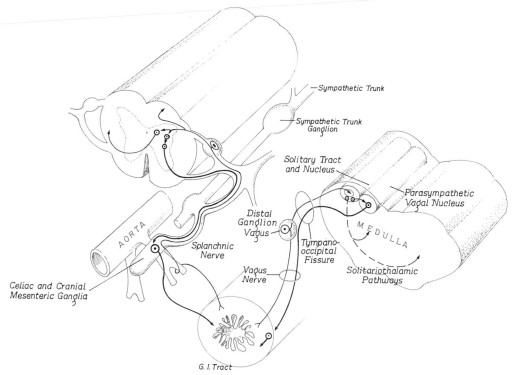

Figure 15–1. General visceral afferent system. Reversal of the GVE sympathetic pathway (conscious perception) and parasympathetic pathway (reflex function).

Brain Stem Nuclei and Tracts

The axons continue from the various ganglia into the central nervous system. Those axons in the facial, glossopharyngeal, and vagus nerves enter the ventrolateral aspect of the medulla and course to a position near the lateral aspect of the fourth ventricle adjacent to the sulcus limitans. There the axons course rostrally and caudally in a column called the solitary tract. This tract is surrounded by neurons forming the nucleus of the solitary tract, in which the axons in the tract terminate. This solitary tract and its nucleus develop in the alar plate adjacent to the motor column of the general visceral efferent system; therefore it is found dorsolateral to the parasympathetic nucleus of the facial, glossopharyngeal, and vagal nerves. The solitary tract stands out in myelin-stained sections as a densely stained cylindrical structure surrounded by the unstained cell bodies of its nucleus. It extends from the level of the facial nucleus (special visceral efferent) rostrally to caudal to the obex. Caudally the gracilic and medial cuneate nuclei are dorsal to it. Rostrally the medial vestibular nucleus is dorsal to it.

The nucleus of the solitary tract probably participates mostly in reflex activity and projects to the cell bodies in the general visceral efferent column directly or indirectly by way of interneurons in the reticular formation that participate in the various metabolic centers regulating visceral function—respiratory, cardiovascular, swallowing, micturition.[8]

Some cell bodies in the nucleus of the solitary tract project axons rostrally in a pathway for conscious projection. These course mostly on the contralateral side of the brain stem in an ill-defined solitariothalamic pathway that closely parallels the medial lemniscus and spinothalamic pathway. These axons terminate at a synapse in the ventral caudal medial nucleus of the thalamus, which in turn projects axons via the internal capsule to the somesthetic cortex.

The axons of the general visceral afferent system receptors in the body cavities that course centrally over the splanchnic nerves follow in a reverse pathway from that taken by the motor neurons of the general visceral efferent system. From the sympathetic trunk the axons course by way of the rami communicantes to the spinal nerve and the dorsal root. The cell body is located in the corresponding spinal ganglion. The axon continues over the dorsal root into the dorsal grey column of the spinal cord, and terminates on a neuronal cell body located there.

Passing through interneurons in the grey matter, the reflex pathway can be completed by synapse on a preganglionic cell body in the intermediate grey column (T1–L5). The pathway for conscious projection involves synapse of the GVA axon in the dorsal root on a cell body in the dorsal grey column whose axon enters the same or opposite lateral funiculus and courses cranially along with the axons of the spinothalamic system. This is probably a multisynaptic system which follows the same course as that of the spinothalamic system (general somatic afferent), including synapse in the ventral caudal lateral thalamic nucleus for projection to the somesthetic cortex.

There is some evidence that from the body cavities, the GVA neurons in the vagus nerve are concerned mostly with reflex activity, and those entering the spinal cord by way of the sympathetic trunk are concerned mostly with the conscious projection of visceral afferent stimuli—the source of "visceral pain."[13]

In addition to these pathways from the dendritic zone to the central nervous system, there is now evidence that some GVA neurons reside entirely within the wall of the viscus in an enteric plexus in which intrinsic reflex activity can occur.

FUNCTIONAL CONCEPTS

Most smooth muscle regulation is involuntary, and occurs at a reflex level not reaching the level of conscious perception. The enteric plexus within the wall of the bowel may function autonomously, independent of its extrinsic nerve supply and the central nervous system. Pacemaker activity has been recognized in selected areas of the bowel. Visceral surfaces are mostly insensitive to many of the stimuli which the surface of the body is sensitive to. There is no conscious perception of touching, pinching, or cutting normal viscera. This is exemplified by the rumenotomy or cesarian section, which are performed with local anesthesia of the body wall and parietal peritoneum. The wall of the rumen or uterus is incised without anesthesia and without discomfort to the patient.

Conscious perception of visceral sensation—visceral pain—occurs following tension or distention of the wall of the viscus or traction on its mesentery. Diseased, inflamed visceral surfaces are sensitive to touching and cutting. Loss of blood supply (ischemia) to the wall of the viscera is a source of visceral pain.

Visceral pain is poorly localized to its specific source, being reflected as a dull, deep pain in the body cavity. This may reflect the fact that compared to the general somatic afferent system there are fewer general visceral afferent neurons, and they are stimulated only occasionally by modalities that are conducted to the level of conscious perception. Thus the cerebrum has little experience with localizing the source of these modalities, which come from structures that cannot be visualized. This provides part of the basis for the phenomenon of referred pain, in which a specific area of the body surface is hypersensitive and seems to be where the pain is coming from.

In referred pain the visceral pain is referred to the surface of the body supplied by sensory neurons whose axons terminate in the same segment of the spinal cord and on the same cells as the visceral afferents. Thus there is a dermatomal distribution to referred visceral pain, and the surface of the body can be mapped to represent the areas of pain referral for the various visceral organs. For example, the diaphragm is referred to the shoulder and neck region innervated by general somatic afferent neurons in cervical nerves 5, 6, and 7. The stomach is referred to the midthorax region (T6–T9). The ureter is referred to the area of the scrotum (L3, L4). Many theories have been proposed to explain this phenomenon. The common pool theory proposes that both the GSA and GVA neurons synapse in the dorsal grey column on the same cell bodies for the conscious projection pathway by way of the spinothalamic system. The GSA system is stimulated frequently, while the GVA system is stimulated only occasionally. The site of the stimulus from the GSA system is recognized easily on the surface of the body, and the brain has "learned" the source of the stimulus. When the same dorsal grey column neurons are stimulated by excessive activity in the GVA system, the brain misinterprets the source and refers it to the origin of the GSA neurons.

The viscerovisceral reflex arc theory proposes that excessive GVA stimulation causes a reflex spasm of peripheral somatic blood vessels by way of GVE sympathetic motor neurons in the same spinal cord segments. Release or accumulation

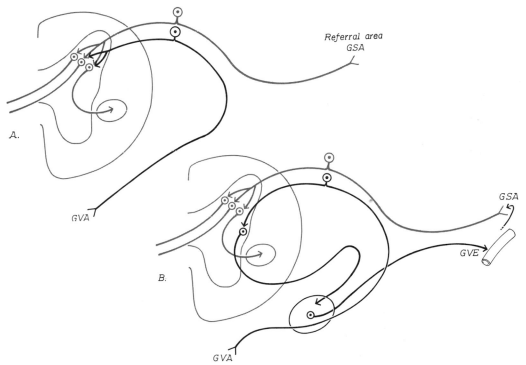

Figure 15–2. Anatomy of the dermatomal rule for referred visceral pain. *A:* Theory of common pool of neurons for GSA and GVA that project to the brain. *B:* Theory of a GVA viscerovisceral reflex arc causing tonic spasm of peripheral blood vessels which alters tissue metabolism with the accumulation of byproducts that stimulate the local GSA receptors.

of abnormal substances at the site of the vasospasm then stimulates the dendritic zone of the GSA neurons in that area of GVE distribution. These impulses are conducted into the segmental dorsal grey column and projected to the somesthetic cortex, which projects the pain to the body surface innervated by the GSA system.

SPECIAL VISCERAL AFFERENT SYSTEM—TASTE

The primary receptors for the sense of taste, the gustatory sense, are responsive to chemical agents taken into the mouth and are organized in the form of small structures, taste buds, associated with the various glossal papillae. Taste buds also occur in the soft palate, pharynx, larynx, lips, and cheeks. The neuroepithelial taste cells surround a pit, the taste pore. Short cytoplasmic processes, taste hairs, protrude into the lumen, in which they are "sensitive" to chemical substances dissolved in the saliva in the pit. There is a rapid turnover of the neuroepithelial receptor cells in the taste bud.[1, 2, 12]

These neuroepithelial receptor cells are in synaptic relationship with the dendritic zone of the special visceral afferent neurons. The cell bodies of these neurons are in the geniculate ganglion of the facial nerve, and the distal ganglia of the glossopharyngeal and vagus nerves. The facial neurons are distributed to the palate and rostral two thirds of the tongue by way of branches of the trigeminal nerve.[14] The glossopharyngeal nerve innervates taste buds in the caudal one third of the tongue and the rostral pharynx. The vagus innervates taste buds in the caudal pharynx and the larynx.

The course and central pathway for reflex activity and conscious perception are the same as those described for the general visceral afferent system neurons in these three cranial nerves. In the cat, taste perception is located primarily in the presylvian gyrus.[4, 9, 10]

The perception of taste is a psychological phenomenon involving the central projection of many afferent systems and the role of higher centers such as the limbic system, which contributes the factors of memory of past experiences. Although the primary afferent is the chemoreceptor in the taste bud, thermoreceptors and mechanoreceptors in the oral cavity and pharynx and olfactory receptors also contribute to the sensation.[7]

SPECIAL VISCERAL AFFERENT SYSTEM—SMELL

The telencephalon can be subdivided on a developmental evolutionary basis into the archipallium, the paleopallium, and the neopallium. The archipallium and paleopallium comprise the rhinencephalon or the "smell brain." On an anatomic and functional basis, the rhinencephalon consists of an olfactory portion (paleopallium) and a nonolfactory portion or limbic system (archipallium). The limbic system has evolved extensively in the higher species of mammals, and in addition to the telencephalon involves nuclei and tracts in the brain stem.

The olfactory (paleopallial) portion of the rhinencephalon is the special visceral afferent system designed for the conscious perception of smell. The nonolfactory portion or limbic system is concerned with the emotional response to afferent stimuli, one of which is the olfactory special visceral afferent system.

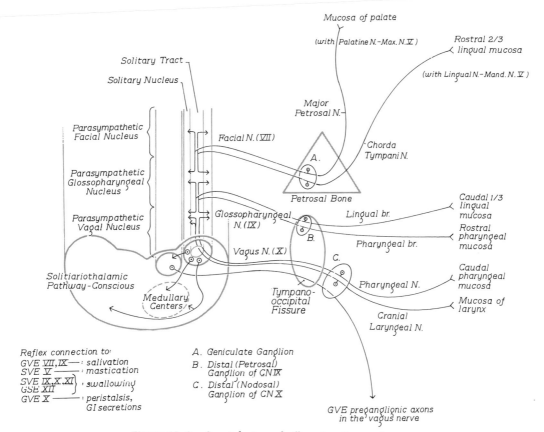

Figure 15–3. Special visceral afferent pathways for taste.

The specialized chemoreceptor of the olfactory rhinencephalon is a bipolar neuron located in the olfactory epithelium of the nasal mucosa of the caudal part of the nasal cavity. The cell body and dendritic zone reside in the epithelium. Six to eight long cilia project from the apex of the olfactory cell and lie in the secretion on the surface of the olfactory epithelium, where they are stimulated by chemical substances dissolved in the secretions.[6, 11] The axon courses away from the cell body into the connective tissue of the nasal mucosa, and joins with the other axons to form the olfactory nerves—cranial nerve I. These pass through the foramina in the cribriform plate of the ethmoid bone and into the olfactory bulbs, in which the telodendria synapse with the dendritic zones of the neurons of the olfactory bulb. These are brush (tufted) and mitral cells. Many olfactory neurons converge on a few neurons of the olfactory bulb.

The axons of the mitral cells of the olfactory bulb project through the olfactory tract and lateral olfactory stria to the ipsilateral olfactory cortex over the pyriform lobe. Synapse may occur with neurons in the cortex of the olfactory peduncle (lateral olfactory gyrus), or lateral stria, or in the olfactory tubercle,

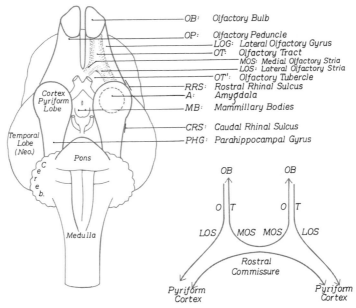

OLFACTORY RHINENCEPHALON

OB: Olfactory Bulb
OP: Olfactory Peduncle
LOG: Lateral Olfactory Gyrus
OT: Olfactory Tract
MOS: Medial Olfactory Stria
LOS: Lateral Olfactory Stria
OT': Olfactory Tubercle
RRS: Rostral Rhinal Sulcus
A: Amygdala
MB: Mammillary Bodies
CRS: Caudal Rhinal Sulcus
PHG: Parahippocampal Gyrus

Figure 15–4.   Anatomy of the special visceral afferent olfactory system.

which is a nucleus located between the lateral and medial olfactory striae. The majority of the central olfactory projections are ipsilateral and project to the pyriform cortex without a relay through a thalamic nucleus.

The functions of the two olfactory bulbs are correlated by axons of the brush neurons in the olfactory bulb that course through ipsilateral olfactory tract and medial olfactory stria, the rostral commissure, and the contralateral medial olfactory stria and olfactory tract to the contralateral olfactory bulb. The olfactory peduncle includes the olfactory tract and the adjacent cortex of the lateral olfactory gyrus ventral to the rostral lateral rhinal sulcus. Commissural fibers in the rostral commissure also pass between the cortices of the two pyriform lobes.

This is the conscious perception pathway for the olfactory—special visceral afferent—system. The so-called reflex pathway involves projections into the nuclear areas of the limbic system. Axons in the medial olfactory stria enter the septal area (septal nuclei and subcallosal area). Axons in the lateral olfactory stria enter the amygdaloid nucleus and hippocampus. These provide pathways for the olfactory system to enter nuclei of the limbic system.

The development of the olfactory portion of the rhinencephalon (the SVA system) varies extensively among species of mammals. In the dog, the sense of smell is highly developed functionally and anatomically, and this is referred to as a macrosmatic species. Primates are microsmatic, lacking a well-developed olfactory system.

Experimental lesions in one olfactory bulb or peduncle produce unilateral anosmia. Bilateral lesions in the olfactory bulbs, peduncles, or pyriform lobes cause complete anosmia. Lesions in any part of the nonolfactory portion of the rhinencephalon, the limbic system, do not interfere with the sense of smell.

Deficiencies in the sense of smell are difficult to verify by clinical testing. The owner's observations of the animal's behavior on sensing the presence of food or game in the field may be more reliable information. Substances such as cloves, cinnamon, perfume, xylol, or benzol can be used, but one must be careful of irritating chemicals that stimulate the general somatic afferent neurons of the trigeminal nerve which are distributed in the nasal mucosa. The most common cause of complete anosmia is severe rhinitis with involvement of the olfactory nasal mucosa. Head injury may cause a shearing off of the olfactory nerves as they pass through the cribriform plate, resulting in anosmia.

REFERENCES

1. Beidler, L. M., and Smallman, R. L.: Renewal of cells within taste buds. J. Cell Biol., 27:263, 1965.
2. Bell, F. R., and Kitchell, R. L.: Taste reception in the goat, sheep, and calf. J. Physiol., 183:145, 1966.
3. Cottle, M. K.: Degeneration studies of primary afferents of the IXth and Xth cranial nerves in the cat. J. Comp. Neurol., 122:329, 1964.
4. Emmers, R.: Localization of thalamic projection of afferents from the tongue in the cat. Anat. Rec., 148:67, 1964.
5. Fletcher, T. F., and Bradley, W. E.: Afferent nerve endings in the urinary bladder of the cat. Am. J. Anat., 128:147, 1970.
6. Graziadei, P. P. C.: The ultrastructure of vertebrate olfactory mucosa. In Friedmann, I., ed., The Ultrastructure of Sensory Organs. Amsterdam, North Holland Publishing Co., 1973, 267–306.
7. Kitchell, R. L.: Newer knowledge on taste in dogs and cats. Gaines Vet. Symp., 14:15, 1964.
8. Morest, D. K.: Experimental study of the projections of the nucleus of the tractus solitarius and the area postrema in the cat. J. Comp. Neurol., 130:277, 1967.
9. Morrison, A. R., Hand, P. J., and Ruderman, M. I.: Cortical gustatory and facial somesthetic areas of the cat as revealed by an anatomicophysiological technique. Anat. Rec., 172:462, 1972.
10. Morrison, A. R., and Tarnecki, R.: A new location for the gustatory cortex of the cat. Anat. Rec., 181:431, 1975.
11. Moulton, D. G., and Beidler, L. M.: Structure and function in the peripheral olfactory system. Physiol. Rev., 47:1, 1967.
12. Murray, R. G.: The ultrastructure of taste buds. In Friedmann, I., ed., The Ultrastructure of Sensory Organs. Amsterdam, North Holland Publishing Co., 1973, 3–81.
13. Paintal, A. S.: Vagal sensory receptors and their reflex effects. Physiol. Rev., 53:159, 1973.
14. Rhoton, A. L., Jr.: Afferent connections of the facial nerve. J. Comp. Neurol., 133:89, 1968.
15. Vemura, E., Fletcher, T. F., and Bradley, W. E.: Distribution of lumbar afferent axons in muscle coat of cat urinary bladder. Am. J. Anat., 139:389, 1974.

Chapter 16

NONOLFACTORY RHINENCEPHALON: LIMBIC SYSTEM

ANATOMY
TELENCEPHALON
DIENCEPHALON

MESENCEPHALON
FUNCTION

The limbic system is the name given for the nonolfactory portion of the rhinencephalon, which includes the archipallium of the telencephalon. The term refers to the anatomic arrangement of the telencephalic nuclei and tracts that are components of this system, and are arranged as two incomplete ring-like structures on the medial aspect of the telencephalon at its border with the diencephalon. Limbus refers to border, and these telencephalic structures border the main mass of the cerebral vesicle. The term has been expanded in usage to include the major nuclei and pathways in the rostral brain stem that are connected with these telencephalic structures anatomically and functionally.

ANATOMY

TELENCEPHALON

The telencephalic components of the limbic system form two "cortical rings" at the border of the diencephalic-telencephalic junction. The inner ring consists of the amygdaloid body, the hippocampus, and the fornix. The outer ring consists of the cingulum, the cingulate gyrus, and the septal area.

The amygdaloid body, one of the basal nuclei of the telencephalon, is a complex of nuclei located in the pyriform lobe deep within the olfactory cortex. A projection pathway, the stria terminalis, passes in the angle between the thalamus and caudate nucleus in a caudal, dorsal, rostral, and ventral direction to terminate in the septal area and rostral hypothalamus. A diagonal band courses on the ventral surface of the cerebrum and connects the amygdaloid body with the septal area.

The hippocampus is a unique gyrus of the cerebrum that has been rolled into the lateral ventricle in which it is found, forming part of the medial and ventral wall of the lateral ventricle dorsally, and the medial and dorsal wall of the ventricle ventrally. The hippocampus extends from the amygdaloid body in each

296

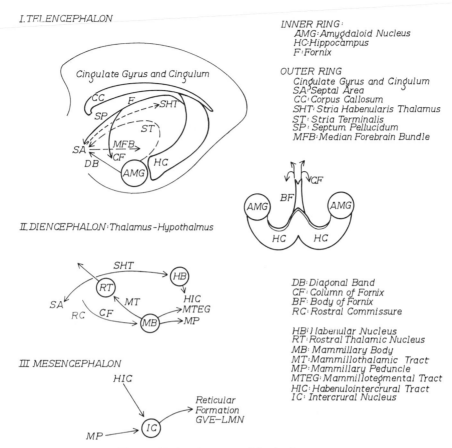

Figure 16–1. Anatomy of the limbic system.

pyriform lobe in a curve, progressing caudally and then dorsally and rostrally over the diencephalon, from which it is separated by meninges. Dorsal to the caudal thalamus the hippocampi from each side meet at the median plane and a commissure is formed there, the hippocampal commissure. Caudal to the pyriform lobe the hippocampus is covered superficially by the parahippocampal gyrus, which is bounded laterally by the caudal lateral rhinal sulcus and medially where it joins the hippocampus by the hippocampal sulcus. The parahippocampal gyrus is continued dorsally, dorsal to the corpus callosum, by the cingulate gyrus.

Axons course to and from the hippocampus along its lateral side, forming the fimbria and crus of the fornix. The two crura meet rostral to the hippocampal commissure and pass rostrally as the bodies of the fornix. After coursing rostrally they turn ventrally at the level of the rostral commissure; here the two bodies separate and form the distinctly cylindrical columns of the fornix. Each column splits at the rostral commissure and a small bundle courses rostrally into the septal area. The larger portion of the column passes caudal to the rostral commissure (postcommissural column) and ventrally through the hypothalamus on either side of the third ventricle to terminate in the mammillary body on either side. The body and proximal column of the fornix are attached dorsally to the corpus callosum by the septum pellucidum. There are leptomeninges ventral to the body of the fornix rostrally to the level of the interventricular foramen.

The cingulum is the long association tract forming the longitudinal fibers in the white matter of the cingulate gyrus. These fibers course from the parahippocampal gyrus caudally to the septal area and frontal lobe gyri rostrally. The cingulate gyrus is the cerebral cortex covering the cingulum that is located dorsal to the corpus callosum and is continuous caudally with the parahippocampal gyrus and rostrally with the septal area.

The septal area consists of the subcallosal area, which is the cerebral cortex ventral to the genu of the corpus callosum and the septal nuclei. These nuclei are nuclear masses in the ventral septum pellucidum protruding into the lateral ventricle from the medial side. The septal area connects with the hippocampus by way of the adjacent columns of the fornix, with the amygdaloid body through the diagonal band and stria terminalis, and with the habenular nuclei via the stria habenularis thalamus. The medial forebrain bundle passes caudally from the septal area into the hypothalamus. By way of this pathway, limbic system efferents can influence the hypothalamic centers that control the activity of the general visceral efferent system.

The function of the limbic system involves visceral motor activation. The hypothalamic nuclei serve as the upper motor neuron that regulates the general visceral efferent system. These hypothalamic nuclei, as well as the brain stem GVE lower motor neuron, receive numerous limbic system efferents.

DIENCEPHALON

In the thalamus the habenular nucleus and the rostral thalamic nucleus function mainly in the limbic system. The habenular nucleus is located adjacent to the third ventricle rostral to the pineal body. It connects with the telencephalic septal area by way of the stria habenularis thalamus located on either side of the dorsal thalamus adjacent to the third ventricle. It connects with the intercrural nucleus of the mesencephalon via the habenulo-intercrural tract. The rostral thalamic nucleus receives afferents from the mammillary body of the hypothalamus through the mamillothalamic tract. The rostral thalamic nucleus projects predominantly to the cingulate gyrus and adjacent neopallium.

The limbic system component of the hypothalamus is the mammillary body. The paired mammillary bodies are located adjacent to the ventral midline caudal to the infundibulum of the hypophysis in the most caudal portion of the hypothalamus. They connect with the hippocampus by way of the columns of the fornix, and with the rostral thalamic nucleus via the mammillothalamic tract. The paired columns of the fornix and mammillothalamic tracts pass through the hypothalamus adjacent to the third ventricle. In addition to these pathways, the mammillary bodies connect with the mesencephalic tegmentum and the visceral motor column in the medulla through the mamillotegmental tract. The mammillary peduncle courses caudally to the mesencephalic intercrural nucleus.

MESENCEPHALON

The intercrural nucleus is the only limbic system nucleus in the mesencephalon. It is located between the two crus cerebri on the ventral surface of the mesencephalon on the floor of the intercrural fossa. It connects with the habenular nucleus by way of the habenulointercrural tract, the mammillary bodies via the mammillary peduncle, and the reticular formation of the brain stem, which in turn influences the visceral motor column—general visceral efferent lower motor neuron in the medulla.

TABLE 16–1. NONOLFACTORY RHINENCEPHALON: LIMBIC SYSTEM. SUMMARY OF MAJOR STRUCTURES

I. Telencephalon:
  A. Inner cortical ring
      Amygdaloid body
      Hippocampus
         Fimbria-fornix—septal area, hypothalamus, mammillary bodies
  B. Outer cortical ring
      Cingulum and gyrus
      Septal area
         Medial forebrain bundle—hypothalamus: brain stem LMN—GVE
II. Diencephalon:
  A. Thalamus
      Habenular nucleus
        Stria habenularis thalamus
        Habenular intercrural tract
      Rostral thalamic nucleus
  B. Hypothalamus
      Mammillary bodies
        Mammillothalamic tract
        Mammillotegmental tract—reticular formation
III. Mesencephalon:
      Intercrural nucleus—reticular formation

FUNCTION

The limbic system receives and associates afferent impulses from the olfactory (SVA), optic (SSA), auditory (SSA), exteroceptive (GSA), and interoceptive (GVA) sensory systems. It projects predominantly on the hypothalamus and caudal brain stem primarily influencing the visceral motor column.

The limbic system is involved with mostly emotional or behavioral patterns. Emotion involves visceral reaction, which is controlled largely by the autonomic nervous system. This system is regulated centrally by the hypothalamus, which accounts for the multitude of connections of the limbic system with the hypothalamus.

The limbic system is considered to function in man as the higher center controlling the psychic and motor aspects of behavior. It is the portion of the brain involved in man's basic drives, sexual activity, emotional experience, memories, and fears and pleasures.[4, 6, 10, 17]

James Papez, professor of neurology at Cornell University, suggested in 1937 that the part of the rhinencephalon now classified as the limbic system was concerned with activity other than the perception of smell.[19] Following his observations of the distribution of the rabies lesion in dogs in these rhinencephalic structures and the bizarre behavior exhibited by the rabid animal, he attributed to these structures a role in the control of normal behavior.

Since then many different experimental procedures and clinical observations have substantiated this role of the limbic system in the control of an animal's behavior. These observations have included the effect of direct stimulation of rhinencephalic structures, the effect of ablation of portions of these structures, and the syndromes produced by diseases causing lesions in these structures.

The specific results have varied even with the use of similar procedures because of the difficulty in the exact placement of stimulating electrodes and the variable spread of electrical excitation to adjacent structures, coupled with the fact that adjacent nuclei may have diametrically opposed functions. Surgical ablations that were repeated often lacked exact specificity. Nevertheless, the general conclusion drawn from all these observations is that the alteration of the animal's behavior suggests either that a basic drive has been satisfied, or that the condition of an unsatisfied basic drive has been created. Some examples of these observations follow.

Self-Stimulation.   Self-stimulation experiments were designed in which electrodes were implanted in various specific areas of the limbic system and stimulation occurred when the experimental animal stepped on a lever or bar in the floor of the cage.[5,18,24] The response observed was assumed to be pleasurable when it was sought and continually repeated by the animal, even to the exclusion of feeding. A painful experience was assumed when the stimulation was actively avoided. Such self-stimulation of the intercrural nucleus, septal area, and rostral hypothalamus in cats and rats was sought so actively that the animal continually pressed the bar to the exclusion of eating. These areas have been called the pleasure centers. Similar stimulation of the lateral hypothalamus and selected mesencephalic areas resulted in complete avoidance of the source of the stimulus. These were referred to as pain centers.

Direct Stimulation.   Direct stimulation of the feline cingulate gyrus, amygdala, or hippocampus results in the production of a psychomotor convulsion, one characterized by a marked abnormal behavior preceding the tonic-clonic somatic motor phase of the convulsion.[8,11,13,14] Expressions of arousal, fear or rage, or both, were observed. Direct stimulation of the temporal lobe in man under local anesthesia has caused individuals to completely recall a past experience, and express the full emotional impact of the event. Upon cessation of the stimulus, the patient does not remember recalling the event.

Experimental Destruction.   Ablation experiments have resulted in variable responses, all of which show alteration in the animal's behavior. In cats, amygdalectomy results in unfriendliness and fear or even a rage response—complete sympathetic response with a tendency to attack animate or inanimate objects.[8,23] Hypersexuality in males and hyperphagia also have been observed. All these behaviors represent unsatisfied basic drives that the animal is attempting to remedy. Amygdalectomy has caused aggressive monkeys to be tame, nonaggressive, sometimes hypersexual, and to show no emotional response when confronted by objects or events that formerly elicited an emotional response. Lesions in the temporal lobe in man often cause psychomotor convulsions. Removal of the temporal lobe may stop the convulsions, but seriously blunts the emotional response of the individual, and memory of past events is often lost. Bilateral lesions have been produced in the amygdala in dogs that showed variable degrees of aggressiveness and viciousness. This has seemed to be helpful only in alleviating the aggressive behavior in nervous, fear-biting dogs.

Diseases.   Destruction of the amygdala or hippocampus in cats using aluminum oxide creme directly applied to the area resulted in psychomotor convulsions.

Diseases that cause lesions in the temporal lobe in man often are the source of psychomotor convulsions. Neonatal or childhood trauma, or infectious diseases that cause encephalitis of this area, such as the measles virus, cause damage to the temporal lobe. The temporal lobe is associated closely with the amygdala and hippocampus. Their functions overlap, and the lesions described as in temporal lobe usually involve the hippocampus as well. Psychomotor convulsions in man are characterized by loss of contact with the external environment and hallucinations of visual events, or often by visceral sensations (smells, tastes) that are pleasing or distasteful. This is accompanied by visceral motor activity such as pupillary dilation, salivation, mastication, fecal and urinary excretions, and a somatic activity consisting of wildly running around as if searching for something, along with a good deal of expression of emotion. It usually culminates in a generalized seizure characterized by falling on one side, opisthotonos, and tonic (rigid extension) and clonic (rapidly alternating contraction and relaxation of a muscle) activity of the limbs, alternating with paddling or running movements of the limbs. Complete recovery follows. The duration may be from 2 to 3 or 10 to 15 minutes.

Psychomotor seizures have been observed in dogs with lesions in the pyriform lobe or hippocampus. When agenized flour is used in dog foods, it causes necrosis in these areas bilaterally and produces this kind of convulsion.[16, 20] Similar necrosis from ischemia of unknown origin produces this behavior, as well as inflammatory lesions caused occasionally by the distemper virus.[21] In dogs psychomotor convulsions have been referred to as "running fits," because before the dog falls on its side and evidences tonic-clonic activity of its extremities along with opisthotonos, it may have a period of running wildly around its environment and barking and growling, completely unaware of anyone or anything. Occasionally, the psychic stage is manifested in what might be called an hallucination. The dog may stand in a corner, barking and growling, with dilated pupils and the hair erect on its back as if it were going to attack an object, although there is nothing there. Extreme fear may be manifested. The dog is usually nonresponsive to the owner during these episodes.

At the present time, the most common cause of convulsions in dogs that are accompanied by a psychic stage with bizarre behavior is lead poisoning. There have not been adequate studies on the distribution of the lesion to determine if limbic system structures are more affected.

Frontal Lobotomy. Frontal lobe structures are connected intimately with the limbic system and hypothalamus, and are involved in the status of an animal's behavior.[7,9] Frontal lobotomies have been performed in man and in animals to alleviate violent aggressive behaviors that are destructive in nature. In man, extensive changes in personality and loss of intellect accompany the loss of aggressive behavior, and therefore the procedure now is seldom used. The results in dogs have been variable.[2,3,15,22]

In one study frontal lobotomies were performed on two groups of aggressive animals.[1] One group consisted of malamutes used as sled dogs that had marked aggression toward one other. The other group of dogs and cats consisted of house pets that had histories of aggressive behavior toward people. The lobotomies performed on the malamutes with interspecies aggression were more successful than those performed on the animals aggressive toward man. In most instances, the lobotomized malamutes were able to return to the sled dog team and to function without attacking the other dogs. However, this surgical procedure is not without serious sequelae and should be performed only as a last resort.

More recently, electroconvulsive shock therapy has been used alone or together with lobotomies on dogs with aggressive behavior.[12]

REFERENCES

1. Allen, B. D., Cummings, J. F., and de Lahunta, A.: The effects of prefrontal lobotomy on aggressive behavior in dogs. Cor. Vet., 64:201, 1974.
2. Andersson, B.: A case of nervous distemper treated with a prefrontal lobectomy. Nord. Vet. Med., 8:17, 1956.
3. Andersson, B., and Olsson, K.: Effects of bilateral amygdaloid lesions in nervous dogs. J. Sm. Anim. Pract., 6:301, 1965.
4. Bandler, R., and Flynn, J. P.: Neural pathways from thalamus associated with regulation of aggressive behavior. Science, 183:96, 1974.
5. Bruner, A.: Self-stimulation in the rabbit: An anatomical map of stimulation effects. J. Comp. Neurol., 131:615, 1967.
6. Brutowski, S.: Functions of prefrontal cortex in animals. Physiol. Rev., 45:721, 1965.
7. Coffey, F. J.: Ethology and canine practice. J. Sm. Anim. Pract., 12:123, 1971.
8. Egger, M. D., and Flynn, J. P.: Further studies on the effects of amygdaloid stimulations and ablation on hypothalamically elicited attack behavior in cats. In Adey, W. R., and Tokizane, T., eds., Progress in Brain Research. Structure and Function of the Limbic System. Amsterdam and New York, Elsevier, 1967.
9. Fox, M. W.: Abnormal Behavior in Animals. Philadelphia, W. B. Saunders Co., 1968.
10. Fulton, J. F.: The Frontal Lobes and Human Behavior. Liverpool, Eng., University Press, 1952.
11. Gol, A.: Relief of pain by electrical stimulation of the septal area. J. Neurol. Sci., 5:115, 1967.
12. Hoerlein, B. F.: Advances in canine neurology. Gaines Vet. Symp., 24:3, 1974.
13. Hunsberger, R. W., and Bucher, V. M.: Affective behavior produced by electrical stimulation in the forebrain and brain stem of the cat. In Adey, W. R., and Tokizane, T., eds., Progress in Brain Research. Structure and Function of the Limbic System. Amsterdam and New York, Elsevier, 1967.
14. Kling, A., and Coustan, D.: Electrical stimulation of the amygdala and hypothalamus in the kitten. Exp. Neurol., 10:81, 1964.
15. Kramer, W., and Beigers, J. D.: Frontale leucotomie bij de hond. Tijdschre. Diergeneesk., 83:589, 1958.
16. Mellanby, E.: Diet and canine hysteria, experimental production by treated flour. Br. Med. J., 2:885, 1946 and 2:288, 1947.
17. Olds, J.: The limbic system and behavioral reinforcement. In Adey, W. R., and Tokizane, T., eds., Progress in Brain Research. Structure and Function of the Limbic System. Amsterdam and New York, Elsevier, 1967.
18. Olds, J.: Pleasure centers in the brain. Sci. Am., 195:105, 1956.
19. Papez, J.: A proposed mechanism of emotion. Arch. Neurol. Psychiatry, 38:725, 1937.
20. Parry, H. B.: Canine hysteria in relation to diet. Vet. Rec., 60:389, 1948.
21. Parry, H. B.: Epileptic states in the dog with special reference to canine hysteria. Vet. Rec., 61:23, 1949.
22. Redding, R. W.: Prefrontal lobotomy of the dog. Proc. Am. Anim. Hosp. Assoc., 39:374, 1972.
23. Summers, T. B., and Kaelber, W. W.: Amygdalectomy: Effect in cats and a survey of its present status. Am. J. Physiol., 203:1117, 1962.
24. Wilkinson, H. A., and Peele, T. L.: Intracranial self-stimulation in cats. J. Comp. Neurol., 121:425, 1963.

Chapter 17

SEIZURES — CONVULSIONS

DEFINITION
CLASSIFICATION
PATHOGENESIS
SEIZURE THRESHOLD
CAUSES OF SEIZURES
EXTRACRANIAL
INTRACRANIAL

IDIOPATHIC EPILEPSY
EXAMINATION OF THE PATIENT
TREATMENT
Anticonvulsants
Recommendations
The Management of Status Epilepticus
NARCOLEPSY AND CATAPLEXY

DEFINITION

The terms *seizure, convulsion, epilepsy,* and *fit* are synonyms for a brain disorder expressed as a paroxysmal cerebral dysrhythmia, a paroxysmal transitory disturbance of brain function that has a sudden onset, ceases spontaneously, and has a tendency to recur. The period of the seizure is referred to as the ictus, or the attack. The manifestation of these seizure disorders is extremely variable. Any unusual involuntary phenomenon that is episodic and recurrent in nature should be evaluated as a seizure disorder. Such phenomena include: loss or derangement of consciousness, excessive or decreased voluntary muscle tone or movement, visceral muscle activity, and altered behavior.

Postictal depression refers to the period of recovery after a seizure when the patient may wander around in confusion, circling or bumping into objects from blindness, or may sleep for a long period. The length and form of postictal depression are variable. There is no correlation between the severity of the seizure and the duration, nature, or severity of the postictal phase. A short, partial seizure may have a longer, more complex postictus than a grand mal seizure. As a rule, this phase lasts less than an hour, but much longer periods up to 1 to 2 days can occur that are not necessarily related to a more severe seizure. This probably represents the severe neuronal disturbance "exhaustion" caused by the excessive neuronal activity throughout the nervous system.

CLASSIFICATION

Seizures may be classified as partial or general. Those that begin as partial seizures may generalize subsequently.

Partial Seizures. Partial seizures have an "epileptogenic" or seizure focus that does not spread. The signs seen indicate the location of the seizure focus in the brain. When the seizure focus is in the motor area of the cerebrum there may be head turning, tonus or clonus of one or more limbs, and flexion of the trunk. In the visual area of the cerebrum there may be light biting and a photogenic seizure, while in the limbic system there may be altered behavior with complex motor activity, including somnolence, confusion, apparent blindness, failure to recognize objects, viciousness, screaming, barking, attacking inanimate objects, voracious or absent appetite, fear behavior, chewing, and licking. Such activity followed by a generalized scizure is referred to as a psychomotor seizure.

The duration of a partial (focal) seizure is variable. At any time it may spread to become a generalized seizure. The electroencephalogram may localize the seizure focus.

A partial seizure that begins in one group of muscles and slowly spreads to other muscles in the same limb and then to the other ipsilateral limb muscles is called a Jacksonian seizure. It may terminate in a generalized seizure. It is caused by a structural lesion in the area of the contralateral motor cerebral cortex, and rarely occurs in domestic animals.

Generalized Seizures. Generalized seizures in veterinary medicine usually are restricted to the grand mal seizure and have no localizing sign. This is the most common form of convulsion in dogs. It is characterized by a variable, brief psychic stage or behavioral alteration in which the dog may become restless, seek attention of its owner, or stare into space. This is then followed by a combination of visceral and somatic motor activity as the dog loses contact with its environment and becomes unconscious. Pupillary dilation, excessive salivation, and chewing activity represent the visceral motor activity. The limbs become tonic and are extended rigidly, and the animal falls on its side. A brief period of opisthotonos, marked tonic limb extension, and apnea is followed by or alternated with clonic limb activity and paddling or running movements. This somatic motor activity usually is bilaterally symmetric from the onset and throughout its course. The entire convulsion generally only lasts 1 to 2 minutes, but this is variable. Occasionally, there are urinary and fecal excretions during or after the convulsion. Petit mal seizures consist of an extremely brief (few seconds) loss of consciousness and generalized loss of muscle tone. The seizure has a characteristic electroencephalographic pattern. True petit mal seizures probably do not occur in domestic animals.

Generalized tetanic convulsions with rigid tonic extension of the limbs, opisthotonos, and apnea are found in strychnine poisoning and are elicited easily by any form of stimulation to the patient. Such convulsions are not accompanied by paddling or running movements, masticatory activity, or salivation, and rarely does the patient lose consciousness.

The degree of partial seizure or the development of a generalized seizure depends on the degree and rate of spread of electrical activity from the initial seizure focus. If the seizure activity remains confined to its initial focus in the motor cortex, the involuntary motor activity is confined to a small muscle group or one limb. If the initial focus is confined to the temporal-pyriform lobe neurons, the seizure manifestation may be limited to episodes of behavior demonstrating fear or hysteria, motor activity such as mastication, or facial muscle twitching.

The seizure generalizes when the electrical activity spreads to the diencephalon, which in turn discharges to both cerebral hemispheres. The ultimate motor activity that is observed results from the upper motor neuron discharge on the entire lower motor neuron of the brain stem and spinal cord.

PATHOGENESIS

Fundamental to all seizures is a small focus of "epileptic" neurons that exhibit some uniquely abnormal characteristics which cause them to intermittently spontaneously depolarize. Neurons utilize oxygen and glucose to generate energy used by the pump mechanism that moves sodium ions out and potassium ions in through the cell membrane. This maintains the membrane potential of the neuron. Interference with this mechanism can generate a seizure. Such disturbances can arise extracranially in the form of metabolic or toxic diseases, or intracranially in the form of organic diseases that alter structure in the brain. Idiopathic seizures occur in individuals who have no definable extra- or intracranial disease. Such individuals have an inherently low seizure threshold and a tendency for neuronal groups to spontaneously depolarize. This may be inherited in some breeds.

In addition to evaluation of carbohydrate metabolism, aerobic respiration, and electrolyte concentrations in studies of seizure disorders, the role of excitatory and inhibitory neurotransmitters is being examined at present. These include the excitatory neurotransmitters acetylcholine, glutamate, and serotonin, and the inhibitory neurotransmitters gamma aminobutyric acid, taurine, and norepinephrine.

SEIZURE THRESHOLD

Each individual has a certain threshold of stimulation; if this threshold is exceeded, a seizure will occur. It varies among individuals, and may be the underlying cause of most idiopathic epilepsies. Presumably, the metabolic and structural bases for this threshold are established genetically.

The so-called normal individual has a seizure threshold that can be exceeded only by stimuli such as certain convulsant drugs and electric shock treatment. Individuals with the lower seizure threshold can be divided into two groups. In the first group are those in whom seizures can be stimulated by conditions such as fatigue, fever, photic stimulation, hyperventilation, or estrus. In the second are those individuals with the lowest seizure threshold, who have spontaneous seizures with no detectable stimulus. This is typical of many idiopathic epileptics.

Seizures can be a sign of serious organic brain disease, or of a genetically determined neuronal morphology and physiology that allow spontaneous depolarization. The prognosis obviously is dependent on the underlying cause. It is the responsibility of the examiner to determine this to the best of his or her ability. Educating the client as to the significance of this clinical sign is also an important responsibility of the clinician, and may determine the survival of the patient and the success of the therapy.

CAUSES OF SEIZURES[5, 12, 17, 18, 25, 29, 30, 33, 35, 36, 37, 51, 53, 56, 61]

Convulsions occur when there is disturbance to the function of the neurons of the prosencephalon. Anything that alters neuronal function in the brain is poten-

TABLE 17–1. CAUSES OF SEIZURES

EXTRACRANIAL
  Hypoglycemia
    Glycogen storage diseases
    Beta cell neoplasm of pancreas
  Hypoxia
    Cardiorespiratory disease
  Hepatoencephalopathy
  Renal disease
  Hypocalcemia
  Hyperkalemia
  Hyperlipoproteinemia
  Gastrointestinal disease
    Parasitism
    "Garbage" toxicity
INTRACRANIAL
  Inflammations
    Canine distemper encephalitis, toxoplasmosis, cryptococcosis
    Other viral encephalitides: rabies, equine
    Feline infectious peritonitis meningoencephalitis in cats
  Neoplasia
    Primary or metastatic
  Malformations
    Hydrocephalus, lissencephaly, pachygyria
  Injury
  Degenerations
    Polioencephalomalacia in ruminants
    Thiamine deficiency in cats
    Salt poisoning in pigs
    Intoxications:
      lead, mercury, arsenic, chlorinated hydrocarbons, organic phosphates, hexachlorophene,
        ethylene glycol
IDIOPATHIC EPILEPSY

tially seizure-producing. The cause of the alteration can be either extracranial or intracranial.

EXTRACRANIAL

A discussion of extracranial causes that alter neuronal metabolism follows. Usually with these diseases there are no clinical neurologic signs apparent in the interictal period (between seizures).

Hypoglycemia.[39] Functional neoplasms of the beta cells of the pancreatic islets may occur in the dog usually at the age of 5 years or older.[7, 15, 16, 41, 48, 71, 79] Typically, the convulsions are grand mal and occur prior to feeding, when the blood glucose level is at its lowest. Convulsions are the most common neurologic abnormality, but occasionally evidences of altered behavior, or mild ataxia or paresis, or both, may be presenting signs. A fasting blood glucose level of less than 60 mg per 100 cc is suspicious, and less than 40 mg per 100 cc is diagnostic for hypoglycemia associated with the neurologic abnormality.

Episodic hypoglycemia occasionally is observed in hunting dogs, and causes convulsions associated with periods of exercise.[39] This is thought to be due to the inability of the dog to mobilize liver glycogen into utilizable glucose. Feeding the animal before hunting, or providing glucose in the form of candy bars while hunting, may allay the condition. Some young dogs of the toy breeds from 6 to 12 weeks old have a predilection for hypoglycemia. A glycogen storage disease that has been related to the von Gierke syndrome in man occurs in puppies and causes hypoglycemia. The clinical signs may be precipitated by stress. Ketones are often present in the urine in high concentrations. Treatment with 4 cc per kg of body weight of a 50 per cent glucose solution should alleviate the immediate neurologic signs. Some dogs grow out of the condition in 3 to 4 months.

Liver Disease. Severe liver disease with excess ammonia in the blood can lead to convulsions. The most common example of this in the dog is the hepatic encephalopathy associated with portacaval anastomosis.[3, 6, 16, 49, 68, 72, 73, 74, 77, 78, 80] In the horse the liver necrosis of Theiler's disease may produce convulsions, along with the other signs of acute hepatic encephalopathy.[28]

Hypocalcemia. Hypocalcemia associated with parturition in the bitch may cause convulsions.[38, 62] It also has been reported in hunting dogs following exercise, and in chronic renal disease. Treatment with 4 cc per kg of a 10 per cent solution of calcium gluconate should alleviate the neurologic signs.

Renal Disease. Occasionally, renal disease associated with prolonged uremia causes convulsions in dogs.[76] The acidosis that accompanies this disease may be the cause of the neurologic disturbance. Hypoglycemia and hypocalcemia also have been incriminated.

Hypoxia. Hypoxia from cardiovascular disease or pulmonary disease may cause periodic episodes of collapse or convulsions.[10, 13, 19, 22, 26, 43, 44, 45, 63, 64, 65, 66] Repeated convulsive episodes lead to hypoxia of nervous tissue and may be self-perpetuating.

Hyperkalemia. Hyperkalemia occurs in adrenocortical insufficiency (Addison's disease), or may follow the sudden withdrawal of steroids after their prolonged use, and convulsions may occur.

Hypomagnesemia. This electrolyte disturbance is more often a cause of convulsive activity in the bovine species referred to as "grass tetany."

Hyperlipoproteinemia. Seizures have been observed in dogs with defective lipid metabolism causing hyperlipoproteinemia. It has occurred most commonly in the miniature schnauzer, with the onset of seizures between 2 and 7 years.[82]

Intestinal Parasitism. Intestinal parasitism in young puppies may be associated with convulsions that may be produced by a concomitant hypocalcemia, or hypoglycemia, or both.

INTRACRANIAL

Intracranial diseases are the more common causes of convulsions. Usually, a thorough neurologic examination detects abnormal neurologic signs in the interictal period. The presence of these signs usually indicates organic brain disease.

Inflammation. Encephalitis from any cause that involves prosencephalic structures can be a source of convulsions. Canine distemper encephalitis is the most common cause of convulsions in the dog associated with encephalitis.[59] The kind of convulsion associated with this disease is not specific, but visceral motor activity is often prominent in the form of clonic masticatory activity and salivation, the so-called "chewing gum fits." In addition to the convulsions there are usually interictal signs of diffuse neurologic deficit, suggesting multifocal disease. The CSF may be abnormal, with mild elevations of mononuclear cells and protein. Toxoplasmosis or cryptococcal meningoencephalitis also may be causes of seizures in dogs or cats.

Neoplasm.   Primary or metastatic neoplasms may cause convulsions.[8, 52, 54] They are more common in older dogs. Other evidence of focal neurologic disease may be apparent from the interictal neurologic examination. However, if a cerebral neoplasm is slow in growing, does not increase intracranial pressure significantly, and does not affect the sensorimotor cortex or its pathway to and from the brain stem, or the optic radiation and visual cortex, no interictal neurologic deficit may be detected. CSF pressure sometimes is elevated and the protein content may be elevated slightly. The signs, including the frequency of the convulsions, are usually progressive.

Malformation.   Hydrocephalus is the most common malformation of the prosencephalon, and occasionally causes convulsions. Electroencephalography usually indicates this diagnosis, and pneumoventriculography confirms it. Visual deficit and behavioral abnormalities may accompany this malformation, but no one set of signs is diagnostic.

Lissencephaly and pachygyria have been observed in the Lhasa apso. Behavioral abnormalities, with an inability to train properly, and visual deficits appear at an early age, but seizures usually do not occur until near the end of the first year of life. This malformation also was observed in a wire-haired terrier that presented with nonprogressive signs of severe cerebellar abnormality from birth. The cerebellum was reduced markedly in size and dysplastic. There was no evidence of degeneration or previous in utero inflammation. A litter mate with similar ataxia was raised to 4½ years of age. The ataxia persisted unchanged. At 1½ years of age this dog began to have seizures. They occurred at the rate of at least four per month for about 2 years, despite anticonvulsant therapy. In the last year they increased in frequency to one to two weekly. The dog died following a seizure at 4½ years old.

Injury.   Trauma to the brain may cause convulsions at the time of the initial damage, but more often the convulsions do not take place until weeks or months after the injury occurred and the tissue has healed. The cerebral scar is somehow thought to serve as the seizure focus in this condition.

Neuronal Degeneration.   Diseases that cause neuronal degeneration often cause convulsions.[1, 23]

Polioencephalomalacia in cattle, sheep, and goats usually is related to abnormal metabolism of the thiamine coenzyme. Convulsions may accompany the marked neurologic deficit typical of this disease that is destructive to the cerebral cortex. Immediate treatment with thiamine early in the course of the disease may reverse the signs.

Thiamine deficiency occasionally occurs in cats on an all-fish diet that contains a thiaminase, or following a prolonged anorexia.[20] Generalized convulsions frequently are elicited by handling the animal. Early treatment with a few mg of thiamine alleviates the condition.

Intoxication with lead in some areas may be a common cause of convulsions in the dog.[81] There are many sources, including paint, linoleum, tarpaper, roofing materials, and batteries. Gastrointestinal and neurologic signs occur together or singly in this disease. The neurologic signs usually involve convulsions or abnormal behavior. The convulsions are often psychomotor, accompanied by bizarre behavioral abnormalities. The results of blood studies are considered to be nearly pathognomonic for this disease when numerous erythrocytes are observed that are nucleated and have basophilic stippling, in the absence of a severe anemia.

Urinary levels of alpha aminolevulinic acid may be elevated. The finding of elevated blood levels of lead is diagnostic. In young growing dogs a radiograph of long bones may show a "lead line" at the metaphysis. Treatment with calcium ethylenediaminetetraacetic acid often results in rapid recovery from the signs.

In calves with lead poisoning the seizures often are associated with propulsive, maniacal activity. Hyperesthesia is pronounced. Odontoprisis and lack of ruminal motility may be noted. Blindness is common.

Intoxication with chlorinated hydrocarbons, hexachlorophene, organic phosphates, and mercury may affect neuronal metabolism and cause convulsions. Cats are especially susceptible to the chlorinated hydrocarbons used in many flea dip preparations. Strychnine poisoning acts predominantly on the spinal cord inhibitory neurons, but the effects of this toxin may be more widespread in the central nervous system.

Salt poisoning occasionally is observed in pigs fed on garbage high in salt content; concomitant with a restriction of their water intake. The toxicity is related to the sodium ion. The convulsions are often characterized by a rapid backward movement, with the pig in a sitting position. Signs of diffuse cerebral disease accompany the convulsions. The laminar cerebral necrosis often is accompanied by a marked infiltration of eosinophils in this disease.

Water intoxication occurs in calves and possibly pigs when a large volume of water is consumed. Convulsions may accompany the other signs of diffuse brain disturbance. In most cases, hemoglobinuria is present. Cardiac arrythmia is common. Hypo-osmolar serum is diagnostic.

IDIOPATHIC EPILEPSY

Idiopathic epilepsy is a syndrome characterized by repeated episodes of convulsions for which there is no known demonstrable clinical or pathologic cause.[2, 9, 31] The diagnosis ultimately is made by ruling out the extracranial and intracranial diseases that cause convulsions on examination of the patient.

Idiopathic epilepsy is seen predominantly in miniature and toy poodles, but also frequently in German shepherds, Saint Bernards, standard poodles, cocker spaniels, beagles, Irish setters, and other breeds, including mongrels. Convulsions usually begin between 1 and 3 years of age, with some exceptions. They may be preceded by a short aura during which the animal acts as if it knows a convulsion is coming. The convulsion is usually grand mal in type, lasting from one half a minute to 2 minutes. In the immediate postictal period the patient usually is depressed and occasionally blind. The convulsions sometimes recur at fairly regular intervals. The interval varies from one or a few weeks to months between convulsions. During the interictal period the patient shows no signs of neurologic disturbance. Often these convulsions can be controlled with proper anticonvulsant therapy.

The cause of idiopathic epilepsy is unknown. Some of these patients show abnormalities in their electroencephalograms recorded in the interictal period. An hereditary basis is suggested by clinical observation of the high incidence in the miniature poodle breed and in certain families of dogs, i.e., dachshunds, German shepherds, Belgian tervurens, and Alaskan huskies. Genetic factors control the developmental mechanisms in the nervous system that regulate the seizure threshold, which is different for each individual. Dogs with idiopathic epilepsy may have a lower threshold as a result of minor alterations of these genetic factors. The frequency of convulsions may increase as the dog ages, and occasionally the patient develops status epilepticus, during which death frequently occurs.

A form of idiopathic epilepsy has been observed in horses that seems to be related to the estrus period when estrogen levels are increased. Seizures only occur during these periods in these mares.

EXAMINATION OF THE PATIENT

The following is an example of an examination of a dog presented with the chief complaint of convulsions. This demonstrates the kind of information the examiner should obtain in attempting to diagnose the cause of convulsions.

Chief Complaint.   Seizure.

Signalment

AGE.   Less than 1 year—canine distemper encephalitis; lead poisoning; hypoglycemia of toy breeds; puppies with severe intestinal parasitism; young dogs with signs of liver disease who may have a portacaval shunt; hydrocephalus; lissencephaly.

One to 3 years—usual onset of idiopathic epilepsy.

Over 5 years—neoplasia in prosencephalon; hypoglycemia from beta cell neoplasm in pancreas.

BREED.   Hypoglycemia of toy breeds; hydrocephalus in toy and brachycephalic breeds; neoplasms in brachycephalic breeds; idiopathic epilepsy in German shepherds, Saint Bernards, standard and miniature poodles, beagles, Irish setters and Belgian tervuren; leukodystrophy in Cairn and West Highland white terriers; lipodystrophy in German short-haired pointers and English setters; lissencephaly in the Lhasa apso; portacaval shunts and hyperlipoproteinemia in miniature schnauzers.

SEX.   Mammary gland adenocarcinomas metastasize to the brain; seizure threshold may be reduced during estrus.

USE.   Hunting dogs may develop hypoglycemia.

History

DESCRIPTION.   Obtain a careful description of the seizure. A consistent focal location in partial seizures may indicate the site of a structural lesion. Seizures from intoxicants and in idiopathic epilepsy usually are symmetric, with no lateralizing focal component. Bizarre behavioral abnormalities that precede a generalized seizure may occur in lead poisoning. Seizures in cats with severe flexion of the trunk and neck occur in thiamine deficiency. Idiopathic epileptics usually have short, generalized, grand mal convulsions.

Transient cerebral ischemia such as from heart worms may produce episodes of transient ataxia and collapse. Episodic collapse may occur in hypoadrenocorticoidism (Addison's disease). These are not seizure disorders.

ONSET AND COURSE.   An explosive onset of continuous seizures, serial or status epilepticus, can occur with neoplasms, intoxicants, or idiopathic epilepsy. A progressive course with more frequent and longer seizures is found with inflammations or neoplasms. Regular intervals are more common in idiopathic epilepsy, but even in that disease they may be progressive. Hypoglycemic seizures often occur consistently prior to feeding.

ENVIRONMENT. Investigate the environment for other dogs or litter mates with signs suggestive of canine distemper. A source of intoxicants should be sought, for example: lead—paint, linoleum, wallboard, tarpaper, roofing materials; metaldehyde—snail bait; hexachlorophene—soap; ethylene glycol—antifreeze; insecticides—chlorinated hydrocarbons, organophosphates; rodenticides—fluoroacetate (1080); mercury—seed treated with fungicide; arsenic—ant poisons, insecticides; phenols—cresol, germicides.

DIET. An all-fish diet may precipitate thiamine deficiency in cats. Engorgement on spoiled garbage may cause seizures in dogs.

PAST MEDICAL HISTORY. Seizures can follow intracranial injuries up to 2 years or longer. Such injuries usually have produced transient signs of cerebral disturbances such as stupor, unconsciousness, and tetraplegia.

Febrile illness may have been caused by the canine distemper virus. The neurologic form can occur days to weeks later.

Difficult, prolonged birth may produce cerebral lesions from hypoxia or trauma.

Diagnosis of neoplastic disease in other organs may herald a metastasis to the brain.

Previous progressive neurologic deficit which culminated in a seizure suggests organic brain disease.

Evidence of behavior change, polyuria and polydipsia, or a voracious, indiscriminate appetite may suggest hypothalamic involvement by a pituitary neoplasm. Signs of hyperadrenocorticoidism (Cushing's disease) may accompany a pituitary adenoma.

Recent changes in behavior often accompany frontal lobe neoplasia. Episodic behavioral alterations in the young dog may accompany hepatic encephalopathy, or the malformations of lissencephaly and pachygyria.

The primary purpose of the examination of the patient is to establish if the disease producing the seizure is *extracranial* or *intracranial*.

Physical Examination. Other organs that may be diseased and occasionally may produce seizures include the liver, kidney, and cardiorespiratory structures. Diffuse systemic disease may accompany the various encephalitides in the dog.

Neurologic Examination. Abnormalities in the interictal neurologic examination suggest intracranial structural brain disease. Focal signs suggest a neoplasm, infarct, or previous injury. Mild hemiparesis and general proprioceptive deficit only observable on postural reaction testing suggest an internal capsule or sensory-motor cortex lesion; hemianopsia suggests an optic tract, radiation or occipital lobe lesion. Circling may occur toward the side of a cerebral lesion. Signs of multifocal central nervous system disease suggest inflammation or multiple neoplastic metastasis. Signs of diffuse neurologic disturbance can occur with inflammatory or degenerative diseases or from metabolic disturbance that is extracranial in origin.

If interictal signs are absent, either extracranial or intracranial disease may be present. A small focal area of injury, neoplasia, or inflammation in a "quiet" area of the brain may produce seizures with no definable interictal signs. Most extracranial diseases do not produce interictal signs. The most common extracranial disease is hypoglycemia, followed by hepatoencephalopathy and hypoxia. Dogs with idiopathic epilepsy do not have interictal signs.

Ancillary Examination

LABORATORY FINDINGS.   CBC: Lead poisoning—presence of nucleated red blood cells, basophilic stippling, and a low normal packed cell volume; may be normal with viral encephalitis; increased WBC with abnormal differential may accompany suppurative meningoencephalitis; leukocytosis occasionally occurs in portacaval anastomoses; polycythemia—greater than 70 to 75 per cent packed cell volume may produce seizures.

BUN: Increased in chronic renal disease; may be decreased in portacaval shunts.

Urinalysis: Signs of renal or liver disease; look for ammonium biurate crystals in hepatic encephalopathy; ketosis occurs in hypoglycemic puppies.

Liver function: BSP—higher than 5 per cent retention of bromsulfalein in 30 minutes suggests diffuse liver dysfunction—most valuable for portacaval anastomoses; serum glutamic pyruvic transaminase and alkaline phosphatase may be increased with focal or diffuse liver lesions; NH3 may increase in blood with diffuse liver disease and seizures.

Fasting blood glucose: A 24-hour fast is usually sufficient to demonstrate the hypoglycemia from pancreatic neoplasms. Forty-eight hours may be necessary in toy breeds with glycogen storage disease. Less than 60 mg of glucose per dl is suspicious. Less than 40 mg per dl is diagnostic.

Calcium: Hypocalcemia may cause tetanic-type convulsions in eclampsia, chronic renal disease, especially if congenital, or following parathyroid gland removal.

Acid-base and electrolyte abnormalities (except calcium) rarely cause seizures in dogs.

CSF: Normal in all idiopathic epileptics, most dogs with extracranial metabolic diseases, and some dogs with intracranial organic diseases.

Mild elevation of protein levels with normal cells or mild mononuclear pleocytosis occurs in viral encephalitis or with neoplasia. Pressure may be elevated with neoplasia.

RADIOGRAPHY.   In suspected cases of cranial injury or neoplasms that may be adjacent to the bony walls of the cranium, causing erosion, radiographs may help to confirm a diagnosis. Pneumoventriculograms may confirm a case of hydrocephalus. Evidence of metastatic neoplasia on thoracic radiographs may help diagnose similar brain neoplasia.

SCINTIGRAPHY.   Radioisotope scanning procedures of the brain may help confirm some space-occupying lesions or large infarcts.

ELECTROENCEPHALOGRAPHY.   EEG is usually helpful in confirming suspicious cases of hydrocephalus, and may help confirm inflammatory and neoplastic diseases.

CEREBRAL ANGIOGRAPHY.   Some have found this useful to diagnose space-occupying lesions.

If the signalment and history are appropriate, and all the results of the physical, neurologic, and ancillary examinations are normal, idiopathic epilepsy can be diagnosed.

TREATMENT

Treatment should be directed at the primary disease if it can be recognized.[50, 58] The convulsions should be controlled by pharmacologic agents.[46, 55, 60] The following anticonvulsants are the most commonly used.

Anticonvulsants

Phenytoin (Dilantin).   This drug does not prevent initiation of a seizure, but stops its spread. It occasionally produces a mild ataxia, and takes about 4 to 7 days to build an effective CNS level.[67, 75, 84] It causes an undesirable level of sedation in cats. It is supplied in 30-, 100-, and 250-mg capsules for oral use. There is no firmly established maximum dosage.[42] The dose used is the amount that will control the seizures. The usual dose to begin with is about 6 to 10 mg per kg tid. As a rule, if control is going to be achieved, it will occur at a dose below 20 mg per kg tid.

Phenobarbital.   The action of this drug is on the nerve cell body, preventing initiation of a seizure but not its propagation. It raises the seizure threshold. This drug is effective rapidly, and is especially useful in treatment of status epilepticus. It is the drug of choice for cats. Its disadvantage is the sedation that often follows moderate doses. It is supplied in 1/8 gr (8 mg), 1/4 gr (16 mg), and 1/2 gr (32 mg) tablets for oral use, and in vials of 1 gr (64 mg) and 2 gr (128 mg) for parenteral use. The dose is 2 mg per kg, bid, or tid.

When a dog presents with recurrent seizures, a combination of phenytoin and phenobarbital often is used for immediate and prolonged therapy. The phenobarbital provides the immediate control, and is decreased over a 1-week period as the phenytoin takes effect. If control continues to be successful, the phenobarbital is stopped. This combination may decrease the effectiveness of the phenytoin.[84]

Some cases may require continued therapy with phenytoin and phenobarbital. These can be purchased mixed in a single capsule with 100 mg of Dilantin and 1/4 or 1/2 gr of phenobarbital.

Phenobarbital is the drug of choice for cats.

Primidone (Mylepsin, Mysoline).   About 25 per cent of this drug is broken down to phenobarbital in the liver. It acts directly on the neurons to prevent initiation of seizure.

Primidone has a rapid anticonvulsant action, but often produces a severe depression and occasionally ataxia. This may be transient as the patient adjusts to the drug. Of all the drugs used for seizures, this may produce the most significant polyphagia, polydipsia, and polyuria.[32] It is not recommended for cats by the manufacturer.

It is supplied in 50-mg and 250-mg tablets. The recommended dose is 50 mg per kg, split in doses bid or tid. This so frequently produces sedation that smaller doses often are used initially.

Diazepam (Valium). Diazepam, a benzodiazepine, is used mostly in cases of status epilepticus.[70] It often produces significant sedation, and has received only limited use as a daily therapeutic drug for generalized seizures. Some have thought it useful as a daily anticonvulsant in combination with primidone in large dogs at a dose of 10 mg bid orally. It is supplied as a tablet in 5- and 10-mg quantities.

Paramethadione.   Experimental data is being obtained at present on the use of paramethadione as an anticonvulsant in dogs.[57] This is a drug used for petit mal seizures in man. Preliminary data indicate that it appears to be as effective as the other canine anticonvulsants, but also that it may be especially helpful in those cases found difficult to control with the usual canine anticonvulsants.

Recommendations

There are no specific dosage levels or guidelines, except for reliance on experience.[36] It is most important that the drug be given exactly as directed, with no lapses in therapy. A lapse in therapy often produces seizures. If seizures remain uncontrolled, the dosage should be increased progressively, or a second drug may be combined with the first. If a change in drug is considered necessary do not stop the drug in use abruptly, but slowly decrease it as the new drug is initiated.

Clients should be instructed thoroughly that a trial with one or more drugs may be necessary to achieve successful control in their animal. Most seizure patients without progressive organic disease can be controlled at least partially.

It is not unusual for relapses to occur, even in well-controlled patients. The exacerbation of a seizure disorder after successful management does not necessarily indicate the presence of a progressive organic lesion, but just may require more vigorous therapy. Similarly, if the seizures change in pattern, this does not necessarily infer the presence of an organic lesion.

There is often no correlation between the severity and duration of the seizure and the underlying disease. Some idiopathic epileptics have much more serious seizures than dogs with large intracranial neoplasms. The prognosis in serious seizure disorders, including status epilepticus, is not necessarily grave if there is no indication of organic brain disease from the examination. Except in status epilepticus, dogs usually do not die from a seizure.

As a rule, anticonvulsants are not administered to a patient that has had a single convulsion and there is no indication of the cause upon complete examination of the patient. Even with short, mild seizures that are infrequent, therapy may not be administered. Sometimes the decision to treat may depend on the concern of the owner.

The Management of Status Epilepticus

Status epilepticus is a condition in which seizures are continual, one after the other, with no recovery between them. These can lead to irreversible coma or death, and should be considered a medical emergency. Death is caused by a combination of hyperthermia, circulatory collapse, and acidosis and hypoxia from muscle exertion and impaired respiration.

The seizures must be stopped. The drugs of choice, in the order of their use, are diazepam, phenobarbital, and barbiturate anesthesia.

Diazepam (Valium) is a tranquilizer that enhances presynaptic inhibitory mechanisms.[4] It is particularly useful in stopping the generalized seizures of a status patient, dog or cat. As mentioned earlier, it has received only limited use as a daily anticonvulsant. It has a relatively short action, and often needs repeated administration. It is supplied in 2-cc vials with 5 mg per cc, and in 5-mg and 10-mg tablets. In status, it usually is given intravenously in 5- to 10-mg doses every 10 to 15 minutes until the seizures stop. The intramuscular route may be used in a violent patient. If 3 or 4 doses are inadequate, intravenous phenobarbital should be administered at a rate of 6 mg per kg. There is no real limit to the amount of medication. Give enough to stop the seizures. As a last resort, anesthetize with sodium pentobarbital to effect.

The ideal management should include the following steps:

1. Be sure the patient's airway is intact and not obstructed.

2. Place an indwelling intravenous catheter in the patient.

3. Draw blood for complete blood count, glucose, and calcium determinations.

4. Administer 50 per cent dextrose intravenously—2 to 25 cc. (toy poodle to German shepherd).

5. If hypocalcemia is suspected, as in eclampsia, administer slowly 5 to 10 cc of 10 per cent or 20 per cent calcium gluconate.

6. Administer the intravenous anticonvulsant—diazepam, phenobarbital, or barbiturate anesthesia.

7. Hyperthermia should be treated with ice-water baths.

8. As soon as the animal can swallow, oral medication with phenobarbital, with or without phenytoin, or primidone should be instituted.

9. Corticosteroids may be administered intravenously (dexamethasone, 1 to 2 mg per kg) to stabilize lysosomes and to prevent catecholamine release.

Narcolepsy and Cataplexy

Narcolepsy is a central nervous system disorder of sleep in which the patient experiences recurrent episodes of uncontrollable sleep that last for a few minutes, and that often occur at inappropriate times. Cataplexy often accompanies narcolepsy, and is a recurrent episode of sudden loss of function of part or all the voluntary muscles, except those for respirations and extraocular muscles, resulting in collapse. In man, these may be stimulated by such emotional events as laughter or fear. In dogs, such episodes have been associated with the onset of eating or with extreme excitement, such as chasing a cat. They are *not* accompanied by tonic or clonic muscle activity of voluntary muscles. Sometimes the attack can be aborted by harsh tactile or auditory stimulation.

Studies in man and animals have shown that these narcoleptic attacks are episodes of rapid eye movement (REM) sleep. This also is referred to as paradoxical sleep because the electroencephalogram shows low voltage, high frequency activity typical of the awake patient, but it is associated with complete loss of detectable motor tone in most muscles except the extraocular muscles and sometimes the facial muscles. Normally, REM or paradoxical sleep occurs for short intervals during regular sleep.[24, 34]

Narcolepsy accompanied by cataplexy can occur with organic lesions of the rostral brain stem. More commonly, it is idiopathic. It is assumed to represent a morphologic or biochemical disturbance in those portions of the brain stem concerned with cerebrocortical depression and arousal (ARAS, raphe system, locus ceruleus) and motor function (upper motor neuron, reticular formation).

The disease has been observed in dogs, cats, and horses, especially in Shetland ponies.[11, 27, 40, 47, 83] In the latter, it has been referred to as fainting disease.[69] This disease is *not* responsive to the usual anticonvulsant drugs, but often can be controlled with stimulants such as dextroamphetamine (Dexedrine, 5 to 10 mg tid) and methylphenidate (Ritalin, 5 to 10 mg bid or tid); an antidepressant, imipramine (Tofranil, 0.4 to 0.8 mg per kg intravenously or per os tid); or a monoamine oxidase inhibitor, phenelzine (Nardil).

REFERENCES

1. Andersson, B., and Olson, S. E.: Epilepsy in a dog with extensive bilateral damage to the hippocampus. Acta. Vet. Scand., *1*:98, 1959.
2. Atkeson, F. W., Ibensen, A., and Eldrige, E.: Inheritance of an epileptic type character in Brown Swiss cattle. J. Hered., *35*:45, 1944.
3. Audell, L., Jönsson, L., and Lannek, B.: Congenital porta-caval shunts in the dog. Zentralbl. Veterinaermed., *21*:797, 1974.
4. Averill, D. A., Jr.: Treatment of status epilepticus in dogs with diazepam sodium. J. Am. Vet. Med. Assoc., *156*:432, 1970.
5. Barker, J.: Epilepsy in the dog—a comparative approach. J. Sm. Anim. Pract., *14*:281, 1973.

6. Barrett, R. E., de Lahunta, A., Roenigk, W. J., Hoffer, R. E., and Coons, F. H.: Five cases of congenital portacaval shunt in the dog. J. Sm. Anim. Pract., 17:71, 1976.
7. Beck, A. M., and Krook, L.: Canine insuloma. Two surgical cases with relapses. Cor. Vet., 55:330, 1965.
8. Berryman, F. C., and de Lahunta, A.: Astrocytoma in a dog causing convulsions. Cor. Vet., 65:212, 1975.
9. Biefelt, S. W., Redman, H. C., and McClellan, R. O.: Sire and sex-related differences in rates of epileptiform seizures in a purebred beagle dog colony. Am. J. Vet. Res., 32:2039, 1971.
10. Bjork, C. A.: Circulostatic cerebral hypoxic epilepsy. Vet. Med./Sm. Anim. Clin., 65:33, 1970.
11. Blauch, B. S., and Cash, W. C.: A brief review of narcolepsy with presentation of two cases of narcolepsy in dogs. J. Am. Anim. Hosp. Assoc., 11:467, 1975.
12. Breazile, J. E.: Convulsive disorders in dogs. In Kirk, R. W., ed., Current Veterinary Therapy, IV. W. B. Saunders Co., Philadelphia, 1971, 478–484.
13. Bush, B. M., and Fankhauser, R.: Polycythemia vera in a bitch. J. Sm. Anim. Pract., 13:75, 1972.
14. Capen, C. C., and Martin, S. L.: Hyperinsulinism in dogs with neoplasia of the pancreatic islets. Pathol. Vet., 6:309, 1969.
15. Cello, R. M., and Kennedy, P. C.: Hyperinsulinism in dogs due to pancreatic islet cell carcinoma. Cor. Vet., 47:538, 1957.
16. Cornelius, L. M., Thrall, D. E., Halliwell, W. H., Frank, G. M., and Kern, A. J.: Anomalous portosystemic anastomoses associated with chronic hepatic insufficiency in six young dogs. J. Am. Vet. Med. Assoc., 167:220, 1975.
17. Croft, P. G.: Fits in dogs: A survey of 260 cases. Vet. Rec., 77:438, 1965.
18. Cunningham, C. G.: Canine seizure disorders. J. Am. Vet. Med. Assoc., 158:589, 1971.
19. Ettinger, S.: Isoproterenol treatment of atrioventricular block in the dog. J. Am. Vet. Med. Assoc., 154:398, 1969.
20. Everett, G. M.: Observations on the behavior and neurophysiology of acute thiamine deficient cats. Am. J. Physiol., 141:439, 1944.
21. Ewing, G. O., Suter, P. F., and Bailey, C. S.: Hepatic insufficiency associated with congenital anomalies of the portal vein in dogs. J. Am. Anim. Hosp. Assoc., 10:463, 1974.
22. Fisher, E. W.: Fainting in boxers—the possibility of vaso-vagal syncope (Adams-Stokes attacks). J. Sm. Anim. Pract., 12:347, 1971.
23. Fisher, K.: Herdförmig symmetrische Hirngewebsnekrosen bei Hunden mit epileptiformen krämpfen. Pathol. Vet., 1:133, 1964.
24. Fox, M. W., and Stanton, G.: A developmental study of sleep and wakefulness in the dog. J. Sm. Anim. Pract., 8:605, 1967.
25. Gastaut, H., Berard-Baider, M., Darraspen, M., and Van Bogaert, L.: Anatomical and clinical study of 19 epileptic dogs. In Baldwin, M., and Bailey P., eds., Springfield, Ill., Temporal Lobe Epilepsy. Charles C Thomas, 1958, 243–267.
26. Hamlin, R. L., Smetzer, D. L., and Breznock, E. M.: Sinoatrial syncope in miniature schnauzers. J. Am. Vet. Med. Assoc., 161:1022, 1972.
27. Hart, B. L.: Behavioral aspects of canine narcolepsy. Canine Pract., 2:8, 1975.
28. Hjerpe, C. A.: Serum hepatitis in the horse. J. Am. Vet. Med. Assoc., 144:734, 1964.
29. Holliday, T. A.: Clinical aspects of some encephalopathies of domestic cats. Vet. Clin. North Am., 1:367, 1971.
30. Holliday, T. A.: Epilepsy in cats. Mod. Vet. Pract., 51:14, 1970.
31. Holliday, T. A., Cunningham, J. G., and Gutnich, M. J.: Comparative clinical and electroencephalographic studies on canine epilepsy. Epilepsia, 11:281, 1970.
32. Jennings, P. B., Utter, W. F., and Fariss, B. L.: Effects of long-term primidone therapy in a dog. J. Am. Vet. Med. Assoc., 164:1123, 1974.
33. Johnson, J. T.: Tonic seizures in a dog. J. Am. Vet. Med. Assoc., 159:427, 1971.
34. Jouvet, M.: The states of sleep. Sci. Am., 216:62, 1967.
35. Kay, W.: Epilepsy. In Kirk, R. W., ed., Current Veterinary Therapy, V. Small Animal Practice. Philadelphia, W. B. Saunders Co., 1974, 686–699.
36. Kay, W. J.: Epilepsy. Proc. Am. Anim. Hosp. Assoc., 40:402, 1973.
37. Kay, W. J.: Epilepsy in cats. J. Am. Anim. Hosp. Assoc., 11:77, 1975.
38. Kirk, G. R., Breazile, J. E., and Kenney, A. D.: Pathogenesis of hypocalcemic tetany in the thyroparathyroidectomized dog. Am. J. Vet. Res., 35:407, 1974.
39. Kirk, R. W.: Hypoglycemia. In Kirk, R. W., ed., Current Veterinary Therapy, III. Philadelphia, W. B. Saunders Co., 1968, 1968, 78–80.
40. Knecht, C. D., Oliver, J., Reading, R., Selcer, R., and Johnson, G.: Narcolepsy in a dog and cat. J. Am. Vet. Med. Assoc., 162:1052, 1973.
41. Krook, L., and Kenney, R. M.: CNS lesions in dogs with metastasizing islet cell carcinoma. Cor. Vet., 52:358, 1962.
42. Lefebvre, E. B., Haining, R. G., and Labbe, R. F.: Coarse facies, calvarial thickening, and hyperphosphatasia associated with long-term anticonvulsant therapy. N. Engl. J. Med., 286:1301, 1972.
43. Legendre, A. M., Appleford, M. D., Eyster, G. E., and Dade, A. W.: Secondary polycythemia and seizures due to right to left shunting patent ductus arteriosus in a dog. J. Am. Vet. Med. Assoc., 164:1198, 1974.

44. Mahaffey, L. W., and Rossdale, P. D.: Convulsive syndrome in newborn foals. Vet. Rec., 69:1277, 1957.
45. McGrath, C. J.: Polycythemia vera in dogs. J. Am. Vet. Med. Assoc., 164:1117, 1974.
46. Millichap, J. G.: Drug treatment of convulsive disorders. N. Engl. J. Med., 286:464, 1972.
47. Mitler, M. M., Boysen, B. G., Campbell, L., and Dement, W. C.: Narcolepsy—cataplexy in a female dog. Exp. Neurol., 45:332, 1974.
48. Njoku, C. O., Strafuss, A. C., and Dennis, S. M.: Canine islet cell neoplasia: A review. J. Am. Anim. Hosp. Assoc., 8:284, 1972.
49. Oliver, J. E.: Hepatic neuropathies—a review. Vet. Med./Sm. Anim. Clin., 60:498, 1965.
50. Oliver, J. E.: Surgical relief of epileptiform seizures in the dog. Vet. Med./Sm. Anim. Clin., 60:367, 1965.
51. Oliver, J. E., and Hoerlein, B. F.: Convulsive disorders of dogs. J. Am. Vet. Med. Assoc., 146:1126, 1965.
52. Palmer, A. C.: Clinical signs associated with intracranial tumors in dogs. Res. Vet. Sci., 2:326, 1961.
53. Palmer, A. C.: Pathological changes in the brain associated with fits in dogs. Vet. Rec., 90:167, 1972.
54. Palmer, A. C., Malinowski, W., and Barnett, K. C.: Clinical signs including papilloedema associated with brain tumours in twenty-one dogs. J. Sm. Anim. Pract., 15:359, 1975.
55. Parker, A. J.: Canine epileptic convulsions: Treatment. Ill. Vet., 16:5, 1973.
56. Parker, A. J.: Epilepsy in the dog. Ill. Vet., 16:5, 1973.
57. Parker, A. J.: A preliminary report on a new anti-epileptic medication for dogs. J. Am. Anim. Hosp. Assoc., 11:437, 1975.
58. Parker, A. J., and Cunningham, J. G.: Successful surgical removal of an epileptogenic focus in a dog. J. Sm. Anim. Pract., 12:513, 1971.
59. Parry, H. B.: Epileptic states in the dog with special reference to canine hysteria. Vet. Rec., 61:23, 1949.
60. Prynn, R. B.: Medical management of the epileptic patient. J. Am. Anim. Hosp. Assoc., 11:435, 1975.
61. Redding, R. W., and Prynn, R. B.: Seizures. In Kirk, R. W., ed., Current Veterinary Therapy, III. Philadelphia, W. B. Saunders Co., 1968, 463–466.
62. Resnick, S.: Hypocalcemia and tetany in the dog. Vet. Med./Sm. Anim. Clin., 67:637, 1972.
63. Robertson, B. T., and Giles, H. D.: Complete heart block associated with vegetative endocarditis in a dog. J. Am. Vet. Med. Assoc., 161:180, 1972.
64. Rogers, W. A., Donovan, E. F., and Kociba, G. J.: Idiopathic hyperlipoproteinemia in dogs. J. Am. Vet. Med. Assoc., 166:1087, 1975.
65. Rossdale, P. D.: Modern concepts of neonatal disease in foals. Equine Vet. J., 4:1, 1972.
66. Rossdale, P. D.: Pulmonary function in the newborn foal. Proc. Am. Assoc. Equine Pract., 18:69, 1972.
67. Roye, D. B., Serrano, E. E., Hammer, R. H., and Wilder, B. J.: Diphenylhydantoin in dogs and cats. Am. J. Vet. Res., 34:947, 1973.
68. Schenker, S., Breen, K. J., and Hoyumpa, A. M.: Hepatic encephalopathy: Current status. Gastroenterology, 66:121, 1974.
69. Sheather, A. L.: Fainting in foals. J. Comp. Pathol. Ther., 37:106, 1924.
70. Spehlmann, R., and Colley, B.: The effect of diazepam (Valium) on experimental seizures in unanesthetized cats. Neurology, 18:52, 1968.
71. Strafuss, A. C., Njoku, C. O., Blauch, B., and Anderson, N. V.: Islet cell neoplasm in four dogs. J. Am. Vet. Med. Assoc., 159:1008, 1971.
72. Strombeck, D. R., Weiser, M. G., and Kaneko, J. J.: Hyperammonemia and hepatic encephalopathy in the dog. J. Am. Vet. Med. Assoc., 166:1105, 1975.
73. Strombeck, D. R., Meyer, D. J., and Freedland, R. A.: Hyperammonemia due to urea cycle enzyme deficiency in two dogs. J. Am. Vet. Med. Assoc., 166:1109, 1975.
74. Suter, P. F.: Portal vein anomalies in the dog: Their angiographic diagnosis. J. Am. Vet. Rad. Soc., 16:84, 1975.
75. Tobin, T., Dirdjosudjono, S., and Baskin, S. I.: Pharmacokinetics and distribution of diphenylhydantoin in kittens. Am. J. Vet. Res., 34:951, 1973.
76. Tyler, H. R.: Neurologic disorders in renal failure. Am. J. Med., 44:734, 1968.
77. Vitums, A.: Portosystemic communications in animals with hepatic cirrhosis and malignant lymphoma. J. Am. Vet. Med. Assoc., 138:31, 1961.
78. Vitums, A.: Portosystemic communications in the dog. Acta Anat., 39:271, 1959.
79. Wilson, J. W., and Hulse, D. A.: Surgical correction of islet cell adenocarcinoma in a dog. J. Am. Vet. Med. Assoc., 164:603, 1974.
80. Zieve, L.: Pathogenesis of hepatic coma. Arch. Int. Med., 118:211, 1966.
81. Zook, B. C., Carpenter, J. L., and Leeds, E. B.: Lead poisoning in dogs. J. Am. Vet. Med. Assoc., 155:1329, 1969.
82. Rogers, W. A., Donovan, E. F., and Kociba, G. J.: Idiopathic hyperlipoproteinemia in dogs. J. Am. Vet. Med. Assoc., 166:1087, 1975.
83. Mitler, M. M., Stowe, O., and Dement, W. C.: Narcolepsy in seven dogs. J. Am. Vet. Med. Assoc., 168:1036, 1976.
84. Pasten, L. J.: Diphenylhydantoin in the canine: Clinical aspects and determination of therapeutic blood levels. J. Am. Anim. Hosp. Assoc., 13:247, 1977.

Chapter 18

DIENCEPHALON

THALAMUS
ANATOMY
FUNCTION
Direct Cortical Projection System — Primary
    Relay Areas
Diffuse Cortical Projection System — Association
    System
Thalamic Reticular System
*ASCENDING RETICULAR ACTIVATING
    SYSTEM*

Summary of Thalamic Function
CLINICAL SIGNS
CLINICAL EVALUATION OF THE
    UNCONSCIOUS ANIMAL
Neurologic Examination
HYPOTHALAMUS
ANATOMY
Hypothalamic Connections
FUNCTION
CLINICAL SYNDROMES

The diencephalon consists of four general regions:[30, 31, 32] the epithalamus — including the habenula, the pineal body, and the stria habenularis thalamus; the thalamus (dorsal thalamus) — the main mass of the organ between the epithalamus and the hypothalamus; the hypothalamus — the ventral and lateral walls of the third ventricle, below the interthalamic adhesion; and the subthalamus (ventral thalamus) — lateral and caudal to the hypothalamus, continuous with the mesencephalic tegmentum, and includes the subthalamic nucleus, the endopeduncular nucleus, and the zona incerta.

THALAMUS

ANATOMY[33, 40]

The thalamus (dorsal thalamus) is related to the hypothalamus ventrally, and to the internal capsule and caudate nucleus laterally and dorsally. It is composed of numerous nuclear masses, partly separated by sheets of myelinated axons, called medullary laminae. These nuclei and laminae are represented bilaterally on either side of the third ventricle. In the following discussion, reference will be made to one side. Keep in mind that this is a bilateral structure, similar to the rest of the nervous system, and that there are two thalami and two hypothalami. The

Median Section

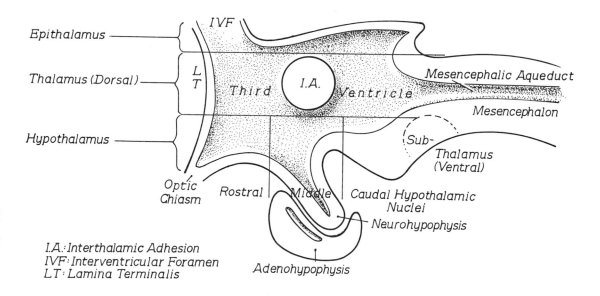

Epithalamus

Thalamus (Dorsal)

Hypothalamus

IVF

LT

Third   I.A.   Ventricle

Mesencephalic Aqueduct

Mesencephalon

Sub-
Thalamus
(Ventral)

Optic
Chiasm

Rostral   Middle   Caudal Hypothalamic
Nuclei

Neurohypophysis

Adenohypophysis

I.A.: Interthalamic Adhesion
IVF: Interventricular Foramen
LT: Lamina Terminalis

Transverse Section Through Optic Tracts and Internal Capsule

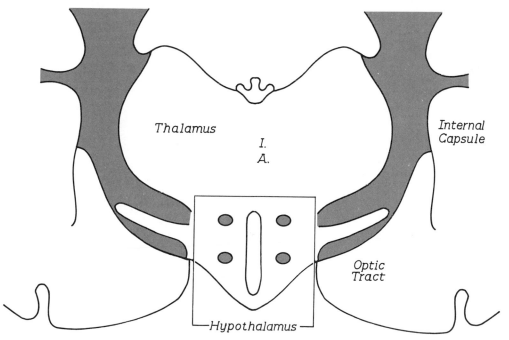

Thalamus

I.
A.

Internal
Capsule

Optic
Tract

Hypothalamus

Figure 18–1.   Divisions of the diencephalon.

internal medullary lamina divides the thalamus on each side into medial and lateral halves, and splits rostrally to enclose a rostral portion, which includes the rostral thalamic nuclei. The lateral half may be subdivided into its nuclei by dividing it into a dorsal and ventral tier by a dorsal plane. The ventral tier produced by this subdivision can be separated further into three nuclear groups from rostral to caudal by two transverse planes. The thin, external medullary lamina forms the external boundary of the lateral half of the thalamus, and is separated from the internal capsule by a narrow nuclear mass, the thalamic reticular nucleus. As a result of these divisions, the following nuclear groups and some examples of their specific nuclei may be listed.[5]

1. Rostral thalamic group—rostral thalamic nucleus (limbic system).
2. Medial thalamic group—medial dorsal nucleus.
3. Lateral thalamic group:

    Dorsal tier—dorsolateral nucleus, caudolateral nucleus, pulvinar.

    Ventral tier—ventral rostral nucleus (extrapyramidal), ventral lateral nucleus (cerebellar), ventral caudal group: ventral caudal medial nucleus (cranial nerve sensory relay), ventral caudal lateral nucleus (spinal nerve sensory relay).

4. Caudal thalamic group—medial geniculate nucleus (auditory), lateral geniculate nucleus (vision).

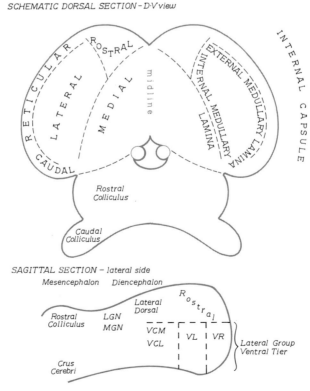

Figure 18–2. Thalamic nuclear groups.

5. Intralaminar—midline thalamic group: central medial nucleus, paraventricular nucleus.

6. Thalamic reticular nucleus (ARAS).

FUNCTION

On a functional basis, the thalamic nuclei can be grouped into three major systems:

Direct Cortical Projection System—Primary Relay Areas

This system has been referred to throughout the text in relation to the conscious perception pathways of sensory systems and thalamic relays of motor systems.

Sensory System. A thalamic relay to the telencephalon occurs in the conscious projection pathway of all sensory systems except olfaction. The thalamic nuclei concerned with this relay are located in the ventral tier of the lateral half of the thalamus and the caudal thalamic group. These are listed below, with a review of the specific sensory pathways afferent to them and the general area of the telencephalon to which each nucleus projects:

VENTRAL CAUDAL LATERAL NUCLEUS. Afferents from spinothalamic tracts (GSA, GVA), medial lemniscus (GP). Efferents to somesthetic cortex (trunk and limbs).

VENTRAL CAUDAL MEDIAL NUCLEUS. Afferents from quintothalamic tract (GSA, GP), solitariothalamic tract (GVA, SVA). Efferents to somesthetic cortex (head).

LATERAL GENICULATE NUCLEUS. Afferents from optic tract.[10] Efferents to visual cortex (occipital lobe).

MEDIAL GENICULATE NUCLEUS. Afferents from brachium of caudal colliculus (auditory). Efferents to auditory cortex (temporal lobe).

Motor System. Axons of extrapyramidal nuclei and the cerebellum have synapses in the thalamus in their circuitry to the telencephalon.

VENTRAL ROSTRAL NUCLEUS. Afferents from the pallidum. Efferents to motor cortex (frontal and parietal lobes).

VENTRAL LATERAL NUCLEUS. Afferents from rostral cerebellar peduncle and the cerebellorubrothalamic tract. Efferents to motor cortex (frontal and parietal lobes).

All these primary relay nuclei also project to other thalamic nuclei.

Diffuse Cortical Projection System—Association System

These thalamic nuclei receive axons only from other diencephalic and telencephalic sources, such as the primary relay thalamic nuclei and the thalamic reticular system nuclei, the hypothalamus, the cingulate gyrus, the frontal cortex, and the striatum. There are no afferents received from the primary afferent pathways in the brain stem. These nuclei project diffusely to all parts of the telencephalon.

Thalamic groups that comprise this system include nuclei in the rostral thalamic group, the medial group, and the dorsal tier of the lateral group.

Thalamic Reticular System

This system is a component of the ascending reticular activating system (ARAS), which receives afferents from lower brain stem levels of the ARAS and collaterals of all ascending conscious sensory pathways. Efferents from this system project to the thalamic nuclei of the association system, which in turn projects diffusely to the telencephalic cortex.

Thalamic groups comprising this system include nuclei in the intralaminar (midline) and reticular groups.

Experimental evidence for the efferent pathways and functions of these systems comes from the following:

1. If the cortex of the telencephalon is removed, retrograde degeneration occurs in those thalamic nuclei that project to the cortex.[24, 25] Such degeneration occurred in the first two systems described (direct cortical projection, diffuse cortical projection) and not in the third system (thalamic reticular).

2. Mild electrical stimulation of nuclei in the direct cortical projection system produces activity only in specific areas of the telencephalic cortex, those to which these nuclei project. Stimulation of any one of the nuclei in the thalamic reticular system produces a slow, spreading, diffuse activity of the entire telencephalic cortex. This is mediated by the nuclei of the thalamic association system.

ASCENDING RETICULAR ACTIVATING SYSTEM

The ARAS is part of the reticular formation, which consists of a network of neurons in the central portion or core of the brain stem from the medulla, through the pons and midbrain, into the diencephalon.[13, 14, 22]

The ARAS receives afferents from all conscious projection pathways of the sensory systems — exteroception, interoception, and proprioception. As these conscious sensory pathways (spinal and cranial) ascend through the brain stem to the primary relay nuclei in the thalamus, collaterals are given off into the reticular formation.

Most of these collaterals synapse in the reticular formation. Neurons of the ARAS then continue the impulse flow rostrally, in a multisynaptic pattern to one of two areas in the diencephalon: the thalamic reticular or hyposubthalamic reticular system. A few collaterals ascend through the ARAS without synaptic interruption to terminate in one of these two diencephalic areas.

The diencephalic portion of the ARAS stimulates the entire cerebral cortex diffusely. The thalamic reticular system affects the cerebral cortex by way of the diffuse telencephalic connections of the nuclei of the association system.

The ARAS functions to "arouse" the cerebral cortex, to awaken the brain to consciousness, to prepare the cortex to receive ascending impulses from any sensory modality. It is responsible for maintaining wakefulness. Decreased activity of the ARAS is associated with sleep. Sleep, a highly complex mechanism, results from diminished activity of brain centers.

Stimulation of dorsal roots, somesthetic tracts, or any part of the ARAS of the sleeping animal arouses it to the awake state. This can be observed in the animal as well as on its electroencephalogram. This does not occur with stimulation of a

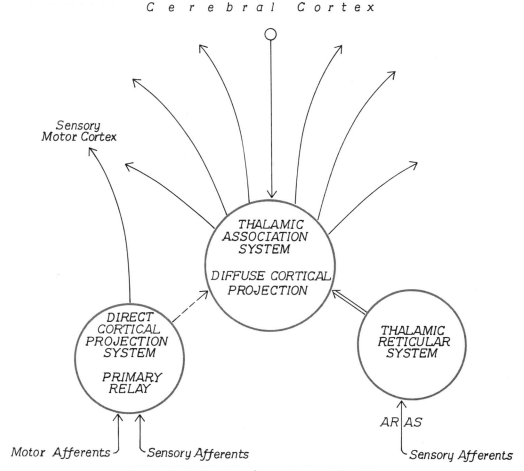

Figure 18–3. Functional organization of the thalamus.

primary relay nucleus in the thalamus. In that case, only the specific projection area of the cerebral cortex shows activity. Conversely, lesions that destroy the ARAS cause a comatose state.

The ARAS is thought to be the seat of consciousness. Both central nervous system depressants and stimulants function on the ARAS. The ARAS may be responsible for the ability to focus attention on particular sources of stimuli, rejecting all others. Thus it monitors the myriad of stimuli that ascend to thalamic levels, accepting what is needed for conscious perception and rejecting what is irrevelant.

Disturbances of consciousness can result from lesions that affect the neuronal

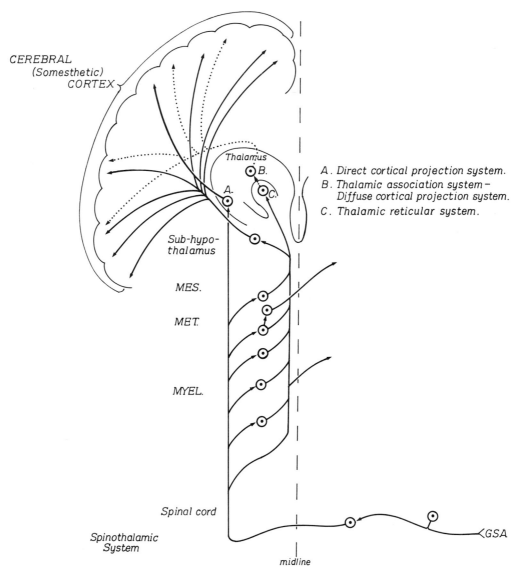

Figure 18–4. Ascending reticular activating system.

activity of the ARAS in the brain stem or the neuronal activity of the cerebral cortex. Based on findings from gross and microscopic examination, the coma that accompanies polioencephalomalacia in ruminants is due to the laminar necrosis in the cerebral cortex. Intracranial injury can produce coma from diffuse cerebral edema or from contusion and hemorrhage in the midbrain and pons of the brain stem. If the semicomatose patient with an intracranial injury has evidence of voluntary limb movements, normal vestibular movements of the eyeballs upon manipulation of the head, no cranial nerve deficits referable to a brain stem lesion, and pupils that may be asymmetric or miotic but respond to light, then the semicoma is probably due to cerebrocortical dysfunction. The prognosis is guarded, but more favorable than for the patient who is semicomatose with clinical evidence of a brain stem lesion that is interfering with the function of the reticular formation in the ARAS.

Summary of Thalamic Function

1. The thalamus is the chief sensory-integrating system of the neuraxis. It functions in the integration and relay of all types of sensory and motor pathways between lower and higher centers.

2. It may serve as the site of conscious perception of some sensory modalities. This is most evident after a lesion destroys the somesthetic cerebral cortex and the perception of some modalities is preserved.

3. It functions in the ARAS as part of the mechanism for maintaining consciousness, for producing a state of attention, or for producing sleep.

CLINICAL SIGNS

Focal thalamic lesions in domestic animals are rare, and would be difficult to localize. Involvement of the direct cortical projection pathways could produce variable degrees of deficits in those systems, such as: lateral geniculate nucleus — contralateral hemianopsia; ventral caudal lateral nucleus — contralateral proprioceptive deficit and hypalgesia; ventral rostral and lateral nuclei — contralateral dysmetria.

Lesions in the limbic system nuclei or tracts result in behavioral changes. Lesions in the thalamic reticular system nuclei result in disturbances of consciousness (depression, semicoma) or convulsions. Rostral thalamic lesions may cause leaning, head turning, circling, or ocular deviation toward the side of the lesion — the adversive syndrome.

CLINICAL EVALUATION OF THE UNCONSCIOUS ANIMAL

Clinical evaluation of the emergency unconscious patient requires a systematic approach, because the time available for appropriate diagnostic and therapeutic decisions may be brief.[26, 27]

Loss of consciousness can occur from either a diffuse or widespread multifocal lesion of both cerebrums, or a lesion affecting the ARAS of the rostral brain stem. Except for traumatic lesions with bilateral cerebral edema and the various diseases that produce diffuse polioencephalomalacia in animals, acute organic diseases that destroy both cerebral hemispheres are rare. Therefore, with these exceptions, most coma caused by structural disease results from brain stem lesions.

The pathophysiologic causes of coma can be grouped into four categories: (1) bilateral diffuse cerebral disease, (2) dorsal tentorial mass lesions that compress or displace the brain stem, (3) ventral tentorial destructive lesions, and (4) metabolic encephalopathy.

Dorsal and ventral tentorial lesions often produce focal neurologic signs. These lesions include neoplasm, abscesses, hemorrhage or contusion or both, localized inflammations, and infarction.

Diffuse brain stem or cerebral destructive lesions may produce symmetric nonlocalizing neurologic signs and coma. These include inflammations, degenerative lesions (polioencephalomalacia, lipodystrophy terminally), injury with or without hemorrhage, and hydrocephalus.

Metabolic encephalopathy, including drug intoxications, usually does not produce focal neurologic signs or alterations of the cerebrospinal fluid.

Be aware of the prolonged postictal coma or stupor that can follow seizures from any cause, including idiopathic epilepsy.

The history of the onset of coma is important. The first fact to establish is whether an injury was observed, or could have happened unobserved. In cases in which an injury could not have occurred, an abrupt onset of coma with structural lesions is more common in ventral tentorial lesions. Space-occupying dorsal tentorial lesions show other evidence of focal signs before the onset of coma. The coma of polioencephalomalacia usually is preceded by ataxia and blindness for at least 6 to 12 hours. Do not overlook drug-induced coma in domestic animals. Drugs used by the owner may have been consumed accidentally in large quantities by the patient.

Neurologic Examination

The neurologic examination may be helpful in defining the site and kind of lesion. Six aspects of the examination should be emphasized.

State of Consciousness. This should be documented carefully, especially to allow one to accurately follow the course of the disease and response to therapy. *Depression or obtundation* are present when an animal responds slowly or inappropriately to verbal stimuli. Some animals may appear disoriented or even act delirious. *Stupor or semicoma* means the patient is generally unresponsive except to vigorous and repeated stimuli that may necessarily be painful. *Coma* means complete unresponsiveness to repeated noxious stimulation.

Vision. Normal response to the menace test determines that the central visual pathway to the visual cerebral cortex is intact. In addition, the pathway from this visual cortex through the brain stem and cerebellum to the facial nucleus and through this cranial nerve to the orbicularis oculi muscle must be intact. If the menace test is absent but pupillary responses to light and facial muscle function are normal, this usually locates the lesion in the cerebral hemispheres. Severe brain stem lesions interfere with the pupillary responses and may depress the cerebral cortex sufficiently to allow no response to the menace test. This is part of the unconscious state from an ARAS lesion. Intact vision in a semicomatose recumbent patient would indicate a brain stem lesion.

Pupillary Size and Response. Structural disease of the rostral brain stem that is severe enough to cause semicoma or coma usually produces fixed pupils either at midpoint or dilated. Metabolic disease that produces the same degree of unconsciousness usually spares the pupillary light reaction. The pupils may be small but reactive in metabolic disease. In acute diffuse cerebrocortical disease, pupils often are symmetrically small. Severe rostral brain stem compression produces dilated, unresponsive pupils. As a unilateral dorsal tentorial (cerebral) lesion herniates and compresses the brain stem, the pupil on the affected side may first become small but remain reactive to light, followed by both pupils becoming small. As the compression increases, the pupils become fixed in midposition or dilation and unresponsive to light.

Extremely small, slit pupils are seen in both metabolic and diffuse cerebrocortical or unilateral dorsal tentorial structural lesions. In the comatose patient reactive pupils imply a metabolic disease, and unreactive pupils strongly suggest structural brain stem disease.

Eye Movements.   In animals, testing eye movements in the semicomatose or comatose patient is limited to moving the head rapidly to detect normal vestibular nystagmus. Caloric testing for vestibulo-ocular reflexes is unreliable in the domestic animal. Loss of any eye movement response to moving the head from side to side in a dorsal plane suggests structural brain stem disease and is a poor prognosis. Asymmetric or abnormal responses may occur if there is damage to the nuclei or nerves of cranial nerves III, IV, and VI. In severe metabolic disease these responses may be absent as well.

Respirations.   Irregularities of respiration may occur with serious brain disease. Cheyne-Stokes respiration may occur with severe bilateral cerebral disease, or diencephalic disease, or both. Mesencephalic lesions may cause a regular sustained hyperventilation referred to as central neurogenic hyperventilation. More caudal brain stem lesions produce bizarre, abnormal breathing patterns often referred to as irregular or ataxic breathing. This usually precedes respiratory arrest.

Traumatic lesions that injure the thorax may produce respiratory abnormalities unrelated to a brain stem lesion.

Motor Responses.   The pattern of spontaneous motor function or the motor response to painful stimuli may aid in the localization of the lesion. In metabolic disease only symmetric deficits occur. Asymmetric deficits suggest structural disease.

In acute disease with mild asymmetric motor responses, the deficient side

TABLE 18–1.   METABOLIC DISEASES THAT MAY PRODUCE COMA

Pancreatic disease:
  Beta cell neoplasia—hypoglycemia
  Diabetes mellitus—hyperglycemia and ketoacidosis
Liver disease: hyperammonemia, hypoglycemia
Renal disease: uremia, acidosis, hypocalcemia
Myocardial disease: ischemic anoxia
Pulmonary disease: anoxic anoxia, acidosis
Adrenal disease:
  Hypoadrenocortical crisis—hyperkalemia
Anemia: carbon monoxide poisoning, hemorrhage
Osmotic abnormalities:
  Water intoxication—hypo-osmolar state
  Salt poisoning—hyperosmolar state, hypernatremia
Nutritional deficiency: thiamine deficiency

TABLE 18–2. POISONS THAT MAY PRODUCE COMA

Hexachlorophene[38]	Lead salts
Cyanide	Dinitrophenol
Barbiturates	Kerosene
Ethylene glycol	Nitrobenzene
Benzene hexachloride, benzene	Turpentine
Amphetamine sulfate	Arsenic
Carbon tetrachloride	Zinc phosphide

may be ipsilateral to a brain stem lesion or contralateral to a cerebral lesion. Shortly after the acute onset of a unilateral cerebral lesion, the animal will be ambulatory and may have a mild contralateral paresis and ataxia. There may be a tendency to turn the head or eyes toward the side of the lesion and to circle in that direction. Any serious deficiency in gait that persists suggests a brain stem lesion. The obtunded, blind animal with a paretic, ataxic gait is more likely to have a bilateral cerebral lesion than a brain stem lesion. Decerebrate rigidity occurs with midbrain lesions, and is characterized by recumbency accompanied by rigid extension of the limbs and opisthotonus.

A comatose patient with decerebrate rigidity and normally reactive pupils probably has a metabolic disease, whereas a similar comatose patient with fixed, unreactive pupils has a structural brain stem lesion.

In metabolic disease, obtundation and semicoma usually precede the motor signs, whereas in dorsal tentorial lesions the opposite occurs.

A list of poisons that may produce coma as the main clinical sign or one of the terminal clinical signs is presented in Table 18–2.[18]

HYPOTHALAMUS

ANATOMY

The hypothalamus is that part of the diencephalon that forms the ventral and lateral walls of the ventral portion of the third ventricle. It extends from the lamina terminalis and optic chiasm rostrally through the mamillary bodies caudally. The ventral surface of the hypothalamus between these areas is the tuber cinereum. A ventral extension of the tuber cinereum is the infundibulum or pituitary stalk. Proximally, the infundibulum widens where it joins the hypothalamus to form the median eminence of the tuber cinereum. Distally, the infundibulum expands to form the distal part of the neurohypophysis, the neural lobe of the hypophysis (pituitary gland).

The hypothalamus may be divided transversely from rostral to caudal into three groups of nuclei. In addition, three longitudinal zones can be recognized throughout each hypothalamus—the periventricular zone, the middle zone, and the lateral zone. Some examples follow:

1. Rostral chiasmatic group—preoptic area (part of telencephalon, fuses with rostral hypothalamus), supraoptic nucleus, paraventricular nucleus, rostral hypothalamic area.

2. Intermediate (tuberal) group—infundibular nucleus (arcuate), dorsomedial nucleus, ventromedial nucleus, lateral hypothalamic area.

3. Caudal (mammillary) group—mammillary body, caudal hypothalamic area.

Hypothalamic Connections

Afferent

TELENCEPHALON (rhinencephalon). Fornix—from hippocampus to mammillary bodies; stria terminalis—from amygdaloid body; medial forebrain bundle—from septal area; pallidohypothalamic fibers—from pallidum (extrapyramidal).

DIENCEPHALON. Thalamic—hypothalamic fibers.

MESENCEPHALON. Mammillary peduncle—collaterals of brain stem afferent pathways—GVA, SVA, from visceral modalities. Dorsal longitudinal fasciculus in the paraventricular central grey substance—collateral from the pathways in the solitary tract—GVA, SVA.

Efferent[9]

MAMMILLOTHALAMIC TRACT. To rostral thalamic nucleus.

HYPOTHALAMOTEGMENTAL PATHWAYS. Mammillotegmental tract—to mesencephalic reticular formation to influence brain stem and spinal cord GVE system; periventricular fibers and dorsal longitudinal fasciculus—to brain stem and spinal cord GVE system.

HYPOTHALAMOHYPOPHYSEAL TRACT. The hypothalamohypophyseal tract courses into the neurohypophysis.[43] Neurosecretory products from the supraoptic and paraventricular nuclei (oxytocin, vasopressin or antidiuretic hormone) course through the supraopticohypophyseal and paraventriculohypophyseal tracts to the neural lobe, in which they are elaborated into the capillary bed and ultimately course to the effector organ to exert their activity.[2] The neurosecretory products from the mediobasal hypothalamic nuclei flow through the axons of the tuberohypophyseal tract, and are released terminally into the capillaries of the neurohypophysis and circulate by way of the portal vessels to the sinusoids of the adenohypophysis to influence the endocrine activity of the cells in the pars distalis. These are the adenohypophyseal releasing factors that are produced in hypothalamic nuclei.

FUNCTION

The hypothalamus serves as a higher center for regulation of visceral motor activity. Its nuclei act as the upper motor neuron for visceral function; therefore, they are considered the upper motor neuron in the autonomic nervous system. Stimulation of the rostral hypothalamus elicits parasympathetic activity, whereas stimulation of the caudal hypothalamus elicits sympathetic activity throughout the body. The hypothalamus functions without voluntary control. The neocortex does not order hypothalamic activity; nevertheless, the hypothalamus is subject to its influence. As an example, consider the gastrointestinal signs that accompany fear, pain, and emotional states. Visceral motor activity associated with the function of the olfactory and limbic systems is mediated through the hypothalamus. In addition, the hypothalamus regulates the activity of a large portion of the body's endocrine system by way of neurosecretory products elaborated from hypothalamic nuclei.

CLINICAL SYNDROMES

Numerous clinical syndromes have been related to lesions that disturb the hypothalamus and adjacent structures.

Abnormal Behavior. Selective ventral hypothalamic lesions in cats produce rage.

Diabetes Insipidus. Diabetes insipidus is the loss of control of water excretion due to the failure of production or transport and release of antidiuretic hormone (ADH) into the blood stream.[28, 29] This failure to resorb water from the kidney tubules causes polyuria, and secondarily polydipsia. The urine specific gravity is consistently very low (1.002 to 1.005) and does not concentrate when water consumption is stopped, but does show response of the kidney to the intramuscular injection of extracts containing ADH.[3] In a study of 26 cases of neoplasms of the adenohypophysis in dogs, 92 per cent had the clinical diagnosis of diabetes insipidus from direct pressure of the neoplasm on the nuclei in the hypothalamus (supraoptic nuclei).[4, 7, 8, 19, 35]

Abnormal Temperature Regulation. Abnormal temperature control may be manifested as hyperthermia, hypothermia, or poikilothermia. A heat loss center is located in the rostral hypothalamic area which normally responds to elevated body temperatures by initiating sweating, increased respirations, vasodilation, and panting. A heat conservation center is located in the caudal and lateral hypothalamic areas that responds to depressed body temperature by initiating piloerection, shivering, vasoconstriction, and increased basal metabolic rate, thereby increasing feeding. Lesions of these centers inhibit their normal regulatory function: in the case of the heat loss center they cause hyperthermia, while in the heat conservation center they cause hypothermia. Hyperhidrosis (excessive sweating) may accompany hyperthermia with disturbances of these centers. Bilateral destruction of the descending hypothalamotegmental tracts concerned with the conservation and dissipation of the body heat may produce poikilothermia, in which the body temperature varies with the environmental temperature.

Abnormal Appetite.[12] Abnormalities in appetite are expressed as hyperphagia and obesity, or anorexia and cachexia. A satiety center resides in the ventromedial hypothalamic nucleus. If destroyed bilaterally, hyperphagia and obesity result, which may be accompanied by savageness. In the lateral hypothalamic area there is a feeding center responsible for the stimulation of appetite. Lesions in this center cause anorexia that is complete, resulting in cachexia and eventual death. The amygdaloid body is also involved in appetite control.

The adiposogenital syndrome (Froelich's syndrome) results from hypothalamic lesions involving the satiety center and the mediobasal nuclei concerned with gonadal stimulation by way of the hypophysis. Such animals become obese and their genitalia atrophy.[34, 35]

Abnormal Carbohydrate Metabolism. The hypothalamus is involved with the regulation of the blood sugar level of the body. The exact mechanism of this control is unknown. Lesions involving the ventral wall of the third ventricle have been associated with hyperglycemia, glycosuria, and abnormal glucose tolerance curves.

There are reports in the veterinary literature of neoplasms of the pars intermedia in horses associated with hyperglycemia and glycosuria that are unresponsive to insulin.[1, 4, 16, 20, 41, 42] These neoplasms usually exert pressure on the hypothalamus as they grow dorsally out of the hypophyseal fossa. In addition, these animals often exhibit a failure to shed their winter hair coat through the warm months of the year.[1, 11] Hyperthermia and hyperhidrosis also have been reported with these neoplasms, and occasionally diabetes insipidus and a ravenous appetite.

Abnormal Heart Rate. Alterations of cardiovascular function have been observed in cattle with abscesses of the hypophysis and involvement of the hypothalamus. The interference with the role of the hypothalamus in autonomic function results in a marked slowing of the heart, or bradycardia.

Abnormal Sensorium. Hypothalamic lesions that interfere with its role in the ARAS may result in variations in the state of consciousness, occasionally producing semicoma.

Hyperadrenocorticoidism. Hyperadrenocorticoidism often accompanies neoplasms of the adenohypophysis that produce adrenocorticotropic hormone or a similar acting polypeptide hormone.[6] This syndrome has been reported with chromophobe adenomas and pars intermedia neoplasms of the canine pituitary. If the hypothalamus is compromised by the neoplasm, various signs of hypothalamic dysfunction may accompany the signs of hyperactivity of the adrenal cortex.

Signs of hyperadrenocorticoidism include:[15, 17, 21, 23, 36, 37, 39] (1). polyuria, polydipsia, polyphagia; (2). bilaterally symmetric alopecia with sparing of the head and distal extremities, thin hypotonic skin, patchy hyperpigmentation, comedones, keratin plugs, petechiae or ecchymoses, and calcinosis cutis; (3) pendulous, flaccid abdomen, enlarged liver; (4) atrophic testicles or prolonged anestrus; and (5) lameness (osteoporosis), skeletal muscle atrophy, and weakness. In laboratory tests, the complete blood count shows stress response (lymphopenia, eosinopenia); there are elevated serum cholesterol, glucose, glutamic pyruvic transaminase, and alkaline phosphatase levels; urinary specific gravity is from 1.008 to 1.014; and there is evidence of glycosuria.

REFERENCES

1. Bäckström, G.: Hirsutism associated with pituitary tumors in horses. Nord. Vet. Med., *15:*778, 1963.
2. Bisset, G. W., Clark, B. J., and Errington, M. L.: The hypothalamic neurosecretory pathways for the release of oxytocin and vasopressin in the cat. J. Physiol., *217:*111, 1971.
3. Bovee, K. C.: Urine osmolarity as a definitive indicator of renal concentrating capacity. J. Am. Vet. Med. Assoc., *155:*30, 1969.
4. Brandt, A. J.: Über Hypophysenadenom bei Hund und Pferd. Skand. Vet. Tidskr., *30:*875, 1940.
5. Cabral, R. J., and Johnson, J. I.: The organization of mechanoreceptive projections in the ventrobasal thalamus of sheep. J. Comp. Neurol., *141:*17, 1971.
6. Capen, C. C., and Koestner, A.: Functional chromophobe adenoma of the canine adenohypophysis. An ultrastructural evaluation of neoplasm of pituitary corticotrophs. Pathol. Vet., *4:*326, 1967.
7. Capen, C. C., Martin, S. L., and Koestner, A.: Neoplasms in the adenohypophysis of dogs. Pathol. Vet., *4:*301, 1967.
8. Capen, C. C., Martin, S. L., and Koestner, A.: The ultrastructure and histopathology of an acidophil adenoma of the canine adenohypophysis. Pathol. Vet., *4:*348, 1967.
9. Cheatham, M. L., and Matzke, H. A.: Descending hypothalamic medullary pathways in the cat. J. Comp. Neurol., *127:*369, 1966.
10. Cummings, J. F., and de Lahunta, A.: An experimental study of the retinal projections in the horse and sheep. Ann. N.Y. Acad. Sci., *167:*293, 1969.

11. Eriksson, K. S., Dyrendahl, S., and Grunfelt, D.: A case of hirsutism in connection with hypophyseal tumor in a horse. Nord. Vet. Med., 8:807, 1956.

12. Fonberg, E.: The effect of hypothalamic and amygdalar lesions on alimentary behavior and thermoregulation. J. Physiol., 63:249, 1971.

13. Jouvet, M.: Biogenic amines and the states of sleep. Science, 163:32, 1969.

14. Jouvet, M.: Neurophysiology of the states of sleep. Physiol. Rev., 47:117, 1967.

15. Kelly, D. F., Siegel, E. T., and Berg, P.: The adrenal glands in dogs with hyperadrenocorticism: A pathologic study. Vet. Pathol., 8:385, 1971.

16. King, J. M., Kavanaugh, J. F., and Bentinck-Smith, J.: Diabetes mellitus with pituitary neoplasms in a horse and a dog. Cor. Vet., 52:133, 1962.

17. Kirk, G. R., Boyer, S., and Hutcheson, D. P.: Effects of o,p′:DDD on plasma cortisol levels and histology of the adrenal gland in the normal dog. J. Am. Anim. Hosp. Assoc., 10:179, 1974.

18. Kirk, R. W., and Bistner, S. I.: Handbook of Veterinary Procedures and Emergency Treatment. 2nd ed., Philadelphia, W. B. Saunders Co., 1975.

19. Koestner, A., and Capen, C. C.: Ultrastructural evaluation of the canine hypothalamic-neurohypophyseal system in diabetes insipidus associated with pituitary neoplasms. Pathol. Vet., 4:513, 1967.

20. Loeb, W. F., Capen, C. C., and Johnson, L. E.: Adenomas of the pars intermedia associated with hyperglycemia and glycosuria in two horses. Cor. Vet., 56:623, 1966.

21. Lorenz, M. D., Scott, D. W., and Pulley, L. T.: Medical treatment of canine hyperadrenocorticoidism with o,p′-DDD. Cor. Vet., 63:646, 1973.

22. Magoun, H. W.: The ascending reticular activating system. Res. Publ. Assoc. Res. Nerv. Ment. Dis., 30:480, 1952.

23. Mulnix, J. A.: Adrenal cortical disease in dogs. Scope, 19:12, 1975.

24. Murray, M.: Degeneration of some intralaminar thalamic nuclei after cortical removals in the cat. J. Comp. Neurol., 127:341, 1966.

25. Peacock, J. H., and Combs, C. M.: Retrograde cell degeneration in adult cat after hemidecortication. J. Comp. Neurol., 125:329, 1965.

26. Plum, F., and Posner, J. B.: The diagnosis of stupor and coma. 2nd ed., Philadelphia, F.A. Davis, 1972.

27. Posner, J. B.: Clinical evaluation of the unconscious patient. Clin. Neurosurg., 22:281, 1975.

28. Richards, M. A.: Polydipsia in the dog. The differential diagnosis of polyuric syndromes in the dog. J. Sm. Anim. Pract., 10:651, 1970.

29. Richards, M. A., and Sloper, J. C.: Diabetes insipidus—the complexity of the syndrome. Acta Endocrinol., 62:627, 1969.

30. Rioch, D. M.: Studies on the diencephalon of carnivora. I. Nuclear configuration of the thalamus, epithalamus, and hypothalamus of the dog and cat. J. Comp. Neurol., 49:1, 1929.

31. Rioch, D. M.: II. Nuclear configuration and fiber connections of subthalamus and midbrain of the dog and cat. J. Comp. Neurol., 49:121, 1929.

32. Rioch, D. M.: III. Certain myelinated fiber connections of the diencephalon of the dog and cat. J. Comp. Neurol., 53:319, 1931.

33. Rose, J. E.: The thalamus of the sheep: Cellular and fibrous structure and comparison with pig, rabbit, and cat. J. Comp. Neurol., 77:469, 1942.

34. Saunders, L. Z., and Rickard, C. G.: Craniopharyngioma in a dog with apparent adiposogenital syndrome and diabetes insipidus. Cor. Vet., 42:490, 1952.

35. Saunders, L. Z., Stephenson, H. C., and McEntee, K.: Diabetes insipidus and adiposogenital syndrome in a dog due to an infundibuloma. Cor. Vet., 41:445, 1951.

36. Schecter, R. D., Stabenfeldt, G. H., Gribble, D. H., and Ling, G. V.: Treatment of Cushing's syndrome in the dog with an adrenocorticolytic agent (o,p′-DDD). J. Am. Vet. Med. Assoc., 162:629, 1973.

37. Scott, D. W.: Cushing's Disease (hyperadrenocorticism). Abstracts, 66th Annual Conference, Ithaca, N.Y., New York State College of Veterinary Medicine, 1974, 36–38.

38. Scott, D. W., Bolton, G. R., and Lorenz, M. D.: Hexachlorophene toxicosis in dogs. J. Am. Vet. Med. Assoc., 162:947, 1973.

39. Siegel, E. T., Kelly, D. F., and Berg, P.: Cushing's syndrome in the dog. J. Am. Vet. Med. Assoc., 157:2081, 1970.

40. Sychowa, B.: The morphology and topography of the thalamic nuclei of the dog. Acta Biol. Exp., 21:101, 1961.

41. Tasker, J. B., Whiteman, C. E., and Martin, B. R.: Diabetes mellitus in the horse. J. Am. Vet. Med. Assoc., 49:393, 1966.

42. Urman, H. K., Ozcan, H. C., and Tekeli, S.: Pituitary neoplasms in two horses. Zentrabl. Veterinaermed., 10:257, 1963.

43. Zambrano, D., and de Robertis, E.: Ultrastructure of the hypothalamic neurosecretory system of the dog. Z. Zellforsch. Mikrosk. Anat., 81:264, 1967.

Chapter 19

DIAGNOSIS AND EVALUATION OF TRAUMATIC LESIONS OF THE NERVOUS SYSTEM

CENTRAL NERVOUS SYSTEM
BRAIN
Medical Treatment
Surgical Treatment
Therapy Guidelines
SPINAL CORD
Lumbar, Sacral, and Caudal Segments
Focal Lesion Between the Third Thoracic and
    Fourth Lumbar Segments

Cervical Spinal Cord
PERIPHERAL NERVOUS SYSTEM
THORACIC LIMB
Radial Nerve
Brachial Plexus — Roots of C6–T2
PELVIC LIMB
Sciatic Nerve
Lumbar, Sacral, and Caudal Roots

CENTRAL NERVOUS SYSTEM[2, 11, 13, 17, 20, 34]

BRAIN

The management of patients who present with intracranial injuries should follow a specific list of priorities which is similar to that for any severe injury.

Establish a Patent Airway. Respiratory hypoxia causes cellular anoxia. Hypercapnia increases the cerebral blood flow in the cranial cavity by vasodilation, and increases cerebral edema, which must be avoided. The unconscious patient should be intubated. If therapy is required in the conscious patient, tracheostomy may be performed. Repeated hyperventilation reduces the partial pressure of carbon dioxide.

Stop Major External Hemorrhage

Treat the Shock.[14] The intracranial injury rarely causes shock. The shock that the patient with intracranial injury often experiences is due to tissue damage and loss of blood from other organs. These should be examined at this time for any life-threatening lesions. The temperature, pulse, and respirations should be recorded for evaluation of the response to treatment and for signs of deterioration from a brain stem lesion.

Evaluate the Neurologic Status. The assessment of the neurologic status of a patient with intracranial injury does not require exhaustive knowledge of the neuroanatomy and neurophysiology of the brain to arrive at a clinical diagnosis, recommend therapy, and determine a baseline for further evaluation. If possible, an eyewitness account of the accident and a description of the patient immediately following the accident should be obtained and compared with the present evaluation. The most important signs to evaluate are similar to those described under coma in Chapter 18.

STATE OF CONSCIOUSNESS. This is the best evaluation for signs of progressive cerebral hypoxia. The various levels of consciousness may be described as coma (unconscious and no response to painful stimuli), semicoma or stupor (unconscious but responsive to painful stimuli), delirium, confusion, depression, and alertness. The important factor is to describe what response you observe.

PUPIL SIZE AND RESPONSE. Bilateral miotic, bilateral mydriatic, or asymmetric pupils all suggest brain stem contusion. Unresponsive mydriatic pupils bilaterally are usually due to an irreversible midbrain lesion. Miotic pupils that become mydriatic and unresponsive suggest a midbrain compression by a progressing lesion; and an indication for more aggressive therapy. Asymmetric and bilaterally miotic pupils also occur with primarily acute cerebral lesions. These may change remarkably in the first few hours following the injury. A favorable prognosis is indicated by a change from pupillary abnormality to normal. Before concluding that the pupillary abnormality is due to a midbrain lesion, the eyeballs should be examined carefully for lesions.

POSTURE AND MOTOR FUNCTION. In the recumbent animal, determine whether there is any voluntary movement of the limbs in response to painful stimuli. If reflexes are absent, this would indicate there was an additional spinal cord lesion present. The posture of decerebrate rigidity, extensor rigidity of all four limbs, may occur with severe brain stem lesions that are usually caudal to the red nucleus. Severe vestibular disturbance peripherally or centrally in the pons and medulla causes head tilt, or neck and body flexion, or both. If the patient is ambulatory, determine any degree of paresis or ataxia that may be present by careful observation of gait and response to the testing of postural reactions.

VISION. In the absence of lesions in the eyeball or postorbital area, visual deficits in patients with intracranial lesions usually are due to cerebral edema of the visual cerebral cortex. Pupillary response is normal if there are no accompanying rostral brain stem lesions. In the recumbent, conscious animal this can only be tested by the palpebral response to menacing gestures toward the eyes.

OTHER CRANIAL NERVE FUNCTION. Initial loss of cranial nerve function suggests laceration of the cranial nerve along its course from the brain stem, or laceration and hemorrhage in the brain stem involving its fibers or nucleus. Loss of cranial nerve function subsequent to the initial examination suggests compression and hypoxia, and a more guarded prognosis. When this occurs, it is helpful in localizing the lesion.

RESPIRATIONS. Serious brain stem injury may cause irregularities of respiration. Cheyne-Stokes respiration occurs with diencephalic lesions, hyperventilation with mesencephalic lesions, and irregular or ataxic respirations with medullary lesions. Ataxic respirations usually precede respiratory arrest. Development of these respiratory irregularities and a slowing of the pulse rate are poor prognostic signs.

Signs of vestibular system disturbance (head tilt, truncal torsion, rolling, abnormal nystagmus) can occur with lesions of the vestibular nuclei in the medulla or of the labyrinth in the inner ear. With a nuclear lesion there should be other signs of involvement of adjacent medullary structures. It is important to determine the source of the vestibular system injury, because the prognosis is better for injuries to the inner ear membranous labyrinth. These labyrinth contusions often are associated with a fracture of the petrosal bone, and hemorrhage often occurs from the external ear canal. If the patient is conscious, with voluntary limb movement, and has no other signs of brain stem involvement, it may recover from the peripheral receptor damage by compensation. This will take from weeks to months, and a residual head tilt and mild ataxia may persist.

Another test of brain stem function is that of vestibular nystagmus. Normally rapid movement of the head from side to side in a dorsal plane elicits a nystagmus, with the quick phase toward the direction of head movement. Lesions that interrupt the medial longitudinal fasciculus or the brain stem portion of neurons in cranial nerves III, IV, or VI prevent this normal vestibular nystagmus in an animal with a normal membranous labyrinth.

Do not overlook the possibility of multiple injuries. For example, a patient may present as recumbent, semicomatose, and in shock, with pain perceived from the thoracic limbs and with mild voluntary thoracic limb withdrawal attempts, but with complete analgesia and paralysis caudal to the thoracolumbar junction. Such a patient has intracranial injury and a transverse injury of the spinal cord.

In order to follow the patient's course, a baseline neurologic assessment must be made as soon as possible, and the neurologic status must be reevaluated continually to determine whether the treatment used should be continued or altered.

Cerebral edema is considered to be the usual sequel to intracranial injury, and the primary lesion for which treatment is instituted. The most common gross lesion in the dog and cat with severe intracranial injury is hemorrhage on the median plane in the midbrain tegmentum. This causes semicoma or coma, tetraplegia with or without torticollis, and abnormal pupillary size or response. Subarachnoid hemorrhage, if present, is minimal and often associated with a focal cerebral laceration and hemorrhage. Subdural and extradural hemorrhages are less common.

Medical Treatment

Medical treatment is instituted to correct and prevent cerebral edema, and should consist of high levels of corticosteroids and hypertonic fluids.[3, 12, 16, 25, 26] Dexamethasone (Azium) should be administered in a dose of 2 to 4 mg per kg repeated at 6- to 8-hour intervals. This is similar to the treatment used for shock, and may already have been instituted. Mannitol (Osmitrol—20 per cent) should be administered intravenously over a 10-minute period at a dose of 2 gm per kg, and repeated once or twice at 3- to 4-hour intervals. In experimental brain injury it has been shown that the increased cerebrospinal fluid pressure responds to intravenous mannitol in 30 minutes, whereas responses to corticosteroids take about 6 hours.

Precautions are necessary in the use of hypertonic fluids. If there is any reason to believe that hemorrhage in the cranial cavity has not been controlled, this treatment is contraindicated.[21] In the absence of bleeding from the nares or external ear canals, and in the absence of palpable skull fractures that could injure venous sinuses or the middle meningeal artery, it may be safe to assume that continual hemorrhage inside the cranial cavity is not a consideration. Large doses of hypertonic solutions should not be used without concomitant maintainence of a near normal fluid volume to prevent severe dehydration that can attend the use of these solutions. If hypovolemic shock is present, the blood volume can be reestablished with isotonic lactated Ringer's solution. Hypertonic solutions can be administered simultaneously, although their efficacy may be decreased. It is important not to overhydrate the patient. This stresses the heart and increases the potential for a rebound effect on the intracranial pressure when the hypertonic fluid therapy is stopped. Monitoring of the central venous pressure and the gum perfusion time should help determine the reestablishment of normal blood volume.

Recently, experimental data have shown that intravenous dimethylsulfoxide (DMSO) has the effect of reducing the increased intracranial pressure produced by intracranial injury.[7] It is given intravenously at the rate of 2 gm per kg of a 40 per cent solution. Limited clinical use in the horse and dog have shown no obvious untoward side effects. More data are necessary to determine if it is as useful clinically as those therapies already accepted. The experimental data do not support an additive effect of DMSO to that of mannitol or corticosteroids.

For a favorable prognosis, a response to medical therapy should be seen in 6 to 8 hours following treatment. The patient must be reevaluated constantly. If there are signs of improvement, continue the therapy and observation. Any sign of deterioration is an indication for surgery.

Having evaluated the patient's neurologic status and instituted medical therapy, skull radiographs may be obtained to determine the presence and severity of fractures of the skull bones that bound the cranial cavity. If there are compound fractures or a depressed fracture that obviously encroaches on the brain, surgery should be performed.

Surgical Treatment[18]

The decision to operate to prevent further compression of nervous tissue from the expanding cerebral edema depends on the results of the neurologic evaluation. A patient who presents as comatose, tetraplegic, and with dilated, unresponsive pupils probably has severe contusion with hemorrhage in the midbrain and is not likely to be helped by surgery, but it is the only therapy to offer and should be done immediately. The prognosis is poor. No improvement in the comatose patient with miotic pupils after 24 to 36 hours of medical therapy is indication for surgery.

A patient whose signs deteriorate from those of the initial assessment is a candidate for surgical decompression. Such signs include progression from depression or delerium to semicoma, or from semicoma with normal or miotic pupils to semicoma or coma with dilated, unresponsive pupils. A decreasing pulse rate and deep irregular respirations are signs of deterioration. Surgical decompression is performed by removing a large portion of the calvaria bilaterally.

If radiographs indicate a fracture involving a venous sinus or the middle meningeal artery, or the signs suggest a unilateral cerebral lesion (contralateral cortical visual deficit, or hemiparesis or both), exploratory surgery may be performed to remove a blood clot. Ultimately, this is the most accurate way to locate extradural hemorrhage.

If the patient slowly returns to consciousness and response to painful stimuli improves, then the medical therapy should be continued but the patient must be reevaluated continually. A patient may go from a few days to a week with minimal signs, and then neurologic signs may slowly deteriorate. This suggests slow extradural or subdural bleeding and cerebral compression.

Occasionally, patients with intracranial injury are presented with convulsions or status epilepticus. Diazepam (Valium) in 5-mg doses, intramuscular or intravenous, should be used to stop the convulsions. If they persist, barbiturates should be administered. When the convulsions have stopped, the patient can be evaluated for further neurologic injury.

Patients that are restless or delerious should be given intravenous chlorpromazine (Thorazine) in a dose of 1 mg per kg slowly, provided that a neurologic assessment of the patient is made prior to administering the drug. This drug also may be part of the therapy for shock in the patient.

Whole body hypothermia has been used to reduce cerebral edema and cellular metabolic demands for oxygen, but the response is too variable to recommend it for routine therapy. However, hyperthermia should be prevented. If the patient is presented hypothermic, attempts should not be made to raise the body temperature, for this may be advantageous to the patient.

Therapy Guidelines

1. Ambulatory, confused, depressed: corticosteroids.
2. Delerious: corticosteroids and chlorpromazine.
3. Convulsions: diazepam.
4. Recumbent, semicomatose, comatose: mannitol, corticosteroids.

Adequate nursing care is essential to prevent death from complications. The bladder and rectum should be evacuated regularly. The recumbent patient should be turned as often as possible.

SPINAL CORD[4, 5, 8, 15, 19, 23, 24, 29]

Spinal cord injuries are also described in Chapter 10.

Lumbar, Sacral, and Caudal Segments

The signs that are seen with injury to the lumbar, sacral, and caudal segments of the spinal cord are the same as those that occur with injury of the roots of the spinal nerves of these segments. These include complete analgesia, areflexia, and atonic muscles in the area innervated by these segments. They are described in detail under the peripheral nervous system injuries. In the dog, the caudal segments usually are located over the body of the sixth lumbar vertebra, the sacral segments over the body of the fifth lumbar vertebra, and the last three lumbar segments over the body of the fourth lumbar vertebra. In the cat the sacral segments are often over the body of the sixth lumbar vertebra, and the last three lumbar segments are over the body of the fifth lumbar vertebra. Injury to these segments of the spinal cord is more serious than injury to the roots, and recovery from malacia and hemorrhage should not be expected.

Focal Lesion Between the Third Thoracic and Fourth Lumbar Segments

Focal lesions in one or more of the spinal cord segments from the third thoracic to the fourth lumbar that cause complete dysfunction of the injured tissue from concussion, contusion, or laceration result in paraplegia with intact pelvic limb spinal reflexes, and analgesia of the trunk and limbs caudal to the lesion.

These lesions usually are associated with vertebral fractures and displacements of the vertebral canal. The most common site is the caudal thoracic and cranial lumbar region. Lesions here often result in the Schiff-Sherrington syndrome, which is characterized by rigidly extended hypertonic thoracic limbs and flaccid, hypotonic, paralyzed analgesic pelvic limbs with intact spinal reflexes. The thoracic limbs have normal voluntary motor function despite their marked hypertonia, can perform all the postural reactions and spinal reflexes, and have intact sensation.

If the vertebral canal is displaced at the site of the injury, decompressive laminectomy and realignment should be performed. If there is complete discontinuity of the vertebral canal, nothing can be done for the patient to recover the lost neurologic function. Displacements between 50 and 100 per cent of the vertebral canal have a more guarded prognosis. The smaller the displacement, the more favorable the prognosis. However, this still must be guarded, for at the time of the injury the displacement of the vertebral canal may have been complete, with the involved vertebrae returning to a position of partial displacement. In addition, the examiner cannot determine clinically whether the damage is contusion or laceration. Functional and organic neurologic deficit cannot be differentiated.

Recovery from concussion occurs spontaneously within a few minutes of the time of the accident. Recovery from contusion caused by compression may be enhanced by laminectomy at the site of the vertebral column injury.[4, 6, 22, 28] This should be performed as soon as possible after the diagnosis has been made. The prognosis is more favorable if there are any indications of the functioning of tracts that pass through the site of the lesion, such as voluntary movement of a pelvic limb, tail wagging in response to the examiner, or the perception of pain.

These focal lesions can occur from traumatic rupture of an intervertebral disk, which is diagnosed as a narrow space between adjacent vertebrae. In some instances, there is no lesion in the vertebral column to associate with the focal lesion in the spinal cord. In the absence of localizing vertebral column injury a myelogram is recommended in order to diagnose if there is significant spinal cord swelling to warrant laminectomy and incision of the dura at the site of the swelling.

Medical therapy for the injured spinal cord should include high doses of corticosteroids and hypertonic fluids, as indicated for the injured brain.[10] These should be administered immediately, followed by surgery if it is indicated. It is essential that following a severe injury surgery be performed at once. The longer the delay, the less efficacious is the decompression.

Cervical Spinal Cord

Injuries to the spinal cord from the sixth cervical to the second thoracic segments cause tetraparesis or tetraplegia, with depressed spinal reflexes from the thoracic limbs and hyperactive spinal reflexes from the pelvic limbs. Horner's syndrome (miosis, protruded third eyelid, smaller palpebral fissure, and enophthalmos) occurs with lesions in the first three thoracic segments. Injuries cranial to the sixth cervical segment cause spastic tetraparesis or tetraplegia with hyperactive reflexes in all four limbs. If the injury is severe, death occurs from respiratory failure. The patient should be assessed for respiratory function and this should be supplemented if necessary.

The rationale for medical and surgical therapy is similar to that for the thoracic and lumbar areas. Be aware that significant displacement may accompany fractures of the atlas or axis or both, and the patient may still be ambulatory. These dogs must be handled with extreme care. Neurologic signs can be expected to be worse following anesthesia for radiography or surgery, but this is temporary if the surgeon has been careful.[30]

Penetrating injuries to the spinal cord are uncommon in domestic animals. Gunshot wounds occasionally occur, and cause varying degrees of neurologic deficit. If one side of the spinal cord is injured, paresis or paralysis is found in the limb or limbs on the same side as the lesion. There is no obvious loss of sensation caudal to the lesion because the ascending sensory pathways for pain are located bilaterally. In all cases the foreign material should be removed, and antibiotics should be administered.

In any case of injury to the nervous system, it is important to ascertain how the animal performed at the site of the accident. The spinal cord and peripheral nerves may be subject to complete transection by injuries. Therefore, it is helpful to know whether the signs of loss of neurologic function occurred immediately or over a period of a few minutes to hours. If a period of time elapsed between the injury and the onset of signs, an anatomic transection did not occur.

When examining an injured dog that is not in shock and has no obvious life-threatening lesions but shows the typical signs of the Schiff-Sherrington syndrome, it is easy to overlook injury to the body cavities in the haste to diagnose the location of the spinal cord lesion. A diaphragmatic hernia may be overlooked and become life-threatening during or following surgery for the spinal cord lesion.

PERIPHERAL NERVOUS SYSTEM

Injuries of peripheral nerves are also described in Chapter 4.

THORACIC LIMB

Radial Nerve

The radial nerve innervates all the extensors of the elbow, carpus, and digits. The elbow extensors (triceps brachii) are innervated at the proximal end of the humerus. These muscles must function for the animal to support its weight normally on the thoracic limb. The carpal and digital extensors are innervated at the proximal end of the radius and ulna. The radial nerve supplies sensory innervation to the cranial and lateral surface of the forearm and dorsal surface of the forepaw.

Injuries to the radial nerve at the level of the elbow usually are associated with fractures of the humerus. The animal cannot extend its carpus and digits, and walks supporting its weight on the dorsal surface of the paw. Hypalgesia or analgesia occurs in the sensory distribution of the nerve.

With injuries to the radial nerve medial to the shoulder or more proximally, the patient is unable to support its weight on that limb because of inability to extend the elbow. In addition, the carpus and digits cannot be extended, and hypalgesia or analgesia occurs in the sensory distribution of the nerve. These rarely take place alone at this site. More commonly, the injury is a root avulsion.

Brachial Plexus—Roots of C6–T2[9]

Although the signs that appear following injuries to the brachial plexus or its roots of origin are predominantly those of radial nerve paralysis at the level of the shoulder, there are frequently deficits of other peripheral nerves that leave the brachial plexus. If the musculocutaneous nerve is injured, the limb will be dragged along the floor because of inability to flex the elbow. If the axillary and/or thoracodorsal nerves that innervate the flexors of the shoulder are injured, the elbow will be dropped. Injury to the median and ulnar nerves that innervate the carpal and digital flexors can be determined only by observing failure to flex these joints on testing the flexor reflex, or analgesia in their area of sensory distribution, including the caudal surface of the forearm and the palmar and lateral surfaces of the forepaw. The thoracic limb flexor reflex requires the function of the muscles innervated by the axillary and radial (shoulder flexors), musculocutaneous (elbow flexors), and median and ulnar (carpal and digital flexors) nerves. Careful observation of this reflex may reveal deficits of one or more of its components.

Multiple peripheral nerve involvement is usually caused by contusion or avulsion of the roots of the brachial plexus. This is the most susceptible portion of the peripheral nerve to trauma. The degree of peripheral nerve injury depends on which roots are avulsed. The C8 and T1 roots are affected most commonly, and present as radial, median, and ulnar paralyses. Avulsion of C6 and C7 is reflected as a musculocutaneous, suprascapular, and sometimes axillary nerve paralysis. Usually when most of these roots are avulsed the line of analgesia is at the level of the elbow. Avulsion of ventral roots with sparing of dorsal roots may account for some obvious disparities in motor and sensory deficits. Ipsilateral Horner's syndrome may accompany root avulsions that involve the first two or three thoracic spinal nerves.

Contusion of the brachial plexus medial to the shoulder is rarely by itself the primary site of injury producing the neurologic deficit in the limb.

There is no specific therapy for these avulsions. The torn ends of the rootlets are widely separated and extremely delicate to handle. At least 2 to 3 weeks should be allowed for recovery from contusion without avulsion or laceration. Following this amputation should be considered. Tendon transplantation and arthrodesis of carpus or both carpus and elbow have been recommended in selected cases. The results are not always satisfactory and depend on careful presurgical neurologic evaluation of the patient.[31-33]

PELVIC LIMB

The sciatic nerve (L6, L7, S1) innervates the caudal thigh muscles (biceps femoris, semimembranosus, and semitendinosus), which are concerned primarily with stifle flexion and extension and hip extension. The tibial nerve from the sciatic innervates the caudal leg muscles (gastrocnemius, and superficial and deep digital flexors), which extend the tarsus and flex the digits. Its sensory distribution is to the caudal surface of the leg and plantar surface of the paw. The peroneal nerve from the sciatic innervates the cranial leg muscles (cranial tibial, long digital extensor, and peroneus longus) that flex the tarsus and extend the digits. Its sensory distribution is to the cranial and lateral surfaces of the leg and the dorsal surface of the paw.

The femoral nerve (L3, L4, L5) innervates part of the iliopsoas muscle, which is a flexor of the hip, and all of the quadriceps muscle, which is an extensor of the stifle and is necessary for the animal to support weight on its pelvic limb. The saphenous branch of the femoral nerve is sensory to the medial side of the thigh, leg, and paw.

The complete flexor reflex in the pelvic limb requires the innervation of the hip flexors (iliopsoas, rectus femoris, sartorius, and tensor fascia lata) by the lumbar spinal nerves 2 to 4, femoral, saphenous, and cranial gluteal nerves; the sciatic nerve innervation of the flexors of the stifle; the peroneal nerve innervation of the tarsal flexors; and the tibial nerve innervation of the digital flexors.

Sciatic Nerve

The sciatic nerve is most commonly injured at the place that it crosses the greater ischiatic notch of the ilium, where it may be involved in a pelvic fracture, and in the caudal thigh, where displaced femoral fractures may affect it. It is also subject to injury by hypodermic injections into the caudal thigh muscles. The prognosis for recovery depends on the nature of the material injected and whether or not it directly entered the nerve.

Sacroiliac luxations may severely contuse the roots that compose the sciatic nerve. The L6 and L7 roots both pass on the ventral surface of the sacrum medial to this articulation, where they are subject to injury.

An animal can have a lacerated sciatic nerve, and still perceive pain from a stimulus to the second digit and withdraw the pelvic limb from the stimulus by flexion of the hip. This occurs because of the saphenous nerve innervation to the medial side of the paw; and the intact innervation to the flexors of the hip. No action is seen in the tarsus and digits. Partial stifle flexion may occur owing to the function of the gracilis (obturator nerve) and caudal part of the sartorius (femoral nerve). Muscle tone should be palpated during this procedure to help evaluate the nerve injury.

When presented with an animal with obvious musculoskeletal injury in an area closely associated with one of the peripheral nerves described, the first responsibility following the treatment of shock, hemorrhage, and other life-threatening injuries is to evaluate the nervous system. The presence of the musculoskeletal injury may prevent evaluation of motor function. Sensory examination determines if the nerve is functioning, and may determine a partial deficit. A failure of response on the part of the peripheral nervous system tested does not determine if a nerve has been lacerated by the contusion.

If no response is obtained, a number of alternatives remain to determine if the nerve is lacerated. The nerve may be explored simultaneously with the surgical repair of the skeletal injury, or as a separate procedure. Another alternative is to wait 3 to 4 days and stimulate the nerve using an electromyographic unit or an ordinary dry cell battery connected to two hypodermic needles that can be inserted in the vicinity of the nerve.[1, 5] This is done between the site of the injury and one or more of the muscles innervated by the nerve. If the nerve has been lacerated, Wallerian degeneration will have occurred in the distal segment, and the nerve will be unable to conduct an impulse. If the nerve is bruised but anatomically intact, response in the muscles should be seen following the stimulus. Because a nerve may be proved to be functional does not necessarily mean that it will return to complete function once the contusion is reduced. There may be partial laceration or disruption of nerve fibers. Physiologic testing does not readily allow quantitation of partial nerve disruption.

At least 2 to 3 weeks should be allowed for recovery of nerve function in contused nerves. The disrupted ends of lacerated nerves should be apposed and sutured.[27] Regeneration occurs at best at the rate of 1 to 4 mm per day. Measurement from the site of the injury to the site of muscle innervation provides an estimate of the time necessary for regeneration.

Lumbar, Sacral, and Caudal Roots

The lumbar, sacral, and caudal spinal nerves and their roots are injured by fractures of the associated vertebrae. Injury to the roots of the spinal nerves L6, L7, and S1 appears an a sciatic nerve paralysis. Injury to the roots of spinal nerves S1, S2, and S3 causes inability to close the anus, analgesia of the anus and perineal region, and distention of the bladder and rectum. Injury to caudal nerves causes analgesia of and inability to move the tail. The level of the vertebral fracture and displacement determines the degree of neurologic deficit.

In most cases these roots and spinal nerves are not lacerated but are severely contused and often compressed by displacement of the vertebral canal. If the displacment cannot be corrected, a laminectomy should be done to free the involved roots. Spinal nerve roots are part of the peripheral nervous system and are subject to the same principles of healing and regeneration.

REFERENCES

1. Allam, M. W., Nulsen, F. E., and Lewey, F. H.: Electrical intraneural bipolar stimulation of peripheral nerves in the dog. J. Am. Vet. Med. Assoc., *114*:87, 1949.
2. Averill, D. R., Jr.: Intracranial injuries. *In* Kirk, R. W., ed., Current Veterinary Therapy, IV. Philadelphia, W. B. Saunders Co., 1971, 473–476.
3. Ballinger, W. F., Rutherford, R. B., and Zuidema, G. D.: The Management of Trauma. 2nd ed., Philadelphia, W. B. Saunders Co., 1973.
4. Brasmer, T. H.: Evaluation and therapy of spinal cord trauma. *In* Kirk, R. W., ed., Current Veterinary Therapy, V. Philadelphia, W. B. Saunders Co., 1975, 662–666.
5. Chrisman, C. L., Burt, J. K., Wood, P. K., and Johnson, E. W.: Electromyography in small animal clinical neurology. J. Am. Vet. Med. Assoc., *160*:311, 1972.
6. Committee on Trauma, American College of Surgeons: The Management of Fractures and Soft Tissue Injuries. Philadelphia, W. B. Saunders Co., 1960.
7. de la Torre, J. C., Kawanaga, H. M., Rowed, D. W., Johnson, C. M., Goode, D. J., Kajihara, K., and Mullan, S.: Dimethyl sulfoxide in central nervous system trauma. Ann. N. Y. Acad. Sci., *243*:362, 1975.
8. Ducker, T. B., and Hamit, H. F.: Experimental treatments of acute spinal cord injury. J. Neurosurg., *30*:693, 1969.
9. Griffiths, I. R.: Avulsion of the brachial plexus in the dog. *In* Kirk, R. W., ed., Current Veterinary Therapy, VI. Philadelphia, W. B. Saunders Co., 1977.
10. Griffiths, I. R.: Vasogenic edema following acute and chronic spinal cord compression in the dog. J. Neurosurg., *42*:155, 1975.
11. Hoerlein, B. F.: Canine Neurology. 2nd ed., Philadelphia, W. B. Saunders Co., 1971.
12. Hooshmand, H., Dove, J., Houff, S., and Suter, C.: Effects of diuretics and steroids on CSF pressure. Arch. Neurol., *21*:499, 1969.
13. Kirk, R. W., and Bistner, S. I.: Handbook of Veterinary Procedures and Emergency Treatment. 2nd ed., Philadelphia, W. B. Saunders Co., 1975.
14. Martin, D. B.: Intensive care of the shock patient. Gaines Vet. Symp., *19*:27, 1969.
15. Martin, S. H., and Bloedel, J. R.: Evaluation of experimental spinal cord injury using cortical evoked potentials. J. Neurosurg., *39*:75, 1973.
16. Miller, J. D., and Leech, P.: Effects of mannitol and steroid therapy on intracranial volume-pressure relationships in patients. J. Neurosurg., *42*:274, 1975.

17. Oliver, J. E., Jr.: Management of the patient with acute head injury. Gaines Vet. Symp., 19:22, 1969.
18. Oliver, J. E., Jr.: Surgical approaches to the canine brain. Am. J. Vet. Res., 29:353, 1968.
19. Osterholm, J. L.: The pathophysiological response to spinal cord injury. J. Neurosurg., 40:5, 1974.
20. Palmer, A. C.: The accident case. IV. The significance and estimation of damage to the central nervous system. J. Sm. Anim. Pract., 5:25, 1964.
21. Parker, A. J.: Blood pressure changes and lethality of mannitol infusions in dogs. Am. J. Vet. Res., 34:1523, 1973.
22. Parker, A. J., and Smith, C. W.: Functional recovery from spinal cord trauma following incision of spinal meninges in dogs. Res. Vet. Sci., 16:276, 1974.
23. Parker, A. J., Marshall, A. E., and Sharp, J. G.: Study of the use of evoked cortical activity for clinical evaluation of spinal cord sensory transmission. Am. J. Vet. Res., 35:673, 1974.
24. Parker, A. J., Park, R. D., and Stowater, J. L.: Traumatic occlusion of segmental spinal veins. Am. J. Vet. Res., 35:857, 1974.
25. Shenkin, H. A., and Bouzarth, W. F.: Clinical methods of reducing intracranial pressure. N. Engl. J. Med., 282:1465, 1970.
26. Sims, M. H., and Redding, R. W.: The use of dexamethasone in the prevention of cerebral edema in dogs. J. Am. Anim. Hosp. Assoc., 11:439, 1975.
27. Swaim, S. F.: Peripheral nerve surgery in the dog. J. Am. Vet. Med. Assoc., 161:905, 1972.
28. Trotter, E. J.: Canine intervertebral disc disease. In Kirk, R. W., ed., Current Veterinary Therapy, V. Philadelphia, W. B. Saunders Co., 1975, 666–674.
29. Vise, W. M., Yaston, D., and Hunt, W. E.: Mechanisms of norepinephrine accumulation within sites of spinal cord injury. J. Neurosurg., 40:76, 1974.
30. Trotter, E. J.: Surgical repair of fractured atlas in a dog. J. Am. Vet. Med. Assoc., 161:303, 1972.
31. Bennett, D., and Vaughan, L. C.: The use of muscle relocation techniques in the treatment of peripheral nerve injuries in dogs and cats. J. Sm. Anim. Pract., 17:99, 1976.
32. Frost, W. W., and Lumb, W. V.: Radiocarpal arthrodesis: A surgical approach to brachial paralysis. J. Am. Vet. Med. Assoc., 149:1073, 1966.
33. Hussain, S., and Pettit, G. D.: Tendon transplantation to compensate for radial nerve paralysis. Am. J. Vet. Res., 28:336, 1967.
34. Oliver, J. E., Jr.: Intracranial injury. In Kirk, R. W., ed., Current Veterinary Therapy, VI. Philadelphia, W. B. Saunders Co., 1977.

Chapter 20

SMALL ANIMAL AND EQUINE NEUROLOGIC EXAMINATIONS

SMALL ANIMAL EXAMINATION
SIGNALMENT
HISTORY
GENERAL PHYSICAL EXAMINATION
NEUROLOGIC EXAMINATION
Gait
Postural Reactions
Spinal Reflexes
Cranial Nerves
Cerebrospinal Fluid
SUMMARY OF SIGNS WITH LESIONS AT
    SPECIFIC LOCATIONS
SPINAL CORD
Lumbosacral: Fourth Lumbar to Fifth Caudal
    Segment
Thoracolumbar: Third Thoracic to Third Lumbar
    Segment
Caudal Cervical: Fifth Cervical to Second
    Thoracic Segment
Cranial Cervical: First Cervical to Fifth
    Cervical Segment
MEDULLA AND PONS
CEREBELLUM
MESENCEPHALON

DIENCEPHALON (THALAMUS AND
    HYPOTHALAMUS)
TELENCEPHALON (CEREBRUM)
EQUINE NEUROLOGIC EXAMINATION
    (METHOD OF A. de LAHUNTA
    AND I. G. MAYHEW)
SIGNALMENT
HISTORY
GENERAL PHYSICAL EXAMINATION
NEUROLOGIC EXAMINATION
Mental Status and Behavior
Gait and Posture
Spinal Reflexes
SUMMARY OF SIGNS WITH LESIONS
    AT SPECIFIC AREAS OF THE
    SPINAL CORD
Lumbosacral Intumescence (L4 through
    Caudal Segments)
Thoracolumbar (T3–L3)
Cervical Intumescence (C6–T2)
Cervical Spinal Cord Cranial to the
    Intumescence (C1–C5)
Cranial Nerve Examination
INTERPRETATION OF CSF ANALYSIS

SMALL ANIMAL EXAMINATION

The proper evaluation of a patient with neurologic disease includes a thorough clinical examination to determine the location of the lesion, and radiographic and cerebrospinal fluid examinations to further define the kind of disease process present and in some instances the cause of the disease. Utilization of a routine procedure provides the examiner with the experience to render an accurate evaluation of these patients. The anatomic diagnosis depends on the recognition of signs resulting from the specific location of lesions in the nervous system. Experience with the distribution of lesions that occur in certain disease entities often leads to a definitive diagnosis. Examination of the patient should include a review of the history, a general physical examination, a neurologic examination, and a radiographic or clinical laboratory examination, or both.

344

SIGNALMENT

The signalment of the patient provides the examiner with the age, sex, breed, and use of the patient. When considered together with the chief complaint, it may help direct the line of questioning in taking the history. For example, patients less than 1 year old that are presented for convulsions are more likely to have an inflammatory than a neoplastic disease. Lead poisoning is more common in dogs less than 1 year of age. Toy breeds with functional hypoglycemia usually have seizures when they are less than 6 months old. Hypoglycemic convulsions caused by functional neoplasms of pancreatic beta cells rarely are seen before 5 years of age. Idiopathic epilepsy often begins between 1 and 3 years of age. Neoplastic disease of the nervous system usually occurs in the older patient, except for neurofibromas and a spinal cord neuroepithelioma, which are not limited by age.

The sex of the patient is an important consideration because mammary gland adenocarcinomas of the female rank high among the more common neoplasms that metastasize to the brain. Estrus may lower the seizure threshold in some individuals prone to idiopathic epilepsy.

Of the various breeds, the brachycephalic breeds are more prone to primary brain neoplasms. Although any breed of dog including mixed breeds can develop idiopathic epilepsy, it is most common in miniature poodles, followed by a high incidence in German shepherds, Saint Bernards, and beagles. There are probably few if any breeds in which this disease has not been reported. Any list of incidence by breed probably will vary according to the location from which it is reported. Although the incidence is much lower, there is a predilection by breed for the degenerative diseases of the nervous system that have been recognized and may be inherited. These include globoid cell leukodystrophy in Cairn and West Highland white terriers, a lipodystrophy in German short-haired pointers and English setters, and a diffuse neuronal abiotrophy that presents as cerebellar disease in Kerry blue terriers. Hyperkinetic episodes occur in Scottish terriers, the so-called "Scotty cramps." Congenital deafness may be familial in Old English sheepdogs. Some puppies of toy breeds and breeds that hunt have abnormalities in glucose metabolism that cause episodic weakness, collapse, or convulsions.

Although there are many causes of weakness and ataxia in the pelvic limbs, intervertebral disk protrusion rarely occurs before 1 year of age in chondrodystrophic breeds and only occasionally before 5 years in the larger breeds. Young Afghan hounds have an hereditary necrosis of spinal cord white matter. A demyelinating myelopathy occurs in young miniature poodles and rapidly produces a spastic tetraplegia. Cervical vertebral malformation occurs in young Basset hounds from C2 to C4 and in young or adult Great Danes and Doberman pinschers from C5 to C7. Older German shepherds have a high incidence of degenerative myelopathy.

HISTORY

The line of questioning followed in taking the history of the patient depends on the chief complaint. In all cases the review should include a summary of the past medical and surgical history unrelated in time to the present complaint.

If the chief complaint is an injury, the questioning will focus on the authenticity of the trauma, when it occurred, when the signs first appeared, and how

they have changed to the present time. By twenty-four hours after an injury the signs usually remain static or improve. Progressive neurologic signs usually are not due to a single episode of trauma.

When a dog presents with convulsions, it is necessary to obtain as thorough a description of the convulsion as possible in order to be certain of its authenticity and to attempt to determine the kind of convulsion. The majority of convulsions seen in veterinary medicine are generalized (grand mal) convulsions. This is the type that occurs with idiopathic epilepsy, intoxications, and many diseases of the prosencephalon with structural lesions. Psychomotor convulsions are more common in cases of lead poisoning and diseases of the limbic system. Descriptions of these convulsions often include activities of the patient that could be described as bizarre behavior or hysteria prior to the generalized convulsion. Partial motor convulsions may occur with or without confusion but with no loss of consciousness. These may be characterized by episodic muscular activity limited to a small group of muscles such as the eyelids, lips, all facial muscles, muscles of mastication, or part or all of the musculature of one limb or both limbs on one side of the body. The consistent onset of partial convulsions in one muscle area may be associated with a focal brain lesion in the contralateral motor cortex. Only rarely do these partial convulsions in dogs slowly spread from the initial muscle group to a wider area of the body in a specific pattern (Jacksonian convulsion). Partial convulsions involving more of a behavioral abnormality occur with limbic system seizure foci. A careful description of a dog that is "collapsing" may help distinguish a seizure disorder from narcolepsy or cataplexy, or syncope from a cardiac lesion.

The history of patients presented with signs of progressive neurologic disease should include careful documentation of each sign the patient has shown, in order to help determine whether the lesion is focal or disseminated in the nervous system. For example, a patient that first showed paresis (weakness) and ataxia of the pelvic limbs that progressed to complete paraplegia and then developed a head tremor, head tilt, and abnormal nystagmus necessarily has lesions in more than one location to explain the signs. A progressive thoracolumbar spinal cord lesion and a lesion in the cerebellomedullary region of the brain would account for these signs. Such a multifocal distribution of lesions is characteristic of an inflammatory lesion such as the encephalomyelitis caused by the canine distemper virus or toxoplasmosis, or cryptococcosis in dogs and cats. The signs of inflammatory disease usually progress faster than those of the familial degenerative diseases. A neurofibroma of a spinal nerve of the brachial plexus that invades the vertebral canal through an intervertebral foramen and compresses the spinal cord often first causes an undiagnosed lameness in the affected thoracic limb, followed by lower motor neuron paresis of that limb with neurogenic muscular atrophy. Following invasion of the vertebral canal by the neoplasm and compression of the spinal cord, a spastic paresis and ataxia appear in the ipsilateral pelvic limb. This is followed by tetraparesis and tetraplegia with hyperreflexia, and spasticity of the pelvic limbs and depressed reflexes in the thoracic limbs. In some instances of what seems to be a sudden onset of disease, thorough questioning of the owner may elicit previous signs that indicate a progressive disorder. As a rule signs that are precipitous in onset are due to injury or loss of vascular integrity. Be aware that neoplastic disease may produce rapidly progressive signs with a fairly sudden onset.

In the young animal, malformation or diseases acquired in utero must be considered, and the patient's history should document whether the signs were present from birth or as soon as the patient was ambulatory enough for the signs to be recognized. This is particularly important in patients with signs of cerebellar disease. In the cat, the panleukopenia virus induces a cerebellar degeneration in utero. The signs when the patient is ambulatory are nonprogressive. A nonprogressive cerebellar degeneration or malformation of unknown cause may occur in utero in the dog. Herpesvirus may cause cerebellar degeneration in the first 2 weeks of life in the dog. Progressive cerebellar signs commencing around 3 months of age may be the onset of a diffuse inflammatory disease such as canine distemper encephalitis or a progressive cerebellar degeneration. In Kerry blue terriers a diffuse neuronal abiotrophy begins in the Purkinje cells of the cerebellum and causes a cerebellar ataxia, usually around 10 to 12 weeks of age. There is evidence for an hereditary basis for this disease. The signs of globoid cell leukodystrophy in Cairn and West Highland white terriers usually begin between 3 and 6 months of age. These often include cerebellar in addition to spinal cord signs.

If intoxication is suspected, a thorough search should be carried out to find a possible source of the intoxicant. Lead may be consumed from lead-based paints, linoleum, tarpaper, and batteries. Many insecticides contain chlorinated hydrocarbons that can cause generalized myoclonus or grand mal convulsions. Others contain organic phosphates that can cause myoclonic activity, or convulsions, or both, in addition to salivation, vomiting, diarrhea, and initially miosis. Dial soap contains hexachlorophene that can produce convulsions, stupor, or coma. Ethylene glycol (antifreeze) may produce similar signs following a brief period of ataxia.

A history of progressive convulsions with increasingly shorter interictal periods is typical of neoplasia of the prosencephalon. The review should include a previous history of the diagnosis of neoplasia in other systems of the body.

GENERAL PHYSICAL EXAMINATION

In all cases in which a neurologic examination is indicated, it should be preceded by a thorough general physical examination of all other body systems. Primary disease of other systems may be manifested by episodes of weakness or collapse. The same episodes can present with hypoadrenocorticoidism. Convulsions may occur in patients with extensive liver or kidney disease or functional pancreatic islet neoplasms. Musculoskeletal diseases often are confused with neurologic disease.

NEUROLOGIC EXAMINATION

The neurologic examination can be divided into four parts: gait, postural reactions, spinal reflexes, and cranial nerves. In this description an intact reflex only requires the function of the peripheral nerves being tested and the segments of the spinal cord or brain stem in which the afferent axon enters and the cell bodies and axons of the efferent neurons are located. A reaction depends on the same components as the reflex, plus the ascending pathways through the white matter of the spinal cord and brain stem to the cerebellum and sensorimotor cortex of the cerebrum, and the descending pathways that return from the cerebrum by way of its internal capsule, and the white matter of the brain stem and spinal cord. The lower motor neuron has its cell body and dendritic zone in the ventral grey column of the spinal cord or specific cranial nerve nucleus in the brain stem. Its axon leaves the central nervous system and courses through peripheral nerves to its telodendron in the group of muscle fibers it innervates. The upper motor neurons have cell bodies and dendritic zones in collections of grey matter in the cerebrum (motor cerebral cortex) or brain stem (red nucleus, reticular nuclei). Their axons descend in tracts through the white matter in the brain and spinal cord to end in telodendria in the vicinity of the lower motor neuron that they ultimately influence.

The precise order in which the parts of a neurologic examination are performed varies with the preference of the examiner and the attitude of the patient. If the patient is resting quietly in a cage at the time of examination, the cranial nerve examination may be done first. If the patient is excited or apprehensive, it may be more convenient to perform the cranial nerve examination after the patient has been handled during the examinations of gait, reactions, and reflexes.

Gait

Examination of the gait should be done in a place where the patient may be allowed to move freely, unleashed, and the ground surface is not slippery. The floor of many examining rooms is too slippery for adequate evaluation of the patient's gait. In some cases of vertebral column injury with spinal cord contusion resulting in paresis and ataxia, moving the patient on a slippery floor may cause a fall, and further injury may result. A carpeted room is ideal.

The degree of functional deficit dictates the necessity for further examination of strength and coordination. A patient that is tetraplegic—unable to support its weight or move its limbs when the weight is borne on them—need not have further tests performed for the postural reactions. A grade 0 paraplegic patient need not be examined for postural reactions in the pelvic limbs, but the thoracic limbs should be examined carefully. Occasionally, a patient with progressive myelitis may present as paraplegic because of an extensive thoracolumbar spinal cord location of the lesion but also have an asymmetric thoracic limb gait because of a less severe focus of the lesion in the cervical spinal cord. An early sign in dogs with ascending myelomalacia associated with an acute intervertebral disk extrusion may be a hesitant, stumbling, awkward gait in the thoracic limbs. The severity of advanced pelvic limb weakness is evaluated best by holding the patient suspended at the base of the tail and observing its gait. The degree of pelvic limb deficit from thoracolumbar spinal cord lesions may be graded according to the following scheme:

0   Absence of purposeful movement—paraplegia.

1 Unable to stand to support; slight movement when supported by the tail—severe paraparesis.

2 Unable to stand to support; when assisted moves limbs readily but stumbles and falls frequently—moderate paraparesis and ataxia.

3 Can stand to support but frequently stumbles and falls—mild paraparesis and ataxia.

4 Can stand to support—minimal paraparesis and ataxia.

5 Normal strength and coordination.

Postural Reactions

Following observation of the gait for strength and coordination, the postural reactions can be tested especially to determine if there are less obvious deficits in strength and coordination when the gait appears to be normal.

Wheelbarrowing. The thoracic limbs may be tested by supporting the patient under the abdomen so that the pelvic limbs are off the ground surface and forcing the patient to walk on its thoracic limbs. The normal animal walks with symmetric movements of both thoracic limbs and the head extended in normal position. Patients with lesions of the peripheral nerves of the thoracic limbs, cervical spinal cord, or brain stem may have asymmetric movements, with stumbling or knuckling over on the dorsum of the paw of the affected limb. Hypermetria occasionally is observed. With more severe lesions in this area, there is a tendency to carry the head flexed with the nose close to and occasionally reaching the ground surface for support. If no deficit is observed, extend the neck while the animal is wheelbarrowed. This sometimes reveals a mild deficit, a tendency to knuckle over on the dorsum of the paw, which was not observed before. This is often helpful to confirm a cervical spinal cord lesion in Great Danes or Doberman pinschers that have a cervical vertebral malformation and show mild pelvic limb paresis and ataxia, but no overt thoracic limb signs.

Hopping—Thoracic Limb. While still supporting the pelvic limbs, hop the animal on one thoracic limb while holding the other off the ground surface so that the entire weight of the body is supported by the limb to be tested. Move the dog forward and to each side but especially laterally, and observe the strength and coordination of the limb. Repeat this on the other thoracic limb and compare the response. Asymmetry occurs with paresis or ataxia. Hypermetria may be seen with general proprioceptive or cerebellar deficits. This is an effective way of determining minor deficits when the gait appears to be normal, as occurs with contralateral cerebral sensorimotor cortex lesions.

Extensor Postural Thrust. The same sequence of tests can be done on the pelvic limbs. The extensor postural thrust reaction is performed by holding the patient off the ground surface by supporting it caudal to the scapulae, lowering it to the ground surface, and observing the patient extend its pelvic limbs to support its weight. Moving the patient forward and backward in this position tests the symmetry of pelvic limb function, strength, and coordination.

Hopping—Pelvic Limb. Continuing to support the patient by the thorax so that the thoracic limbs are not in contact with the ground surface, one pelvic limb can be held up and the patient forced to hop laterally or forward on the supporting limb. Both pelvic limbs should be tested this way and the response compared.

Hemistanding and Hemiwalking. The patient's ability to stand and walk with the thoracic and pelvic limbs on one side can be tested by holding the opposite thoracic and pelvic limbs off the ground surface and forcing the patient to walk forward or to the side. These are referred to as the hemistanding and hemiwalking reactions.

A patient with a unilateral lesion of the sensorimotor cortex or internal capsule may have a normal gait but show deficits in its postural reactions on the side opposite the lesion. Attempts to hemiwalk on the contralateral side are exaggerated (hypermetric) and spastic, and stumbling may occur. With unilateral cervical spinal cord lesions, the limbs on the same side as the lesion show a deficiency in the gait and are unresponsive on postural reaction testing, including inability to support the animal in the hemiwalking reaction.

Placing. Other postural reactions that can be tested include placing with the thoracic limbs. The patient is supported off the ground surface and its thoracic limbs are brought to the edge of a table or similar surface so that the dorsal surface of the paws makes contact. This test should be performed on both thoracic limbs simultaneously and individually, with and without blindfolding the patient. Vision can compensate for the sense of position when the general proprioceptive system is abnormal.

Tonic Neck Reaction. The tonic neck reaction involves extension of the head and neck so that the nose is directed dorsally. The normal patient responds by extension of all the joints of both thoracic limbs. A patient with disease of the general proprioceptive system in the cervical spinal nerves, cervical spinal cord, or medulla fails to extend its carpus or digits or both, and these joints passively flex so that the weight is borne on the dorsal surface of the paw. The same response may occur if a patient is paretic either as a result of disease of the motor neurons that innervate the thoracic limb, or in the white matter of the spinal cord that influences these motor neurons.

Proprioceptive Positioning. Proprioceptive positioning tests this afferent system by determining the patient's ability to recognize when the paw has been flexed so that the weight is borne on its dorsal surface. The normal animal returns the paw to its usual position. In patients with severe paresis, this test may also be deficient.

Spinal Reflexes

Muscle tone and spinal reflexes are evaluated best when the patient is in lateral recumbency and as relaxed as possible. It is important to test muscle tone, tendon reflexes, and the flexor reflex to noxious stimuli, in that order, to maintain the cooperation of the patient.

Muscle Tone. Muscle tone is evaluated by passive manipulation of the limbs individually. The degree of resistance is determined to be less than normal (hypotonic), normal, or more than normal (hypertonic). The latter may be referred to as spasticity. The degree of spasticity varies from a mild increased resistance to passive manipulation, to a marked increase that may be "clasp knife" in character. It is referred to as "clasp knife" because as attempts are made to flex a limb, the degree of extension of the limb increases, until suddenly it gives way to complete flexion without resistance.

Hypotonia usually occurs with lower motor neuron disease, whereas upper motor neuron disease is characterized by hypertonia or spasticity. The functional integrity of the lower motor neuron is necessary to cause muscle cell contraction in order to maintain muscle tone. It is also necessary to maintain the normal health of the muscle cell it innervates. When denervated, these cells degenerate. This is observed clinically as neurogenic atrophy, and can be detected electromyographically by the production of abnormal potentials in resting muscle. The upper motor neuron influences the activity of the lower motor neuron to produce voluntary motor activity and to maintain muscle tone for support of the body against gravity. Although the upper motor neuron includes both facilitatory and inhibitory functions on the activity of the lower motor neuron, when the upper motor neuron is diseased the result usually observed is a release of the lower motor neuron from inhibition and overactivity of the facilitatory mechanism. This release is seen as hypertonia or spasticity.

Patellar Reflexes. The most reliable tendon reflex is the patellar reflex. It is obtained by lightly tapping the patellar tendon with the patient in lateral recumbency and as relaxed as possible for proper evaluation. A pediatric neurologic hammer is the most useful instrument, but any hard object such as scissor handles can be used. The reflex can be elicited in all normal dogs and is mediated by the femoral nerve through the third to fifth lumbar spinal cord segments. The degree of normal response varies with the breed. Large breeds of dogs have a brisker reflex than the short-legged breeds like the dachshund. The response should be evaluated as absent (0), hyporeflexic (+1), normal (+2), hyperreflexic (+3), or clonic (+4). An absent reflex or hyporeflexia occurs when there is disease of a portion of the reflex arc. Hyperreflexia or clonus is often present in upper motor neuron disease.

Biceps and Triceps Reflex. In the thoracic limb, the biceps and triceps reflexes can be elicited in most dogs that are relaxed and in lateral recumbency. Lightly tapping the tendon of insertion of the triceps proximal to the olecranon elicits a slight extension of the elbow. The reflex is mediated by the radial nerve through the seventh and eighth cervical and first and second thoracic spinal cord segments. The biceps reflex is elicited by placing a finger on the distal ends of the biceps and brachialis muscles at the level of the elbow. Tapping this finger with the hammer elicits a slight flexion of the elbow. The muscle contraction can be palpated in some instances when no movement of the joint is seen. The musculocutaneous nerve mediates this reflex through the sixth, seventh and the eighth cervical spinal cord segments. The normal patient has a mild reflex response to these stimuli. In a few normal patients they are difficult to elicit. They are absent when there is disease of some portion of the reflex arc. They may be hyperactive in some cases with disease of the upper motor neuron.

Flexor Reflex—Pelvic Limb. The flexor reflexes to painful stimuli determine the integrity of the reflex arc as well as the pathway in the central nervous system that is concerned with the patient's response to painful stimuli. The most reliable stimulus is pressure exerted on the base of the toenail with hemostats. Many normal animals do not respond to the stimulus of a pin. In the pelvic limb, the flexor reflex is mediated by the sciatic nerve through the sixth and seventh lumbar spinal cord segments and the first sacral segment. Abnormality of the motor portion of the sciatic nerve distal to the pelvis causes paralysis, hypotonia, and atrophy of the flexors of the stifle, tarsus, and digits as well as of the extensors of the tarsus and digits. There is no resistance to flexion or extension of the tarsus. On walking with a sciatic nerve paralysis, the tarsus is lower on the affected side and the paw may be placed on its dorsal surface; however, the limb is able to support weight as long as the femoral nerve is intact.

Sensory branches of the peroneal nerves supply the dorsal surface of the paw. The plantar surface is supplied by tibial nerve sensory branches. The medial side of the paw is supplied by the saphenous nerve, a branch of the femoral nerve at the femoral triangle. This enters the spinal cord through the third to fifth lumbar segments. A patient may have a contused sciatic nerve from a pelvic fracture and have no function of the muscles innervated by this nerve and analgesia of the lateral, dorsal, and plantar surfaces of the paw. However, the intact saphenous nerve provides sensation to the medial surface of the paw. If this area is stimulated the patient will flex the hip with the intact innervation of the iliopsoas muscle, but the stifle, tarsus, and digits fail to flex. For this reason both the medial and lateral surfaces of the paw should be tested for reflex responses as well as pain perception.

Pain Perception.　The patient shows signs of pain when the impulses generated by a noxious stimulus have entered the spinal cord over the peripheral nerves and dorsal roots and are relayed to tracts in the lateral funiculi of the spinal cord bilaterally. These tracts ascend the spinal cord in the lateral funiculi, and continue through the medulla, pons, and mesencephalon to specific nuclei in the thalamus for relay to the somatic sensory cerebral cortex. Pain may be evidenced when the impulses reach the thalamus or cerebrum.

Flexor Reflex—Thoracic Limb.　In the thoracic limb the thoracodorsal, axillary, musculocutaneous, median, ulnar, and radial nerves are responsible for flexion of the shoulder, elbow, carpus, and digits when a painful stimulus is applied to the paw. These arise from the sixth cervical to the second thoracic spinal cord segments. The specific sensory nerve stimulated depends on the location of the stimulus. The median and ulnar nerves innervate the skin of the palmar surface of the paw; the radial nerve supplies the dorsal surface. In the forearm the radial nerve supplies the skin on the cranial and lateral surfaces. The ulnar nerve supplies the caudal surface and the musculocutaneous nerve the medial surface.

Crossed Extensor Reflex.　In patients with upper motor neuron disease and release of the lower motor neuron, a crossed extensor reflex may be elicited in the recumbent animal when the flexor reflex is stimulated. This occurs in the limb opposite the one being tested for a flexor reflex. To avoid voluntary extension of the contralateral limb as a response to pain, the flexor reflex first should be elicited with as mild a stimulus as is necessary and the opposite limb observed for extension. When elicited in a patient in lateral recumbency this is an abnormal reflex, indicative of upper motor neuron disease.

Perineal Reflex.　The perineal reflex is elicited by stimulating the anus with a noxious stimulus and observing contraction of the anal sphincter and flexion of the tail. It is mediated by branches of the sacral and caudal nerves through the sacral and caudal segments of the spinal cord.

Panniculus Reflex.　The panniculus reflex is the contraction of the cutaneous trunci in response to mild stimulation of the skin of the trunk. It can be elicited from the thoracic and most of the lumbar region. The regional segmental spinal nerves contain the sensory neurons that are stimulated. The impulses are carried into the related spinal cord segments and then relayed through the white matter of the spinal cord cranially to the eighth cervical spinal cord segment. Here synapse occurs on lower motor neurons of the lateral thoracic nerve that innervates the cutaneous trunci. This reflex may be useful in diagnosing the level of a complete thoracolumbar spinal cord lesion.

Cranial Nerves

The cranial nerve examination should be performed at the time that the patient is in the most cooperative attitude. The procedure for examining the cranial nerves is described here, with the specific cranial nerves being examined indicated in parentheses.

Observe the head for any evidence of a head tilt (vestibular VIII), facial muscle weakness or contracture (VII), or atrophy of the muscles of mastication (motor V). Palpate these muscles for tone and atrophy. With one eye of the patient covered, menace the opposite eye with threatening gestures of the hand, being careful to avoid striking the patient or stimulating the hair with air currents (II–VII). Repeat this on the opposite side. If the response is absent, check the eyelids for ability to close (VII). Observe the symmetry of the pupils and their reaction to light in either eyeball (II–III). Observe the eyes for evidence of abnormal position, strabismus (III, VI, vestibular VIII), or abnormal nystagmus (vestibular VIII). Test the corneal and palpebral reflexes (sensory V–VII), ear movement (VII), and the position of the philtrum (VII). Examine the commissure of the lips for hypotonia that exposes mucosa and allows saliva to escape (VII). Check the skin sensation from the entire surface of the head with a safety pin (sensory V). If evaluation is difficult and a deficit is suspected, the most sensitive area to test is the mucosa of the nasal septum inside each naris. Observe the jaws for normal closure (motor V). Open the mouth and observe whether resistance is normal (motor V). Observe the position of the tongue, its movements and size (atrophy), and pull on it to test its strength (XII). Check the gag reflex by probing the pharynx with a finger (IX, X).

Additional Tests: Visual. Additional tests may be performed for certain of the cranial nerves if an abnormality is suspected. If a visual deficit is suspected from the menace test, the patient should be walked through a maze with the lights both on and off. After observing the patient without a blindfold, cover one eye and repeat the maneuver through the maze. Observe this for each eye. These tests for vision test not only the eyeball and second cranial nerve, but also the central visual pathway to the visual cerebral cortex. Because approximately 65 per cent (cat) to 75 per cent (dog) of the optic nerve axons cross in the optic chiasm, clinically a patient will show a unilateral blindness with an ipsilateral optic nerve lesion or a contralateral lesion in the optic tract, lateral geniculate nucleus, optic radiation, or visual cerebral cortex. The deficit is more complete with optic nerve lesions, and the pupil on the affected side will be more dilated than the pupil in the normal eyeball and unresponsive to light directed to the affected eyeball. The dilated pupil in the affected eyeball will respond to light directed to the normal eyeball as long as the oculomotor nerve (III) is intact. With unilateral lesions in the central visual pathway from the optic tract to the visual cerebral cortex, pupillary function is normal. This occurs because some of the optic nerve axons concerned with pupillary control cross in the optic chiasm as well as in the pretectal area, so that impulses stimulated by light in one retina reach both oculomotor nuclei.

Cerebellar lesions may cause a failure of the menace response, but visual function and facial muscle function are normal in all other tests.

Additional Tests: Vestibular. For further examination of the vestibular system (vestibular VIII), the head should be held laterally over each shoulder with the exposed eyeball covered except for the limbus. Observe the eyeball for the development of a positional nystagmus. Make a similar observation with the head and neck extended and both eyeballs covered with the lower eyelids except for the limbus at the superior portion of the eyeball. In the normal patient no nystagmus develops and the corneas remain in the center of the palpebral fissure. In patients with unilateral disease of the vestibular system, the eye on the affected side is depressed and does not elevate into the center of the fissure. and nystagmus may be observed. The head should be moved from side to side and the normal vestibular nystagmus elicited should be observed. In bilateral peripheral vestibular disease or severe lesions in the brain stem, this response may be absent. This lack of normal eye movement is a poor prognosis in animals with intracranial injury. In unilateral vestibular lesions the rapidity of the response may not be equal in both directions of head movement.

The nystagmus elicited by spinning the patient should be observed, and the rapidity and duration compared following spinning both to the left and the right. An assistant is needed to hold the patient in a normal standing position and spin it rapidly six or seven times. The postrotatory nystagmus elicited is observed immediately upon stopping the spin.

The presence of a spontaneous or positional nystagmus or a postrotatory nystagmus that is markedly different on each side is evidence of disturbance of the vestibular system. With disturbance of the peripheral portion of this system (the eighth cranial nerve), the abnormal spontaneous or positional nystagmus is either horizontal or rotatory, with the quick phase directed toward the side opposite the lesion. The postrotatory nystagmus developed after spinning the patient to the opposite side from the lesion is depressed when compared to the response observed on spinning the patient toward the side of the lesion. With extensive bilateral peripheral vestibular disease the examiner may not be able to elicit nystagmus.

A horizontal, rotatory, or vertical spontaneous or positional nystagmus occurs with disturbance of the central portion of the vestibular system. In addition, with central vestibular lesions the direction of the nystagmus may vary with changes in the position of the head. A rapid pendular congenital nystagmus may occur in puppies with abnormalities of the visual system.

The sense of smell (I) and hearing (cochlear VIII) are difficult to evaluate unless the deficit is complete. Usually the owner's observations of the patient in its natural environment are more reliable for determination of these sensations.

Cerebrospinal Fluid

Following completion of the general physical and neurologic examinations, radiographic or clinical laboratory procedures or both may be performed, depending on the differential diagnosis that has been made. In any case of suspected brain or spinal cord disease, with the exception of some cases of authentic injury, the cerebrospinal fluid should be obtained from the cerebellomedullary cistern and examined for its pressure, total cell count, percentage distribution of the types of cells present, and total protein content. This provides information on the kind of lesion present and occasionally on its cause. In some instances it may confirm the presence of a central nervous system lesion when only equivocal signs are present. One example of this is distinguishing central from peripheral vestibular disease when the signs are mild and the lesion is not advanced.

Canine cerebrospinal fluid normally has an opening pressure of less than 170 mm. It is clear and colorless and contains no red blood cells, less than 5 mononuclear cells per cubic millimeter, and less than 25 mg of protein per dl (tricarboxylic acid precipitation and turbidometric analysis).

Both the total cell count and the protein level may be increased in inflammation of the central nervous system. In viral disease these increases are slight to moderate and the cell increase is mostly in mononuclear cells. Occasionally only the protein content is increased in nonsuppurative encephalitis. In bacterial inflammation the increase in cells and protein is moderate to large. Neutrophils predominate in the cell increase. Inflammation of the meninges causes larger increases in cells and protein than inflammation confined to the parenchyma. Space-occupying lesions cause elevations in the cerebrospinal fluid pressure, and mild to moderate increases in protein with or without a cell increase. Parenchymal necrosis may cause protein elevations without significant pleocytosis. The organisms may be visible in the fluid in cryptococcosis. Organisms may be cultured from the fluid in bacterial disease. In canine distemper infected cells in the cerebrospinal fluid may fluoresce when stained with specific antibodies conjugated with fluorescein.

A copy of the neurologic examination form routinely used at the New York State College of Veterinary Medicine follows:

Neurologic Examination

Signalment:	Clinic No. _____ ___
History:	Date _____
	Clinician _____

Mental Status:
Gait and Posture:

Cranial Nerves:

II	Menace			
	Pupils			
	Ophthalmoscopic			
III	Pupillary OS	OD	Strabismus	
V	Motor: Mand.			
	Sensory: Ophth.	Max.	Mand.	
VI	Strabismus			

Muscle Tone

VII
VIII Cochlear
      Vestibular: Head tilt
      Nystagmus: Resting
              Positional
              Postrotatory
              Vestibular

IX, X
XII

Spinal Reflexes:

Patellar	LH	RH	
Biceps	L	R	
Triceps	L	R	
Perineal		Tail	
Flexor	LF	RF	Crossed
	LH	RH	Extensor
Pain Perception			

Additional Tests:
  Lesion(s) location:

Differential diagnosis:

Postural Reactions:
  Wheelbarrowing

Hopping:		LF	RF
		LH	RH
Extensor postural thrust			
		LH	RH
Hemistand		L	R
Hemiwalk		L	R
Proprioceptive positioning			
		LF	RF
		LH	RH
Tonic neck and eye			
Placing: Optic		tactile	

SUMMARY OF SIGNS WITH LESIONS AT SPECIFIC LOCATIONS

SPINAL CORD

Lumbosacral: Fourth Lumbar to Fifth Caudal Segment

With *complete destruction* from the fourth lumbar through the fifth caudal segments, there is flaccid paraplegia—no support, gait, or movement of pelvic limbs and tail, no postural reactions in the pelvic limbs, areflexia of the flexor, patellar, and perineal reflexes, atonia or soft muscles, with no resistance to manipulation of pelvic limbs or tail, neurogenic atrophy in chronic lesions, a dilated anus, and analgesia from the pelvic limbs, tail, and perineum.

With *partial destruction* of grey and white matter between the fourth lumbar and fifth caudal segments, there is found flaccid paraparesis and ataxia of pelvic limbs with normal thoracic limbs; postural reactions of pelvic limbs are attempted but poorly accomplished; hyporeflexia or areflexia of flexor, perineal, and patellar reflexes; hypotonia—normal or weak resistance to manipulation of pelvic limbs, and hypotonic anus; slight neurogenic atrophy in chronic lesions; and normal or depressed pain perception (hypalgesia) from pelvic limbs, tail, and perineum.

Thoracolumbar: Third Thoracic to Third Lumbar Segment

With *complete destruction* or *dysfunction*, when the focal site is between the third thoracic and third lumbar segments, there occurs spastic paraplegia, with no voluntary support, gait, or movement of pelvic limbs, no postural reactions in the pelvic limbs, and normal or hyperactive flexor and patellar reflexes. Crossed extensor reflex may occur, muscle tone is normal or hypertonic, but occasionally hypotonic, and there is analgesia from the area caudal to the lesion.

With *partial destruction* or *dysfunction*, when the focal site is between the third thoracic and third lumbar segments, there is spastic paraparesis and ataxia of pelvic limbs with normal thoracic limbs. All postural reactions are poorly performed in the pelvic limbs, flexor and patellar reflexes are normal or hyperactive, crossed extensor reflex may occur, muscle tone is normal or hypertonic, and pain perception is normal or depressed from the area caudal to the lesion.

Caudal Cervical: Fifth Cervical to Second Thoracic Segment

With *partial destruction* of grey matter between the fifth cervical and the second thoracic segments, tetraparesis and ataxia of all four limbs are found, with the thoracic limb deficit worse than that of the pelvic limb, or there is tetraplegia with the patient in lateral recumbency. Thoracic limbs are hyporeflexic or areflexic, have normal tone or are hypotonic, and neurogenic atrophy occurs if there is a chronic lesion. The pelvic limbs show normal reflexes or are hyperreflexic, have normal tone or are hypertonic, and there is no atrophy. Pain perception is normal or depressed from all four limbs, or depressed from thoracic limbs only. All postural reactions are performed poorly, with the thoracic limb function worse than that of the pelvic limb. There is miosis, protruded third eyelid, ptosis, and enophthalmos (T1–T3 lesion).

Cranial Cervical: First Cervical to Fifth Cervical Segment

With *partial destruction* or *dysfunction*, when the focal site is between the first and fifth cervical segments, spastic tetraplegia is observed, with the patient in lateral recumbency. No postural reactions are present, reflexes are normal or hyperactive in all four limbs, crossed extensor reflexes may occur, muscle tone is normal or hypertonic; and there is hypalgesia from the area caudal to the lesion. With spastic tetraparesis and ataxia of all four limbs, the deficit in the pelvic limbs is usually worse than that in the thoracic limbs. Postural reactions are performed poorly, reflexes are normal or hyperactive, crossed extensor reflexes may occur, muscle tone is normal or hypertonic, and pain perception is normal or depressed from the area caudal to the lesion.

MEDULLA AND PONS

Lesions in the medulla and pons result in spastic tetraparesis and ataxia of all four limbs or tetraplegia, ipsilateral spastic hemiparesis and ataxia (unilateral lesions), central vestibular signs, depression and irregular respirations, and hypalgesia of the trunk and limbs.

Signs of cranial nerve deficit are as follows: facial hypalgesia or analgesia (sensory V), paresis or paralysis of masticatory muscles (motor V), medial strabismus (VI), facial paresis or paralysis (VII), pharyngeal paresis (IX, X), and tongue paresis (XII).

CEREBELLUM

With diffuse lesions the signs are: symmetric ataxia with preservation of strength, dysmetric gait (hypometria or hypermetria), truncal ataxia, head tremor, muscle hypertonia, occasional abnormal nystagmus, and bilateral menace deficit.

With unilateral lesions the signs are usually ipsilateral, occasionally contralateral. The body and the head tilt toward the side of the lesion, occasionally away from side of lesion, and there is ipsilateral menace deficit.

MESENCEPHALON (Midbrain)

With lesions in this area, the following signs occur: spastic tetraparesis and ataxia of all four limbs or tetraplegia, spastic hemiparesis if the lesion is unilateral (usually contralateral), depression, stupor (semicoma), or coma, and hypalgesia of the head, trunk, and limbs. Signs of cranial nerve deficit are ventrolateral strabismus (III) and mydriasis and nonreactive pupil (III). There is deviation of the eyeballs in certain positions of the head, and the head and neck are flexed laterally, with the nose directed toward the shoulder with severe midline or unilateral lesions in the tegmentum.

DIENCEPHALON (Thalamus and Hypothalamus)

Bilateral lesions of the diencephalon produce the following signs: mildly spastic tetraparesis and ataxia, bilateral visual deficit with dilated unresponsive pupils (optic tracts), and bilateral hypalgesia (ventral caudal lateral and medial nuclei).

Unilateral lesions are indicated by mildly spastic contralateral hemiparesis and ataxia, which may be observed only as deficient postural reactions, contralateral visual deficit with normal pupils, contralateral hypalgesia (most noticeable in the head), and the adversive syndrome—circling, and head and eye deviation toward the side of lesion.

With lesions which are either bilateral or unilateral the manifestations are: depression, stupor (semicoma), or coma, behavioral changes, convulsions, and the following hypothalamo-hypophyseal disorders: body temperature, glucose metabolism, appetite control, autonomic nervous system, water balance, gonadal function, and thyroid and adrenal function.

TELENCEPHALON (Cerebrum)

Lesions in this area are evidenced by changes in a number of ways. Changes in behavior or temperament include depression (lethargy, obtundation), stupor (semicoma), or coma, lack of recognition of owner or environment and bewilderment, loss of trained habits, and irritable, hysterical, maniacal, or aggressive behavior. In propulsion the animal often paces and circles in one direction, and turns the head and eyes in one direction; this direction is toward a unilateral lesion, called the "adversive" syndrome (turn to). This may require a rostral thalamic involvement in the lesion. Seizures are partial (contralateral face or limbs or both) or generalized (grand mal, psychomotor). The gait usually is normal, but contralateral postural reactions are deficient. Bilateral lesions produce blindness. Unilateral lesions produce contralateral visual deficit with normal pupil responses to light. Occasionally contralateral facial hypalgesia occurs. Acute diffuse lesions may produce bilateral miosis. Pseudobulbar paralysis is observed only on voluntary movement: contralateral lower facial paralysis (lip and nose), pharyngeal paresis, and tongue paresis.

EQUINE NEUROLOGIC EXAMINATION (Method of A. de Lahunta and I. G. Mayhew)

Neurologic evaluation of an animal with a suspected problem must follow or be incorporated into a complete physical examination. The aims of a neurologic examination are: (1) determining the presence of a lesion or lesions, (2) locating the lesion.

It is only *after* the neurologic examination that a complete list of the problems can be formulated based on the patient history, the physical examination, and ancillary aids. Experience with the location and extent of lesions in specific diseases then allows the compilation of a differential list of etiologies, leading to a prognosis and suggested therapy.

The logical order of events is thus: (1) history, (2) general physical exam, (3) neurologic examination (**presence and location of lesion**), (4) radiography, (5) CSF study results, (6) other ancillary aids, and (7) problem list, resulting in **pathogenesis, prognosis,** and **therapy.**

Results of a neurologic examination should always be recorded. Subtle changes often make a great difference in prognosis and therapy, and these must not be left to memory.

SIGNALMENT

The signalment should include a description of the breed, sex, age, color, and use of the patient. A few neurologic diseases are specific to particular breeds. The young Arabian foal has a presumed hereditary cerebellar cortical abiotrophy. A somewhat similar condition exists in the Gotland pony breed. Signs are present at birth or usually occur prior to 4 to 6 months of age. An atlanto-occipital malformation has been seen only in Arabians or Arabian cross foals. Some are born showing severe spasticity of the limbs and tetraparesis, while others do not show signs, according to the owners, until several months of age. Narcolepsy has been observed in Shetland ponies and may begin prior to 6 months of age. Night blindness (stumbling and falling while being ridden during and after dusk) has been seen in the Appaloosa breed. Neurologic signs due to congenital malformations usually are present at birth and are nonprogressive. The true wobbler syndrome is not breed-specific but is more common in the younger animals from 6 months to about 2 years of age. The literature suggests it is more common in the rapidly growing male thoroughbred. A recently observed diffuse spinal cord degeneration of unknown pathogenesis usually causes signs prior to 6 months of age. A similar disease has been described as familial in zebras. Acute hepatoencephalopathy (Theiler's disease) is not usually seen in foals less than 1 year old. Melanomas are common in the grey horse. More cases of myelitis syndrome associated with a protozoal agent have been seen in mature standardbred horses.

HISTORY

In addition to the data applicable to the present illness, the history should include a summary of all past medical and surgical events. The line of questioning referable to the chief complaint depends on the nature of the complaint.

Careful documentation of the onset and course of a neurologic disorder is important in order to distinguish between a traumatic or acute vascular disorder and a disorder of a progressive nature such as inflammation, degeneration, or neoplasia. As a rule, 24 hours after an injury the neurologic signs are static or improved. Progressive neurologic signs are not usually caused by a single episode of trauma. It is not uncommon for an owner to blame a neurologic disorder on an injury from a fall when in fact the underlying progressive neurologic disorder caused the fall. Be aware that neoplastic involvement of the nervous system occasionally may occur suddenly and progress rapidly. The wobbler syndrome may have a slow insidious onset and progress, or occur suddenly without obvious evidence of progression. Thus any neurologic signs caused by a space-occupying type of lesion may appear suddenly even though the primary lesion is slowly progressive.

If the neurologic disorder has been progressive, the examiner should carefully document the occurrence of each sign to determine if the lesion is focal or diffuse in the nervous system. A patient with progressive paresis and ataxia of the pelvic limbs with normal thoracic limb function that subsequently develops a facial paresis and hemiatrophy of the tongue must have more than one lesion to explain the signs. Such a multifocal distribution of lesions is characteristic of an inflammatory lesion such as protozoal encephalomyelitis in horses. By careful questioning of an owner concerning the onset of neurologic signs, it may become apparent that there were previous signs, suggesting a progressive problem.

The history of previous or concurrent diseases affecting other body systems should be investigated in the patient as well as in the rest of the herd. Upper respiratory disease, abortions, or minor illness with fever may have occurred in a herd in which one or more horses have neurologic signs caused by equine herpesvirus I (rhinopneumonitis). In this disease, a history of other horses affected with a mild transient ataxia may be found on examination of a patient that became recumbent in a 24- to 48-hour period. A history of strangles infection in the patient or in the herd may accompany the signs of a brain abscess due to *Streptococcus equi*. Determine if there is a present or past history of a problem similar to that shown by the patient in other related or unrelated animals. Evidence of a family history may help document an hereditary disease.

The environment should be examined directly or indirectly for a source of toxins or possible poisonous vegetation. A *Fusarium* species of mold infecting corn has been implicated in equine leukoencephalomalacia, a rare disease today. *Centaurea* species (yellow star thistle and Russian knapweed) are involved in the pathogenesis of nigropallidal encephalomalacia. The pyrrolizidine alkaloids from species of *Senecio* (ragwort and common groundsel), *Amsinckia* (fiddleneck), or *Crotalaria* (wild pea) produce a chronic hepatic cirrhosis that may result in hepatic encephalopathy. A syndrome of episodic ataxia and muscle spasms—"staggers"—may occur in horses consuming rye grass, or paspallum grasses infected with ergot (*Claviceps paspali*). Ataxia and cystitis have been associated with feeding on *Sorghum* grasses (sorghum, sudan, Johnson grass). Locoweed poisoning has been reported in horses grazing on *Oxytropis* and *Astragalus* herbs. They showed wasting, abnormal gait, and hypersensitivity during handling.

Horses grazing in fields in which lead fallout has occurred from industrial wastes have been poisoned. A source of growth of *Clostridium botulinum* is often difficult to document. Wound infections with this organism should be considered as a source of toxin in cases of suspected botulism.

The vaccination history of the animal is important in evaluating differential diagnosis for the various viral encephalitides, equine infectious anemia, and strangles infection. Rhinopneumonitis titers apparently are not necessarily protective against the neurologic form of this disease. Biologics of equine origin such as tetanus antitoxin may be implicated as the source of an agent causing acute hepatic necrosis and encephalopathy.

GENERAL PHYSICAL EXAMINATION

The complete general examination of all body systems other than the nervous system should precede the neurologic examination. Primary disease of other systems may be manifested by neurologic signs. The severe cerebral disorder of hepatic encephalopathy is a common example of this in the horse. Other extracranial encephalopathies include neonatal septicemia and maladjustment syndrome (respiratory distress syndrome), neonatal hypoglycemia, transit tetany, and hypomagnesemia. In such cases the signs are often intermittent. Patients with cardiac malformations may present with episodes of weakness or collapse (syncope). The same can occur with hypoadrenocorticoidism. Musculoskeletal disorders most frequently are confused with signs of neurologic disease. Palpation of limbs and joints sometimes aided by simultaneous auscultation may reveal fractures that are the cause of the clinical signs. A rectal examination should be included and can assist in defining sublumbar muscle tenderness (myositis). A grossly distended bladder can be expected in most recumbent horses, but in a standing horse usually is suggestive of paralysis of the bladder. Palpable crepitus associated with the pelvic cavity and hip area in a horse with a severe lameness, muscle atrophy, or pelvic limb paresis should be studied carefully. Often these apparently abnormal findings are not associated with a bony lesion. Palpation may reveal firm muscles and cold skin in aortic-iliac thrombosis. Neuritis of the cauda equina may present because of dysuria or obstipation. Epistaxis often accompanies cranial nerve deficits caused by guttural pouch mycosis. Surface wounds should be looked for in consideration of tetanus, botulism, or rabies. Ticks may be implicated in producing a flaccid paralysis of foals.

NEUROLOGIC EXAMINATION

The neurologic examination should include the areas of mental status, gait and posture, spinal reflexes, cranial nerve reflexes, and sensation. The order in which the parts of a neurologic examination are performed is unimportant; however, those procedures that will upset the patient the least should be performed first. Complete spinal reflexes cannot be assessed in most horses that are ambulatory; however, in such cases it is reasonable to assume that they are present even if they possibly are exaggerated (spastic).

Mental Status and Behavior

The owner should be questioned regarding the behavior of the patient. He or she can best judge if it has changed and can inform you of how the patient normally responds. The breed and age may influence the behavior. It is especially important to judge the mental status carefully in the recumbent patient. Cervical spinal cord disease may produce recumbency without altering the animal's behavior.

If its behavior is unchanged, the animal will remain alert and responsive. Horses with suspected botulism may be recumbent and too weak to move but usually respond to the examiner. Occasionally, some depression is observed. A recumbent animal that is obtunded, semicomatose, convulsing, or delirious probably has a brain lesion. Sometimes a horse that is down due to spinal cord disease, aortic thrombosis, myositis, or acute vestibular disease will act delirious in its frantic struggle to get up. The most remarkable alterations in behavior usually occur with hepatic encephalopathy.

Gait and Posture

The horse should be moved at the walk and trot in a straight line, walked in large and small circles in both directions, and backed. It may help to observe subtle deficits if this is also done on a gentle slope or while the head is elevated. Blindfolding may exacerbate an ataxia if it is cerebellar or vestibular in origin. It has little effect on the ataxia caused by spinal cord lesions. Slight asymmetry in length of strides may be detected by walking next to the horse stride for stride. Allowing the horse to move freely without a lead in a paddock also may be helpful. The horse with mild general proprioceptive ataxia from spinal cord disease may gait fairly well in a straight path but show ataxia on quickly turning at the end of a paddock.

Signs of weakness, or ataxia, or both may be elicited by gently pushing the hindquarters or pulling the patient by the tail to one side as it is standing and walking (the sway response). The normal horse resists these movements, or steps briskly to the side as it is pushed or pulled. The weak horse can be pulled easily to the side and may stumble or fall. The weak horse also may tend to buckle or collapse when strong pressure is applied with the fingers to the withers and loin region. The ataxic horse may sway to one side, be slow to protract a limb, cross its limbs, or step on its opposite limb. The ataxic animal may abduct the outside pelvic limb too far as it is pushed to one side or moved in a small circle. This may appear as a hypermetric movement similar to the stringhalt action, and is assumed to be a sign of a general proprioceptive tract lesion. The animal that is pushed or circled may keep a clinically affected pelvic limb fixed in one position on the ground and pivot around it without moving it. The same failure to protract the limb may be seen on backing. It may even force the horse into a "dog-sitting" posture. This is assumed to be caused by a lesion in the general proprioceptive tracts, or the upper motor neuron tracts, or both. It usually occurs in the more severely affected patient. Walking the patient with the neck held extended may cause a thoracic limb to scuff the ground when there is mild cervical spinal cord disease. It is often difficult to distinguish paresis from ataxia, but in most instances it is unimportant because of the close anatomic relationship of the ascending general proprioceptive and descending upper motor neuron tracts in the white matter of the spinal cord.

Occasionally, with general proprioceptive tract lesions the animal may hold an affected limb longer in an abnormal position (crossed or abducted) when placed there by the examiner.

As a rule mild lesions of the tracts in the cervical spinal cord cause a more obvious deficit in the pelvic limbs but usually some thoracic limb deficit can be detected. If no thoracic limb deficit is observed and the pelvic limb signs are mild, the lesion either could be in the thoracolumbar spinal cord or in the cervical spinal cord. If the pelvic limb signs are moderate or severe with normal thoracic limbs, the lesion causing the signs is limited to the thoracolumbar spinal cord. When the pelvic limb signs are very severe but the thoracic limb signs are very subtle, then the possibility of a thoracolumbar lesion *and* a mild cervical lesion, or a diffuse spinal cord lesion, should be considered. Similarly, a moderate thoracic limb deficit with mild pelvic limb signs may be due to multifocal or diffuse lesions and is unlikely to be caused by a focal cervical spinal cord contusion. Most multifocal myelopathies in horses are inflammatory or infectious (myelitis) and most diffuse diseases are equine degenerative myeloencephalopathy.

Signs of upper motor neuron tract disease may produce muscle hypertonia (spasticity) in addition to paresis. This may be manifested as a stiff, short-strided gait with little carpal flexion, and may be the most salient feature of the thoracic limb deficit in cervical spinal cord disease.

The same hypertonic, spastic, short-strided gait may occur with cerebellar disease with or without obvious hypermetria. This gait, which is seen in Arabians with cerebellar cortical abiotrophy, can best be described as an apparent delay in the onset of the voluntary movement followed by an exaggerated response. The exaggerated response may produce a quick, short stride with limited joint movement (hypermetria). In the disease in Arabians these signs are symmetric in all four limbs but may be more obvious in the thoracic limbs. Strength is normal and there is no general proprioceptive ataxia in cerebellar disease. A head tremor and an abnormal menace response consistently accompany the gait abnormality. In unilateral cerebellar disease the abnormal gait usually is observed in the ipsilateral limbs.

Unilateral cerebral lesions generally do not interfere with the gait unless accompanied by increased intracranial pressure. Extensive manipulations that require extra coordinated efforts (hopping, righting, standing up) may elicit some minimal abnormalities in the contralateral limbs. If circling occurs, it is usually toward the side of the cerebral lesion. These lesions may be localized best by a visual deficit in the contralateral eyeball with normal pupillary response bilaterally. If increased intracranial pressure also is present, however, the pupillary responses also may be deficient. A dilated, unresponsive pupil may occur on the ipsilateral side from oculomotor nerve compression.

When lesions affect the vestibular system peripherally (otitis media), or centrally in the vestibular nuclei or vestibular portions of the cerebellum, there is usually a head and body tilt toward the side of the lesion. If the lesion is peripheral, strength and general proprioception are normal and the animal drifts or lurches toward the affected side. Although such an animal shows no weakness or lack of knowledge as to where its limbs are located, it may show a slightly wide base stance, presumably for better balance. Blindfolding accentuates this loss of balance and may cause the animal to fall to the affected side. Further examination of the eyeballs may elicit other abnormalities due to lesions in this system (see section on cranial nerve examination).

Spinal Reflexes

It should be remembered that an intact reflex only requires the muscles, their peripheral nerves, and the segments of brain stem or spinal cord from which the afferent neurons enter and the efferent neurons leave the CNS. A sensory (pain) response on the part of the patient requires the afferent peripheral nerve and the white matter of the spinal cord and brain stem to the grey matter of the sensory cortex. Such a response usually is seen as a reaction on the part of the patient that also requires an intact pathway from the sensory motor cortex of the cerebrum through the white matter of the brain and spinal cord to efferent neurons and their axons in peripheral nerves. These efferent neurons of such reflex arcs and reactions, along with their terminal neuromuscular junctions, are the final common pathway of all motor function and are termed the lower motor neuron. All descending connections of neurons that help regulate the function of these LMNs are termed upper motor neurons. Thus the UMN includes the grey matter of the cerebral motor cortex, cerebellum, and brain stem nuclei (red nucleus, substantia nigra, reticular formation) and their descending tracts.

The upper motor neuron contains tracts that are both facilitatory and inhibitory to the function of the lower motor neuron; however, when upper motor neuron lesions exist there is usually a resulting "release" of the lower motor neuron from inhibition. Thus upper motor neuron signs are classically those of hypertonia of muscles and hyperreflexia of reflex arcs. If the lower motor neuron is affected, passive manipulation of the appropriate limb will reveal decreased or absent tone (flaccidity). Muscle tone cannot be assessed in a limb that the horse is lying on. Such lower motor neuron lesions also affect the local reflex arcs and thus cause depressed or absent reflexes. The last characteristic of lower motor neuron lesions is rapid muscle atrophy that results from denervation of peripheral muscles. Myelitis (i.e., protozoal) that affects the grey matter as well as the white matter produces observable atrophy of pelvic limb muscles if the lesion involves segments L4 through S1, and of the thoracic limb muscles if it is in segments C6 through T2. This is often asymmetric. In tetanus, the remarkable hypertonia results from neurotoxin interference with interneurons in the spinal cord that normally inhibit lower motor neuron reflex function.

The tendon reflexes should be examined first because they do not elicit a pain response. As a rule, these require a recumbent animal and can only be tested adequately in the limbs the animal is not lying on. Lower motor neuron lesions or lesions anywhere in the reflex arc cause hyporeflexia or areflexia, whereas upper motor neuron lesions result in reflexes that at least are present and may be hyperreflexic.

Patellar Reflex. This is elicited by holding the limb relaxed in a partially flexed position and tapping the intermediate patellar ligament that normally produces stifle extension. This reflex is mediated through the femoral nerve and primarily the L4 and L5 segments of the spinal cord. The femoral nerve is also sensory to the medial side of the limb through its saphenous nerve branch.

Triceps Reflex. Hold the relaxed limb in partial flexion, tap the triceps tendon at the olecranon, and observe for a mild elbow extension. This is mediated through the radial nerve and the cervical intumescence (C7, C8, T1). This nerve is also sensory to the midlateral surface of the arm and forearm. If this nerve is injured proximal to the triceps innervations the animal will drag or stand on the dorsum of the hoof and cannot support weight on the limb. This would also occur if the cell bodies in the cervical intumescence were affected. If the nerve is injured in the arm distal to the triceps innervation, weight can be supported but the digit cannot be extended; therefore the patient stands on the dorsum of the hoof.

Flexor Reflex—Pelvic Limb. Use fingers, forceps, or an electric prod on the coronary band or heel bulb, depending on the severity of the neurologic deficit. Use whatever is necessary to determine the reflex as well as the response to pain without upsetting the patient any more than is necessary.

The flexor reflex response requires the sciatic nerve and spinal cord segments L6, S1, and S2. If the sensory stimulation is restricted to the dorsal metatarsal region, the peroneal nerve will be stimulated. The plantar metatarsal region is innervated by the tibial nerve branch of the sciatic nerve. The coronary band and heel bulb receive both tibial and peroneal nerve innervation. Flexion of the stifle, hock, and digit is mediated by the sciatic nerve and its peroneal and tibial branches. Hip flexion is mediated by the entire lumbar spinal cord and the segmental innervation of the psoas major muscle.

When this reflex is performed, *two* observations should be made: first, the amount of reflex initiated, and second, the animal's cerebral response to the painful stimulus. The reflex only requires the sciatic nerve and the sixth lumbar and first and second sacral spinal cord segments. The cerebral response to pain requires that the sensory portion of these components *plus* the ascending spinal cord tracts that transmit sensory information to the rostral brain stem and cerebral cortex be intact. The cerebral response to pain may be manifested by one or more of the following: pupillary dilation, altered respirations, head, ear, eyeball, and trunk movements, or kicking if the limb stimulated is not paralyzed. Lesions in the peripheral nerve being tested produce hypalgesia or analgesia and a depressed or absent reflex response. Lesions in the ascending spinal cord tracts for the sensory modalities perceived as pain produce hypalgesia or analgesia without any loss of the reflex function. Transverse spinal cord lesions that produce paresis or paralysis caudal to the lesion may be localized by finding a line of hypalgesia or analgesia along the body wall.

The panniculus reflex also may be helpful in localizing a thoracolumbar spinal cord lesion. Gentle pin pricking of the skin along the dorsal and lateral aspects of the body wall elicits a quivering of the skin of the trunk from contraction of the cutaneous trunci muscle. The sensory stimulation is carried to the spinal cord segments by the dorsal branches of the segmental spinal nerves at the level of the stimulation. The sensory information is relayed cranially from that point through the spinal cord white matter to the first thoracic and eighth cervical segments, where it initiates action in the lower motor neuron cell bodies of the lateral thoracic nerve which innervates the cutaneous trunci. A lesion anywhere along this pathway may interfere with this reflex.

Flexor Reflex—Thoracic Limb. Stimulation of the coronary band or heel bulb stimulates the dendritic zone of neurons in the median nerve (and ulnar nerve laterally). The response of flexion of the digit, carpus, elbow, and shoulder requires the function of the last three cervical and first two thoracic spinal cord segments and the axillary, musculocutaneous, median, ulnar, and radial nerves.

A lesion that involves the spinal cord at the level of the cervical intumescence produces tetraparesis with lower motor neuron signs in the thoracic limbs (atonia, areflexia, atrophy) owing to the disturbance of the grey matter from C6 to T2, and upper motor neuron signs in the pelvic limbs (normal or exaggerated reflexes, and hypertonia without atrophy) due to the disturbance to the upper motor neuron tracts in the spinal cord white matter at C6 to T2.

A local cervical reflex similar to the panniculus reflex of the trunk can be elicited by gently pricking the skin of the lateral neck and observing flicking of the skin of the neck due to contractions of the cutaneous coli and brachiocephalicus muscles. Some severe cervical lesions involving grey matter (myelitis) can result in a depressed or absent local cervical reflex.

Perineal Reflex. Mild stimulation of the skin of the perineum elicits reflex closure of the anus and tail flexion if the pudendal, caudal rectal and caudal nerves and the last three sacral and caudal segments of the spinal cord are intact. In horses with rabies the tail and anus may be hypotonic and hypalgesic.

Be sure to observe and differentiate both the reflex response and the cerebral response or reaction to the painful stimuli used. Occasionally, a severe spinal cord lesion has been found to result in hypalgesia confined to the ipsilateral limb or including a portion of the trunk if the grey matter lesion is diffuse. However, this is not common and the other findings in neurologic evaluation best define the site.

The axial musculature and vertebral spines should be palpated for deformities, or focal pain, or both. The few cases of equine myotonia that have been seen could be detected easily by palpation of tense hypertrophied muscles that are hypersensitive to mechanical stimulus resulting in a prolonged (less than 2 minutes) tight muscle "knotting" (myotonic dimple) upon percussion. These foals do have a stiff, choppy gait in the pelvic and occasionally the thoracic limbs, especially after a period of rest. Acute extensive midcervical myelitis may result in a visual and palpable deformity (scoliosis) of the cervial vertebral column that mimics vertebral fracture or luxation.

SUMMARY OF SIGNS WITH LESIONS AT SPECIFIC AREAS OF THE SPINAL CORD

Lumbosacral Intumescence (L4 through Caudal Segments)

1. Thoracic limbs normal.
2. Ataxic and paretic pelvic limbs, with decreased ability to support weight to paraplegia (total pelvic limb paralysis).
3. Decreased or absent tail, anus, and pelvic limb tone and reflexes. Atrophy of pelvic limb muscles.
4. Hypalgesia or analgesia of the same areas with a line at the cranial edge of the lesion.
5. Urinary incontinence and obstipation.

Thoracolumbar (T3–L3)

1. Thoracic limbs normal.
2. Pelvic limb ataxia and paresis to paraplegia.
3. Normal tail and anal tone and reflexes and normal or exaggerated pelvic limb reflexes with normal tone or hypertonia.
4. Hypalgesia or analgesia caudal to the lesion.
5. Urinary incontinence.

Cervical Intumescence (C6–T2)

1. Paresis (tetraparesis) and ataxia of all four limbs to tetraplegia.
2. Depressed or absent thoracic limb reflexes and tone with atrophy.
3. Normal or exaggerated pelvic limb reflexes and tone.
4. Hypalgesia or analgesia caudal to the cranial edge of the lesion. Hypalgesia may be more pronounced in the thoracic limbs.

Cervical Spinal Cord Cranial to the Intumescence (C1–C5)

1. Ataxia and paresis (tetraparesis) of all four limbs to tetraplegia. Ataxia and paresis may be more obvious in the pelvic limbs.
2. Normal or exaggerated reflexes and tone in all four limbs.
3. Hypalgesia caudal to the lesion.

Cranial Nerve Examination

I. Olfactory Nerve.   Clinical deficit in smell rarely is encountered in the horse. Normal function may be observed by the patient's ability to smell the hand of the examiner or its feed.

II. Optic Nerve.   Visual deficits may be seen as the animal maneuvers in its environment or through a maze. In the normal animal a sudden gesture of the hand toward the eye elicits immediate closure of the palpebral fissure and the head may jerk away from the movement. It is imperative to perform this maneuver far enough from the animal that contact is not made and air currents cannot be felt. The afferent component of this pathway includes the ipsilateral refractive media of the eyeball, retina, optic nerve, and chiasm and primarily the contralateral optic tract, lateral geniculate nucleus (thalamus), and the optic radiation and occipital cortex of the cerebrum. The latter structures are contralateral to the eyeball being tested because 80 to 90 per cent of the optic nerve axons cross in the optic chiasm in the horse. The lower motor neuron involved is the facial nucleus in the medulla and facial nerve to the orbicularis oculi. There is indirect evidence that the pathway between the visual cerebral cortex and the facial nucleus involves the cerebellum. Young Arabians with cerebellar cortical abiotrophy do not respond to the menace gesture with eyelid closure, yet they have no facial palsy or visual deficit. Very young foals also may not respond, or become refractory during repeated testing. Thus, in horses with a poor or absent menace response it is important to determine whether they can see by other means.

Space-occupying or necrotic lesions in one cerebrum produce a contralateral visual deficit which can be observed by the failure to respond to the menace gesture, and by walking the patient through a maze, especially with the normal eye blindfolded. Bilateral lesions of the optic radiation (leukoencephalomalacia) or visual cortex (hepatic encephalopathy, viral encephalitides) produce a bilateral visual deficit. Pupillary responses to light are normal. Only if the lesion is in the eyeball or optic nerve or chiasm are pupillary light responses abnormal. Bilateral optic tract lesions also interfere with this but unilateral lesions may not. The afferent pathway to light directed into the eyeball is the same as for the menace gesture to the level of the lateral geniculate nucleus. The axons for this function pass by the neurons in this thalamic nucleus and synapse in the pretectal region of the brain stem. These second neurons in the afferent pathway in turn synapse on neurons in both oculomotor nuclei. Crossing can occur at the optic chiasm, as well as at the pretectal and oculomotor nuclear levels. Therefore shining the light in one eyeball produces reflex pupillary constriction in both eyeballs. The efferent lower motor neuron is the parasympathetic preganglionic neuron in the oculomotor nucleus and its axon in cranial nerve III (oculomotor nerve). Synapse occurs in the ciliary ganglion just caudal to the eyeball and postganglionic axons innervate the constrictor muscle of the pupil in the iris. This pupillary constriction pathway is limited to the brain stem and is spared by lesions affecting the visual pathways in the cerebrum.

In severely depressed animals the amount of pupil closure to light may be minimal, but the pupil usually is not mydriatic. An excited animal may have very widely dilated pupils that respond poorly to light. Prior to directing the light through the pupil for this reflex, pupillary apertures should be checked for size and symmetry. A widely dilated pupil in a normal eyeball suggests an oculomotor nerve deficit. It is unresponsive to light directed into either eyeball. The normal pupil responds when light is directed into the mydriatic pupil only if the optic nerve of the affected eyeball is intact. A partially dilated pupil may occur in severe unilateral retinal or optic nerve lesions and only responds to light directed into the normal eyeball. Bilateral severe miosis may occur with acute diffuse cerebral lesions. Severe brain stem contusions can produce a range of pupillary abnormalities that may change rapidly in the first few hours after the injury. Progressive bilateral dilation is a grave sign and suggests progressive edema in the mesencephalon.

Although a partially miotic pupil that contracts well to light is an easily recognized part of Horner's syndrome in other species, it can be difficult to detect in the horse. The most striking features of Horner's syndrome in the horse are ipsilateral hyperhidrosis, hyperthermia of the head, and cranial neck and ipsilateral ptosis of the upper eyelid. Other findings include mild miosis, congestion of nasal and conjunctival membranes, and increased lacrimation. This syndrome is seen in guttural pouch mycosis and surgery (postganglionic), deep cervical injections, space-occupying cervical lesions, and experimental section of the cervical sympathetic trunk (preganglionic). This is because the sympathetic supply for the eye and blood vessels of the head is carried in the cervical sympathetic trunk adjacent to the cervical vagus nerve. These fibers pass up the neck to the cranial cervical ganglion on the wall of the guttural pouch adjacent to the internal carotid artery, and the postganglionic fibers follow other vessels and nerves to all parts of the head.

The optic nerve should be observed with the ophthalmoscope as part of the neurologic examination. It occasionally may reflect increased intracranial pressure by the appearance of swelling at the optic disk.

III. Oculomotor Nerve (to Dorsal, Ventral and Medial Recti, Ventral Oblique, and Levator Palpebrae). The parasympathetic component of the oculomotor nerve is tested along with the optic nerve and visual pathway examination.

IV. Trochlear Nerve (to Dorsal Oblique)

VI. Abducens Nerve (to Lateral Rectus and Retractor Bulbi). The function of the extraocular muscles and their innervation by cranial nerves III, IV, and VI are tested simultaneously by observing the position of the eyeballs in the orbits and their movements. An abnormal position (strabismus) occurs if there is interference with the innervation of these muscles.

Without experimental or direct clinicopathologic correlation, the specific position of the strabismus in the horse for paralysis of each of these three cranial nerves is unknown. Comparing with other species and with man, an oculomotor palsy should produce a lateral and ventral strabismus. Ptosis and mydriasis may accompany this due to paralysis of the levator palpebrae and pupillary constrictor muscles, respectively. A trochlear nerve palsy should cause the medial aspect of the pupil to rotate dorsally.

An abducens nerve palsy should cause a medial strabismus and possible lack of eyeball retraction (with protrusion of the third eyelid) when the corneal reflex is tested. These forms of strabismus should be present in all positions of the head because of the muscle paralysis.

Be aware of the strabismus associated with disturbances of the vestibular system. There is a direct anatomic connection between the vestibular system (cranial nerve VIII, vestibular nuclei, and vestibular part of cerebellum) and these extraocular muscle neurons by way of the medial longitudinal fasciculus (MLF) in the brain stem. Vestibular abnormalities may interfere with the normal tonic mechanism controlling eyeball position relative to head position and a strabismus may result. This is usually ventral and sometimes medial and may correct itself in certain positions of the head. The affected eyeball will abduct and adduct (normal vestibular nystagmus) if the head is moved from side to side. With unilateral vestibular disorders this vestibular strabismus occurs on the ipsilateral side.

If there is bilateral disturbance of the vestibular system or the MLF, then moving the head from side to side does not induce a normal eyeball movement (vestibular nystagmus). This is a grave sign in intracranial injuries, because it indicates that a brain stem lesion has occurred to interfere with the MLF.

V. Trigeminal (to Muscles of Mastication and Sensation to Most of Head). Lesions that affect the mandibular nerve innervation of the muscles of mastication bilaterally cause a dropped jaw and inability to close it. Unilateral lesions can be detected best by the atrophy of the temporal and masseter muscles that can be palpated.

The sensory function of this cranial nerve can be tested by gentle palpation of the eyelids medially (ophthalmic nerve) and laterally (maxillary nerve), which causes the palpebral fissure to be closed (facial nerve). This is the palpebral reflex. Gentle palpation of the cornea with the lids held open tests the sensory function of the ophthalmic nerve and the extraocular muscle innervation that causes the eyeballs to be retracted (oculomotor and abducens) and the third eyelid to protrude passively. This is the corneal reflex. Gentle palpation or light pin pricking of the upper lip, nostrils, and nasal septum tests the maxillary nerve, and of the lower lip and cheek tests the mandibular nerve response. In a depressed animal palpation of the nasal septum with a blunt probe may be required to elicit a hypalgesia.

Idiopathic hyperesthesia, referred to as trigeminal neuralgia, has been assumed in horses that continually rub one side of their faces.

Lesions that involve the spinal tract of the trigeminal nerve on the side of the medulla can produce a sensory deficit without paresis of the masticatory muscles.

Cerebral lesions that interfere with the somesthetic cortex of the parietal lobe can produce a mild contralateral hypalgesia, most evident in the sensitive nasal septum.

VII. Facial Nerve (to Muscles of Facial Expression). This is the lower motor neuron of many of the reflexes that have been tested that produce closure of the palpebral fissure (menace, corneal, palpebral). Paresis or paralysis of these facial muscles causes the ear, upper eyelid, and the lower lip to droop, and the upper lip and nose to be pulled toward the normal side. A mild paresis may be detected by careful observation of the use of the lips on prehension and the lack of action of the nostrils on inspiration.

Injury to the buccal branches on the side of the face (recumbency, facial trauma) causes signs of paresis in the lips and nostrils only.

The facial nucleus can be affected by lesions in the medulla. The nerve can be involved in meningitis, otitis media, guttural pouch mycosis, or presumably by a selective transient neuritits (idiopathic facial paralysis). The diffuse neuropathy that primarily affects the cauda equina (neuritis of the cauda equina) also may affect other spinal and cranial nerves, including the facial nerve.

VIII. Vestibulocochlear Nerve

1. The cochlear division mediates the sensory modality interpreted as sound. Deafness most often is due to lesions of this nerve or the receptor in the cochlear duct. Congenital deafness is caused by aplasia or degeneration of this receptor end organ. Bilateral otitis media and otitis interna cause deafness. Unilateral deafness associated with otitis media and otitis interna may be difficult to detect.

2. The vestibular division innervates the receptor end organs in the semicircular ducts, macula, and utricle that function in the orientation of the head with

the body, limbs, and the eyes. Vestibular system abnormalities can occur with lesions in the eighth cranial nerve, vestibular nuclei in the medulla, or vestibular components of the cerebellum. The abnormal posture of head, body, and eyes and the abnormal gait have been described. In addition, abnormal nystagmus may be observed. With peripheral nerve disorders (injury, otitis media or interna) the quick phase of the nystagmus always is directed to the opposite side from the lesion (head tilt), and may be horizontal or rotatory. In the first few days after the onset of the signs the nystagmus may be spontaneous—visible at all times. After this it may be elicited only by holding the head in different positions—positional nystagmus. With lesions in the central components of the vestibular system, the positional nystagmus may change direction with different positions of the head.

Remember that in pure vestibular system abnormalities such as cerebellar disease there is no loss of strength. With diffuse cerebellar cortical disease (e.g., as occurs in Arabian foals) the remarkable hypertonic dysmetria is symmetric. With unilateral vestibular disorders (otitis media or interna) the ataxia is asymmetric with tilting of the head and leaning, falling, or rolling of the body toward the side of the lesion.

Cases of otitis media or interna may present with a sudden onset of clinical signs, and a frantic patient.

IX, X, XI. Glossopharyngeal, Vagus, and Spinal Accessory Nerves. The most important clinical deficits of one or more components of these nerves are laryngeal and pharyngeal paralysis. The cell bodies of the neurons that innervate these muscles are in the nucleus ambiguus of the medulla. The peripheral nerves are associated closely with the portion of the guttural pouch often affected by mycotic infections, and dysphagia often occurs with this disease and with diffuse pouch empyema (catarrh).

Pharyngeal paralysis can be detected by observing the appearance of food and water at the nostrils, inability to swallow food or water, and inadequate swallowing of a stomach tube. The degree of difficulty depends on whether the lesion is unilateral or bilateral. Dysphagia is a common sign in rabies, probably due to lesions in the medulla. Be aware that severe diffuse cerebral disease may cause swallowing difficulties even though there is no primary lesion in the nucleus ambiguus. Also remember that myositis of the pharyngeal and lingual muscles may interfere with the swallowing function. Dysphagia is also one of the most prominent signs of the diffuse lower motor neuron paralysis in suspected botulism.

Laryngeal paralysis can be detected by the characteristic inspiratory dyspnea (roaring) that is audible on respiration. Neuropathy of these cranial nerves associated with chronic lead poisoning may cause pharyngeal and laryngeal paralysis.

XII. Hypoglossal Nerve (Motor to Tongue Muscles). Paralysis of one nerve produces atrophy of the ipsilateral half of the tongue but does not interfere much with its function. Bilateral palsy interferes with swallowing. The normal tongue resists attempts to pull it from the mouth. The paretic tongue can be pulled from the mouth easily and is slow to return. In a severely depressed horse the tongue may be pulled from the mouth easily, and it will hang out for a while before being returned to the mouth. Occasionally the tip may be chewed on. This can occur without a hypoglossal neuron lesion. The upper motor neuron (extrapyramidal nuclear) lesions in yellow star thistle poisoning may cause sudden dystonia of the masticatory (V), facial (VII), and tongue (XII) muscles that interferes with prehension and swallowing functions, occasionally accompanied by behavior changes and leaning and/or circling tendencies.

Palpate the skull for any deformities.

INTERPRETATION OF CSF ANALYSIS

Normal values for equine CSF analysis are: cisternal pressure—161 to 456 mm H_2O; protein—0 to 92 (mean 37) mg per dl; RBC—0; WBC—0 to 5 mm^3; creatine phosphokinase 0 to 7 (mean 1) international units; glutamic-oxalacetic transaminase 18 to 43 (mean 30) Sigma-Frankel units; and lactic dehydrogenase 0 to 5 (mean 1.5) international units. There is no significant difference in cytology or protein and enzyme levels between fluid from the cerebellomedullary cistern and the lumbosacral subarachnoid space. It should be clear and colorless.[8]

As a general rule injury to the CNS results in an xanthochromic (yellow) CSF with slightly elevated protein (80 to 150 mg per dl) or occasionally a definitely bloody sample. However, large hemorrhages may be present epidurally with very little change in CSF. This can depend partly on the site of collection. If a brain or cranial cervical lesion is suspected, then an atlanto-occipital sample should be taken. A lumbosacral sample should be taken for all spinal cord problems caudal to this. Other diseases that can result in xanthochromic CSF with elevated protein and a few mononuclear cells (10 to 30 per mm^3) are intracarotid injections of drugs such as promazine, deep cerebral abscess (*Streptococcus equi*), vertebral osteomyelitis, and acute wobbler syndrome. Classically equine herpesvirus I (rhinopneumonitis) vasculitis/myelopathy results in an xanthochromic fluid with elevated protein (80 to 200 mg per dl) and little or no cellular response. The CSF changes with protozoal myelitis are variable. Although a moderately elevated protein (100 to 200 mg per dl) and mononuclear pleocytosis (50 to 100 per mm^3) can be expected, the CSF is often normal. The arboviral encephalitides produce a pleocytosis that can vary in nature. In Venezuelan equine encephalomyelitis and eastern equine encephalomyelitis during the acute phase, a high neutrophil count (<100 to $500 +$ per mm^3) can be expected that will change to a predominantly small mononuclear pleocytosis over several days. Western equine encephalomyelitis produces a less marked pleocytosis (50 to 200 per mm^3) that is predominantly (> 50 per cent) small mononuclear cells. In all cases the protein content also is elevated to about 100 to 300 mg per dl. Rabies virus encephalomyelitis alters the CSF results in a manner similar to that in western equine encephalomyelitis. The most common diffuse cerebral disease, hepatoencephalopathy, does not effectively alter the CSF findings; although a slight yellow discoloration may be apparent as a result of the profound dehydration and icterus.

REFERENCES

1. Adams, L. G., Dollahite, J. W., Romane, W. M., Bullard, T. L., and Bridges, C. H.: Cystitis and ataxia associated with sorghum ingestion by horses. J. Am. Vet. Med. Assoc., 155:518, 1969.
2. de Lahunta, A.: Neurological problems of the horse. Proceedings 19th Annual Convention Am. Assoc. Equine Pract., 19:25, 1973.
3. Ferris, D. H., and Beamer, P. D.: Comparative studies of equine encephalomyelitis caused by nematodes, viruses, and mycotoxins. Proceedings 17th Annual Convention Am. Assoc. Equine Pract., 17:173, 1971.

4. Gabel, A. A., and Koestner, A.: The effects of intracarotid artery injection of drugs in domestic animals. J. Am. Vet. Med. Assoc., *162*:1397, 1963.

5. Harries, W. N., Baker, F. P., and Johnston, A.: An outbreak of locoweed poisoning in horses in southwestern Alberta. Can. Vet. J., *13*:141, 1972.

6. Harrington, D. D.: Pathologic features of magnesium deficiency in young horses fed purified rations. Am. J. Vet. Res., *35*:503, 1974.

7. Holliday, T. A.: The nervous system—examination. *In* Catcott, E. J., and Smithcors, J. F., eds., Equine Medicine and Surgery. 2nd ed., Wheaton, Ill., American Veterinary Publications, Inc., 1972, 459–463.

8. Mayhew, I. G., Whitlock, R. H., and Tasker, J. B.: Equine cerebrospinal fluid: A study of normal values. Am. J. Vet. Res., in press.

Chapter 21

CASE DESCRIPTIONS

Each case description has three parts: the first part is the description of the neurologic disorder; the second part includes the neuroanatomic diagnosis and how this was determined, the differential diagnosis, and the ancillary data available in the case; and the third part includes the course of the disease, the final clinical or necropsy diagnosis, and a brief discussion of the syndrome.

Case 1: Case Description

Signalment. A 4-year-old female mongrel Great Dane.

Chief Complaint. Weakness and ataxia.

History. Starting 5 months prior to examination, this dog had episodes of coughing and gasping. Numerous examinations during this time did not result in a definite diagnosis. The owner commented that the dog's eyes looked different during this period of time. One month prior to examination, a veterinarian observed anisocoria from a small left pupil. About 10 days prior to examination, the dog began to lose coordination in the pelvic limbs and a head tilt was apparent. The ataxia progressed to the thoracic limbs.

Examination. The dog was alert and responsive but seemed disoriented in space. Its head was tilted to the left. It was reluctant to stand but could do so unassisted, and it continually leaned against the wall on its left side. When excited, the dog nearly tipped over toward its left side. Its strength seemed to be normal.

    Postural reactions were difficult to test because of the animal's disorientation. It frantically grasped for support when picked up to perform postural tests. There was a suggestion that the left pelvic limb hopped poorly.

    Hypertonia was marked in the thoracic limbs and mild in the pelvic limbs. There was no atrophy. Patellar reflexes were hyperactive (plus 3) bilaterally. Biceps and triceps reflexes were present. Flexor reflexes and the perineal reflex were all normal and pain perception was normal.

    On cranial nerve examination there was observed in the left eye a small pupil, protruded third eyelid, and smaller palpebral fissure. The head was tilted to the left (left ear more ventral). On holding the head and neck in extension the left eyeball did not elevate normally in the fissure. A positional abnormal nystagmus occurred that was mostly rotatory to the right. There was a moderate atrophy of the tongue muscles on the left side. The gag reflex was normal.

Diagnosis

Neuroanatomic Diagnosis. These signs indicated a caudal brain stem lesion on the left side. The vestibular signs (head tilt, tipping of the body to the left, strabismus, and abnormal nystagmus) were severe. The degree of severity suggested central vestibular involvement. The tongue atrophy indicated hypoglossal nucleus or nerve involvement, which could not occur with otitis media or other middle and inner ear disease. The signs of Horner's syndrome (miosis, protruded third eyelid, and smaller palpebral fissure) were due to sympathetic nerve paralysis to the orbital structures. This can occur with middle ear disease. It would be unlikely with medullary disease without more evidence of medullary involvement accompanied by ipsilateral severe hemiparesis. The history of gagging and coughing suggested paresis of pharyngeal muscles and could occur with disease of the pharyngeal branches of the ninth and tenth cranial nerves on one side. This also would not accompany an otitis media.

If the earliest observations of gagging and anisocoria were reliable, they suggest involvement of these nerves long before any vestibular signs or other signs of brain stem involvement. The latter occurred later and would be best explained by an extramedullary or extracranial mass involving the pharyngeal branches of the ninth and tenth cranial nerves and the sympathetic trunk or the cranial cervical ganglion, which later grew into the cranial cavity and compressed the left side of the medulla. The failure to observe any facial paresis indicated that the lesion should be caudal to the internal acoustic meatus. Within the medulla the vestibular nuclei extend further caudal than the facial nucleus and could be affected by a compressing mass at that point.

Differential Diagnosis. As suggested, an extramedullary mass lesion would best explain the development of this syndrome. An inflammatory lesion of the middle ear was excluded on anatomic grounds. Inflammations of the medulla in the dog rarely produce such specific cranial nerve deficits. An exception could be an extramedullary abscess, but these are rare in the dog. In most animals they are associated with otitis media and petrosal bone abscesses. The progression of signs, with vestibular signs coming late in onset, did not suggest this pathogenesis. A chronic meningitis or diffuse meningeal neoplastic process possibly could produce these signs if it was concentrated on the left side of the medulla. However, this would not explain the Horner's syndrome. The signs were too progressive for any traumatic or ischemic degenerative lesion. Most other degenerations would not be this focal in nature. Progression and age ruled out malformation.

Ancillary Studies. Cerebrospinal fluid had an opening pressure of 140 mm CSF. After removing 2 cc of clear, colorless fluid the closing pressure was 60 mm CSF. It contained 3 RBC and no WBC per cmm, and 71 mg of protein per dl.

Plain radiographs were normal. A scintiscan only slightly suggested increased uptake of radioisotope on the left side of the caudal fossa.

Outcome

The ancillary studies supported the diagnosis of an extramedullary mass. The brain-CSF barrier had been disturbed and the protein was moderately elevated. There was no indication of a primary suppurative inflammatory lesion. Following anesthesia for the ancillary studies the vestibular signs were remarkably exacerbated, and the dog continually attempted to roll to the left side.

In the dog this form of vestibular disturbance has only been seen with vestibular nuclear lesions or lesions of the vestibular components of the cerebellum.

The dog was still difficult to evaluate for postural reactions but did show evidence of more difficulty manipulating the paws on the left side, which was further indication of involvement of the left side of the medulla.

Prognosis for recovery was poor without surgical intervention and guarded with it. It was difficult to keep the dog from injuring itself when it rolled. The owner elected to have euthanasia performed.

Necropsy Findings. Four days after these studies necropsy revealed massive enlargement of the vagosympathetic trunk in the cranial cervical region. It included the distal ganglion of the vagus and extended into the cranial cavity through the tympanooccipital fissure and jugular foramen. Within the cranial cavity this mass measured 14 mm in diameter and compressed the medulla caudal to the trapezoid body and seventh and eighth cranial nerves (Fig. 21–1). The intracranial portion of the hypoglossal neurons was distended with

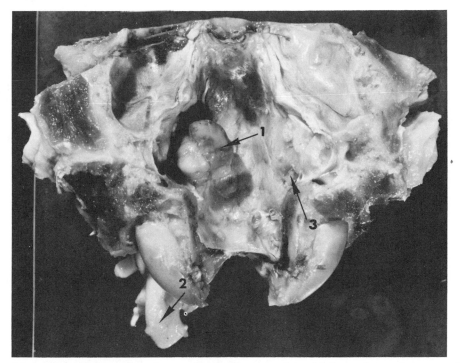

Figure 21–1. Case 1: Dorsoventral view of ventral aspect of caudal fossa of cranial cavity with the brain removed. The mass on the left (*1*) is continuous through the jugular foramen and tympanooccipital fissure with a similar mass in the vagosympathetic trunk (*2*). The normal right jugular foramen is indicated (*3*).

neoplastic tissue, as was the spinal portion of the eleventh cranial nerve. The glossopharyngeal and vagal neurons were directly involved in the large intracranial mass. Although the mass spared the cranial cervical ganglion, the adjacent sympathetic trunk was involved. On microscopic examination this neoplasm was diagnosed as a neurofibroma.

The course of the disease, with sympathetic and pharyngeal areas being the first presumed to be involved, is highly suggestive that the mass began outside the cranial cavity in the region of the tympanooccipital fissure. This is further supported by the late onset of the vestibular signs. There is no indication of when the hypoglossal involvement began, since this would have required visualization of the hemiatrophy of the tongue.

Remember that Horner's syndrome can be produced by lesions in a wide range of anatomic locations. The presence of other signs of neurologic disturbance usually determines the site of the lesion in the sympathetic nervous system. Dogs with persistent choking, gagging, or coughing for which no explanation can be found in the pharynx should be evaluated for a possible partial paralysis of the pharyngeal muscles.

Case 2: Case Description

Signalment. A 5-year-old male Great Dane.

Chief Complaint. Inability to use the pelvic limbs.

History. Two days prior to examination the dog had been out walking with its owner and on returning to the house developed difficulty using its pelvic limbs. Within a few minutes it collapsed on these limbs and could not get up.

Examination by a veterinarian the next morning revealed paraplegia with a normal patellar reflex, absent flexor reflex, and depressed perineal reflex. There was also urinary incontinence.

Examination. On examination two days after the onset of symptoms the dog was alert and responsive, but had no voluntary use of the pelvic limbs — grade 0 paraplegia. Occasionally a mild degree of hip flexion occurred on walking the dog on its thoracic limbs with the pelvic limbs held up by the tail. Thoracic limbs and trunk function were normal.

The pelvic limbs were hypotonic to manipulate. Both patellar reflexes were brisk (plus 3). Pelvic limb flexor reflexes were both absent. No pain was perceived from digits three through five or the dorsal, lateral, or plantar aspects of the paws. Stimulation of the medial side of the paw elicited pain and excited mild hip flexion. The anus was dilated, atonic, and areflexic. The tail was atonic and unresponsive to the perineal reflex. Pain was absent from the tail, perineum, caudal thigh, and skin distal to the stifle, except on the medial side of the leg and paw. Sensation was normal from the cranial thigh region. There was a line of analgesia at about the L6 vertebra. No pain was elicited on manipulation of the caudal lumbar and sacral vertebrae.

The bladder was distended and urine often was dribbled involuntarily.

Diagnosis

Neuroanatomic Diagnosis. These clinical signs indicated that there had been complete destruction of the caudal, sacral, and last two lumbar segments. The preserved patellar reflex and pain on the medial side of the leg and paw indicated that segments L4 and L5 and the femoral and saphenous nerves were intact. Normal sensation in the cranial thigh region indicated that the L4 segment and lateral cutaneous femoral nerve were intact. The dorsal branches of the emerging spinal nerves course caudally to supply the skin one to two vertebral lengths caudal to their site of origin from the vertebral canal. Therefore the line of analgesia is often one to two vertebrae caudal to the spinal nerve that emerges from the intervertebral foramen and supplies the skin up to the line of analgesia. When the stimulus from the medial side of the paw entered the spinal cord over the L4 and L5 dorsal rootlets, the reflex disseminated to the L5 through L1 segments to initiate contraction of the psoas major and iliacus muscles and hip flexion was observed. Destruction of the L6, L7, and S1 segments prevented stimulation of alpha motoneurons of the sciatic nerves. Therefore no flexion of the stifle, tarsus, or digits occurred. Bladder paralysis was due to the lesion of the sacral segments.

Differential Diagnosis. The acute onset without recognized signs of progression suggested an acute traumatic lesion or sudden vascular compromise. There was no history to support external trauma. A severe acute intervertebral disk extrusion at L4–L5 or L5–L6 could produce these signs. This is not unreasonable in a 5-year-old Great Dane. There was no associated pain on manipulation of the caudal lumbar vertebra. Sudden infarction of these spinal cord segments from fibrocartilaginous emboli would produce this sort of onset and clinical signs. The acute onset and total sudden destruction are not compatible with either intra- or extramedullary neoplasm, or inflammatory lesions or malformations.

Ancillary Studies. Plain radiographs were normal. A myelogram indicated a slight intramedullary swelling from the middle of the fourth lumbar vertebra to the L5–L6 articulation.

Cisternal cerebrospinal fluid was clear and colorless and contained normal cells and 68 mg of protein per dl.

Outcome

The ancillary studies supported an ischemic myelopathy of the involved spinal cord segments. Hemorrhage, or edema, or both may occur in this lesion and could account for the intramedullary swelling that was observed on the myelogram. Elevated CSF protein levels often occur from the tissue destruction that accompanies this lesion. It may be much more apparent if the CSF is sampled closer to the lesion. An intramedullary neoplasm would not produce such a sudden onset of signs.

No change occurred over 1 week's observation and the owner elected to have euthanasia performed on the dog.

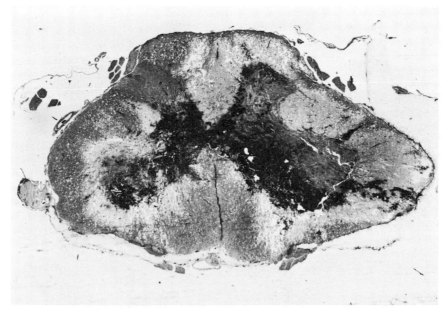

Figure 21–2. Case 2: Transverse section of L7 spinal cord segment with extensive hemorrhagic necrosis of grey matter and ischemic necrosis of white matter. Hematoxylin and eosin.

Necropsy Findings. At necropsy the lumbosacral intumescence appeared slightly swollen, and on opening the dura there was a brownish-yellow discoloration on the surface of the caudal lumbar and sacral segments, along with small hemorrhages. On transverse sections there was a gross lesion from the fifth lumbar segment caudally. In the caudal part of the L5 segment there was a mild brown discoloration of the grey matter. The L6, L7, sacral, and caudal segments were soft and most of the grey matter and a variable amount of the adjacent white matter were distinctly hemorrhagic or discolored grey. On microscopic examination this was a severe hemorrhagic necrotizing myelopathy—a hemorrhagic infarct. (Fig. 21–2). Fibrocartilaginous embolic material was present in arteries and veins. There was no apparent degeneration of associated intervertebral disks.

The final diagnosis was fibrocartilaginous embolic ischemic myelopathy bilaterally from the caudal portion of the L5 segment through the caudal segments.

Fifteen cases of this disease have been observed by the author in many different breeds at all levels of the spinal cord. Spontaneous recovery, compensation, or both occurred in seven of these cases. The prognosis for recovery is better if the paresis is incomplete and the lesion spares the grey matter of the cervical or lumbar intumescences. If recovery is going to occur there usually will be some evidence of this within 1 week after the onset of the neurologic signs. Although degenerate intervertebral disks that rupture into vertebral bodies are presumed to be the source of this fibrocartilaginous embolic material in the leptomeningeal and parenchymal vessels in man, there is no evidence yet to support this in the dog. One study revealed intervertebral disk material herniated into the ventral internal vertebral plexus and proposed this as the source of the emboli.[14]

Case 3: Case Description

Signalment. An 11-year-old female collie.

Chief Complaint. Unable to use the pelvic limbs.

History. Ten days prior to examination this dog became lame in the left thoracic limb. One week later the dog began to drag the left pelvic limb, and within 3 days it went down in the pelvic limbs and could not get up.

Examination. The dog had been recumbent for 1 day when it was examined. It lay in lateral recumbency and could not assume a sternal position. If picked up and supported by the trunk and tail, it would walk on the thoracic limbs with short, stiff strides. The pelvic limbs were paraplegic, grade 0. The trunk had to be supported or it would swing to the side, causing the dog to fall.

There were no postural reactions present in the pelvic limbs. The right thoracic limb was stiff but responded normally to hopping. The left thoracic limb was slow in hopping. Both pelvic limbs and the right thoracic limb were hypertonic on passive manipulation. The left thoracic limb was hypotonic and mild atrophy was apparent in most muscles of that limb. No pain was elicited on neck manipulation.

Patellar reflexes were both brisk (plus 3). Both triceps reflexes were brisk, as was the right biceps reflex. No biceps reflex was elicited on the left. Flexor reflexes were normal in all four limbs. There was normal pain perception from the thoracic limbs but distinct hypalgesia in the pelvic limbs. A line of hypalgesia was detected in the cranial thoracic region.

Cranial nerve examination was normal. However, the left pupil was consistently smaller than the right. The left third eyelid protruded and the eyeball seemed depressed in the orbit. The left palpebral fissure was smaller than the right.

Diagnosis

Neuroanatomic Diagnosis.   These signs indicated that there was a focal spinal cord lesion in the cranial thoracic region. A transverse lesion at the third thoracic segment would cause a spastic paraplegia and loss of trunk strength. Partial involvement of T2 and T1 on the left along with T3 would cause a complete left Horner's syndrome if the grey matter or ventral roots were affected. Partial involvement of T1 and C8 grey matter or roots on the left would account for the mild left thoracic limb signs and atrophy that were observed. The asymmetry suggested by the course described in the history, the left thoracic limb signs, and Horner's syndrome would indicate that a progressive lesion had grown on the left side, compressing the spinal cord from left to right.

Differential Diagnosis.   The localizing signs, signs of asymmetry, progressive course, and age of the dog all indicated a diagnosis of a neoplasm compressing the spinal cord. Extramedullary neoplasms are more common and cause more evidence of asymmetry than intramedullary lesions. Neurofibromas are common in the dog. They occasionally occur in the sympathetic trunk and invade the vertebral canal via the rami communicantes, spinal nerves, and roots. If the trunk was involved at the level of the cervicothoracic ganglion, the Horner's syndrome would have preceded the spinal cord signs. An epidural metastasis at this site could also explain these signs. Extramedullary neoplasms may grow slowly to substantial size with concomitant spinal cord compression without obvious neurologic signs if the displacement is slow. However, it seems that when a critical point in the ability of the compressed vasculature to supply the spinal cord is passed, then ischemia occurs and clinical signs are rapidly progressive even over a few days, as observed in this case. Anesthesia for ancillary studies of these cases may precipitate further ischemia if it decreases cardiac outflow and normal blood flow with proper oxygenation to this compromised section of the spinal cord.

The lack of history and the presence of progressive signs excluded external trauma. Intervertebral disk extrusion could not be excluded, but this is an unusual site for it to occur. The rate of speed of progression and localizing signs were unusual for an inflammatory lesion. Ischemic degeneration would be unlikely to take this long to develop if the initial onset of left thoracic limb lameness is considered pertinent.

Ancillary Studies.   Plain radiographs were normal. The dye column on the myelogram stopped abruptly over the caudal aspect of the body of T2, and, in fact, a small amount of dye escaped from the vertebral canal and was seen dorsally adjacent to the spine of T3 and ventrally along the ventral aspect of the vertebral body of T2 (Fig. 21–3).

Cisternal CSF was clear, colorless, and contained no cells and 31 mg of protein per dl. The pressure was normal.

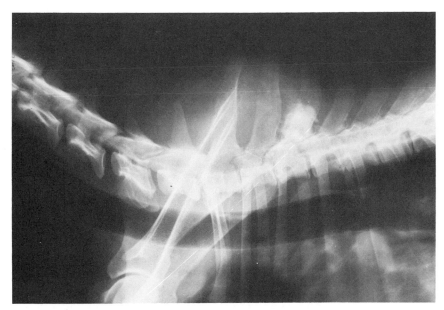

Figure 21–3. Case 3: Lumbar Skiodan myelogram demonstrating a block to normal flow at the T2–T3 articulation and leakage of dye into the epaxial area beside the spine of T3.

Outcome

The ancillary studies supported the clinical diagnosis of an extramedullary cranial thoracic space-occupying lesion. Exploratory surgery was recommended but because of the age of the dog and severity of the signs, the owner elected to have euthanasia performed.

Necropsy Findings. At necropsy a large, firm nodular mass was found located in the thorax

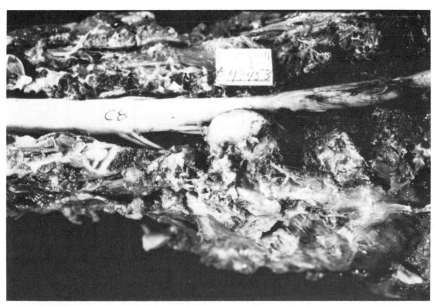

Figure 21–4. Case 3: Necropsy exposure of neurofibroma in the epidural space compressing the left first thoracic spinal roots and the second thoracic spinal cord segment.

on the left longus colli muscle involving the cranial aspect of the left thoracic sympathetic trunk and left cervicothoracic ganglion. This mass extended dorsally between the first two ribs and entered the vertebral canal through the intervertebral foramen between T1 and T2. It compressed the left first thoracic spinal nerve and expanded into the epidural space, where it compressed the spinal cord to the right (Fig. 21–4). The second and especially the third spinal cord segments were the most compressed. The third thoracic segment was reduced to less than one-half its normal width. The mass was diagnosed as a neurofibroma.

This case emphasizes the value of Horner's syndrome in the localization and interpretation of lesions. This syndrome probably occurred before the gait deficit if it can be assumed that the sympathetic trunk and cervicothoracic ganglion were affected initially before the mass expanded into the vertebral canal. Most spinal cord neoplasms are extramedullary and therefore are amenable to surgical removal if they can be diagnosed before the spinal cord compromise and the associated clinical deficit are marked.

Case 4: Case Description

Signalment.   An 8-year-old male coonhound.

Chief Complaint.   Weakness and ataxia.

History.   About 4 weeks prior to examination this dog was noticed to be slow on treeing a raccoon. This occurred 1 month after the dog had been bitten by a raccoon. The dog continued to "slow down" when hunting. Six days prior to examination it could not stand unassisted. The pelvic limbs seemed more affected than the thoracic limbs.

Examination.   The dog was reasonably alert and responsive. It could not stand unassisted. If supported it veered off to the right and walked slowly with stiff, awkward movements, tipping to the right. The limbs appeared markedly hypertonic. The animal's strength seemed good but it was very disoriented. The head was tilted to the right and the neck was curved to the right (concave right). Along with this posture the head and neck were extended more than normal. The trunk often weaved from side to side and a head tremor was evident.

On postural reaction testing there was greater deficit on the left than on the right side. Postural reactions were difficult to test because of the dog's disorientation. The deficit was especially evident in the hopping responses. The dog would fall on attempting to hemiwalk on the left side. Proprioceptive positioning was absent on the left side.

The dog preferred left lateral recumbency and with little stimulation would assume a position of opisthotonos. The thoracic limbs would extend rigidly. The pelvic limbs often were flexed.

There was marked hypertonia in the limbs. This was more apparent in the left limbs when the dog was in right lateral recumbency. No atrophy was evident. Patellar reflexes were both brisk (plus 3). Of the thoracic limb tendon reflexes only the left triceps reflex was apparent. Perineal and flexor reflexes were all present. Pain was intact and no significant hypalgesia could be detected.

On cranial nerve examination the only abnormalities were referable to the vestibular system. The head was tilted to the right. On neck extension a positional nystagmus was induced that was rotatory to the right side. On the same maneuver the right eye was noted to drift ventrally and laterally. However, in some positions of the head it was in a normal position, and both eyes abducted and adducted well on moving the head from side to side.

Diagnosis

Neuroanatomic Diagnosis.   The signs of vestibular disturbance were prominent in this case —the right head tilt, leaning and falling to the right, vestibular strabismus of the right eye, and abnormal nystagmus. With disturbance of the peripheral nerve or receptor portions of the vestibular system the abnormal nystagmus would be directed away from the side of the disturbance, which is denoted by the direction of the head and body tilt. In this case the abnormal nystagmus was directed to the same side as the head tilt, which indicates disturbance of the central portions of the vestibular system.

Even more obvious were the signs of other systems being affected that only occur in the brain stem. The marked degree of bilateral thoracic limb hypertonia, the truncal ataxia and tendency to opisthotonic posture would only be expected with central involvement of the descending upper motor neuron portion of the reticular formation, or possibly the rostral vermal portion of the cerebellum, or both. These signs suggested a tendency toward decerebration. Experimental rostral cerebellar lesions may produce opisthotonos with flexion instead of extension of the pelvic limbs. The deficit in postural reactions which was most pronounced on the left in the hopping, hemiwalking, and proprioceptive positioning responses implicated lesion of the upper motor neuron and general proprioception tracts in the brain stem.

Cerebellar, vestibular, and UMN-GP deficits could well be explained by a caudal fossa lesion. The predominantly left-sided postural reaction deficit should be explained by a predominantly left-sided pontine or medullary lesion. This reflected damage to the left rubrospinal and reticulospinal tracts which mostly cross at their origin in brain stem nuclei rostral to the lesion, and damage to the left spinocerebellar and cuneocerebellar tracts that project mostly to the cerebellum from the trunk and limbs on the same side.

The predominance of right-sided central vestibular signs may reflect a multifocal lesion in the cerebellum or medulla with disturbance of these structures on the right side, or these may be paradoxical vestibular signs from a left-sided cerebellar medullary lesion.

The remarkable preservation in strength and sensorium in the face of severe cerebellar-vestibular disturbance suggested that the lesion might be extramedullary and compressing these structures rather than intramedullary, unless it was predominantly in the cerebellar medulla.

Although the history implicated a raccoon bite 1 month prior to the onset of neurologic signs, all the signs observed were the antithesis of coonhound paralysis, which produces profound paresis with loss of tone and reflexes, and muscle atrophy. Further, the onset of this disease usually follows the incriminating bite by 7 to 10 days.

Differential Diagnosis. The signs of a progressive focal lesion in the caudal fossa of an aged dog are suggestive of a neoplastic disease.

A focal inflammatory lesion that was proliferative and space-occupying could produce these signs. Granulomatous encephalitis (reticulosis) would be the most common lesion of this type. Toxoplasmosis occasionally may produce a focal granulomatous lesion. A bacte-

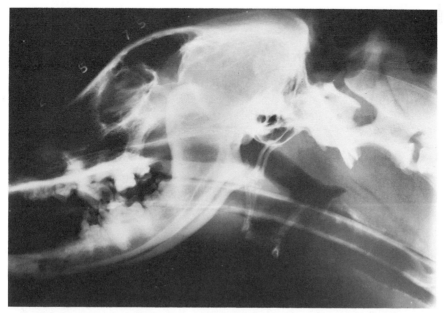

Figure 21–5. Case 4: Lateral radiograph of skull showing an oval area of opacity in the position of the tentorium cerebelli.

rial abscess, although rare in the dog, also should be considered. These are most commonly associated with the extension of a suppurative lesion in the middle and inner ear to the meninges and occur more commonly in pigs and cats. Such a focal lesion with space-occupying signs would not be compatible with canine distemper encephalitis. Cryptococcal leptomeningitis usually produces more diffuse signs, although cerebellar-vestibular signs are common.

Traumatic lesions would be excluded by the history and progressive course. Degenerative lesions are more diffuse except for vascular accidents. The latter are not associated with a progressive course. Malformations were excluded by the age of the patient.

Ancillary Studies. Two cisternal cerebrospinal fluid samples were obtained. The first was on the second day of hospitalization and contained 40 RBC and 14 mononuclear cells per cmm, and 98 mg of protein per dl. The second sample was obtained on the fourth day. The opening pressure was 265 mm CSF; closing pressure was 120 mm CSF. The fluid was clear and colorless but contained 8 RBC and 40 WBC per cmm. The latter were mostly mononuclear cells. There were 176 mg of protein per dl.

Plain radiographs revealed an oval area of abnormal mineralization on either side of the tentorium cerebelli within the cranial cavity (Fig. 21–5).

Outcome

On the second day of hospitalization all the signs were slightly worse. In addition, the left pupil was slightly larger than the right, although both still responded to light. On the third day the signs of decerebration seemed more profound. The dog could make no effort to get up. When held in a standing position the thoracic limbs extended caudally and the neck extended in an opisthotonic posture. Voluntary limb movement could still be induced. The dog would struggle to maintain some semblance of balance but to no avail.

The cerebrospinal fluid abnormality confirmed the central location of a lesion and helped to substantiate a neoplasm as the cause, as indicated by the increased intracranial pressure, the mild elevation in cells, and moderate elevation of protein. Radiography further substantiated the extramedullary neoplastic nature of the lesion. The degree of mineralization suggested an osseous neoplasm and not a meningioma.

With a poor prognosis for survival more than a few days and a guarded prognosis for surgical recovery, the owner elected euthanasia.

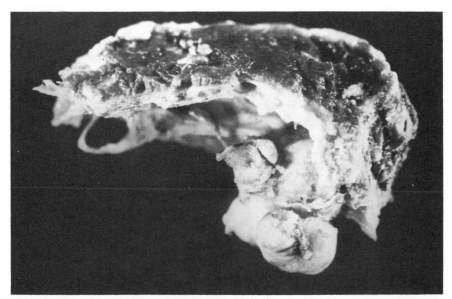

Figure 21–6. Case 4: Lateral view of the calvaria removed at necropsy with the mass at the site of the tentorium cerebelli.

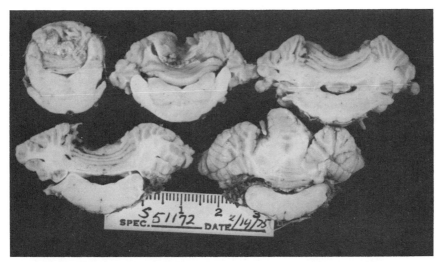

Figure 21–7. Case 4: Transverse sections at the level of the pons and medulla, showing the compression of the cerebellum and brain stem caused by the tentorial mass.

Necropsy Findings. A large, firm nodular mass completely enveloped the tentorium cerebelli and projected ventrally, severely compressing the middle and rostral portions of the cerebellar vermis and paravermal lobules (Fig. 21–6). At the most compressed portion of the cerebellum it measured only 7 mm thick (Fig. 21–7). The caudal vermis projected caudally into the foramen magnum. The entire pons and medulla were compressed by the mass growing into the cerebellum. Dorsal to the tentorium the mass compressed the medial side of each occipital lobe.

On microscopic examination the mass was an osteogenic sarcoma.

The kind of lesion and its location clearly explain the clinical signs and results of the ancillary studies. It was not possible to determine if the predominance of right-sided vestibular signs resulted from a left- or right-sided lesion. There was bilateral involvement of the vestibular portions of the cerebellum as well as the vestibular nuclei. There was no clinical evidence of visual disturbance from the mild compression of each occipital lobe.

Case 5: Case Description

Signalment. A 6-year-old spayed female Boston terrier.

Chief Complaint. Seizures.

History. Seven weeks prior to examination the first seizure was observed. Three seizures occurred over a 2-hour period, each lasting 1 to 2 minutes. It was reported that these began with the dog shaking all over, salivating, then falling on its side and they alternated between severe rigidity and shaking. The animal appeared to lose consciousness. A veterinarian had prescribed primidone therapy. A number of seizures occurred over the 7-week period, but their exact occurrence was not well documented. Seizures did occur the day before admission.

Examination. On initial examination the dog appeared to be blind. The pupils were dilated and unresponsive to light. The dog stumbled from side to side on walking.

Thorough neurologic examination the following day revealed a reasonably alert and responsive dog. The gait was essentially normal. Occasionally the right forepaw was slow to protract on turning left and would almost turn over onto its dorsal surface.

On wheelbarrowing the right thoracic limb occasionally stumbled. The hopping response was slow in the right limbs, especially the right pelvic limb. The right pelvic limb was slower to respond on walking backward with the pelvic limbs. Hemistanding was normal. Hemiwalking was slow and awkward on the right side. The proprioceptive positioning response was slow in both right limbs. Placing was normal. On extending the neck, the right thoracic limb occasionally flexed distally so that the dorsal surface was on the ground.

Muscle tone was normal. No atrophy was observed. Patellar reflexes were both brisk. Biceps and triceps reflexes were absent. Perineal and flexor reflexes were normal, as was pain perception.

On cranial nerve examination the menace response appeared to be slightly slower from the right lateral field. On walking the dog through a maze to the left no object was bumped but on walking to the right occasionally an object was hit. Pupils were normal in size and responsive to light. There was a suggestion that there was less response to mild stimulation of the nasal mucosa with a blunt instrument on the right side. The rest of the cranial nerves were normal.

Diagnosis

Neuroanatomic Diagnosis.   The clinical signs observed on the day following hospital admission all suggested a left cerebral lesion. A lesion in the centrum semiovale would interfere with ascending conscious proprioceptive neurons from the thalamus and descending upper motor neuron projections from the motor cortex, explaining the essentially normal gait but deficient contralateral postural reactions. If the lesion was confined to the sensorimotor cortex the same systems would be affected and cause the same signs. The slight right facial hypalgesia could result from a lesion in the same location affecting the general somatic afferent neuronal projection from the thalamus. Although pain perception pathways ascend bilaterally from the limbs, trunk, and face on one side, the predominance of the contralateral projection has only been detected for the face with unilateral thalamic or cerebral lesions. Involvement of the optic radiation in the left centrum semiovale would account for the observed visual deficit on the right side.

Similarly, the same systems could be affected on the left side of the diencephalon in a fairly small area. The GP and UMN systems are together in the internal capsule or could be affected separately in the ventrocaudolateral thalamic nucleus and crus cerebri, respectively. The left optic tract and left ventrocaudomedial thalamic nucleus involvement would explain the visual deficit and facial hypalgesia, respectively.

Why did the initial examination indicate blindness with dilated unresponsive pupils and a paretic-ataxic gait that were absent on the following day? These signs can be explained by a bilateral optic nerve or chiasm lesion such as occurs most commonly with optic neuritis, plus a more diffuse mild lesion, probably in the brain stem, that would cause the generalized paresis and ataxia. These lesions would be unlikely to appear suddenly and resolve in a 36- to 48-hour period. The blindness with paresis and ataxia could be a prolonged postictal depression. The dog was observed to seizure the day before admission and had been blind and ataxic since then. These signs commonly are seen for a short period of time, (usually less than 3 hours) following a seizure, and then they completely disappear. However, occasionally they last for 1 to 2 days after a seizure. The presence of dilated unresponsive pupils is unusual as a sign of postictal depression.

A third explanation is that these signs were the result of fairly severe intracranial pressure elevation associated with a mass lesion. The blindness reflected bilateral cerebral compression or edema. The dilated unresponsive pupils were due to the cerebral mass compressing the mesencephalon and ventrally located oculomotor neurons. Such lesions frequently cause pupillary dilation (general visceral efferent deficiency) without strabismus (general somatic efferent deficiency). The same brain stem compression could cause the paresis and ataxia. This is probably the best explanation in view of the results of the neurologic examination performed after these signs resolved, which indicated a primary left cerebral lesion. However, the more typical sign that results from an expanding cerebral mass is ipsilateral pupillary dilation from the asymmetric ipsilateral cerebral herniation and compression of the midbrain.

There is no obvious answer to this dilemma, except that an organic lesion involving these other structures is not compatible with the signs observed. Postictal depression or increased intracranial pressure or both may be involved.

Differential Diagnosis. Progressive seizures in an aged dog associated with interictal signs of a focal cerebral lesion are highly suggestive of a neoplasm. Brachycephalic breeds are thought to be especially prone to gliomas, which further adds to this diagnosis. A focal inflammatory lesion such as a toxoplasma granuloma, bacterial abscess, or granulomatous encephalitis (reticulosis) could produce these signs. Canine cerebral abscesses are rare. All three of these should produce abnormalities in the cerebrospinal fluid.

With no immediate or past history of trauma and the presence of progressive signs this would be unlikely. Posttraumatic seizures occasionally occur but require a history of injury associated with signs of significant intracranial injury.

Malformation at this age would be unlikely. Most degenerative disorders are diffuse and do not produce focal signs. Vascular injuries are the exception, but the signs should be sudden in onset and not progressive. Extracranial metabolic diseases are excluded because of the presence of a focal neurologic deficit. Idiopathic epilepsy would be excluded by the age of onset and the interictal neurologic abnormality.

Ancillary Studies. The CBC, BUN, serum glucose, and electrolytes were normal. The cisternal cerebrospinal fluid opening pressure was 160 mm CSF. Three cc of a clear colorless fluid were withdrawn. The closing pressure was less than 30 mm CSF. The fluid contained 4 RBC and 2 WBC per cmm, and 39 mg of protein per dl.

Plain radiographs of the skull and thorax were normal.

Outcome

Elevated CSF protein levels with normal color and cells commonly occur with intracranial neoplastic disease. Although the opening pressure was in the high normal range, the drop to below 30 after the sampling (the lowest number that can be recorded) suggested a decreased total size of the CSF-containing space. This would be more significant if only 2 cc were removed—the standard amount—and would not cause such a large drop in pressure. Ordinarily on removal of 2 cc from the cerebellomedullary cistern the closing pressure is not less than one-half of the opening pressure. If it is, this suggests a smaller total volume of CSF from a subarachnoid space compromised by a space-occupying lesion.

Plain radiographs are only helpful if a neoplastic lesion is adjacent to the skull and has eroded it, or if the neoplasm is of cartilage or bone that has mineralized. Primary and most metastatic brain neoplasms cannot be visualized. Even meningiomas that may be mineralized usually are not visualized.

For the next week of hospitalization, no seizures were observed in the animal. The dog's neurologic status remained unchanged except that the right menace deficit and facial hypalgesia no longer could be detected. All signs were referable to a left frontal lobe location.

Because of the poor prognosis for recovery and guarded prognosis if the suspected mass could be localized further by scintiscan and operated on, the owner elected euthanasia.

Necropsy Findings. The rostral pole of the left frontal lobe was distended. The cortical surface was thin and fluctuated on palpation. The affected gyri included the prorean, precruciate, rostral ectomarginal, and rostral compositus. On transverse section there was a well-demarcated mass in the center of the left frontal lobe. It was soft, grey, gelatinous, and contained numerous fluid-filled cystic spaces (Fig. 21–8). The white matter of the left parietal lobe caudal to the mass was swollen. No other lesions were observed. On microscopic examination this mass was an astrocytoma.

The necropsy confirmed a left cerebral astrocytoma as the cause of the focal neurologic signs and presumably the cause of the progressive seizures in this aged Boston terrier. This does not solve the dilemma of an exact explanation for the presenting signs that had resolved by the following day. There was no evidence at the time of necropsy of cerebral herniation, or direct compression of the optic nerves or chiasm. Postictal depression with atypical pupillary dilation remains the best explanation.

This case exemplifies the value of careful neurologic examination of the patient with seizures. Observation of interictal deficits strongly supports an organic brain lesion and would not occur in idiopathic epilepsy or most extracranial and metabolic disease.

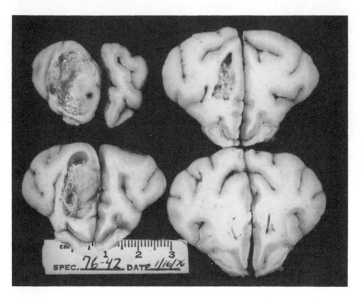

Figure 21-8. Case 5: Transverse sections of astrocytoma in left frontal lobe.

Case 6: Case Description

Signalment.   A 3-year-old female mongrel setter.

Chief Complaint.   Abnormal pelvic limb function.

History.   Five days prior to examination this dog left its home. Four days later it was found lying alongside a road unable to get up.

Examination.   On initial examination the dog was alert and responsive. It sat in sternal recumbency but refused to get up on its pelvic limbs. If assisted, thoracic limb function was normal. The right pelvic limb seemed to have normal neurologic function but the dog was reluctant to bear weight on the limb. The left pelvic limb was less functional and stood with the dorsal aspect of the paw turned over on the ground.

Tone, reflexes, and pain perception were normal in the right pelvic limb. Voluntary motion was readily induced. The left pelvic limb would flex slightly at the hip when handled, but even on noxious stimulation there was no flexion of the stifle or tarsus and no pain was perceived from the paw, leg, or caudal thigh except along the medial aspect. The patellar reflex was normal.

The tail was atonic, areflexic, and analgesic. The anus was partly dilated. Slight response to perineal stimulation occurred on the right side. Pain was perceived from the right side of the perineum and not the left. The left proximal caudal thigh region was also analgesic. The bladder was distended and had to be expressed manually.

Diagnosis

Neuroanatomic Diagnosis.   Neurologic deficit was limited to the left sciatic nerve or its roots of origin, the left sacral nerves or roots, and the caudal nerves bilaterally. The L4 and L5 roots and spinal nerves were preserved on the left because of the intact patellar reflex (femoral nerve) and intact pain sensation on the medial aspect of the limb (saphenous nerve). Hip flexion was normal because of the intact L1-L5 roots and spinal nerves to the psoas major muscle. Sensation was normal over the cranial thigh region because of the intact L4 roots and spinal nerves (lateral cutaneous femoral nerve). The deficit of the left sacral roots or nerves was reflected in the atonic, areflexic, analgesic left anus and perineum (pedundal nerve) and analgesic proximal caudal thigh area (caudal cutaneous femoral nerve). The bladder paralysis was due to bilateral pelvic nerve paralysis or bilateral sacral nerve paralysis. The total tail deficit reflected a bilateral caudal nerve lesion. The lesion must explain a left L6 through S3 spinal nerve lesion and bilateral pelvic and caudal nerve lesion.

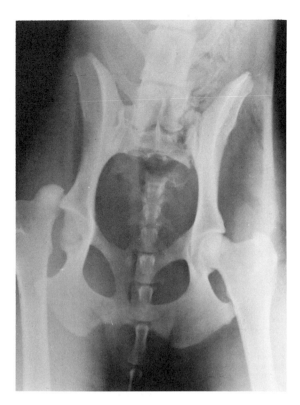

Figure 21-9. Case 6: Ventrodorsal radiograph showing right coxofemoral luxation and left fracture of sacrum with sacroiliac subluxation.

Differential Diagnosis. The presumed acute onset, along with the history of finding this dog beside the road, and the pain and abnormality palpated in the skeletal structures of the pelvic region, were highly presumptive of a traumatic lesion of external origin. The signs of neurologic deficit can be explained readily by contusion of roots and spinal branches of peripheral nerves.

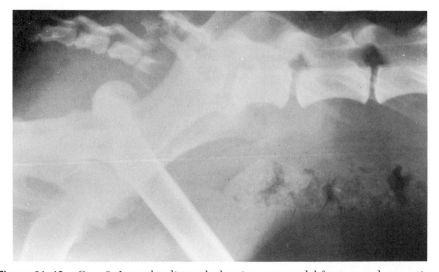

Figure 21-10. Case 6: Lateral radiograph showing sacrocaudal fracture and separation.

A sacrocaudal fracture and luxation could account for the total dysfunction of the caudal nerves. The left sciatic palsy could have occurred from fracture of the ischium with medial displacement of the cranial portion and hip, which contused the nerve as it passed distally medial to the greater trochanter of the femur. Fracture of the body of the ilium at the greater ischiatic notch with displacement of the bone fragments may have contused the sciatic nerve as it passed over this notch. Sacral fractures with sacroiliac luxation will contuse the ventral branches of L6 and L7 spinal nerves that must course caudally on the ventromedial aspect of this joint to form the sciatic nerve. The same traumatic lesion can easily contuse the sacral nerve ventral branches as they emerge from the pelvic sacral foramina.

Ancillary Studies.   Radiography revealed a craniodorsal dislocation of the right hip, a sacrocaudal fracture with ventral displacement of the caudal vertebrae, and a fracture of the sacrum at the left sacroiliac joint which was subluxed (Figs. 21–9, 21–10).

Outcome

Within a few days the dog recovered sensation in the distribution of the left sciatic nerve but motor function remained absent. Within the next 10 days the dog began to get up and walk. Neurologic function of the right pelvic limb was normal. The left pelvic limb could support weight normally (femoral nerve). The limb was advanced by hip flexion (iliopsoas muscle—lumbar nerves), but the animal walked with the stifle extended and the paw placed with its dorsal surface on the ground due to the persistent sciatic palsy. Incontinence persisted from the pelvic nerve injury. The tail remained paralyzed and analgesic.

Necropsy Findings.   After 1 month with no improvement, euthanasia was performed. At necropsy the skeletal injuries were observed that were diagnosed radiographically. The caudal nerves were torn and fibrosed at the sacrocaudal fracture. The left L7 spinal nerve ventral branch was discolored and entirely embedded in fibrous tissue ventromedial to the sacroiliac joint. A portion of the left L6 spinal nerve ventral branch was involved in the same fibrous adhesion. The ventral branches of the sacral nerves were embedded in hemorrhage and fibrous tissue. No spinal cord lesions were observed.

Case 7: Case Description

Signalment.   An 8-year-old small female mongrel.

Chief Complaint.   Head tilt.

History.   Six weeks prior to examination this dog fairly suddenly developed a mild right head tilt. This sign slowly became worse, although some days it seemed better. For the preceding week or two some difficulty in the dog's gait had been observed.

Examination.   The dog was alert and responsive. Its head was constantly tipped to the right to a marked degree. Occasionally the dog drifted to the right as it walked. Strength and general proprioception seemed normal in the gait.

On postural reaction testing there was a slight asymmetry with a slower response with the right limbs, especially the right pelvic limb. This was only observed in the hopping response. Muscle tone and all spinal reflexes were normal. No atrophy was evident. Pain perception was normal.

On cranial nerve examination there was anisocoria, with the right pupil slightly larger than the left. The pupillary light reflex responses were intact, but the right pupil never contracted as much as the left. Frequently the right eyeball assumed a ventrolateral position. However, this was not constant in all positions of the head. When the head was moved from side to side to observe vestibular nystagmus, both eyeballs were able to fully adduct and abduct. There was no spontaneous nystagmus at rest. With the head held flexed to the left a vertical to slightly rotatory left nystagmus occurred. This rotatory left nystagmus was exacerbated after the dog was rolled over once. The normal nystagmus induced by moving the head from side to side was slower than normal, especially on moving the head to the left. No other cranial nerve deficits were observed.

Diagnosis

Neuroanatomic Diagnosis. These signs, which are predominantly vestibular, indicated a lesion in the right side of the brain in the caudal fossa. The reason for locating the lesion in the central and not peripheral portion of the vestibular system is because of the postural reaction deficit. Nothing about the vestibular signs indicated a central lesion. All were compatible with a disturbance of the peripheral receptor. The only possible exception was the occasional vertical component of the abnormal nystagmus. If this were consistently only vertical, it should indicate a central lesion. A variation from vertical to rotatory has been seen in peripheral diseases. However, in peripheral disease the direction of the rotation is away from the side of the head tilt. This is determined by the direction of movement of the 12 o'clock point on the limbus of the eyeball in relation to the dog's left or right side.

Peripheral vestibular disturbances may accompany otitis media or otitis interna. The only additional neuroanatomic structures that can be affected by this disease are the facial nerve (facial paralysis), cochlear nerve (deafness), and postganglionic sympathetic nerves (Horner's syndrome). Postural reactions are not directly interfered with by vestibular system disorders. Lesions in the medulla that interfere with the upper motor neuron, or general proprioceptive system, or both cause a slowing of the postural reaction responses. A severe lesion in these tracts in the medulla causes an ipsilateral spastic hemiparesis and ataxia. A mild lesion may produce only a postural reaction deficit. A lesion in the cerebellar peduncles that disturbs the general proprioceptive system in the spinocerebellar and cuneocerebellar tracts produces an ipsilateral hemiataxia if severe or only a deficit in ipsilateral postural reactions.

The ventrolateral strabismus that was inconstant and easily elicited by head and neck extension is a common finding in the eye on the same side as the other signs of a vestibular disturbance. It results from the disturbance in normal tonic input from the vestibular system to the nuclei of the cranial nerves that innervate the extraocular muscles. To differentiate this from the strabismus of an oculomotor nerve paralysis, in the latter the strabismus is constant and the ability to adduct the eyeball is impaired.

The larger right pupil was not explained by ocular examination. It could have reflected mild oculomotor nerve compression on the floor of the cranial cavity. However, there were no associated clinical signs of increased intracranial pressure.

Differential Diagnosis. Progressive signs of a focal right cerebellomedullary lesion in an aged dog are most suggestive of a mass lesion. Neoplasia, granulomatous encephalitis, reticulosis, or abscess must be considered. This is a common clinical presentation in a dog with a papilloma or carcinoma of the choroid plexus of the fourth ventricle. The white matter of the cerebellar medulla and peduncles is the most common site affected by the inflammatory form of the reticulosis lesion. An abscess of the right cerebellomedullary angle from a similar lesion in the petrosal bone usually produces a facial paresis or paralysis along with the central vestibular signs. These are rare in dogs. The inflammatory disease caused by canine distemper, toxoplasmosis, or cryptococcosis usually produces multifocal or diffuse lesions and signs. Injury and ischemic lesions produce sudden onset of signs and nonprogression.

Ancillary Studies. Plain radiographs of the skull, including the tympanic bullae, were normal.

Cerebrospinal fluid had an opening pressure of 90 mm CSF. It was clear and colorless and contained 166 RBC and 103 WBC per cmm. All the latter were mononuclear cells. There were 286 mg of protein per dl and the closing pressure was 80 mm CSF.

Outcome

The ancillary studies supported a focal granulomatous inflammation or reticulosis as the cause of the clinical signs. Space-occupying lesions in the caudal fossa often do not elevate CSF pressure. If the meninges are involved in the reticulosis lesion it is not uncommon for the protein and leukocytes to be moderately increased, as in this case.

This is a lesion that occurs within the parenchyma and would not be amenable to surgery. It usually continues to progress in its development, although the rate may be slow.

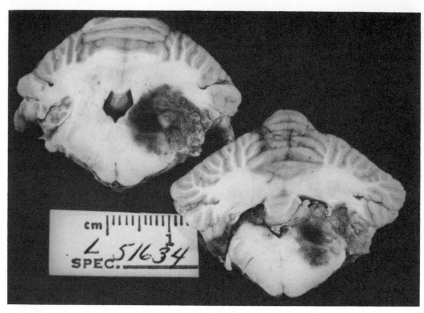

Figure 21–11. Case 7: Transverse sections of granuloma in the right side of the cerebellum and medulla.

In some instances corticosteroid therapy has been thought to slow its progression, but only temporarily. The owner elected to have euthanasia performed.

Necropsy Findings. At necropsy the area of the right choroid plexus was enlarged and a grey-brown color. On transverse section three lesions were observed. At the right cerebello-medullary angle there was a large area of brown discoloration with a whorled appearance that blended with the adjacent parenchyma (Fig. 21–11). It involved all the right cerebellar peduncles and adjacent cerebellar medulla. It extended into the adjacent medulla, where it involved the caudal cerebellar peduncle, vestibular nuclei, and the spinal tract and nucleus of the trigeminal nerve. No signs of facial hypalgesia were observed to relate to the involvement of the central projections of the trigeminal nerve. The rest of the lesion distribution explained the clinical signs observed.

Two additional smaller focal whorled brown lesions were observed. One occupied a portion of the ventral septal nuclei, caudate nucleus, rostral commissure, column of the fornix, and adjacent rostral diencephalon, all on the left side. The other was smaller and located in the right parahippocampal gyrus and adjacent hippocampus. No signs were related to these areas. The only signs that could be predicted to occur from the areas disturbed by these lesions are changes in behavior and attitude, or seizures, or both.

On microscopic examination all these lesions were diagnosed as granulomatous encephalitis. No organism was identified.

Case 8: Case Description

Signalment. A 5-year-old gelded Thoroughbred.

Chief Complaint. Muscle atrophy and weak pelvic limbs.

History. Two months prior to initial examination atrophy occurred in the horse's left masseter muscle. The onset was rapid, over a one-week period. The horse continued to race well. One week prior to examination, while the animal was being rested for a sesamoid problem, atrophy was observed in the right gluteal region and an altered gait occurred.

Examination. The gelding was alert and responsive. The pelvic limb gait was abnormal. There was a slight delay in the onset of the protraction phase of the right pelvic limb.

On the horse's turning to the left the hind quarters swayed left, and it had difficulty co-ordinating the right pelvic limb with the left. When the hindquarters were pushed to the right the right pelvic limb was slow to abduct. On backing, it was slow to retract from the supporting position. There was distinct atrophy of the right middle gluteal and tensor fascia lata muscles. Tail and anal tone and the perineal reflex were normal. No hypalgesia was detected.

The left masseter muscle was severely atrophied. The left temporal muscle was mildly atrophied. There was no lack of jaw tone or strength and no deviation was observed. The remainder of the cranial nerve examination was normal.

Diagnosis

Neuroanatomic Diagnosis. These clinical signs suggested a primary lesion of the muscles that were atrophied, a peripheral neuropathy of the left mandibular and right cranial gluteal nerves, or a multifocal lesion of the central nervous system with lesions in the left trigeminal motor nucleus in the pons and right side of the spinal cord segments L5, L6, and S1 primarily affecting the ventral grey column.

Although the right pelvic limb gait was the most abnormal, the left was not normal and the overall pelvic limb disturbance seemed greater than would be expected if the lesion was confined to the right cranial gluteal nerve or the muscles it innervates. A similar delay in the onset of protraction with forward gait and retraction with backing is seen with spinal cord lesions affecting the white matter cranial to the lumbosacral intumescence. It is not clear whether this is a sign of motor or proprioceptive deficiency. For this reason a spinal cord lesion with white matter and ventral grey column involvement from L5 to S1 was most suspect.

Peripheral neuropathy or primary myopathy with such a distribution as this has not been reported in the horse. A myopathy of the masseter muscles has been reported in debilitated young horses but the involvement is bilateral.

Differential Diagnosis. An inflammatory disease would best explain the multifocal, asymmetric, and progressive nervous system signs. The progressive signs would be untoward for a single episode of trauma, as would the lesion distribution. The repeated contusions that may occur with the cervical malarticulation in the wobbler syndrome may give progressive signs but they are fairly symmetric and reflect a cervical spinal cord location. Degenerative myeloencephalopathy produces symmetric signs of white matter disease in all four limbs and occurs in the young horse. Multifocal metastatic neoplasia is rare but conceivably could explain the asymmetry and progression of signs.

The possible inflammatory lesions that should be considered include protozoal encephalomyelitis, parasitic encephalomyelitis, multifocal bacterial encephalomyelitis, and equine polyneuritis (neuritis of the cauda equina). Although cranial nerve signs do occur in some cases of equine polyneuritis, the signs of neuritis of the cauda equina are most profound at that time, with symmetric paralysis and analgesia of the tail, anus, perineum, bladder, and rectum. Similarly, when pelvic limb gait abnormality accompanies the neuritis of the cauda equina there is usually complete loss of function of the caudal and sacral nerves, as just described. *Streptococcus equi* abscesses may occur in the central nervous system of horses and may be multiple, but usually are in the brain. The lesion distribution seen in this case would be unusual for embolic bacterial disease. Migrating larvae of *Strongylus vulgaris* may affect any part of the central nervous system. If this was the cause of the lesion in the motor nucleus of the trigeminal nerve, it would be unusual not to have more signs of damage to adjacent structures in the pons and medulla. The same could be said for embolic bacterial disease or the lesion produced by protozoa. Nevertheless, multi-focal grey matter lesions such as these in the horse are most commonly caused by an unidentified protozoan.

Although the viral-induced equine encephalitides produce an encephalomyelitis, the signs are mostly of diffuse brain disease, and focal cranial nerve nuclear signs or asymmetric lumbosacral spinal cord signs would be most unusual.

Ancillary Studies. Repeated studies of the complete blood count, electrolytes, and serum enzymes revealed no significant abnormality. Lumbosacral cerebrospinal fluid was slightly xanthochromic but contained no cells and 70 mg of protein per dl.

Muscle biopsy of the atrophied left masseter muscle revealed neurogenic atrophy. Radiographs of the temporomandibular joints were normal.

Outcome

After 3 weeks of hospitalization and treatment with corticosteroids, the pelvic limb gait abnormality was slightly worse. The horse was discharged but the rapid deterioration of pelvic limb function required rehospitalization 1 week later.

On reexamination the horse was recumbent and could not get up unassisted. It would sit like a dog on its paretic pelvic limbs when it attempted to stand. The hair was worn off the skin over the thigh muscles, where there was severe bruising from struggling to get up. When assisted its thoracic limbs functioned normally. The pelvic limbs were both paretic and ataxic and took short, weak strides. The right limb was worse and would cross under the body or overflex in an exaggerated protraction phase.

There was severe atrophy of the right middle gluteal and tensor fascia lata muscles. There was mild atrophy of the right biceps femoris, semitendinosus, semimembranosus, and gastrocnemius muscles. The right patellar reflex was brisk. The tail and anal tone were reduced, although the perineal reflex was still intact and no hypalgesia could be detected.

On cranial nerve examination the only abnormalities observed were atrophy. There was severe atrophy of the left masseter and temporal muscles and the entire right half of the tongue. Prehension and swallowing were normal except that occasionally a bolus of hay fell out of the mouth.

The neuroanatomic and differential diagnosis remained essentially the same, only now the disease involved the right hypoglossal nucleus or nerve, or both, and more of the lumbosacral intumescence. A protozoan-induced encephalomyelitis remained the most likely disease producing these signs.

Ancillary Studies.   Normal CSF usually contains less than 30 Sigma Frankel (SF) units of glutamic oxalacetic transaminase. A CBC performed on two occasions revealed a leukocytosis with an absolute neutrophilia. Cisternal cerebrospinal fluid was slightly xanthochromic and contained 29 RBC and no WBC per cmm, 29 mg of protein per dl, 55 SF units of glutamic oxalacetic transaminase, and no creatine phosphokinase. Lumbosacral CSF was xanthochromic and contained 24 RBC and 31 mononuclear cells per cmm and 166 mg of protein per dl, 87 SF units of glutamic oxalacetic transaminase, and 2 international units of creatine phosphokinase.

Because of the progressive signs, and the horse's inability to get up, the owner elected euthanasia.

Necropsy Findings.   At necropsy lesions were confined to the nervous system. On transverse section of the lumbosacral intumescence there were bilateral discolorations and softening from L5 through S2 (Fig. 21–12). The softening was more prominent on the left side. These lesions involved the lateral funiculi and adjacent ventral grey columns. The associated ventral rootlets from L5 through S2 showed a brown discoloration. On microscopic examination this consisted of a severe necrotizing nonsuppurative inflammation of grey and white matter with some hemorrhage. Protozoal organisms were present in the lesion (Fig. 21–13). The lesion in the right ventral grey column was more chronic and correlated with the chronic atrophy of the right middle gluteal and tensor fascia lata muscles. In this lesion the neuronal cell bodies were absent and were replaced by numerous hypertrophied astrocytes.

The right hypoglossal nerve was discolored grey. On transverse sections there was a reddish-brown discoloration in the medulla limited to the site of the right hypoglossal nucleus. On microscopic examination there was degeneration of myelin and axons in the right hypoglossal nerve and the nucleus was entirely devoid of neurons and filled with numerous hypertrophied astrocytes. The same microscopic lesion was found in the pons limited to the motor nucleus of the left trigeminal nerve. A group of protozoal organisms was found adjacent to the hypoglossal nuclear lesion. No other lesions were present in the brain.

The cranial nerve nuclear lesion was presumed to be related to the protozoal agent. In other cases the same lesion has been accompanied by inflammation. Possibly the protozoa

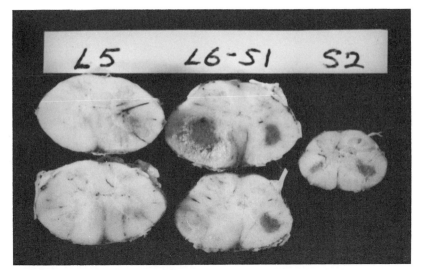

Figure 21–12. Case 8: Transverse sections of the necrotizing inflammatory spinal cord lesion in the lumbosacral intumescence.

gain entry to the central nervous system from muscle over its motoneurons and destroy the cell bodies of these motoneurons.

The active inflammatory lesion in the spinal cord that was presumed to be related to the protozoal organisms that were present previously has been seen confined to the medulla, cerebellum, or cerebrum of horses with signs directly related to the extensive area of destruction that occurs in this disease.

Even with the lack of cranial nerve signs, the signs that related to the spinal cord involvement in this case are characteristic of this protozoal disease in the horse. The progressive course, asymmetric signs, signs of grey matter involvement, and abnormal cerebrospinal fluid suggest this diagnosis over the others discussed.

Although this protozoan has many structural characteristics of *Toxoplasma gondii* and

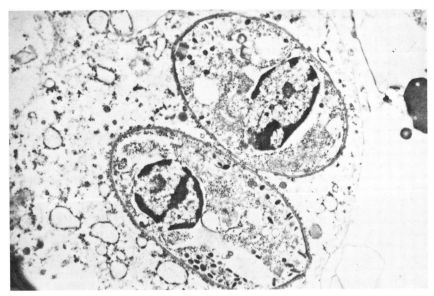

Figure 21–13. Case 8: Electron photomicrograph of two protozoa in cytoplasm of a macrophage in the spinal cord lesion.

belongs in the same subphylum, Apicomplexa, it has some different features. On rare occasion this parasite occurs in neuronal cell body cytoplasm and often a number of organisms appear arranged like a rosette. These features have not been reported in toxoplasmosis. Histochemical studies also have shown differences. Horses with this disease often have no antibody against *Toxoplasma gondii.*

In a retrospective study of equine spinal cord disease at the New York State College of Veterinary Medicine, it was found that this disease predominated in standardbreds from 1 to 3 years of age. It has been observed in most all breeds from 1 to 10 years of age and at all times of the year, but especially in the warmer months. The exact identity and life cycle of this protozoan remain to be determined.

Case 9: Case Description

Signalment.   A 10-month-old female German shepherd.

Chief Complaint.   Weak, incoordinated pelvic limbs.

History.   The signs of pelvic limb abnormality began fairly suddenly 1 week prior to examination. There was no opportunity for external injury. The signs of pelvic limb weakness and incoordination progressed during the week before examination.

The only other previous medical illness occurred two months before when the dog had diarrhea for a few days. This responded to antibacterial therapy.

The dog had received canine distemper vaccine as a puppy. The age of the dog when vaccinated and the number of vaccinations had not been recorded.

Examination.   The dog was alert and responsive and showed a grade 1 paraparesis and ataxia. It was unable to get up on its pelvic limbs unassisted. If helped by holding the base of the tail both limbs moved voluntarily, but with little effect on support or locomotion. The right pelvic limb moved slightly more than the left. There were no responses of either limb to postural reaction testing. Thoracic limb gait and response to postural reaction testing were normal.

Pelvic limb tone was normal. Both patellar reflexes were slightly brisk. Perineal and pelvic limb flexor reflexes were normal. Hypalgesia was evident in both pelvic limbs, perineum, tail, and trunk caudal to the thoracolumbar junction.

Cranial nerve examination was normal.

Diagnosis

Neuroanatomic Diagnosis.   These signs of severe UMN paresis and GP ataxia of the pelvic limbs could be caused by a focal or diffuse white matter lesion caudal to T3. The normal or hyperactive pelvic limb reflexes suggested that the lesion was cranial to the L4 segment. The stability of the trunk shown when the dog was walked supported by the tail suggested a lesion caudal to the midthoracic segments. The line of hypalgesia suggested a lesion near the thoracolumbar junction. There were no signs that could not be explained by a focal lesion at this site.

Differential Diagnosis.   Progressive spinal cord disease in young dogs of less than 1 year most commonly is caused by canine distemper myelitis. Usually there is some evidence of the multifocal nature of that disease, such as mild thoracic limb signs, or cerebellar-vestibular signs, or both, in addition to the severe paraparesis. Cerebrospinal fluid is often abnormal with a mild elevation of protein and occasionally a pleocytosis.

Although spinal cord neoplasms usually are not considered in the young animal, there is one that has a predilection for young dogs and especially German shepherds. A neuroepithelioma has been observed in 7 dogs between the ages of 6 months and 3 years and 2 months. Four were German shepherds. All occurred in an intradural extramedullary position at a site between the T10 and L1 spinal cord segments. Myelography is required to confirm this diagnosis.

Occasionally a multiple cartilaginous exostosis that involves a vertebra grows into the vertebral canal and compresses the spinal cord. This occurs in young dogs less than 1 year, but readily can be palpated in the long bones and ribs. The vertebral lesions can be observed on radiographs.

Similar signs are seen in older German shepherds with degenerative myelopathy. This rarely is seen before 4 or 5 years of age, and is a slow, insidiously progressive disease that takes months to reach the stage of paraparesis and ataxia manifested by this dog.

Intervertebral disk extrusions produce similar signs; however, they are rarely seen before 4 or 5 years of age in breeds such as the German shepherd and are rare before 18 months in the chondrodystrophic breeds.

Thoracolumbar vertebral malformations often produce signs similar to these in dogs less than 1 year of age. Usually the malformation can be palpated but it can always be observed on radiographs.

Osteomyelitis with spinal cord compression causes severe pain and usually a leukocytosis and fever. It also can be observed on radiographs.

Although paraparesis and ataxia may reflect the onset of an inherited metabolic degeneration of white or grey matter in young dogs, as the lesion progresses the signs reflect the diffuse involvement of the spinal cord and brain. There has been no such lesion reported in German shepherds.

There was no history of trauma, and the progression of signs did not agree with this diagnosis.

Ancillary Studies. The complete blood count was normal. Cerebrospinal fluid pressure was 110 mm CSF and contained 0 RBC and 1 WBC per cmm, and 18 mg of protein per dl. Plain radiographs were normal.

Outcome

The dog was treated with corticosteroids for a 6-day period. At the end of this period the dog was much improved and walked unassisted with a grade 3 to 4 paraparesis and ataxia. The pelvic limbs were partly flexed on standing and walking, and the left hind paw was frequently dragged on protraction.

The dog was discharged. Three weeks later it returned because the signs had regressed to those observed at the initial examination—a severe grade 1 paraparesis and pelvic limb

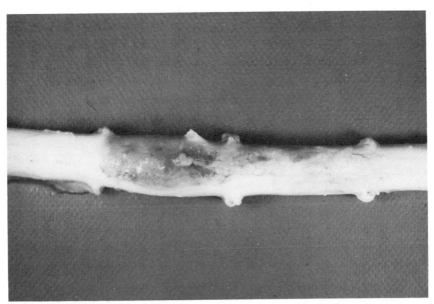

Figure 21–14. Case 9: Intradural spinal cord neoplasm located between the spinal roots of segments T12 and T13 on the left side.

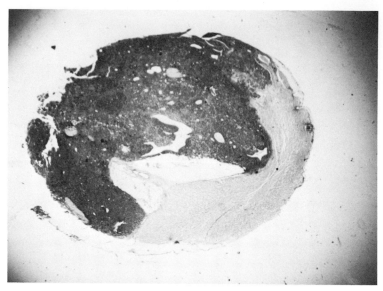

Figure 21–15. Case 9: Transverse section of intradural-extramedullary spinal cord neoplasm at the T12 segment. Hematoxylin and eosin.

ataxia. There was still a line of hypalgesia at the thoracolumbar junction. The degree of hypalgesia was worse.

A second cerebrospinal fluid examination revealed 8 RBC and 0 WBC per cmm, and 13 mg of protein per dl.

Because of the severity of the signs and poor prognosis, euthanasia was requested.

Necropsy Findings. At gross necropsy a red-colored swelling was present in an intra-dural location, mostly on the left side of the T12 spinal cord segment (Fig. 21–14). It meas-ured 15 mm long × 6 mm wide. At its widest point it compressed the spinal cord to a 1 mm-thick band of tissue curved over the right side of the intradural, extramedullary mass (Fig. 21–15). Nerve rootlets coursed through the mass and it was not attached to the dura.

On microscopic examination the mass was extremely cellular, with minimal supporting tissue. The neoplastic cells mostly appeared to be epithelial cells arranged at random, in sheets or around an oval or elongate lumen. It was diagnosed as a neuroepithelioma.

This was one of the first of these neoplasms observed. In retrospect a myelogram should have been done to confirm the diagnosis and locate the lesion for surgical removal. Of the seven cases observed one was surgically removed from an Old English sheepdog. The dog's clinical signs improved and have not regressed over an 18-month period.

During the course of progressive spinal cord signs from compression by a neoplasm, intervertebral disk, or malformed vertebrae it is not uncommon for brief periods of clinical improvement to occur. These often follow corticosteroid therapy, as was observed in this patient in this report.

Case 10: Case Description

Signalment. A 10-month-old female Arabian horse.

Chief Complaint. Incoordination.

History. At 3 to 4 weeks of age this filly was noticed to stumble occasionally and even fall when running in a paddock. The pelvic limbs splayed out at times. There was no history of any difficulty at birth. These signs of a gait abnormality slowly worsened. They were more noticeable in the pelvic limbs, the hooves of which sometimes were dragged on their dor-sal surface.

Examination. This filly was alert and responsive but had a remarkably abnormal gait with paresis and ataxia in all four limbs. The abnormal signs were symmetric in the thoracic and pelvic limbs but were worse in the pelvic limbs.

The filly walked with basewide pelvic limbs that had a longer stride than normal, causing the animal to sway from one side to the other. Occasionally the hooves were dragged on their dorsal surface at the onset of the protraction phase of the stride. On turns the hindquarters swayed to the side. The outside pelvic limb often was abducted excessively during protraction. The thoracic limbs appeared to be hypertonic and spastic, as manifested by a short-strided gait with limited motion of the joints. Occasionally the dorsal surface of the hooves scuffed at the onset of protraction.

Turning the filly in a tight circle exaggerated the ataxia. The pelvic limb on the outside of the turn overflexed or abducted excessively during protraction. The pelvic limb on the inside of the circle occasionally was slow to begin protraction and would remain in one position on the ground, being used as a support for the animal to pivot around. When it did protract it was ataxic and sometimes stepped on the opposite hoof. The thoracic limbs only occasionally were slow to begin protraction or stepped on each other as the animal turned.

Gentle pulling of the filly by the tail to the side as it walked, the sway response, caused it to stumble. There was much less resistance than normal to this tail pressure. Finger pressure applied to the withers or loin caused the filly to sink and almost collapse on the ground.

When allowed to run free in a paddock, the filly showed less gait deficit as it ran in a straight line but remarkable ataxia and some paresis when forced to turn quickly at the end of the paddock.

Muscle tone and size appeared to be normal. The perineal and tail tone and reflexes were normal. No hypalgesia could be detected. Cervical vertebral palpation and manipulation were normal. No abnormal pain was elicited.

Cranial nerve examination was normal.

Diagnosis

Neuroanatomic Diagnosis. The clinical signs of spastic paresis and ataxia reflect a deficit in function of the upper motor neuron and general proprioceptive systems, respectively. The symmetry of signs and abnormality of all four limbs indicate a focal cervical or diffuse spinal cord white matter lesion.

Differential Diagnosis. A diffuse degenerative myeloencephalopathy occurs in young horses of many breeds and causes slowly progressive signs. The onset is prior to 2 years and often prior to 6 months. The signs reflect the diffuse degeneration of neurons in all funiculi. It predominates in the thoracic spinal cord and in the spinocerebellar tracts. This was considered the most likely presumptive diagnosis for this case.

An atlanto-occipital malformation occurs in Arabian horses and causes cranial cervical spinal cord compression that produces signs at birth or usually by a few months of age. The signs are often quite severe. This malformation can be detected by the abnormal posture of the neck with limited flexion of the atlanto-occipital joint. This immobility, as well as the abnormal vertebra, can be palpated. Radiography will confirm the diagnosis.

The cervical vertebral malarticulation-malformation that is the cause of cervical spinal cord compression referred to as the wobbler syndrome can produce these signs. It usually does not produce signs before 6 months of age and would not be expected to produce signs before 1 month of age, as in this patient. Physical and neurologic examination cannot differentiate this disease from degenerative myeloencephalopathy. Radiographic study with careful measurement of the cranial and caudal orifices of each vertebral foramen may reveal the malformation in this wobbler syndrome.

Spinal cord compression from an epidural abscess with or without osteomyelitis is uncommon in the horse. The prolonged course and the absence of other signs of infection and pain on cervical vertebral manipulation would not suggest this diagnosis.

The early age of onset and the long, slowly progressive course would not be expected from the various equine spinal cord inflammatory diseases. Protozoal myelitis is the most common cause of a focal, segmental, cervical spinal cord lesion of an inflammatory nature. It is rare in horses under 1 year of age and usually produces more rapidly progressive signs, although some have been observed to remain unchanged over fairly long periods of time. There was no asymmetry of signs or focal areas of hypalgesia, reflex loss, or atrophy to suggest this diagnosis. Equine herpesvirus type I (rhinopneumonitis), encephalomyelopathy, and vasculitis can produce similar signs owing to the diffuse nature of the spinal cord ischemic leukomyelopathy. However, the signs are always sudden in onset and not progressive, as in this case. *Streptococcus equi* produces parenchymal abscesses in the brain of horses but rarely in the spinal cord. Such a lesion in the spinal cord would most likely produce more severe or asymmetric signs. Similarly, parasitic myelitis would be expected to produce more asymmetric signs and either no progression following one excursion through the parenchyma or more rapid progression from subsequent migration than was observed here.

The slow onset and progression of signs would not be compatible with a traumatic lesion of external origin. The short period of normal posture and gait and the slowly progressive signs would not occur with a spinal cord malformation.

Ancillary Studies. Plain radiographs of the cervical vertebrae from full extension to full flexion were normal. A cervical venogram following the introduction of radiopaque dye into the marrow of the body of the axis revealed no obstruction to flow in the vertebral ventral internal venous plexus.

Lumbosacral and cisternal cerebrospinal fluids were normal.

Prior to necropsy a myelogram was made following the introduction of sodium iodide into the cerebellomedullary cistern. Although with the neck in full flexion there was interruption but not obstruction to the flow in the ventral aspect of the subarachnoid space over the craniodorsal aspects of each vertebral body, normal flow occcured along the dorsal aspect of the spinal cord. This is a normal phenomenon in the horse.

Outcome

Because of the slowly progressive signs and poor prognosis for normal use of this animal, the owner requested euthanasia.

Necropsy Findings. No gross lesions were apparent in the central nervous system. When the cervical vertebrae were disarticulated no compression of the spinal cord was apparent when it was observed through the interarcuate space as each vertebral articulation was

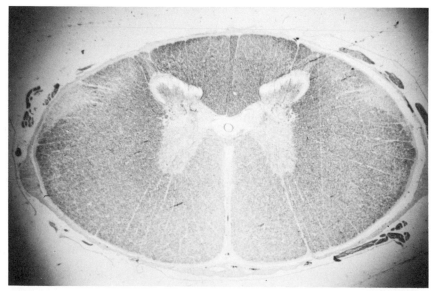

Figure 21–16. Case 10: Transverse section of spinal cord at the T15 segment. Note severity of myelin degeneration in spinocerebellar tracts (dorsolateral funiculi) and in ventral funiculi. Luxol fast blue and cresyl echt violet.

flexed and extended. There were no significant abnormalities in the disarticulated cervical vertebrae.

On microscopic examination there was a diffuse degenerative lesion in the central nervous system that was most apparent in the spinal cord white matter. Myelin degeneration was apparent in all spinal cord segments. This lesion predominated in the lateral and ventral funiculi of the thoracic spinal cord. The spinocerebellar tracts were the most completely involved (Fig. 21–16). Astrocytosis accompanied this lesion. There was axonal degeneration scattered through the white and grey matter of almost all segments, but it was especially pronounced in the nuclei of the dorsal spinocerebellar tracts. It also occurred in various nuclear areas in the brain stem, especially the caudal medullary proprioceptive nuclei.

These lesions are compatible with the diagnosis of degenerative myeloencephalopathy. This disease has been reported in horses and zebras. One study of a closely related group of zebras suggested a genetic basis for this disease. The affected horses have included 13 males, nine females, and many breeds: seven Arabians, five quarter horses, four thoroughbreds, two Morgans, one standardbred, one Appaloosa, and two mixed breeds. The mean onset of signs was 6 months, with a range of from near birth to 24 months. There was a chronic progression of signs from the time of onset in most horses. The disease is presumed to be a form of progressive neuronal degeneration. A nutritional pathogenesis is being investigated.

Case 11: Case Description

Signalment.   A 7-year-old female domestic cat.

Chief Complaint.   Seizures, behavioral change.

History.   The cat experienced a sudden onset of depression, lack of normal responsiveness to its owners, and episodes of jerky movements in the face and left thoracic limb. The following day it was presented to a veterinarian who observed two of the episodes and described the cat as turning its head with jerky shaking movements to the left, and extending the left thoracic limb caudally along the trunk in a series of clonic movements. Similar clonic movements occurred in the left pelvic limb. These were accompanied by facial muscle twitching, excessive salivation, and pupillary dilation. They each lasted about 1 minute, after which the cat seemed to act normally except for expressing resentment at being handled.

The seizures were treated with phenobarbital and thiamine. No more occurred over the next 2 days, and the cat was discharged.

Two weeks later the cat was returned because of a persistent aggressive behavior that made it unmanageable and no longer compatible as a pet.

Examination.   The cat was alert and responsive and well oriented to its environment. It resented prolonged handling and would growl and strike without provocation. No seizures or circling was observed.

The gait was normal, but a mild postural reaction deficit occurred on the left side. The left pelvic limb did not respond as readily as the right with flexion when the cat was backed up in the extensor thrust position. Hopping was also slower in the left pelvic limb. Hopping on each thoracic limb showed only an equivocal deficit in the left thoracic limb, but when the animal was walked forward only on the thoracic limbs (wheelbarrowing) with the neck extended, the left thoracic limb was slower and often adducted and brushed the medial side of the right limb. Normal tone and mass were determined on passive manipulation and palpation of the limb. Patellar and flexor reflexes were normal, as was pain perception. No asymmetry was detected.

There was a persistent menace deficit in the left lateral visual field of the left eyeball. Pupillary responses to light were normal. The remaining cranial nerve functions were normal.

Diagnosis

Neuroanatomic Diagnosis.   These signs are compatible with a right cerebral lesion. The partial seizure described consistently on the left side of the trunk and left limbs reflects a seizure focus in the contralateral motor cortex. Disturbance of the function of this right sensorimotor cortex or its afferent and efferent processes in the internal capsule does not affect the gait but interferes with the contralateral postural reactions, as seen in this case. The menace deficit in the left side of the visual field of the left eye with normal pupillary responses to light can be explained by a lesion in the right optic tract, lateral geniculate nucleus, optic radiation, or visual cortex. The latter two would be affected by a right cerebral lesion.

Differential Diagnosis.   The most common cause of an acute onset of predominantly unilateral cerebral signs in a cat, followed by partial resolution and often leaving a persistent change in behavior, is an ischemic encephalopathy—cerebral infarction—due to vascular compromise of unknown origin.

External injury could produce similar signs. Accurate documentation of the history should contribute to this diagnosis. Careful observation and palpation of the surface of the head, including the conjunctival surfaces, may show evidence of external injury. Usually following external trauma the cat initially has more severe signs of cerebral disturbance and is slower to resolve than following the cerebral infarction syndrome. Radiography may reveal evidence of an external injury.

One of the most common causes of seizures in cats is thiamine deficiency secondary to prolonged anorexia or all-fish diets with significant thiaminase content. Seizures usually are generalized and often grand mal. Ataxia and pupillary dilation may be observed on interictal examination, but not the entirely unilateral deficits observed in this case. The lesion is a diffuse metabolic encephalopathy that ultimately results in a bilateral degenerative lesion in the brain stem. The lack of appropriate history and the presence of focal, lateralizing cerebral signs in this cat would not warrant this diagnosis.

Of the various inflammatory diseases that affect the brain of the cat, a toxoplasma granuloma or bacterial abscess in one cerebrum would best comply with the focal signs observed. In either case the acute onset followed by partial resolution of signs would be unlikely. The agent of feline infectious peritonitis and *Cryptococcus neoformans* produces diffuse meningitis or ependymitis, or both, and diffuse, less localizing signs. Usually if the signs of these diseases reflect a focal area of involvement, it is referable to the caudal fossa and cerebellomedullary regions, and not the cerebrum. Cerebrospinal fluid should reflect the nature of these inflammatory diseases.

Meningiomas and gliomas occasionally occur in older cats and could produce these focal signs, but the sudden onset and nonprogression of the clinical disorder would be unlikely.

Similarly, the acute onset and lack of progression, as well as the age of onset, would eliminate brain malformation or the degenerative diseases caused by the inborn errors of metabolism. Signs of a unilateral cerebral malformation would be present at birth, or if seizures were the first indication of this lesion they would be expected to occur before a year of age. The feline leukodystrophies and lipodystrophies that have been described have produced signs in young cats less than 6 months old. Although toxic encephalopathy from such chemicals as lead, ethylene glycol, organophosphates, or chlorinated hydrocarbons may produce a sudden onset of seizures, residual signs of a unilateral cerebral lesion or the spontaneous resolution of signs would not be expected.

Ancillary Studies.   Radiographs of the skull were normal. Cisternal cerebrospinal fluid contained 1634 RBC per cmm without crenation or xanthochromia, 9 mononuclear cells per cmm, and 18 mg per dl of protein. Tests for feline leukemia virus were negative.

Outcome

The cerebrospinal fluid abnormality was consistent with an ischemic lesion and the inflammatory response to the tissue damage. The red bood cells presumably resulted from the procedure for obtaining the fluid. Erythrocytes from previous hemorrhage usually are crenated and the fluid may be xanthochromic after the cells are removed by centrifugation. Usually the protein also is mildly elevated following the parenchymal destruction that occurs in cerebral infarction.

Because this cat's change in behavior made it incompatible as a pet, euthanasia was requested.

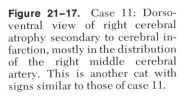

Figure 21–17. Case 11: Dorso-ventral view of right cerebral atrophy secondary to cerebral infarction, mostly in the distribution of the right middle cerebral artery. This is another cat with signs similar to those of case 11.

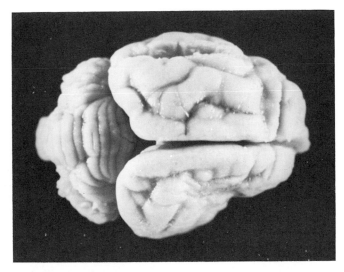

Necropsy Findings. The only gross lesion observed on removal of the brain was a yellow discoloration and softness of the right temporal lobe. On palpation of the transverse sections of the formalin-fixed brain there was softening evident in both pyriform lobes and the adjacent parahippocampal gyri.

Microscopic examination revealed an extensive encephalopathy bilaterally in the parahippocampal gyri and the hippocampus. On the right side the lesion extended into the cerebral cortex of the gyri of the frontal and parietal lobes located laterally. The lesion consisted of parenchymal degeneration with extensive astrocyte proliferation and hypertrophy. These hyperplastic gemistocytes completely filled areas of cortex, with varying degrees of neuron loss and degeneration. Occasionally small areas of cavitation occurred in the hippocampus and parahippocampal gyrus. Small blood vessels were prominent in these areas. A few vessels in the lesion and in the leptomeninges were surrounded by lymphocytes. No primary vessel lesion was observed. These lesions are compatible with an ischemic pathogenesis. The degenerate areas mostly are supplied by branches of the middle cerebral arteries.

These lesions confirmed the diagnosis of feline ischemic encephalopathy or cerebral infarction. The disease has been observed in adult cats of all breeds and ages at all times of the year but primarily in the late summer. Although the cerebral lesion is ischemic in nature, the cause of the ischemia is not known. Vascular lesions have only been observed in four of 27 necropsies. Viral isolation procedures on tissue culture and electron microscopy on brain tissue have not revealed any agent.

Although the lesion is usually most profound in the distribution of one middle cerebral artery (Fig. 21–17), it is not limited to the area of brain supplied by that vessel. Although the signs reflect a unilateral cerebral lesion, the lesions are often bilateral but worse in one cerebrum. In addition, occasionally lesions occur in the brain stem but to a lesser extent and usually without associated clinical signs.

The prognosis for life in these cats is usually good. Only one death has been observed associated with this lesion, and that occurred within the first 24 hours of recognized signs. Residual signs that may affect the animal's compatibility as a companion include propulsive pacing or circling, seizures, and a change in behavior to aggressiveness.

Case 12: Case Description

Signalment. An 8-month-old female Cairn terrier.

Chief Complaint. Depression and ataxia.

History. At 6 months of age this dog was presented to a veterinarian for lethargy, frequent urination, increased water consumption, and carrying the tail flexed between the pelvic limbs. A granular yellow discharge was noted at the vulva. The dog was treated for cystitis and these signs resolved after 4 days of hospitalization. The vaccination status was considered adequate.

At 8 months old the animal was reexamined for depression, circling, standing with its head pressed against the wall, and abnormal use of the pelvic limbs that had been present for 24 hours. The owner recalled that there were other brief periods when the dog stood quietly staring off into space, seemingly oblivious of the environment.

After 24 hours of hospitalization and treatment with fluids, antibiotics, and steroids the dog's behavior was normal.

Laboratory tests performed at this time revealed a leukocytosis (23,800 per cmm) and neutrophilia (19,278 per cmm). The total plasma protein was low at 4.5 gm per dl (normal: 6.0–7.8). The blood urea nitrogen was slightly low at 9 mg per dl (normal: 10–20). The serum glutamic pyruvate transaminase was significantly elevated at 192 Sigma-Frankel units (normal: < 50), as was the serum alkaline phosphatase at 263 international units (normal: < 30). Subsequently, during similar episodes of depression the animal responded to removal of food.

Examination. The dog was small for its breed and age. No physical or neurologic abnormalities were observed.

Diagnosis

Neuroanatomic Diagnosis. Although no signs were observed during the examination, the signs described in the history were suggestive of a diffuse neurologic disorder with cerebral involvement. The depression and change in behavior reflected decreased cerebrocortical or ascending reticular activating system function and limbic system disturbance. The pelvic limb ataxia may reflect mild diffuse brain stem dysfunction, or spinal cord dysfunction, or both.

Differential Diagnosis. Neurologic abnormalities that consist of a transient disturbance of brain function that ceases spontaneously but has a tendency to recur are suggestive of a metabolic abnormality.

Major structural brain lesions rarely produce the signs described with periods of complete recovery, except for seizures. For this reason it would be unlikely that these signs were due to lesions caused by inflammation, injury, malformation, or neoplasia. Minor structural lesions in an area of the brain that does not produce signs of neurologic deficit may initiate seizures, but examination in the interictal period is normal.

Lead poisoning, which is more common in the young dog and may produce signs of gastrointestinal disturbance along with neurologic signs, usually causes seizures. If the encephalopathy is severe, persistent signs of structural disease may occur and produce lethargy, visual deficits, and ataxia. However, these would not be expected to resolve spontaneously.

Extracranial diseases that may produce metabolic encephalopathy include pancreatic beta cell neoplasms or metabolic abnormalities in glycogenolysis that produce hypoglycemia, hepatic disease leading to significant hyperammonemia, renal disease with chronic uremia, and cardiovascular disease that causes cerebral hypoxia.

Beta cell pancreatic neoplasms occur in older dogs and would be unlikely at this age. The metabolic aberration in glycogenolysis that is found in toy breeds usually occurs around 3 months of age. Chronic uremia with encephalopathy at this age could result from renal hypoplasia. The most common cardiovascular diseases that result in decreased cardiac output and cerebral hypoxia are arrhythmias such as ventricular tachycardia and atrial fibrillation, severe heart block, or rarely, dirofilariasis. Hepatic encephalopathy at this age is most commonly due to an abnormal portacaval anastomosis.

Ancillary Studies. Clinical laboratory studies revealed a mild leukocytosis (18, 500 per cmm) with neutrophilia (13, 300 per cmm), monocytosis (2, 600 per cmm), and band cells (600 per cmm). A mild anemia was present (PCV 33; 1.1 per cent reticulocytes). Total serum protein was reduced to 3.2 gm per dl (normal: 5.0–6.7) with both albumin and globulin less than normal: albumin 1.7 gm per dl (normal: 2.6–3.4); globulin 1.5 gm per dl (normal: 2.0–3.9). Liver enzymes were elevated in the serum: alkaline phosphatase 98 international units ($<$ 30), glutamic pyruvate transaminase 220 Sigma-Frankel units ($<$ 50). Bromsulphalein was retained longer than normal — 19.5 per cent at 30 minutes ($<$ 5). Blood urea nitrogen was normal (13 mg per dl) on one occasion and below normal (5 mg per dl) on another (normal: 10–20 mg per dl). Blood glucose levels varied excessively. On three occasions levels were determined at 201, 56, and 53 mg per dl (normal: 70–110). Urate crystals were found in the urine on one of five urinalyses. Fasting and 2-hour postprandial serum ammonia values were significantly elevated. The patient's levels were 0.27 and 0.24 micromoles per L respectively, while in the control animal they were .02 and .02 micromoles per L.

Plain radiographs revealed a small liver shadow. This was confirmed at laparotomy when a catheter was placed in an intestinal vein of the jejunum. A portogram showed simultaneous opacification of the caudal vena cava and portal vein and liver. A single vessel looped ventrally and then dorsally as it coursed from the portal vein to the caudal vena cava caudal at the diaphragm. This anastomosis left the portal vein just caudal to its right hepatic branch. This represents a reversal of flow through the gastrosplenic and left gastric vein, entering the caudal vena cava at the diaphragm.

Outcome

The ancillary studies confirmed the diagnosis of hepatic encephalopathy due to portacaval shunt. Even though the anastomosis consisted of a single vessel that was accessible to ligation, previous experience has shown that this usually results in death, presumably from portal hypertension.

Conservative therapy was instituted, which consisted of a low protein, high carbohydrate diet that was fed in small amounts at short intervals. An intestinal antibiotic (neomycin sulfate) also was administered for varying periods of time. This dog was alive at 2 years of age, functioning well as a pet 15 months after this diagnosis.

Although this disease more commonly is seen in the young dog, occasionally it has not

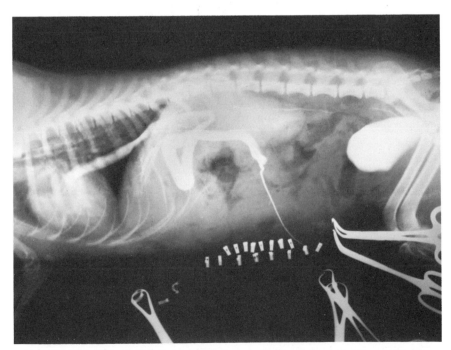

Figure 21–18. Case 12: Portagram following celiotomy and cannulation of a jejunal vein. Two seconds following injection, dye is apparent in the portal vein, its branches in the atrophic liver, a large single portacaval shunt caudal to the liver, and the caudal vena cava. Dye in the kidneys, ureters, and bladder is from a previous injection.

been diagnosed in a dog until 6 years of age. Although the disease has been reported in numerous breeds, there is some indication that it may be familial in miniature schnauzers. The clinical signs can be extremely variable and reflect involvement of one or more systems including hepatic, gastrointestinal, renal, and nervous systems. Stunting and weight loss are common. Clinical complaints often include anorexia, vomiting, polyuria, polydypsia, depression, weakness, ataxia, seizures, pacing, disorientation and staring, head pressing, blindness, stupor, and coma.

Hepatic encephalopathy also has been reported associated with urea cycle enzyme deficiencies and advanced liver disease that includes chronic cirrhosis and diffuse neoplastic infiltration.

REFERENCES

1. Barrett, R. E.: Canine hepatic encephalopathy. *In* Kirk, R. W., ed., Current Veterinary Therapy, VI, in preparation.
2. Barrett, R. E., de Lahunta, A., Roenigk, W. J., Hoffer, R. E., and Coons, F. H.: Four cases of congenital portacaval shunt in the dog. J. Sm. Anim. Pract., *17*:71, 1976.
3. Berryman, F. C., and de Lahunta, A.: Astrocytoma in a dog causing convulsions. Cor. Vet., *65*:212, 1975.
4. de Lahunta, A.: Feline ischemic encephalopathy—a cerebral infarction syndrome. *In* Kirk, R. W., ed., Current Veterinary Therapy, VI, in preparation.
5. de Lahunta, A., and Alexander, J. W.: Ischemic myelopathy secondary to presumed fibrocartilaginous embolism in nine dogs. J. Am. Anim. Hosp. Assoc., *12*:37, 1976.
6. Dubey, J. P., Davis, G. W., Koestner, A., and Kiryu, K.: Equine encephalomyelitis due to a protozoan parasite resembling *Toxoplasma gondii.* J. Am. Vet. Med. Assoc., *165*:249, 1974.
7. Fankhauser, R., Fatzer, R., Luginbühl, H., and McGrath, J. T.: III. Primary reticulosis of the CNS in animals. Adv. Vet. Sci. Comp. Med., *16*:40, 1972.
8. Koestner, A., and Zeman, W.: Primary reticuloses of the central nervous system in dogs. Am. J. Vet. Res., *23*:381, 1962.
9. Mayhew, I. G., de Lahunta, A., Whitlock, R. H., and Geary, J. C.: Equine degenerative myeloencephalopathy. J. Am. Vet. Med. Assoc. (in press).
10. Montali, R. J., Bush, M., Sauer, R. M., Gray, C. W., and Xanten, W. A.: Spinal ataxia in zebras. Vet. Pathol., *11*:68, 1974.
11. Schiefer, B., and Dahme, E.: Primäre Geschwülste des ZNS bei Tieren. Acta Neuropathol., *2*:202, 1962.
12. Teuscher, E., and Cherrstrom, E. C.: Ependymoma of the spinal cord in a young dog. Schweiz. Arch. Tierheilk., *116*:461, 1974.
13. Zaki, F. A., Prata, R. G., and Kay, W. J.: Necrotizing myelopathy in five Great Danes. J. Am. Vet. Med. Assoc., *165*:1080, 1974.
14. Zaki, F. A., and Prata, R. G.: Necrotizing myelopathy secondary to embolization of herniated intervertebral disk material in the dog. J. Am. Vet. Med. Assoc., *169*:222, 1976.

APPENDIX

TRANSVERSE BRAIN SECTIONS

Approximate Levels of 16 Plates of Dog Brain

The following transverse sections are arranged from caudal to rostral through the brain. The white matter is stained and appears black, whereas the grey matter is relatively unstained.

Dorsal view of brain stem.

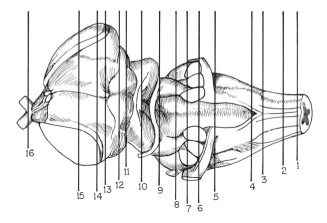

Left lateral surface of the brain stem. (After Evans, H. E., and de Lahunta, A.: Miller's Guide to the Dissection of the Dog. Philadelphia, W. B. Saunders Co., 1971.)

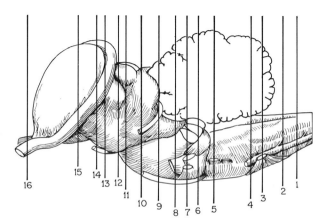

405

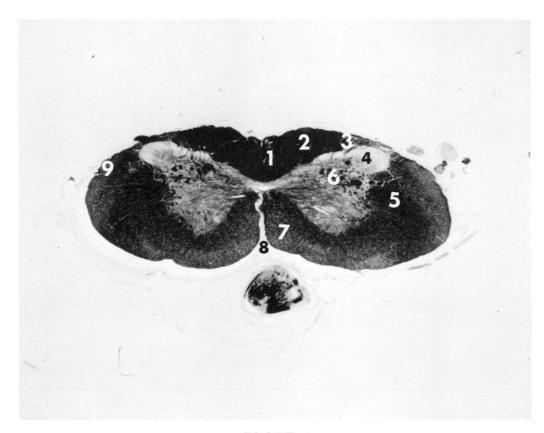

PLATE 1

1. Fasciculus gracilis
2. Fasciculus cuneatus
3. Spinal tract of trigeminal nerve
4. Nucleus of spinal tract of trigeminal nerve—
   dorsal grey column, first cervical segment
5. Rubrospinal tract
6. Lateral pyramidal (corticospinal) tract
7. Vestibulospinal tract
8. Ventral median fissure
9. Spinocerebellar tracts

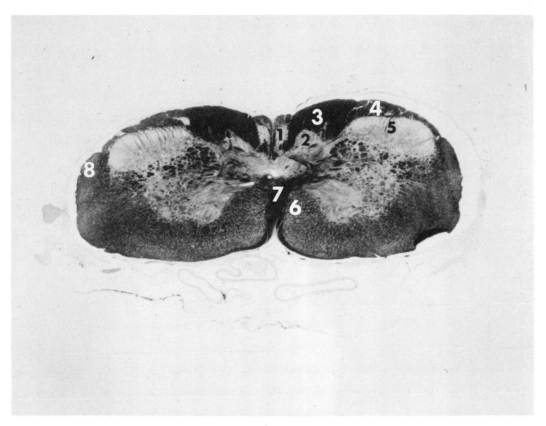

PLATE 2

1. Nucleus gracilis
2. Medial cuneate nucleus
3. Fasciculus cuneatus
4. Spinal tract of trigeminal nerve

5. Nucleus of spinal tract of trigeminal nerve
6. Medial longitudinal fasciculus — tectospinal part
7. Pyramidal decussation
8. Spinocerebellar tracts

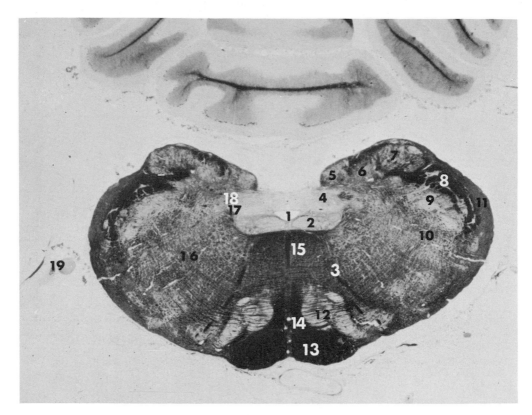

PLATE 3

1. Central canal
2. Hypoglossal motor nucleus
3. Radix of hypoglossal nerve
4. Parasympathetic nucleus of vagus nerve
5. Nucleus gracilis
6. Medial cuneate nucleus
7. Lateral cuneate nucleus
8. Spinal tract of trigeminal nerve
9. Nucleus of spinal tract of trigeminal nerve
10. Nucleus ambiguus
11. Dorsal spinocerebellar tract
12. Olivary nucleus
13. Pyramidal tract
14. Medial lemniscus
15. Medial longitudinal fasciculus — tectospinal part
16. Reticular formation
17. Nucleus of solitary tract
18. Solitary tract
19. Accessory nerve

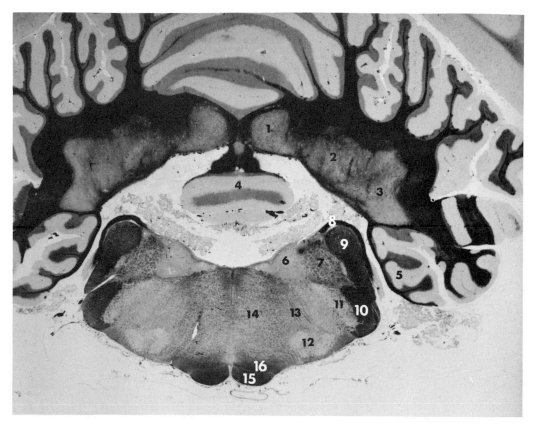

PLATE 5

1. Fastigial cerebellar nucleus
2. Interposital cerebellar nucleus
3. Lateral cerebellar nucleus
4. Nodulus
5. Flocculus
6. Medial vestibular nucleus
7. Caudal (descending) vestibular nucleus
8. Acoustic stria

9. Caudal cerebellar peduncle
10. Spinal tract of trigeminal nerve
11. Nucleus of spinal tract of trigeminal nerve
12. Facial motor nucleus
13. Ascending facial nerve fibers
14. Reticular formation
15. Pyramidal tract
16. Medial lemniscus

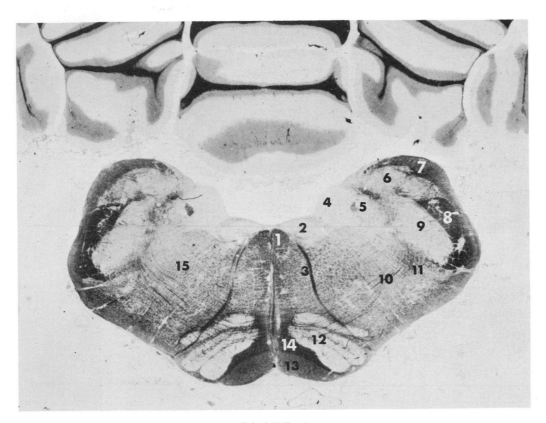

PLATE 4

1. Medial longitudinal fasciculus
2. Hypoglossal motor nucleus
3. Radix of hypoglossal nerve
4. Parasympathetic nucleus of vagus nerve
5. Nucleus of solitary tract
6. Lateral cuneate nucleus
7. Caudal cerebellar peduncle
8. Spinal tract of trigeminal nerve
9. Nucleus of spinal tract of trigeminal nerve
10. Deep arcuate fibers
11. Nucleus ambiguus
12. Olivary nucleus
13. Pyramidal tract
14. Medial lemniscus
15. Reticular formation

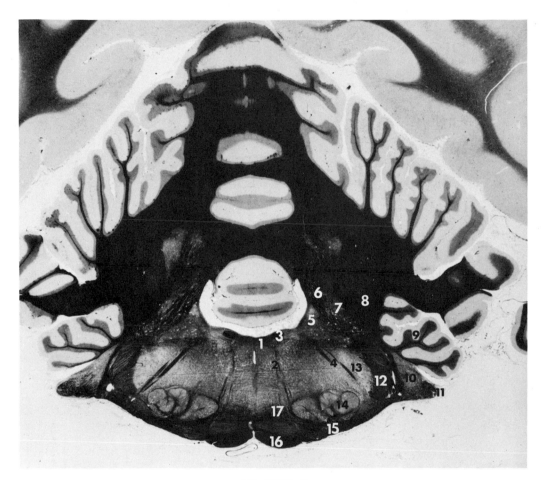

PLATE 6

1. Medial longitudinal fasciculus	10. Cochlear nuclei
2. Abducens nerve fibers	11. Vestibulocochlear nerve
3. Genu of facial nerve	12. Spinal tract of trigeminal nerve
4. Descending facial nerve fibers	13. Nucleus of spinal tract of trigeminal nerve
5. Medial vestibular nucleus	14. Dorsal nucleus of trapezoid body
6. Vestibulocerebellar fibers	15. Trapezoid body
7. Lateral vestibular nucleus	16. Pyramidal tract
8. Caudal cerebellar peduncle	17. Medial lemniscus
9. Flocculus	

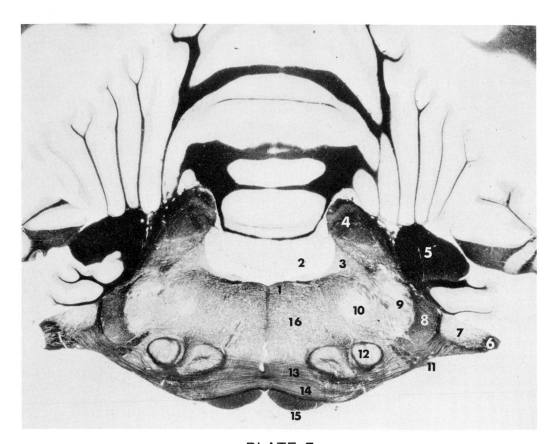

PLATE 7

1. Medial longitudinal fasciculus
2. Rostral medullary velum
3. Rostral vestibular nucleus
4. Rostral cerebellar peduncle
5. Middle cerebellar peduncle
6. Vestibulocochlear nerve
7. Cochlear nuclei
8. Trigeminal nerve

9. Sensory pontine nucleus of trigeminal nerve
10. Motor nucleus of trigeminal nerve
11. Facial nerve
12. Dorsal nucleus of trapezoid body
13. Medial lemniscus
14. Trapezoid body
15. Pyramid
16. Reticular formation

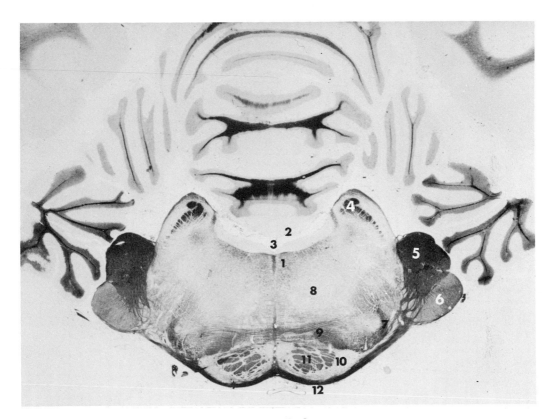

PLATE 8

1. Medial longitudinal fasciculus
2. Rostral medullary velum
3. Fourth ventricle
4. Rostral cerebellar peduncle
5. Middle cerebellar peduncle
6. Trigeminal nerve
7. Lateral lemniscus
8. Reticular formation
9. Medial lemniscus
10. Pontine nuclei
11. Longitudinal fibers of pons
12. Transverse fibers of pons

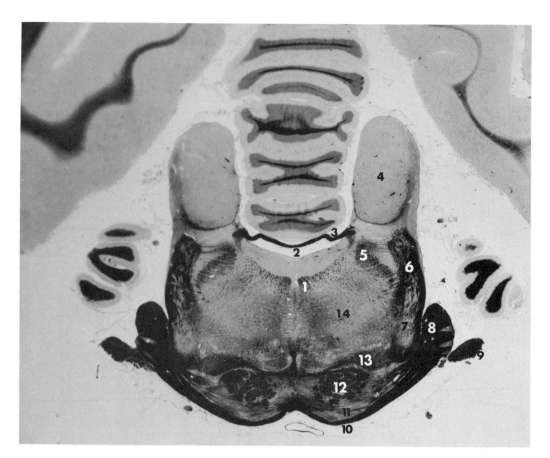

PLATE 9

1. Medial longitudinal fasciculus
2. Fourth ventricle
3. Trochlear nerve
4. Caudal colliculus
5. Rostral cerebellar peduncle
6. Lateral lemniscus
7. Nucleus of lateral lemniscus

8. Middle cerebellar peduncle
9. Trigeminal nerve
10. Transverse fibers of pons
11. Pontine nuclei
12. Longitudinal fibers of pons
13. Medial lemniscus
14. Reticular formation

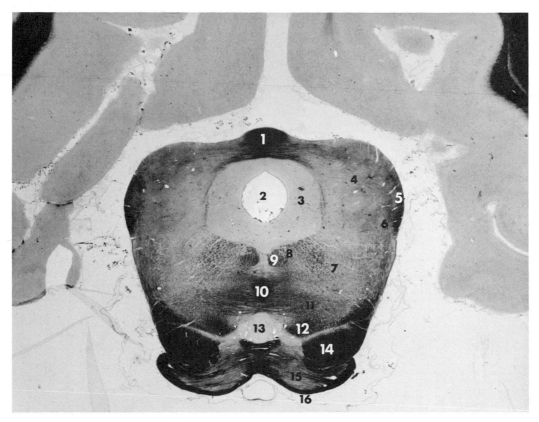

PLATE 10

1. Commissure of caudal colliculus
2. Mesencephalic aqueduct
3. Central grey substance
4. Caudal colliculus
5. Brachium of caudal colliculus
6. Lateral lemniscus
7. Reticular formation
8. Motor nucleus of trochlear nerve
9. Medial longitudinal fasciculus
10. Decussation of rostral cerebellar peduncle
11. Rubrospinal tract
12. Medial lemniscus
13. Intercrural nucleus
14. Crus cerebri
15. Pontine nuclei
16. Transverse fibers of pons

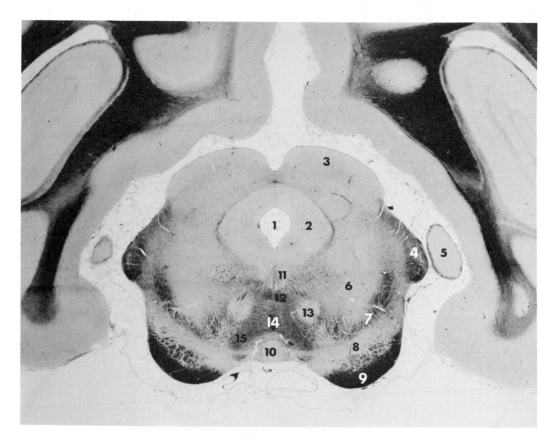

PLATE 11

1. Mesencephalic aqueduct
2. Central grey substance
3. Rostral colliculus
4. Brachium of caudal colliculus
5. Medial geniculate nucleus
6. Reticular formation (deep mesencephalic nucleus)
7. Medial lemniscus
8. Substantia nigra
9. Crus cerebri
10. Intercrural nucleus
11. Oculomotor motor nucleus
12. Medial longitudinal fasciculus
13. Red nucleus
14. Ventral tegmental decussation (rubrospinal neurons)
15. Rubrospinal tract

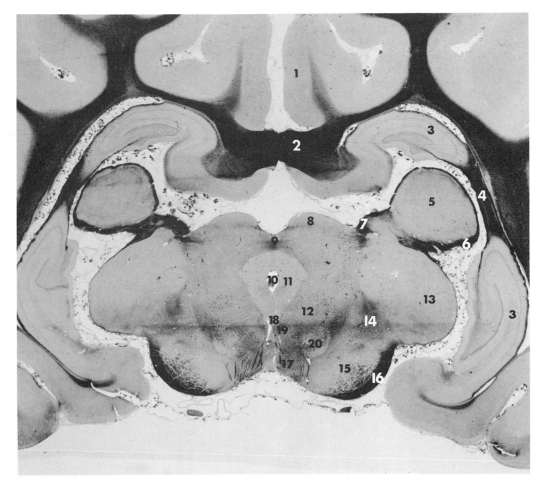

PLATE 12

1. Cingulate gyrus
2. Splenium of corpus callosum
3. Hippocampus
4. Crus of fornix
5. Thalamic nucleus—lateral geniculate
6. Optic tract
7. Brachium of rostral colliculus
8. Rostral colliculus
9. Commissure of rostral colliculus
10. Mesencephalic aqueduct
11. Central grey substance
12. Reticular formation (deep mesencephalic nucleus)
13. Thalamic nucleus—medial geniculate
14. Medial lemniscus
15. Substantia nigra
16. Crus cerebri
17. Oculomotor nerve fibers
18. Parasympathetic nucleus of oculomotor nerve
19. Medial longitudinal fasciculus
20. Red nucleus

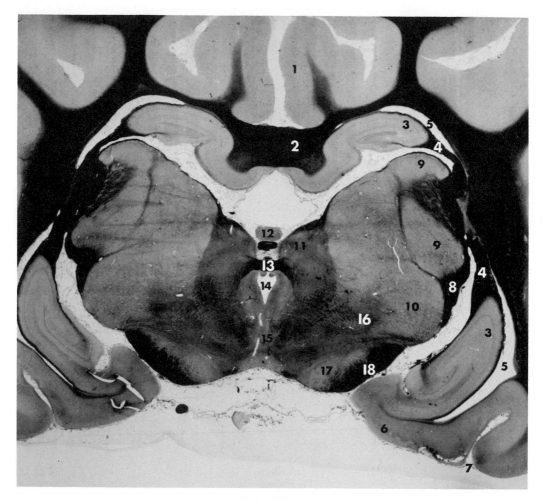

PLATE 13

1. Cingulate gyrus
2. Splenium of corpus callosum
3. Hippocampus
4. Crus of fornix
5. Lateral ventricle
6. Parahippocampal gyrus
7. Lateral rhinal sulcus—caudal part
8. Optic tract
9. Thalamic nucleus—lateral geniculate

10. Thalamic nucleus—medial geniculate
11. Pretectal nuclei
12. Pineal body
13. Caudal commissure
14. Mesencephalic aqueduct
15. Parasympathetic nucleus of oculomotor nerve
16. Medial lemniscus
17. Substantia nigra
18. Crus cerebri

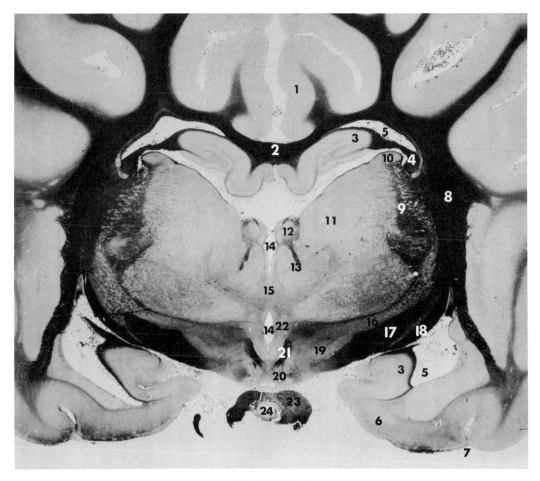

PLATE 14

1. Cingulate gyrus
2. Corpus callosum
3. Hippocampus
4. Crus of fornix
5. Lateral ventricle
6. Parahippocampal gyrus
7. Lateral rhinal sulcus — caudal part
8. Internal capsule
9. Thalamocortical projection fibers
10. Thalamic nucleus — lateral geniculate
11. Thalamic nuclei
12. Habenular nucleus
13. Fasciculus retroflexus (habenulointercrural tract)
14. Third ventricle
15. Interthalamic adhesion
16. Zona incerta
17. Crus cerebri
18. Optic tract
19. Subthalamic nucleus
20. Mammillary nucleus
21. Mammillothalamic tract
22. Caudal hypothalamic region
23. Adenohypophysis
24. Neurohypophysis

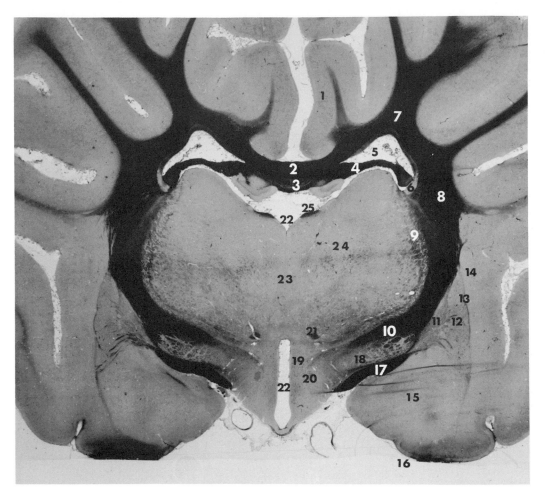

PLATE 15

1. Cingulate gyrus
2. Corpus callosum
3. Body of fornix
4. Crus of fornix
5. Lateral ventricle
6. Caudal caudate nucleus
7. Corona radiata (centrum semiovale)
8. Internal capsule
9. Thalamocortical projection fibers
10. Corticopontine − nuclear − spinal projection fibers
11. Pallidum ⎱ Lentiform nucleus
12. Putamen ⎰
13. External capsule

14. Claustrum
15. Amygdaloid body
16. Pyriform lobe
17. Optic tract
18. Endopeduncular nucleus
19. Hypothalamic nuclei
20. Column of fornix
21. Mammillothalamic tract
22. Third ventricle
23. Interthalamic adhesion
24. Thalamic nuclei
25. Stria habenularis thalami

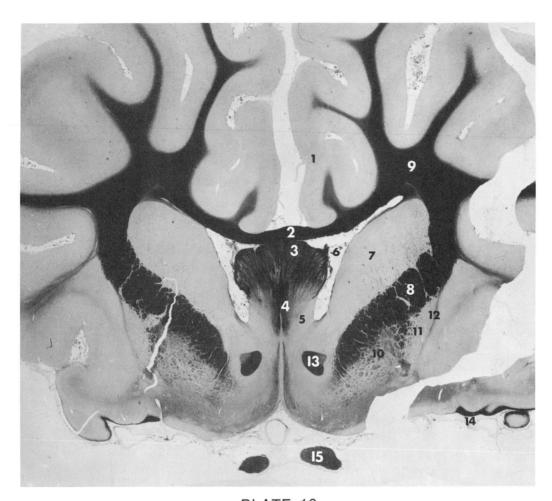

PLATE 16

1. Cingulate gyrus
2. Corpus callosum
3. Body of fornix
4. Column of fornix
5. Telencephalic septum—cellular part (septal nuclei)
6. Lateral ventricle
7. Rostral caudate nucleus
8. Internal capsule

9. Corona radiata (centrum semiovale)
10. Pallidum ⎫
11. Putamen ⎬ Lentiform nucleus
12. External capsule
13. Rostral commissure
14. Lateral olfactory tract
15. Optic nerve

INDEX

Note: Page numbers in *italics* indicate illustrations; numbers followed by "t" refer to tabular material. The preposition "vs." denotes differential diagnosis.

Abducens nerve, evaluation of, in horse, 368
Abducens nerve fibers, 91, *411*
Abiotrophy
    cerebellar cortical, in cattle, 249
        in dogs, 247
        in horses, 250
        in pigs, 251
    definition of, 2
    diffuse neuronal, 345, 347
    hereditary, in Swedish Lapland dogs, 83
    hereditary cerebellar cortical and extrapyramidal nuclear, 247, 248
    Purkinje cell, 247, 249, 251
Abscess
    bacterial, vs. feline ischemic encephalopathy, 400
        vs. osteogenic sarcoma, 382
    cerebral, effect of, on optic radiation, 273
    Corynebacterium pyogenes, 274
    epidural, and spinal cord compression, 397
    extramedullary, vs. extramedullary mass lesion, 374
    spinal cord, in cattle, 210
    Streptococcus equi, 273, 360, 391
Accessory nerve, 100, *408*
    spinal, evaluation of, 370
Acetylcholine, source of, 60
Achalasia, 123
Acoustic stria, *410*
Adenocarcinoma, prostatic metastasis, cerebrospinal fluid in, 51t
Adenohypophysis, *419*
    neoplasms of, 330
Adhesion, interthalamic, *419*, 420
Adiposogenital syndrome, 330
Adrenal medulla, formation of, *16*, 17
Adventitious movements, 142
Adverse syndrome, 358
Afghan hound, acute leukodystropy in, 189, 200
Age
    and hearing loss, 286
    and seizures, 385
    and vestibular disease, 232
    significance of, in neurologic examination, 345, 359
Akabane virus, and hydranencephaly, 29
Amphibian, cerebrum of, 25
Amygdaloid body, 296, *420*

Analgesia, facial, 168, 357, 358
Anencephaly, vs. prosencephalic hypoplasia, 28
Angiography, cerebral, in epilepsy, 312
Animal, small. See *Small animal.*
Anisocoria, diseases associated with, 117
Anophthalmia, 271
Anosmia, 294, 295
Anticonvulsants, 313
Appetite, abnormal, hypothalamic lesions and, 330
Aqueduct, mesencephalic, 10, *11*, *415–418*
    in development of midbrain, 21
    malformation of, and hydrocephalus, 52
Arabian horse
    atlanto-occipital malformation of, 209
    cerebellar cortical abiotrophy in, 250, 359
    gait in, 362
    menace response in, 367
Arachnoid villus, 37, *37*
    malformation of, and hydrocephalus, 52
Archicerebellum, 240
Archipallium, 25, *25*
Arcuate fibers, deep, *409*
Area centralis, of retina, 264, *265*
Artery, hyaloid, 259
Association fibers, of telencephalon, 26
Association system, of thalamic nuclei, 321
Astrocyte, formation of, 10, *12*
Astrocytoma, cerebral, case description, 383–385, *386*
    cerebrospinal fluid in, 51t
    in optic radiation, 275–277
Ataxia
    and cerebellar deficiency, 247
    and vestibular deficiency, 228
    cerebellar, 250
    equine sensory, 206
        testing for, 362
    in hydrocephalus, 53
    in spinal cord disease, 170
    lesions of general proprioception system and, 157
Athetosis, 143
Atlantoaxial subluxation, 192
Atonia, lower motor neuron disease and, 68
Atrophy, neurogenic, spinal reflex depression and, 68
    progressive retinal, 271
Auditory pathway, 284, *285*

Auditory system, 281–287, *282*
Autonomic nervous system, 110
Avulsion, of spinal roots, 76
Axolemma, in motor end-plate, 59, *60*
Axon
    definition of, 2
    destruction of, and degeneration, 69, *70*
    in general somatic afferent system, 160
    in optic chiasm, 266, 267
    of general somatic efferent neuron, 58, *59*
    of telencephalic cortical neurons, 26, *27*

Bacterial inflammation, cerebrospinal fluid in, 49t, 50t, 355
Ballism, 143
Basset hound, malformation of cervical vertebra in, 198
Behavior, abnormal, hypothalamic lesions and, 330
    and limbic system, 299–301
    evaluation of, in neurologic examination, 361
Belgian sheepdog, congenital nystagmus in, 236
Beta cell pancreatic neoplasm, 306, 402
Betz's cells, 126
Biceps reflex
    evaluation of, 351
    in spinal cord disease, 173
    in thoracic limb, 64, *66*
    testing of, topographic anatomy of, 68t
Bladder, automatic, 121
    autonomous, 121
    paralysis of, 361
Bladder function, neuroanatomy of, 119, *120*
Blindness, 270–277
    in hydrocephalus, 53
    night, 359
Bluetongue virus, and hydrocephalus, 51
    and hydranencephaly, 29
Bone, diseases of, vs. neurologic disease, 194
Border disease, 146, 250
Boston terrier, cerebral astrocytoma in, 383–385, *386*
    hydrocephalus in, 53
Botulism, 71, 72
    and cranial nerve lower motor neuron disease, 102
Brachial plexus, avulsion of roots of, 76
    injury to, 340
    spinal nerve, 64, *66*
Brachial plexus neuritis, 79
Brachium, of caudal colliculus, *415, 416*
    of rostral colliculus, *417*
Brain
    transverse sections of, *405–421*
    injury to, and convulsions, 308
    malformations of, 28
    traumatic lesions of, 333
        treatment of, medical, 335
        surgical, 336
Brain disease, acute, pupils in, 117
Brain stem, 22, *156, 405*
    cranial nerve nuclei in, *90*
    cochlear nuclei of, 283
    disease of, 107
    in general visceral afferent system, 289
    vestibular nuclei projections to, 227

Brain stem function, tests for, 334, 335
Brain vesicles, development of, 8, *11*
Breed, significance of, in neurologic examination, 345, 359
Brown-Séquard syndrome, 163
Bulldog, English, meningomyelocele in, 30
Bunny hopping, in spinal dysraphism, 30

Cairn terrier, hepatic encephalopathy in, 401–404, *403*
    leukodystrophy in, 275
Calf
    bluetongue virus in, 29
    dummy, 29
    femoral nerve paralysis in, 75
    hydranencephaly in, 29
    Jersey, hereditary leukodysplasia in, 146
    myelodysplasia in, 215
    obturator nerve paralysis in, 75
    polioencephalomalacia in, 274, 308, 325
    radial paralysis in, 74
    tibial nerve paralysis in, 75
    ulnar paralysis in, 74
Canal, central, *408*
Capsule, external, *420, 421*
    internal, *419–421*
    of telencephalon, 25, *25*
Carbohydrate metabolism, abnormal, hypothalamic lesions and, 330
Carcinoma. See also *Neoplasm.*
    choroid plexus, cerebrospinal fluid in, 51t
Cardiac malformation, neurologic signs of, 360
Cardiorespiratory disease, episodic weakness in, 86
Cardiovascular function, alterations in, hypothalamic lesions and, 331
Cat
    aortic thrombosis in, 76
    cerebral infarction in, 141, 273, 399–401, *401*
    cranium bifidum in, 28
    cuterebra encephalitis in, 51t
    exencephaly in, 28
    Manx, meningomyelocele in, 30
    normal cerebrospinal fluid value in, 48t
    panleukopenia virus in, 347
    spinal root avulsion in, 77
    spinal cord segments in, 61
    taste perception in, 292
    vestibular disease in, 231
Cataplexy, 315
Cattle
    botulism in, 72
    cerebellar syndromes in, 249
    peroneal nerve paralysis in, 75
    spastic syndrome in, 144
    viral diarrhea virus in, 249
Cauda equina, neuritis of, in horse, 80, 391
Cells. See also specific names.
    deterioration of, 2
    in neural tube, differentiation of, 10, *12, 13*
Cell body, of neuron, 2
Centaurea solstitialis, and equine nigropallidal encephalomalacia, 143, 360
Central nervous system, inflammation of, cerebrospinal fluid in, 355

Central nervous system (*Continued*)
  traumatic lesions of, 333–339
    in brain, 333
    in spinal cord, 337
Centrum semiovale, 26, *420, 421*
Cerebellar cortex, anatomy of, 240
  layers of, 239
Cerebellar medulla, 240
Cerebellar nuclei, 243
Cerebellar peduncle, 240
Cerebellum, 238–254
  anatomy of, 240–244, *241*
  degeneration of, diffuse, 252
  herpesvirus and, 347
  development of, 20–21, *20, 21*, 238–240, *239*
  diseases of, signs of, 245–246
  extrapyramidal system projection to, 135, *135*
  function of, 244–245, *244*
  general proprioceptive pathway to, 151, *153*
  inflammation of, 252
  injury to, 253
  lesions of, clinical signs of, 357
  neoplasms of, 252
  Purkinje cell of, 3, *239*
  reticulosis lesion in, 234, 388–390, *390*
  syndromes involving, 246–253
  vestibular nuclei projections to, 227
Cerebral cortex
  anatomic division of, 25, *25*
  histology of, 127–128, *129*
  motor area of, 126, *126*
  projection of sensory systems to, 155
  visual, 268
    disorders of, 273
Cerebral edema, in intracranial injury, 335
Cerebral hemispheres, formation of, 10, *11*
Cerebral infarction, and vascular disease in cat,
  141, 273, 399–401
Cerebrospinal fluid, 33–56
  abnormal, clinical examples of, 50t
  absorption of, 37–38
  circulation of, 35–37
  clinical application of, 38–41
  evaluation of, 354, 371
  examination of, 48–50
  function of, 38
  in epilepsy, 312
  method of obtaining, 42–47
    in horse, 43, 45, *44, 45, 47*
    in small animal, 42
  normal values of, 48t
  production of, 33–35, *34*
Cerebrum
  amphibian, 25
  development of, 22–28, *24–27*
  extrapyramidal system projection to, 135, *135*
  infarction of, 399–401, *401*
  ischemic necrosis of, and blindness, 274
  lesions of, clinical signs of, 358
  malformation of, virus and, 28
  mammalian, 26
  reptilian, 25
  visual pathways in, lesions of, 116
Ceroid lipofuscinosis, 252
Cervical reflex, evaluation of, in horse, 365
Cervical spinal cord. See *Spinal cord, cervical.*
Charolais cattle, myelin disorder of, 215

Chewing gum fit, 307
Cheyne-Stokes respiration, 334
  in unconscious state, 327
Chihuahua, hydrocephalus in, 53
Chloropromazine, 337
Chorea, 143
  and cerebrospinal fluid flow, 35
  formation of, 19, *19*
  of diencephalon, development of, 22, *23, 24*
  of telencephalon, development of, *24*
Choroid plexus papilloma-carcinoma, 184, 235
  cerebrospinal fluid in, 51t
Chromatolysis, central, in Wallerian
  degeneration, 69
Cingulate gyrus, *417–421*
  definition of, 298
Cingulum, of limbic system, 298
Circling, 228, 358
Cirrhosis, hepatic, equine, 360
Clarke's nucleus, 151
Clasp knife reaction, 350
  in spinal cord disease, 173
Claustrum, *420*
Claviceps paspali, and staggers, 360
  and tremors, 145
Clonus, 141, 351
Clostridium botulinum, 72, 102, 108
  and wound infections, 360
Clostridium tetani, 138
Cochlea, 281
Cochlear duct, 281
Colliculus, caudal, *414–416*
  of auditory system, 284
  rostral, *416, 417*
    in pupillary reflex pathway, 268
Collie, extramedullary cranial lesion in,
  377–380, *379*
Collie eye syndrome, 271
Color vision, initiation of, 262
Coma
  clinical evaluation of, 325–328, 357
  definition of, 326
  intracranial injury and, 325, 334
  metabolic diseases and, 327t
  poisons and, 328t
Commissural fibers, of telencephalon, 26, *27*
Conduction deafness, 286
Conscious perception
  general somatic afferent pathway for,
    161, *162*, 165
  pathway for, *266, 268*
  somesthetic cortex for, proprioceptive
    pathway to, 152, *154*
  trigeminal nerve in, 157, 165
Consciousness
  disturbances of, 324
  levels of, 334
  loss of, clinical evaluation of, 325–328
    hypothalamic lesions and, 331
Convulsions. See *Seizures.*
Coonhound, osteogenic sarcoma of tentorium
  cerebelli in, 380–383, *382, 383*
Coonhound paralysis, 68, 77
  raccoon bite and, 78, 381
Corneal reflex, 99
  in dog, 353
  in horse, 369

Corona radiata, *420, 421*
Corpus callosum, 26, *26*, 298, *419–421*
  splenium of, *417*
Corpus striatum, of extrapyramidal system, 129
Cortex
  auditory sensory, 284
  cerebellar. See *Cerebellar cortex.*
  cerebral. See *Cerebral cortex.*
  somesthetic, for conscious perception, 152,
    154
    location of, 155
  visual, 268
    disorders of, 273
Corti, organ of, 283
Cortical projection system, diffuse, thalamic
    nuclei in, 321
Corticopontine spinal projection fibers, *420*
Cow, cerebrospinal fluid collection in, 42
  obturator nerve paralysis in, 75
  polioencephalomalacia in, 51t, 274, 308, 325
  spastic syndrome in, 144
Cramps, Scotty, 144, 345
Cranial cavity, 35
Cranial gluteal nerve paralysis, 76
Cranial nerves
  evaluation of, in intracranial injury, 334
    in spinal cord disease, 175
  examination of, 352
    in horse, examination of, 366
  general proprioception system for, 155, *156*
  in general somatic afferent system, 164–165
  in myelencephalon, functional organization
    of, 17, *18*
  of lower motor neuron, 89–109
    diseases affecting, 102
Cranial nerve II, formation of, 22, 265
Cranial nerve III, 92, *93*, 115
  in development of midbrain, 22, *21*
Cranial nerve IV, 92, *93*
  in development of midbrain, 22, *21*
Cranial nerve V, 97, *97*
  and development of metencephalon, 20, *20*
Cranial nerve VI, 91, *91*
Cranial nerve VII, 98, *99*, 122
Cranial nerve VIII, cochlear division of, 283
  vestibular division, 225
Cranial nerve IX, 100, 122
Cranial nerve X, 100, 122
Cranial nerve XI, 100, 122
Cranial nerve XII, 89
Cranial placodes, 19
Cranioschisis, 28
Cranium bifidum, 28
Creatine phosphokinase, in cerebrospinal fluid,
    49
  in muscle disease, 84
Crista ampullaris, 223
Crus cerebri, *21*, 22, *415–419*
Cryptococcosis, and thoracolumbar spinal cord
    disease, 187
  cerebrospinal fluid in, 50, 355
Cryptococcus neoformans, in cerebrospinal
    fluid, 50
Cryptococcus neoformans infection, vs. feline
    ischemic encephalopathy, 400
Cupula, 223

Cuterebra encephalitis, 234, 252
  cerebrospinal fluid in, 51t
Cyclopic malformation, 257

Dallis grass poisoning, 145
Deafness, 285–286
  congenital, 345
Decerebrate rigidity, 138, 328
Decompression, cerebral, 336
Defecation, control of, 121
Degeneration
  cerebellar, 246
    diffuse, 252
    in pigs, 251
  definition of, 2
  Wallerian, 69, *70*
Dendritic zone, of neuron, 2
  of Purkinje cell, 241
Depression, 326, 334
  postictal, 303
Dermacentor variabilis, 73
Dermatome, in general somatic afferent system,
    161
Devic's syndrome, 272
Dexamethasone, 335
Diabetes insipidus, hypothalamic lesions and,
    330
Diarrhea virus, bovine viral, 249
  and hydrocephalus, 51
Diazepam, in treatment of seizures, 313, 337
Diencephalon, 10, *11*, 318–332
  development of, 22, *23*
  extrapyramidal nuclei of, 132, 133
  hypothalamus, 328–331
  in limbic system, 298
  lesions of, clinical signs of, 357
  relationship of mesencephalon to, *23*
  thalamus, 318–325
Dimethylsulfoxide, 336
Dimpling, myotonic, 85
Diplomyelia, 30
Disease. See specific names.
Disk disease, intervertebral, 181, 345
  and contusion of cervical intumescence, 201
    cervical, 192
    in German shepherd, 395
    in lumbar vertebral column, 177
    protruded-proliferated, *40*
  vs. extramedullary spinal lesion, 378
Diskospondylitis, 186
Distemper chorea, 143
Distemper encephalitis, canine, 234, 252, 272,
    274
  and convulsions, 307
    cerebrospinal fluid in, 50t, 355
Distemper myelitis
  and spinal cord disease, 394
    thoracolumbar 187
  of cervical intumescence, 203
  vs. cervical spinal cord lesion, 195
Distemper virus, and blindness, 274
  and spinal cord destruction, 83
Doberman pinscher, cervical vertebral
    malformation in, 193

Dummy calf, 29
Dummy lamb, 29
Dysphagia, in horse, 104, 107, 370
Dysraphism, spinal, 190
    clinical signs of, 30
Dystonia, 143

Ear, injury to, vestibular signs of, 233
    inner, membranous labyrinth contusions of,
        335
Eastern equine encephalomyelitis, cerebrospinal
    fluid in, 371
Ectosylvian gyrus, 284
Edema, cerebral, cerebrospinal fluid in, 35
    in intracranial injury, 335
Edinger-Westphal nucleus, 116
Electroencephalography, in epilepsy, 312
    in hydrocephalus, 54
Electromyography, in neuromuscular disease, 70
Ellipsoid, 263
Embolism, aortic, 76
Embolus, fibrocartilaginous, and ischemic
    myelopathy, 81, 198, *199*, 203, 375–377
Encephalitis
    and convulsions, 307
    arboviral, 108
        cerebrospinal fluid in, 371
    bluetongue virus and, 29
    cuterebra, cerebrospinal fluid in, 51t
    diffuse, cerebrospinal fluid in, 50t
    distemper, canine, 234, 252, 272, 274, 307
        cerebrospinal fluid in, 50t
    granulomatous, vs. osteogenic sarcoma, 381
    nonsuppurative, cerebrospinal fluid in, 355
    toxoplasma, cerebrospinal fluid in, 50t
        effect of, on optic radiation, 274
Encephalomalacia, equine nigropallidal, 143
Encephalomyelitis, protozoal, 107, 211, 390–394,
    393
    rabies, and lower motor neuron paralysis, 82
Encephalopathy, feline ischemic, 141, 273
Ending, neuromuscular, diseases of, 71
Endomysium, in motor end-plate, 59, *60*
Endoneurium, in motor end-plate, 59, *60*
End-plate, motor, 58, *60*
    neuromuscular junction of, 59, *60*
English bulldog, hydrocephalus in, 53
English setter, ceroid lipofuscinosis in, 275
Ependymoblastoma, cerebrospinal fluid in, 51t
Ependymoma, and hydrocephalus, 52
    cerebrospinal fluid in, 51t
Epilepsy. See also *Seizures.*
    idiopathic, 309, 345
Epithalamus, 318
Equine. See *Horse.*
Esophagus, dysfunction of, 123
    innervation of, 122
Examination, neurologic, 169–177, 344–372
Exencephaly, 28
Exostosis, cartilaginous, 185, 394
Extensor postural thrust, 171, 349
    evaluation of, 173
Extensor reflex, crossed, evaluation of, 352
        in spinal cord disease, 175
        in upper motor neuron disease, 141

Extrapyramidal system, of upper motor neuron,
    128–136, *130–133, 135, 136*
    disturbances to, and involuntary
        adventitious movements, 142
    function of, 136
Eye, movement of, in unconscious state, 327
    sympathetic general visceral efferent lower
        motor neuron innervation of, 111
Eyeball
    embryology of, 257–261, *258*
    innervation of, by parasympathetic general
        visceral efferent system, 115
        by sympathetic general visceral efferent
            system, 111
    malformation of, 271
Eyeball anophthalmia, 271
Eyeball hypoplasia, 271
Eyelid, third, protrusion of, 118

Facial hypalgesia, 168, 357, 358
Facial nerve, 98–100, 122, *412*
    in horse, evaluation of, 369
    lesions of, 98
Facial paralysis, idiopathic, 106
Fasciculus, medial longitudinal, *407–409,*
    411–417
Fasciculus cuneatus, *406, 407*
    in proprioceptive pathway, 152
Fasciculus, gracilis, *406*
    in proprioceptive pathway, 152
Fasciculus retroflexus, *419*
Femoral nerve, function of, 340
    paralysis of, 75
Fibers
    corticopontine spinal projection, 420
    intrafusal, of neuromuscular spindle, 136, *137*
    thalamocortical projection, *419, 420*
    vestibulocerebellar, *411*
Fibrin clot, in cerebrospinal fluid, 48
Fibrocartilaginous ischemic myelopathy, case
    description of, 375–377
    cervical, 198, 203
    lumbosacral, 81
    thoracolumbar, 189
Fissure, ventral medial, *406*
Fit. See *Seizures.*
Flexor-reflex
    in pelvic limb, 66, 67
        evaluation of, 351
            in horse, 364
            in spinal cord disease, 174
        test for, topographic anatomy of, 68t
    in thoracic limb, 64, 352
        evaluation of, in horse, 365
            in spinal cord disease, 174
        test for, topographic anatomy of, 68t
Flexor spasm, 143
Flexor withdrawal response, 161
Flocculus, *410, 411*
Foal, myotonia in, 85, 365
    neuromuscular paresis in, 73
Fornix, 297
    body of, *420, 421*
    column of, *420, 421*
    crus of, *417–420*

Fornix system, 25, *25*
Fovea, 264
Fractures
    of cranial cervical vertebrae, 191
    of hyoid bone, and hypoglossal nerve injury,
        103
    of lumbosacral vertebrae, 76
    of pelvis and tail, case description of, 386–388
    of thoracolumbar vertebrae, 179
    of vertebral column, in large animal, 205
    sacrocaudal, *386, 387*
Froelich's syndrome, 330
Functional classification, 3
Fungal inflammation, cerebrospinal fluid in, 50t
Funiculus, of spinal cord, formation of, 14, *16*
Fusarum species intoxication, 360

Gait, evaluation of, in neurologic examination,
        348, 361
    in spinal cord disease, 170
Ganglion
    abdominal autonomic plexus, formation of, *16,*
        17
    of sympathetic trunk, formation of, *16,* 17
    segmental spinal, 61, *62*
    spinal, formation of, 14, *15*
Gangliosidosis, 275
Genu, of facial nerve, *411*
German shepherd, degenerative myelopathy in,
        188
    eosinophilic myositis in, 83
    neuroepithelioma in, 394–396, *395, 396*
German short-haired pointer, lipodystrophy in,
        275
Glioma, in brachycephalic breeds, 385
    of spinal cord, 190
    vs. feline ischemic encephalopathy, 400
Glossopharyngeal nerve, 100, 122
    lesions of, clinical signs of, 102
    in horse, evaluation of, 370
Glucose, in cerebrospinal fluid, 35
Glucose metabolism, abnormalities in, 306, 345
Glutamic-oxaloacetic transaminase, in
        cerebrospinal fluid, 49
Glycogenolysis, metabolic aberration in, 307, 402
Goat
    cerebrospinal fluid collection in, 42
    myotonia congenita in, 85
    Parelaphostrongylus tenuis in, 51t, 213, 234
    polioencephalomalacia in, 51t, 308, 325
    viral leukoencephalomyelitis in, 213
Golden retriever, hereditary myotonic
        myopathy in, 84
Golgi neurons, 242
Granuloma, cerebral, cerebrospinal fluid in, 50t
    toxoplasma, vs. feline ischemic
        encephalopathy, 400
Grass tetany, 145, 307
Great Dane
    cervical vertebral malformation in, 193
    fibrocartilaginous embolic ischemic
        myelopathy in, 375–377, *377*
    lesion of tympanoccipital fissure in, 373–375,
        375

Great Dane (*Continued*)
    serum neuritis in, 79
    wheelbarrowing in, 349
Grey substance, central, *415–417*
Griseofulvin, effect on visual system, 271
Gunshot wound, to spinal cord, 339
Gustatory sense, special visceral afferent system
        and, 292, *293*
Guttural pouch mycosis, 104, *104,* 370
Gyrus
    cingulate, *417–421*
        definition of, 298
    ectosylvian, 284
    parahippocampal, *418*

Hairy shaker disease, 146
Haloxon neurotoxicity, in sheep, 215
Head tilt, 228
Hearing, evaluation of, 354
    loss of, 285–286
Heart rate, abnormal, hypothalamic lesions and,
        331
Helicotrema, 281
Hematomyelia, 82
Hemifacial spasm, 105–106
Hemistanding reaction, 349
    as test for spinal cord disease, 172
Hemiwalking reaction, 349
    as test for spinal cord disease, 172
Hemophilus somnus, 274
Hemorrhage, subarachnoid, 335
    subdural, 335
Hepatic encephalopathy, 307, 401–404, *403*
    acute, 359
    cerebrospinal fluid in, 371
Hereford syndrome, hereditary, 31
Herniation, of cerebrum, 274
Herpesvirus, and cerebellar degeneration, 347
    canine, effect of, on cerebellum, 246
Herpesvirus I, equine, 212
        cerebrospinal fluid in, 371
        effect of, on herd, 360
        vs. degenerative myeloencephalopathy, 398
Hexachlorophene intoxication, and coma, 328t
    and convulsions, 309
Hippocampus, 25, *25,* 296, *417–419*
History, importance of, in neurologic
        examination, 345, 359
Holstein, cerebellar abiotrophy in, 249
Hopping, in limb testing, 171, 172, 349
Horner's syndrome, 77, 113
    extramedullary lesion and, 374, 380
    in diffuse myelomalacia, 82
    in horse, 113, 368
    lesions producing, 115t
Horse
    aortic thrombosis in, 76
    ataxia in, 362
    botulism in, 72, 108
    cerebellar syndromes in, 250
    cerebrospinal fluid collection in, 43, 45, *44
        45, 47*
    cerebrospinal fluid evaluation in, 371
        normal values, 48t

Horse (*Continued*)
  cervical vertebral malarticulation-malformation
    in, 206
  chronic polyneuritis in, 80
  degenerative myeloencephalopathy in, 214
  femoral nerve paralysis in, 75
  guttural pouch mycosis in, 104
  Horner's syndrome in, 113, 368
  leukoencephalomalacia in, 107, 360
  myotonia congenita in, 85
  neurologic examination in, 358–371
    behavior, 361
    gait, 361
    history, 359
    mental status, 361
    physical examination, 360
    posture, 361
    signalment, 359
    spinal reflexes, 363
  pars intermedia of, neoplasms of, 331
  pectoral paralysis in, 75
  pharyngeal paralysis in, differential diagnosis
    of, 107
  protozoal encephalomyelitis in, 390–394, *393*
  rabies in, 83
  spinal cord disease in, 394
  Strongylus vulgaris in, 214
  viral encephalomyelitis in, 108
  weakness in, 362
Husky, spinal dysraphism in, 30
Hyaloid artery, 259
Hydranencephaly, 28
Hydrocarbon, chlorinated, and convulsions, 309
Hydrocephalus, *41,* 50–54
  ancillary examination in, 53
  and convulsions, 308
  clinical signs of, 53
  compensatory, 51
  definition of, 28
  normal-pressure, 53
  obstructive, 51, 274
  treatment of, 54
Hydromyelia, 30
Hypalgesia, facial, 168, 357, 358
Hyperadrenocorticoidism, 331
Hypercapnia, 333
Hyperesthesia, idiopathic, in horse, 369
Hyperglycemia, 331
Hyperkalemia, and convulsions, 307
  episodic weakness in, 86
Hyperlipoproteinemia, and convulsions, 307
Hypermetria, with general proprioceptive
    deficit, 157
  with cerebellar deficit, 245
Hyperreflexia, 351
Hypersensitivity, denervation, 114
Hyperthermia, 330
Hypertonia, upper motor neuron disease and,
    350, 351
Hyperventilation, 327
Hypoadrenocorticoidism, neurologic signs of,
    360
Hypocalcemia, and convulsions, 307
Hypoderma bovis, 252
Hypoglossal motor neurons, 89
Hypoglossal motor nucleus, *409*

Hypoglossal nerve, in horse, evaluation of, 370
  radix of, *408, 409*
Hypoglycemia, age in, 345
  convulsions in, 306
  episodic weakness in, 86
Hypokalemia, episodic weakness in, 86
Hypomagnesemia, and convulsions, 307
Hypomyelinogenesis, hereditary, in cattle, 250
  in pigs, 251
Hypophyseal pouch, 22
Hypophysis, formation of, 22, 23
Hypoplasia
  cerebellar, primary, 246
  eyeball, 271
  of prosencephalon, 28, 274
  Purkinje cell, 247
Hypothalamic region, caudal, *419*
Hypothalamohypophyseal tract, 329
Hypothalamotegmental tract, hypothalamic
    connections to, 329
Hypothalamus, 328–331
  anatomy of, 328
  formation of, 22, *23*
  function of, 329
  in autonomic nervous system, 110
  lesions of, clinical signs of, 330, 357
Hypothermia, whole body, 337
Hypotonia, in spinal cord disease, 173
  lower motor neuron disease and, 68, 350
Hypoxia and convulsions, 307

Idiopathic epilepsy, 309, 345
Infarction, cerebral, 141, 273, 399–401, *401*
Inflammation
  bacterial, cerebrospinal fluid in, 355
  cerebellar, 252
  definition of, 2
  nonsuppurative, 2
  suppurative, 2
Infundibulum, 328
Injury, cerebral, 333–337
  spinal cord, 337–339
    cervical, 191
    lumbosacral, 177
    of peripheral nerves, 74, 339–342
    thoracolumbar, 179, 205
Interbrain, development of, 22, 23
Interthalamic adhesion, *419, 420*
  in development of diencephalon, 22, 23
Intestines, parasites in, and convulsions, 307
Intoxication, and coma, 328t
  and convulsions, 309
Intracranial injury
  and coma, 325
  diagnosis and evaluation of, 333
  effect of, on vestibular pathway, 236
  pupil size in, 118t
Iodopsin, 262
Irish setter, hereditary myotonic myopathy in, 84
Ixodes holocyclus, 73

Jacksonian seizure, 304, 346
Jugular compression maneuver, 37

Keratitis, neurotrophic, 168
Kerry blue terrier, hereditary cerebellar cortical
    and extrapyramidal nuclear abiotrophy in,
    247, 347
Kidneys, disease of, and convulsions, 307
Kyphosis, 191

L7, fracture of, and spinal root injury, 76
    injury to, 177
Labyrinth, of vestibular system, 222, 222
    degeneration of, 234
Lactic dehydrogenase, in cerebrospinal fluid, 49
Lamb, border disease in, 146, 250
    dummy, 29
Lamina, spiral, of auditory system, 281
Lamina terminalis, of diencephalon, 22, 24
Landry-Guillain-Barré syndrome, 79
Lapland dog, Swedish, hereditary abiotrophy in,
    83
Laryngeal hemiplegia, and roarer horse, 103
Laryngeal paralysis, in horse, 370
Lead posioning, 402
    age in, 345
    and convulsions, 308
Lemmocyte, 59
    proliferation of, in Wallerian degeneration, 69
Lemniscus, lateral, 413–415
    composition of, 284
    medial, 408–418
    in proprioceptive pathway, 153
Lens placode, 258
Lens vesicle, 259
Leptomeninges, formation of, 19
Leptomeningitis, cryptococcal, vs. osteogenic
    sarcoma, 382
Lesions. See under specific system.
Leukodysplasia, in Jersey calves, 146
Leukodystrophy, blindness in, 275
    globoid cell, 345, 347
    in Afghan hounds, 189, 200
Leukoencephalomalacia, equine, 107, 360
Leukoencephalomyelitis, viral, in goat, 213
Lhasa apso, lissencephaly and pachygyria in, 308
Light reflex response, pupillary, 116, 270
Limbic system, 296–302
    anatomy of, 296–299, 297
    function of, 299–301
    major structures of, 299t
Limbs, pelvic. See Pelvic limbs.
    thoracic. See Thoracic limbs.
Lipidosis, sphingomyelin, 275
Lipodystrophy, 252, 345
    blindness in, 275
Lissauer's tract, 160
Lissencephaly, and convulsions, 308
Listeriosis, 107, 235
    cerebrospinal fluid in, 51t
Liver, disease of, and convulsions, 307
Lobe, pyriform, 420
Locoweed poisoning, 360
Lumbosacral plexus, spinal nerve, 67
Lymphosarcoma, lactic dehydrogenase in, 49
    spinal cord, in the cat and dog, 184
        in cattle, 210

Macula, 224, 264
Malformation, definition of, 2
    of spinal cord, 30, 190, 200
Mammal, cerebrum of, 26
Mammillary body, in limbic system, 298
Mammillothalamic tract, 420
    hypothalamic connection to, 329
Mandibular nerve, in horse, evaluation of, 369
Mannitol, 335
Mapping, dermatomal, 161
Medulla
    adrenal, formation of, 16, 17
    and nucleus ambiguus, 101
    cerebellar, 240
    cranial nerve, lower motor neurons, anatomy
        of, 89–102
        diseases of, 102–108
    focal protozoal encephalitis of, 107
    inflammation of, vs. extramedullary mass
        lesion, 374
    lesions of, clinical signs of, 357
    parasympathetic general visceral efferent
        lower motor neuron of, 122–124, 123
    reticulosis lesion in, 388–390, 390
Medulla oblongata, 10, 11
    formation of, 17–19, 18, 19
Megaesophagus, canine, 123
Melanoblast, formation of, 16, 17
Melanoma, in horse, 359
Membrana nictitans, protrusion of, 118
Membrane, otolithic, 224
    tectorial, 283
Menace response, anatomic pathway of, 269
Menace test, 269
    in cerebellar disease, 246
Meninges, cerebral, 34
    inflammation of, and hydrocephalus, 52
        cerebrospinal fluid in, 355
Meningioma
    of cervical spinal cord, 192
    of lower motor neuron cranial nerves, 105
    of thoracolumbar spinal cord, 184
    vs. feline ischemic encephalopathy, 400
Meningitis, cerebrospinal fluid in, 38, 49t
    chronic, vs. extramedullary mass lesion, 374
Meningocele, cerebral, 28
Meningoencephalitis, and central vestibular
        syndrome, 234
    bacterial, cerebrospinal fluid, in 50t
    cryptococcal, and convulsions, 307
Meningoencephalocele, cerebral, 28
Meningoencephalomyelitis, cryptococcal,
        cerebrospinal fluid in, 50t
Meningomyelocele, clinical signs of, 30
    spina bifida and, 179
Mental status, evaluation of, in neurologic
        examination, 361
Mercury poisoning, and blindness, 274
    and convulsions, 309
Mesencephalic aqueduct, 10, 11, 415–418
    in development of midbrain, 21
    malformation of, and hydrocephalus, 52
Mesencephalon, 8, 11, 298
    cranial nerve lower motor neuron, anatomy of,
        92–95
    development of, 21–22, 21

Mesencephalon (*Continued*)
  extrapyramidal nuclei of, 132, *133*
  hypothalamic connection to, 329
  lesions of, clinical signs of, 357
  relationship of diencephalon to, *23*
Mesoderm, in development of eyeball, 259
Metabolism, diseases of, and coma, 327t
  episodic weakness in, 86
Metencephalon, 10, *11*
  development of, 20–21, *20, 21*
Microphthalmia, 271
Micturition, control of, 119
  dysfunction of, 121–122
Midbrain, development of, 21–22, *21*
  lesions of, clinical signs of, 357
  See also *Mesencephalon.*
Miosis, in Horner's syndrome, 113
  spinal root avulsion and, 77
Mitosis, in neural tube cells, 10, *12*
Modiolus, 281
Motoneuron, 58
Motor end-plate, 58, *60*
  neuromuscular junction of, 59, *60*
Motor neuron
  in peripheral nervous system, 2
  lower, 57–88
    cranial nerves of, 89–109
    definition of, 5
    disease of, 68–70
    electromyography in, 71
    general somatic efferent system of, 57–109
      diseases of, 71, 72t
    general visceral efferent system of, 110–124
    location of, 348
    parasympathetic, of medulla, 122
    sacral parasympathetic, 119
    special visceral efferent system of, 89–109
    sympathetic, of eye, 111–113
  upper, 125–148
    and voluntary movement, 139, *139*
    definition of, 125
    disease of, clinical signs of, 140
      in horse, 362
    extrapyramidal system, 128–136
    function of, 136, 363
    location of, 348
    pyramidal system, 125–127
Motor response in, unconscious state, 327
Motor unit, in general somatic efferent system, 58
Müller, cells of, 263
Muscle, diseases of, 83
  extraocular, function of, 93, *94*
  innervation of, *66, 67*
  smooth, in orbital structures, 113, *113*
Muscle tone
  evaluation of, 350
    in spinal cord disease, 172
  in cerebellar disease, 245
  spinal reflexes and, 68
Musculoskeletal disorders, vs. neurologic disease, 360
Myasthenia gravis, 71, 73, 102
  episodic weakness in, 85
Mycosis, guttural pouch, 104, 370

Myelencephalon, 10, *11*
  formation of, 17–19, *18, 19*
  See also *Medulla.*
Myelin, disintegration of, in Wallerian degeneration, 69
  in motor end-plate, 59, *60*
Myelin formation, congenital failure of, and tremors, 146
Myelitis
  distemper, and spinal cord disease, 187, 394
  equine, nonsuppurative, 213
  gait in, 348
  parasitic, vs. degenerative myeloencephalopathy, 398
  protozoal, in horse, 359
    and spinal cord lesion, 211, 397
      cerebrospinal fluid in, 50t, 371
  suppurative, and thoracolumbar spinal cord disease, 187
Myelodysplasia
  canine, 190
  clinical signs of, 30
  in calf, 215
  of cervical spinal cord, 200
  spina bifida and, 179
Myeloencephalopathy, degenerative, in horse, 214, 396–399, *398*
Myelography, cisternal, in horse, 208
  procedure in, 39, *39, 40*
Myelomalacia, diffuse, 82
  focal, cerebrospinal fluid in, 51t
  with intervertebral disk extrusion, 348
Myelopathy
  degenerative, in German shepherd, 188, 395
  demyelinating, 345
    in miniature poodle, 189, 200
  fibrocartilaginous embolic ischemic, 81, 375–377, *377*
  focal, compression and, 81
  ischemic, 81
    and lesions of cervical intumescence, 203
    case description of, 375–377
    of cervical spinal cord, 198, *199*
    vascular emboli and, 189
Myoclonia congenita, in pig, 251
Myoclonus, canine, 143
Myopathy, myotonic, hereditary, 84
Myopathy-myositis, 83
Myositis, eosinophilic, in German shepherd, 83
Myositis-myopathy, masticatory, 83
Myotatic reflex, 136
  in upper motor neuron disease, 141
Myotonia, electromyography in, 71
  equine, 365
Myotonia congenita, 85

Narcolepsy, 315
  in Shetland pony, 359
Necrosis, parenchymal, cerebrospinal fluid in, 49t, 355
Neocortex, and hypothalamus, 329
Neopallium, 25, *25*
Neoplasm,
  and hydrocephalus, 51

Neoplasm (*Continued*)
  and visual deficit, 273, 274
  astrocytoma, 51t, 275–277, 383–385
  at cerebellomedullary angle, and vestibular
    disorder, 235, 388–390
  cerebrospinal fluid in, 49t, 51t
  cervical spinal cord, 192
    in horse, 210
  choroid plexus papilloma-carcinoma, 51t, 235
  definition of, 2
  effect of, on spinal roots, 77
  extramedullary in horse, 210
  intracranial, and convulsions, 308
  intramedullary, in large animals, 215
    of spinal cord, 190
  of adenohypophysis, 330
  of brain stem, 107
  of cerebellum, 252
  of cervical intumescence, 201
  of cranial nerves of lower motor neuron, 105
  of general somatic efferent peripheral
    nerve, 76
  of prosencephalon, 347
  of tentorium cerebelli, case description of,
    380–383
  of thoracolumbar spinal cord, 184
  of vestibulocochlear nerve, 234
  pituitary, effect of, on vision, 272
Nerve
  abducens, 91, *411*
  accessory, 100, *408*
  facial, 98–100, 122, 410, *412*
  glossopharyngeal, 100, 122
  hypoglossal, 89, *408, 409*
  oculomotor, 92, 115, *417*
  olfactory, 293
  optic, 265, *421*
  peripheral, of lower motor neuron, with spinal
    roots, *66, 67*
    diseases affecting, 74
      destruction of, 69
  trigeminal, 97, 98, *413, 414*
  trochlear, 92, *414*
  vagus, 100, 122
  vestibulocochlear, 225, *411*, 412
Nerve deafness, 286
Nervous system
  central. See *Central nervous system.*
  clinical disorders of, diagnosis of, 1–2
  development of, 8–31
  functional classification of, 3t
  peripheral. See *Peripheral nervous system.*
  traumatic lesions of, diagnosis and evaluation
    of, 333–343
Neural canal, 8, *9*
Neural crest cells, 8, *9*
  differentiation in, 14, *15, 16*
Neural folds, 8, *9*
Neural groove, 8, *9*
Neural plate, 8, *9*
Neural tube
  cellular layers of, 10, *13*
  development of, 8–12, *9*
  differentiation of, vs. differentiation of optic
    cup, 260
  functional organization of, *13*
Neuritis
  facial, vestibulocochlear, 233

Neuritis (*Continued*)
  of cauda equina, 391
  optic, 270, 272
  serum, 79
  trigeminal, 106
Neurobiotaxis, definition of, 17
Neuroblast, formation of, 10, *12*
Neuroectoderm, 8, *9*
  in development of eyeball, 257
Neuroepithelioma, *40*, 184
  age in, 345
  in German shepherd, 394–396, *395, 396*
Neuroepithelium, of crista ampullaris, 223
Neurofibroma
  age in, 345
  case description of, 373–375, 377–380
  effect of, on spinal root, 77
  in cattle, 210
  of cervical intumescence, 201
  of thoracolumbar spinal cord, 184
  of thorax, 377–380, *379*
Neuroglia, 10
Neurohypophysis, 10, *11, 419*
  formation of, 22, *23*
Neuroma, following Wallerian degeneration,
  69
Neuromuscular disease, electrodiagnostic
    techniques in, 70
  episodic weakness in, 85
Neuromuscular ending, 59
  diseases affecting, 71
Neuromuscular esophageal defect, 123
Neuromuscular spindle, 136, *137*
Neuromyelitis optica, 272
Neurons
  abducent, 91, *91, 94, 411*
  accessory, 100, *408*
  definition of, 2–3
  epileptic, 305
  extrapyramidal, of telencephalon, 129
  facial, 98, *99*
    lesions of, clinical signs, 98–100
  general proprioceptive, 150
  general somatic afferent, 160
  general somatic efferent, 57
  glossopharyngeal, 100
  Golgi, 242
  hypoglossal, 89, *91*
    lesions of, clinical signs, 90
  motor. See *Motor neuron.*
  oculomotor, 92, *93, 94*, 115
  of auditory system, 284
  of cerebral cortex, 128
  of special visceral afferent system, 292
  of general visceral efferent system, 111
  of pyramidal system, 126
  of special visceral efferent system, 96
  Purkinje, 239
  photoreceptor, development of, 260
  rubrospinal, *416*
  sensory. See *Sensory neuron.*
  trigeminal, 97, *97*
    lesions of, clinical signs, 98
  trochlear, 92, *93, 94*
  vagus, 100
    lesions of, clinical signs, 102
  vestibular, 224
Neuropathy, idiopathic-vestibular, 231

Neuro-ophthalmology, clinical signs in, 277t
Neuropore, 8, *9*
Night blindness, in Appaloosa, 271
Nigropallidal encephalomalacia, 143
Nociceptor, 150
Nodulus, *410*
Nonolfactory rhinencephalon, 296–302
  major structures of, 299t
Norepinephrine, from adrenal medulla, 17
Notochord, 8, *9*
Nucleus (i)
  abducent, 91, *91, 94*
    lesions of, 95
  caudate, caudal, *420*
    rostral, *421*
  cerebellar, 240
    fastigial, 243, *410*
    interpositial, 243, *410*
    lateral, 243, *410*
  cervical, in proprioceptive pathway, 155
  Clarke's, 151
  cochlear, of brain stem, 283, *411, 412*
  cuneate, lateral, *408, 409*
    medial, *407, 408*
      in proprioceptive pathway, 152
  endopenduncular, *420*
  extrapyramidal, of diencephalon, 132, *133*
    of mesencephalon, 132, *133*
    of telencephalon, 129, *131*
  facial motor, *410*
  geniculate, lateral, *417–419*
      disorders of, 273
      in central visual pathway, 268
    medial, *416–418*
  habenular, *419*
    definition of, 298
  hypoglossal motor, *408, 409*
  hypothalamic, 110, 328, *420*
  intercrural, *415, 416*
  lentiform, *420, 421*
  mammillary, *419*
  mesencephalic, deep, *417*
  motor, of trochlear nerve, *415*
  oculomotor, *416*
    lesions of, 95
  of solitary tract, *408, 409*
  olivary, *408, 409*
    as cerebellar afferent, 242
    composition of, 135
  pontine, *413–415*
    as cerebellar afferent, 243
  pontine sensory, of trigeminal nerve, 157
  pretectal, *418*
  red, 132, *416, 417*
    as cerebellar afferent, 243
  subthalamic, *419*
  thalamic, 320, 321, *417–420*
    ventral caudal lateral, 153
    ventral caudal medial, 165
    ventral lateral, 243
    ventral rostral, 131
  thalamic reticular, 320
  trochlear, lesions of, 95
  vestibular, 225, *226, 410–412*
Nucleus ambiguus, 100, *408, 409*
Nucleus gracilis, *407, 408*
  in proprioceptive pathway, 152

Nucleus thoracicus, 151
Nystagmus
  abnormal, 229
  caloric, 229
  congenital, 236
  in examination of vestibular system, 353
  normal, 96
  postrotatory, 229

Obtundation, 326
Obturator nerve, paralysis of, 75
Oculomotor nerve
  anatomy of, 92, 115
  clinical signs, 95, 116
  compression of, and ventrolateral strabismus, 107
  function of, 93
  olfactory bulb, 293
  parasympathetic nucleus of, *417, 418*
Olfactory nerve, 293
  in horse, examination of, 366
Olfactory system, special visceral afferent, 292, *294*
Olfactory tract, lateral, *421*
Olfactory tubercle, 293
Oligodendrocyte, formation of, 10, *12*
Olivary nucleus, *408, 409*
  as cerebellar afferent, 242
  definition of, 135
Olivopontocerebellar degeneration, 249
Ontario disease, 82
Opisthotonus, 245
Optic chiasm, 266
  diseases of, 272
  of telencephalon, 22, *27*
Optic cup, 258
Optic disk, 264, *265*
  injury to, 271
Optic nerve, 265, *421*
  diseases of, 271
  formation of, 265
  in horse, examination of, 366
Optic neuritis, 272
Optic radiation, disorders of, 273
Optic stalk, 258
Optic tract, *417–420*
Optic tracts, diseases of, 272
Optic vesicle, development of, 8, *11,* 257
  in development of diencephalon, 22, *23*
Ossification, dural, 186
Osteogenic sarcoma
  and cranial nerves, 105
  of sacrum, 76
  of tentorium cerebelli, 380–383, *382, 383*
Osteoma, vertebral, 185
Osteomyelitis, vertebral, 186, 198
  with spinal cord compression, 395
Otic placode, 221
Otitis interna, vestibular signs in, 232
Otitis media, and facial nerve paralysis, 105
  vestibular signs in, 232
Otocyst, 221
Ototoxicity, 286
Ox, normal cerebrospinal fluid value in, 48t

Pachygyria, and convulsions, 308
Pachymeningitis, 186
Pain
  as test for general somatic afferent system, 165
  in intervertebral disk disease, 182
  nociceptors and, 150
  perception of, evaluation of, 352
    in spinal cord disease, 174
    vs. spinal reflex response, 169
  referred, 291, *291*
  visceral, 290
Pain pathway, 161, *162*
Paleopallium, 25, *25*
Pallidum, 129, *420, 421*
Palpebral reflex in dog, 353
  in horse, 369
Pancreas, beta cell neoplasm of, 402
Panleukopenia virus, in cat, 246, 347
Panniculus reflex, 64
  evaluation of, 352
  in horse, 365
Papilloma, choroid plexus, 235
  cerebrospinal fluid in, 51t
Parahippocampal gyrus, 296, *418, 419*
Parakeet, renal adenocarcinoma in, 76
Paralysis, coonhound, 68
  tick, 71, 73
Paramethadione, in treatment of seizures, 313
Parasitic inflammation, 213, 234
  cerebrospinal fluid in, 51t
Parasitism, intestinal, and convulsions, 307
Parelaphostrongylus tenuis, in goats and sheep,
    213
    cerebrospinal fluid in, 51t
Parenchymal disease, cerebrospinal fluid in, 38,
    49t, 355
Paresis, in upper motor neuron disease, 140
Pars ciliaris retinae, 260
Pars intermedia, in horse, neoplasms of, 331
Pars iridia retinae, 260
Pars optica retinae, histology of, 261–265, *262*
Paspalum staggers, 145, 360
Patellar reflex, *66, 67*
  evaluation of, 351
    in horse, 364
    in spinal cord disease, 173
  topographic anatomy of, 68t
Paw, nerves supplying, 351
Peduncle, cerebellar, 240
    caudal, *409–411*
    middle, *412–414*
  olfactory, 293, 294
  rostal, *412–415*
Pelvic limbs
  flexor reflex in, evaluation of, 351
    in dog, 174
    in horse, 364
  paralysis of, 75
  paraplegia in, in fibrocartilaginous embolic
    ischemic myelopathy, 375
  reflexes, 65–68
  skin of, peripheral nerve innervation of, *166*
  tests for, 349
  traumatic lesions of, 340
  weakness in, evaluation of, 171t, 348
Pelvic limb reflexes, 65, *67*
Penicillium, and tremors, 145

Perineal reflex
  evaluation of, 352
    in horse, 365
  in spinal cord disease, 175
  topographic anatomy of, 68t
Peripheral nervous system
  afferent portion of, classification of, 3t, 4
  efferent portion of, classification of, 3t, 5
  motor neuron of, 2
  sensory neuron of, 2
  traumatic lesions of, 339–342
Peritonitis, feline infectious, and hydrocephalus, 52
    and vestibular disease, 234
    cerebrospinal fluid in, 50t
    vs. feline ischemic encephalopathy, 400
Peroneal nerve, paralysis of, 75
Petrosal bone, injury to, and ear hemorrhage, 106
pH, of cerebrospinal fluid, 38
Phalaris staggers, 145
Pharyngeal paralysis, in horse, 370
    differential diagnosis of, 107
Phenobarbital, in treatment of seizures, 313
Phenytoin, in treatment of seizures, 313
Phosphate, organic, and convulsions, 309
Physical examination
  equine, 361
  small animal, 347
Pigs
  cerebellar syndromes in, 251
  cerebral meningocele in, 28
  cerebrospinal fluid collection in, 42
    normal values in, 48t
Pineal body, *418*
Pituitary gland, formation of, 22, *23*
Pituitary neoplasms, effect of, on vision, 272
Pituitary stalk, 328
Placing, as test for spinal cord disease, 172
  with thoracic limbs, 350
Pneumoventriculography, in hydrocephalus, 54
  procedure in, 39, *41*
Poikilothermia, 330
Poisons, and coma, 328t
Poisoning
  dallis grass, 145
  lead, 402
    and convulsions, 308
  mercury, and blindness, 274
    and convulsions, 309
  organophosphate, vs. botulism, 73
  salt, and convulsions, 309
  strychnine, and convulsions, 304, 309
  yellow star thistle, in horse, 370
Polioencephalomalacia
  and blindness, 274
  and coma, 325
  and convulsions, 308
  and strabismus, 107
  cerebrospinal fluid in, 51t
Polioencephalomyelitis, in pigs, 82
Polymyopathy, myotonic, 84
Polymyositis, 83
  episodic weakness in, 85
Polyneuritis
  acute, 77
  chronic, 79
    and laryngeal paresis, 103
  equine, cranial nerve signs in, 391

Polyneuropathy, vestibular signs in, 233
Polyradiculoneuritis, acu.
    idiopathic, 68, 77
Pons, 10, *11*
    cranial nerve, lower motor neuron, 97–98
    development of, 20–21, *20, 21*
    fibers of, longitudinal, 243, *413, 414*
        transverse, 243, *413–415*
        transverse, 243, *413–415*
    lesions of, clinical signs of, 357
Pontine nucleus, as cerebellar afferent, 243
Poodle, miniature, demyelinating myelopathy in,
    189, 200
    hydranencephaly in, 29
Porencephaly, bluetongue virus and, 29
Portacaval shunt, 401–404
Postural reactions, in neurologic examination,
    349
    in spinal cord disease, 171
    proprioceptive system lesions and, 157
Postural tremor, 142
Posture
    abnormal, in vestibular disease, 228
    evaluation of, in intracranial injury, 334
        in neurologic examination, 361
    reactions in, evaluation of, 349
Primidone, in treatment of seizures, 313
Progressive retinal atrophy, 271
Projection system, thalamic, diffuse cortical, 321
Proprioception, classification of, 5
    general, 149
    special, 221–237
Proprioceptive positioning, 157, 172, 350
Proprioception system, general, 149–159
    composition of, 64
    diseases affecting, 158
    lesions of, clinical signs of, 157
    special, 221–237
Propriospinal fiber system, 151
Propulsion, 358
Prosencephalon, 8, *11*
    extrapyramidal neurons of, *132*
    hypoplasia of, 274
        definition of, 28
    malformation of, and convulsions, 308
    neoplasia of, 347
Protein, in cerebrospinal fluid, 35, 49
Protozoal equine encephalomyelitis, 107, 211,
    390–394, *393*
    cerebrospinal fluid in, 50t
Pupils, control of, 111–119
    neuroanatomic pathway for, *112*
    evaluation of, in intracranial injury, 334
    in acute brain disease, 117
    reaction of, in unconscious state, 326
Pupillary light reflex response, 270
Pupillary membrane, 259
Pupillary reflex pathway, 268
Purkinje cell, *21*
    abiotrophy of, 247, 249, 251
    formation of, 239
    hypoplasia of, 247
    of cerebellum, 3
Putamen, of extrapyramidal system, 129, *420,
    421*
Pyramid, *412*
Pyramidal system, of upper motor neuron,
    125–127

Pyriform lobe, 294, 297, *420*
Pyrrolizidine alkaloids, 360

Queckenstedt maneuver, 37

Rabies, 107, 108
Rabies encephalomyelitis, and lower motor
    neuron paralysis, 82
    cerebrospinal fluid in, 371
Raccoon bite, and coonhound paralysis, 78, 381
Radial nerve, injury to, 339
Radial nerve paralysis, trauma to peripheral
    nerve and, 74
Radiography, contrast, in epilepsy, 312
    in hydrocephalus, 40
    in spinal cord disease, 38
    with air, in hydrocephalus, 41, 53
Rathke's pouch, 22
Reaction, axonal, in Wallerian degeneration, 69
Reflex. See also specific names.
    patellar tendon, 64, 65, 173
    pelvic limb, 65, 67
    perineal, 175
    thoracic limb, 64, 66
Reflex general somatic afferent pathway, 160,
    162, 164
Reflex pathway, of general visceral afferent
    system, *289, 290*
    pupillary, 268
Renal disease, and convulsions, 307
Reptile, advanced, cerebrum of, 25
Respiration, in unconscious state, 327
Reticular activating system, ascending, 322
Reticular formation, 322, *408–417*
    as cerebellar afferent, 243
    definition of, 134
Reticulosarcoma, cerebrospinal fluid in, 51t
Reticulosis, in cerebellum and medulla, 234,
    388–390, *390*
    primary, cerebrospinal fluid in, 51t
    vs. osteogenic sarcoma, 381
Retina
    diseases of, 271
    histology of, 261–265, *262*
    lesions of, and blindness, 270
    pigment epithelium of, 261
Rhinencephalon, nonolfactory, 296–302
    major structures of, 299t
    olfactory, and smell, 292, *294*
Rhinopneumonitis, 212
    cerebrospinal fluid in, 50t, 371
    effect of, on herd, 360
    vs. degenerative myeloencephalopathy, 398
Rhodopsin, 261
Rhombencephalon, 8, *11*
    in extrapyramidal system, 134
Rhombic lip, in development of cerebellum, 238
Rigidity, decerebrate, 138, 328
Roarer horse, 103
Roof plate, of fourth ventricle, development of,
    17, *19, 21*
    of third ventricle, in development of
        diencephalon, 22, *23*
Rye grass staggers, 146

Salt poisoning, and convulsions, 309
Samoyed, cerebellar abiotrophy in, 247
Sarcolemma, in motor end-plate, 59, *60*
Sarcoma, osteogenic, cranial nerves, and, 105
    of sacrum, 76
    of tentorium cerebelli, 380–383, *382, 383*
Sarcoplasmic trough, in motor end-plate, 60, *60*
Scala tympani, 281
Scala vestibuli, 281
Scar, cerebral, and convulsions, 308
Schiff-Sherrington syndrome, 180, 338
Schwann cell, in motor end-plate, 59, *60*
Sciatic nerve, function of, 66, 174
    injury to, 341
    paralysis of, 75, 351
Scintigraphy, in epilepsy, 312
Sclera, development of, 259
Scoliosis, 191
Scotty cramps, 144, 345
Seizures, 303–317
    causes of, 305–310, 306t
        extracranial, 306
        idiopathic, 309
        intracranial, 307
    cerebral astrocytoma and, 383–385, *386*
    cerebral infarction and, 399–401
    classification of, 303–305
    definition of, 303
    examination of patient with, 310–312
    pathogenesis of, 305
    psychomotor, 301
    significance of, in neurologic examination, 346
    stimulation of limbic system and, 300, 301
    threshold for, 305
    treatment of, 312–315
Semicoma, definition of, 326
    hypothalamic lesions and, 331
    in intracranial injury, 334
Senses. See specific names.
Sensorium, abnormal, hypothalamic lesions and,
    331
Sensory ataxia, equine, 206
Sensory neuron, in central nervous system, 3
    in peripheral nervous system, 2
    to cerebellum, 3
Sensory systems, characteristics of, 149–150
Septum, telencephalic, *421*
Septum pellucidum, *27, 28,* 298
Sex, significance of, in neurologic examination,
    345
Shaker foal, 73
Sheep,
    bluetongue virus in, 29
    border disease in, 146
    cerebrospinal fluid collection in, 42
        normal values in, 48t
    haloxon neurotoxicity in, 215
    Parelaphostrongylus tenuis in, 213, 234
Shivering, 146
Shock, in intracranial injury, 333
    spinal cord, 180
    treatment of, 335
Siamese cat, visual system in, 273
Signalment, in examination, small animal, 345
    equine, 359
Skeleton, diseases of, vs. neurologic disease, 194

Small animals
    neurologic examination in, 344–357
        cerebrospinal fluid, 354
        cranial nerves in, 352
        gait in, 348
        history in, 345
        physical examination in, 347
        postural reactions in, 349
        signalment, 345
        spinal reflexes in, 350
Smell, evaluation of, 354
    special visceral afferent system and, 292, *294*
Sole plate, in motor end-plate, 60, *60*
Somatic afferent system
    classification of, 4
    general, 160–168
        composition of, 64
        diseases affecting, 168
    special, 257–280, 281–287, *282*
    testing, 165
Somatic efferent system
    classification of, 5
    cranial nerves in, 89
    general, 57–88
        definition of, 57
        diseases of, 71, 72t
Spastic syndrome, 144
Spasticity, 350, 351
    in spinal cord disease, 172, 176
Spina bifida, and myelodysplasia, 179
    with meningocele, 30
Spinal cord
    arterial vasculature of, *199*
    cervical, *208*
        compression of, cervical vertebral
            malformation and, 206
        disease of, 191
        injury to, 338
        with spinal root of accessory nerve, *101*
    cervical intumescence, disease of, 201
    development of, 12–17, *13, 15, 16*
        vertebra in, 61
    disease of, 169–220
        equine, 394
        in large animals, 205–216
        in small animals, 177–205
        lower motor neuron, 81
        lumbosacral, 177
        neurologic examination in, 169–177
            cranial nerves in, 175
            gait in, 170
            postural reactions in, 171
            spinal reflexes in, 172
            thoracolumbar, 179
    functional organization of, *13*
    inflammation of, 82
    injury of, 177, 179
    lesions of, clinical signs of, 175, 356
        in horse, 366
        vs. botulism, 72
        traumatic, 337
    malformations of, 30
    neuroepithelioma of, 184, 394–396, *395, 396*
    topography of, 57, *58, 62, 63*
    vestibular nuclei projections in, 225
Spinal cord segments, 61

Spinal cord segments (*Continued*)
  ischemic myelopathy of, 375–377, *377*
  injury to, 337
  lesion of, and spinal cord degeneration, 196, *197*
Spinal cord shock, 180
Spinal dysraphism, clinical signs of, 30
Spinal ganglion, formation of, 14, *15*
Spinal nerves
  destruction of, vs. peripheral nerve destruction, 69
  division of, 57–68
  function of, 61
  general proprioceptive system for, 150
  in general somatic afferent system, 160–164
  injury to, 76, 177, 342
Spinal reflexes, 64, *65*
  depression of, 68
  evaluation of, 350
    in neurologic examination, 172, 350, 363
  in spinal cord disease, 172
  topographic anatomy of, 68t
Spinal root, of brachial plexus, avulsion of, 76
  injury to, 76, 177
Spindle, neuromuscular, 136, *137*
Splenium, of corpus callosum, *417*, 418
Spondylolisthesis, 196
Spondylosis deformans, 186
Spongioblast, formation of, 10, *12*
Staggers, 145
  Claviceps paspali and, 360
Standing sway test, 207
Status epilepticus, management of, 314
Stereocilia, in auditory system, 283
  in vestibular system, 224
Strabismus, 95
  vestibular, 290
Strangles, *Streptococcus equi* and, 270, 360
Streptococcus equi, and parenchymal abscess, 273, 360, 391, 398
Stria, acoustic, *410*
Stria habenularis thalami, *420*
Stria terminalis, of limbic system, 296
"Stroke," 232
Strongylus vulgaris, in horse, 214
  migrating larvae of, 391
Strychnine poisoning, convulsions in, 304, 309
  tetany in, 138
Stupor, 357
  definition of, 326
Subarachnoid space, *34*
Subependymal zone, 28
Subluxation, atlantoaxial, 192
Substantia nigra, *416–418*
  of extrapyramidal system, 132
  lesions in, 143, 248
Subthalamus, 318
Sulcus, lateral rhinal, *418*, *419*
Sulcus limitans, in neural, canal, 12, *13*
Sway, response, in horse, 362
Swedish Lapland dog, hereditary abiotrophy in, 83
Swimmer syndrome, 200
Synapse, 2
Syndrome. See specific names.
Syringomyelia, 30

Talfan's disease, 82
Taste, special visceral afferent system and, 292, *293*
Tectum, of midbrain, 21, *22*
Tegmentum, of midbrain, *21*
Telencephalic septum, *421*
Telencephalon, 10, *11*, 296
  development of, 22–28, *24–27*
  extrapyramidal nuclei of, 129, *131*
  hypothalamic connection to, 329
  in hydranencephaly, 29
  lesions of, clinical signs of, 358
  thalamic relay to, 321
  ventricular system of, development of, *24*
Telodendron, of neuron, 2
Temperature, abnormal, hypothalamic lesions and, 330
Teschen's disease, 82
Tests. See specific names.
Tetanus, 138
  in horse, hypertonia in, 364
  protrusion of third eyelid in, 119
Tetany, 138, 144
Thalamic reticular system, 321
Thalamocortical projection fibers, 284, *419*, *420*
Thalamus, 318–325
  anatomy of, 318
  ascending reticular activating system, 322
  formation of, 22, *23*
  function of, 321, 325
  lesions of, clinical signs of, 325, 357
  ventral caudal lateral nucleus of, in proprioceptive pathway, 153
Theiler's disease, 359
  and convulsions, 307
Thiamine deficiency, 235, 400
  and convulsions, 308
Thomsen's disease, 85
Thoracic limbs
  flexor reflex in, 352
    evaluation of, in horse, 365
  paralysis of, 74
  skin of, peripheral nerve innervation of, *167*
  tests for, 349
    wheelbarrowing, 349
  traumatic lesions of, 339
Thoracic limb pathway, for general proprioception, 152
Thoracic limb reflexes, 64, *66*
Thoracodorsal nerve paralysis, trauma to peripheral nerve and, 74
Thrombosis, aortic, in cat, 76
Tibial nerve, paralysis of, 75
Tick paralysis, 71, 73
Tissue necrosis, cerebrospinal fluid in, 49t
Tongue disorders of, 370
  manipulation of, and paralysis, 103
Tonic neck reaction, 350
  in spinal cord disease, 172
Toxoplasma encephalitis, cerebrospinal fluid in, 50t
Toxoplasma gondii, and neuritis in spinal roots, 77
  and spinal cord destruction, 83
Toxoplasma granuloma, vs. feline ischemic encephalopathy, 400

Toxoplasmosis, 84
  and convulsions, 307
  and thoracolumbar spinal cord disease, 187
  vs. osteogenic sarcoma, 381
Tract
  habenulointercrural, 298, *419*
  mammillothalamic, 298, *419, 420*
  olfactory, 293, *421*
  optic, 267, *417–420*
    diseases of, 272
  pyramidal, *408–411*
  reticulospinal, 134
  rubrosacral, *406*
  rubrospinal, 132, *415, 416*
  solitary, *408*
    nucleus of, *409*
    of general visceral afferent system, 289
  spinocerebellar, *151*, 151, 152, *153, 407*, 408
    lesions of, 158
  spinothalamic, 161
  vestibulospinal, 226, *406*
Transport tetany, 145
Trapezoid body, 283, *411, 412*
Trauma, 2
  diagnosis and evaluation of nervous system in, 333–342
  spinal cord, 177, 179, 191
Tremetol, and tremors, 146
Tremors, in large animals, 145
  in small animals, 146
  postural, 142
  intentional, 245
Tremor syndrome, 143
Triceps reflex, 64, *66*
  evaluation of, 351
  in horse, 364
  in spinal cord disease, 173
  topographic anatomy of, 68t
Trigeminal nerve, 97–98, *413, 414*
  in general somatic afferent system, *163*, 164
  in horse, evaluation of, 369
  in proprioceptive pathway, 155, *156*
  motor nucleus of, *412*
  sensory pontine nucleus of, *412*
  spinal tract of, *406–411*
Trigeminal neuralgia, in horse, 369
Trigeminal neuritis, 106
Trochlear nerve, 92
  motor nucleus of, *415*
Tuber cinereum, 328
Tympano-occipital fissure, lesion of, 373–375
Tyrosine, neural crest cell differentiation and, 17

Ulnar nerve paralysis, trauma to peripheral
  nerve and, 74
Unconsciousness, clinical evaluation of, 325–328
Uvea, 259

Vagus nerve, 100, 122
  disease of, 102, 123
  in horse, evaluation of, 370
  parasympathetic nucleus of, *408, 409*
Velum, rostral medullary, *412, 413*

Venezuelan equine encephalomyelitis, cerebrospinal fluid in, 371
Venography, cervical, in horse, 208
Ventricles, *36*
  fourth, *413, 414*
    choroid plexus papilloma of, 51t
    velum of, *20*
  lateral, *418–421*
    of telencephalon, development of, *24*
  third, *419, 420*
    in development of diencephalon, 22, *23*
Ventriculography, contrast, procedure in, 40, *41*
Vermis, of cerebellum, 240
Vertebra
  cartilaginous exostosis involving, 394
  cervical, malarticulation of, 195
  fractured, and spinal root injury, 76
  in development of spinal cord segments, 61,
    62, 63
  malformation of, 185
Vesicles
  brain, development of, 8, *11*
  lens, 259
  optic, development of, 8, *11*, 257
    in development of diencephalon, 22, *23*
Vestibular cerebellum, 240
  degeneration of, 234
  injury of, 233
Vestibular disease, feline, 231
  canine geriatric, 232
  congenital peripheral, 233
  paradoxical, 290
Vestibular system, 221–237
  anatomy and physiology of, 221–228, *223, 226,*
    227
  diseases of, 231–236
    signs of, 228–231
  disturbances of, in horse, 368
  evaluation of, in intracranial injury, 334
  examination of, 353
  paradoxical signs in, 230
Vestibulocochlear nerve, composition of, 283
  evaluation of, in horse, 369
  vestibular division, 225
Villus; arachnoid, malformation of, and hydrocephalus, 52
Viral disease, cerebrospinal fluid in, 49t, 355
Viral inflammation, cerebrospinal fluid in, 50t
Virus
  Akabane, and hydranencephaly, 29
  and cerebral malformation, 28
  bluetongue and hydranencephaly, 29
    and hydrocephalus, 51
  canine distemper, 143, 187, 234, 252
  diarrhea, bovine, and hydrocephalus, 51
    and cerebellar atrophy, 249
  feline infectious peritonitis, 52, 234
  herpes I, equine rhinopneumonitis, 212
  hog cholera, and cerebellar degeneration, 251
  panleukopenia, in cat, 246, 347
Visceral afferent systems, 288–295
  anatomy of, 288
  classification of, 4
  general, 288–292, *289*
    functional concepts of, 290
  special, 292–295

Visceral efferent system, classification of, 5
  general, 110–124
    diseases affecting, 113
    sacral parasympathetic, 119–122
  special, 96–102
Visceral pain, 290
Vision
  clinical tests for, 269, 269t, 353, 367
  deficient, clinical signs of, 270
    in horse, 367
    in hydrocephalus, 53
    test for, 353
  evaluation of, in intracranial injury, 334
  in unconscious state, 326
Visual cortex, 268
  disorders of, 273
Visual deficit, clinical signs in, 271t
Visual field, definition of, 267
Visual pathway, central, 265–271, 266
Visual system, 257–280
  diseases of, 271–277
Vitamin E, deficiency of, vs. hereditary myotonic
  myopathy, 84
Vitreous chamber, development of, 259

Wallerian degeneration, of lower motor neuron,
  69, 70
Water intoxication, and convulsions, 309

Weakness
  episodic, 85
  in horse, tests for, 362
  in upper motor neuron disease, 140
  pelvic limb, evaluation of, 348
Weimaraner, spinal dysraphism in, 30
West Highland white terrier, leukodystrophy in,
  275
Western equine encephalomyelitis, cerebrospinal
  fluid in, 371
Wheelbarrowing, as test of postural reaction, 349
  as test in spinal cord disease, 171
Withdrawal response, flexor, 161
Wobbler syndrome, 193, 206
  breed and age in, 359
  cervical vertebral malarticulation-malforma-
    tion in, 193, 397
  vs. protozoal encephalomyelitis, 391

Xanthochromic cerebrospinal fluid, 48

Yellow star thistle poisoning, in horse, 370
Yorkshire terrier, hydrocephalus in, 53

Zona incerta, 132, 419